Valvular Heart Disease

Valvular Heart Disease

Catherine M. Otto, MD

Associate Professor of Medicine
Division of Cardiology
University of Washington
Seattle, Washington

W.B. SAUNDERS COMPANY
A Division of Harcourt Brace & Company
Philadelphia   London   Toronto   Montreal   Sydney   Tokyo

W.B. SAUNDERS COMPANY
A Division of Harcourt Brace & Company

The Curtis Center
Independence Square West
Philadelphia, Pennsylvania 19106

Library of Congress Cataloging-in-Publication Data

Otto, Catherine M.
    Valvular heart disease/Catherine M. Otto—1st ed.

        p.   cm.

    ISBN 0–7216–7139–X

    1. Heart valves—Diseases.   I. Title.
    [DNLM: 1. Heart Valve Diseases—therapy.   2. Heart Valve Diseases—
diagnosis.   3. Heart Valve Diseases—pathology.   WG 260 091v 1999]

RC685.V2078   1999   616.1′25—dc21

DNLM/DLC   98-47450

VALVULAR HEART DISEASE   ISBN 0–7216–7139–X

Last digit is the print number: 9   8   7   6   5   4   3   2   1

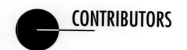

CONTRIBUTORS

R. Pat Cochran, MD
Professor of Surgery
Chair, Division of Cardiothoracic Surgery
University of Wisconsin Medical School
Madison, Wisconsin
Valvular Heart Disease: The Surgical Approach

Corinne L. Fligner, MD
Associate Professor
Department of Pathology
Adjunct Associate Professor
Department of Laboratory Medicine
University of Washington School of Medicine
Seattle, Washington
Pathology and Etiology of Heart Disease

Dennis D. Reichenbach, MD
Professor of Pathology
University of Washington School of Medicine
Seattle, Washington
Pathology and Etiology of Heart Disease

Edward D. Verrier, MD
Professor of Surgery
Chief, Cardiothoracic Surgery Division
University of Washington School of Medicine
Seattle, Washington
Valvular Heart Disease: The Surgical Approach

PREFACE

Worldwide, valvular heart disease remains a major cause of morbidity and mortality. In the United States, valve disease accounts for about 5 to 10% of all cardiac surgical cases, and a far greater number of patients have valve disease that is managed medically. Recognition of a heart murmur remains central to the practice of medicine, especially now that primary care physicians are increasingly responsible for the initial diagnosis of valvular heart disease and referral to a subspecialist.

Over the past several years, noninvasive methods for diagnosis and evaluation of disease severity have greatly increased our knowledge of valvular heart disease. First, the ability to monitor stenosis severity with varying flow rates has broadened our understanding of the complex hemodynamics of valvular stenosis and regurgitation. Second, serial noninvasive studies in patients with mild or moderate degrees of valve dysfunction have improved our understanding of the natural history of valvular disease. Third, these noninvasive methods now allow precise assessment of the changes in valvular and ventricular function after medical or surgical interventions. In addition, better surgical options now are available, including percutaneous interventions, improved valve substitutes, and the increasing use of valve repair procedures. Earlier surgical intervention is being considered more often as the risk-benefit ratio for surgical intervention improves and as the potential long-term adverse consequences of valve disease are more clearly defined.

Optimal care of the patient with valvular heart disease requires knowledgeable collaboration among several different types of health professionals. The diagnosis often is suspected by the primary care physician or nurse practitioner based on auscultation of a cardiac murmur or recognition of symptoms that might be due to valvular disease. Further evaluation by a cardiologist typically involves subspecialists in echocardiography and interventional cardiology, as well as the skilled assistance of cardiac sonographers and cardiac catheterization laboratory technologists. In patients undergoing surgical intervention, patient care is provided not only by the cardiac surgeon but also by cardiovascular anesthesiologists, cardiac perfusionists, and coronary care unit nurses. In addition, interactions with other medical specialties often are needed, for example, in the pregnant patient with valvular heart disease.

This book integrates the diverse knowledge required for optimal care of the patient with valvular heart disease by each of these health professionals, with a comprehensive list of references for each topic. The initial two chapters provide an overview of the prevalence and etiology of valvular heart disease, with detailed illustrations of valvular pathology. The next six chapters provide the background for diagnosis and therapy of patients with valvular heart disease. Chapters on echocardiography, cardiac catheterization, and other diagnostic approaches provide an introduction to each of these diagnostic modalities, focusing specifically on evaluation of valvular disease. Subsequent chapters outline the basic principles of medical therapy and the surgical approach to patients with valvular disease. A chapter on the left ventricular response to pressure and/or volume overload is included, as this is a key factor in the decision-making process regarding the optimal timing of surgical intervention.

The core of the book consists of detailed chapters on aortic stenosis, aortic regurgitation, mitral stenosis, mitral regurgitation, and right-sided valve disease. Each of the chapters on the major valve lesions provides a summary of the pathophysiology, clinical presentation, and natural history of the disease process along with a discussion of medical therapy and surgical intervention, including postoperative outcome. Each chapter is extensively illustrated, and the major clinical trials are summarized in tables whenever possible. Separate chapters are provided for newer, more controversial interventions, such as treatment of mitral stenosis and surgical intervention for mitral regurgitation. The final two chapters of the book cover the areas of prosthetic valves and endocarditis.

While every attempt has been made to provide accurate and up-to-date information, medicine is an ever-changing field, so that readers always should check the recent literature for any changes in diagnostic approaches or therapy. In addition, professional organizations such as the American Heart Association and American College of Cardiology periodically develop consensus guidelines for patient management that should be used when available. Chapters on specific diagnostic techniques and the basic surgical approach are provided as background information. Of course, expertise in these areas requires appropriate education and experience as defined by the relevant accreditation and credentialing bodies and professional organizations. Valvular heart disease in children is not covered in this book, as clinical management requires special expertise due to the additional diagnostic and therapeutic considerations in this population and due to the concurrent presence of complex congenital heart disease in many of these patients.

Valvular heart disease historically has been an interest for many physicians and continues to be an area of fascination for some of us, with the initial stimulus for learning often being the appreciation of a cardiac murmur on physical examination as a medical student. Now that we are on the verge of understanding the cellular and molecular mechanisms of valve disease, it is important to consolidate our current knowledge in order to focus on the possibility of preventing disease initiation and progression in the future.

Catherine M. Otto, M.D.

ACKNOWLEDGMENTS

Sincere thanks are due to the many individuals who helped make this book a reality. In particular, R. Pat Cochran, M.D., and Edward D. Verrier, M.D., provided an excellent chapter on the surgical approach that provides a concise but comprehensive overview for physicians caring for patients with valvular heart disease. The chapter by Corrine L. Fligner, M.D., and Dennis D. Reichenbach, M.D., on the pathology of valvular heart disease has an outstanding and complete set of photographs illustrating the anatomic and histologic abnormalities. My thanks are extended to J. David Godwin, M.D., for providing chest radiographs, and to Kenneth G. Lehmann, M.D., for providing hemodynamic tracings and angiograms in patients with valvular heart disease. In addition, Kenneth G. Lehmann, M.D., and Michael A. Brown, M.D., each provided a thoughtful review and constructive criticism of one of the book chapters. Starr Kaplan deserves special thanks for her insight into the details of valvular anatomy and her skill in making clear drawings of valve anatomy for Chapters 3 and 13.

Although not direct contributors to this book, my research fellows over the past several years (Ian G. Burwash, M.D., Malcolm E. Legget, M.D., and Brad Munt, M.D.) were not only active participants in my research endeavors but also constantly challenged me to learn more about valvular heart disease by their continued inquisitiveness and enthusiasm. As my Division Chief for many years, J. Ward Kennedy, M.D., stimulated my interest in valve disease and provided support and guidance in my pursuit of further knowledge in this area. Sharon Kemp, my program coordinator, earns my deepest thanks for her persistent patience and efficiency in helping with manuscript preparation despite her numerous other responsibilities.

My thanks to the editorial staff at W.B. Saunders, in particular Richard Zorab, for bringing this book to completion, and to the production team for their excellent illustration support and careful work in preparation of the final book.

Finally, as always, I would like to thank my family for their constant encouragement and support.

Catherine M. Otto, M.D.

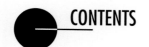

CONTENTS

Color Plates

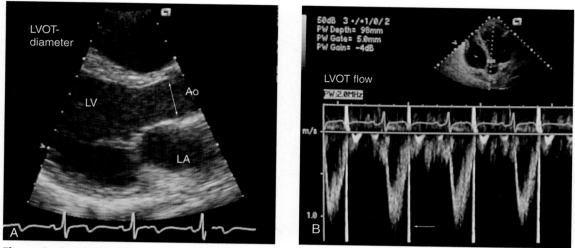

Figure 3•9 This example shows the data needed to calculate stroke volume in the left ventricular (LV) outflow tract. *A*, Outflow tract diameter is measured in a parasternal long-axis view to take advantage of the axial resolution of the ultrasound system. *B*, The flow velocity curve at this site is measured from an apical approach using pulsed Doppler echocardiography with a sample volume length of 5 to 10 mm. Care is taken to ensure the velocity and diameter data are from the same anatomic site by including the aortic valve closing click *(arrow)* in the Doppler recording. Ao, aorta; LA, left atrium.

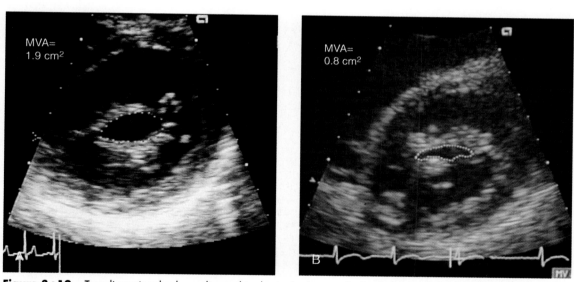

Figure 3•12 Two-dimensional echocardiographic short-axis views at the level of the mitral valve orifice in mid-diastole in a patient with moderate mitral stenosis *(A)* and in a patient with severe mitral stenosis *(B)*. Minimal orifice area is identified by scanning slowing from the apex toward the base, with the valve area (MVA) calculated directly by planimetry of the white-black interface. More severe commissural fusion is evident in the patient with severe stenosis.

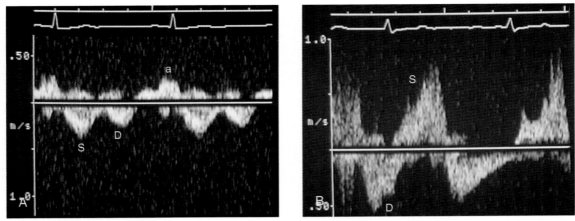

Figure 3•18   *A,* Normal hepatic vein flow shows systolic (S) and diastolic (D) atrial filling, with a small flow reversal after atrial contraction (a). *B,* With severe tricuspid regurgitation, systolic flow reversal is observed.

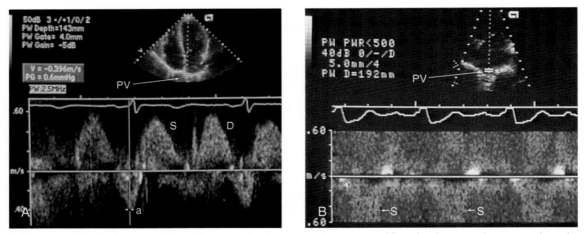

Figure 3•19   *A,* Pulmonary vein (PV) flow recorded from a transthoracic apical four-chamber view shows normal systolic (S) and diastolic (D) atrial filling, with reversal of flow after atrial contraction (a). *B,* With severe mitral regurgitation, systolic flow reversal *(arrow)* is observed, even though the signal strength is suboptimal.

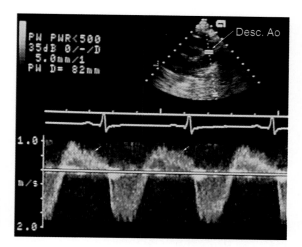

Figure 3 • 20   From a suprasternal notch window, holo-diastolic flow reversal *(arrows)* is seen in the descending thoracic aorta (Desc. Ao) in a patient with severe aortic regurgitation.

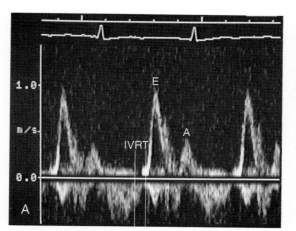

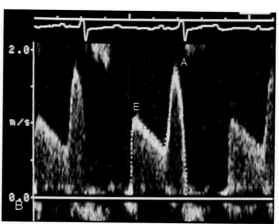

Figure 3 • 23   *A,* Normal left ventricular diastolic filling is characterized by rapid early diastolic filling (E), with a steep deceleration slope and a small atrial contribution to ventricular filling (A). The isovolumic relaxation time (IVRT) is measured as the interval from aortic valve closure to mitral valve opening. *B,* With impaired ventricular relaxation, as is seen in patients with concentric hypertrophy, the early diastolic filling velocity is diminished, the deceleration slope is prolonged, and the atrial contribution to filling is more prominent.

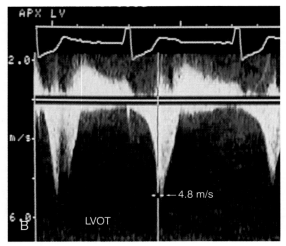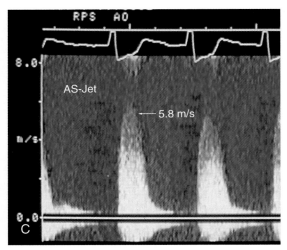

Figure 9•17   *B*, Concurrent severe left ventricular (LV) hypertrophy and hyperdynamic systolic function resulted in mid-cavity obliteration with a late peaking velocity (maximum, 4.8 m/s) at the midventricular level. *C*, The maximum jet velocity across the aortic valve, recorded from a right parasternal approach, was 5.8 m/s. Dynamic midcavity obstruction persisted in the early postoperative period but decreased as left ventricular hypertrophy regressed. Ao, aorta; LA, left atrium. LVOT, left ventricular outflow tract.

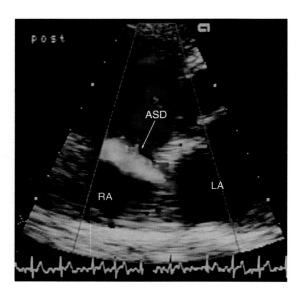

Figure 11•9   Parasternal short-axis echocardiographic image shows the small atrial septal defect (ASD) with left to right flow typically seen after balloon mitral valvuloplasty. LA, left atrium; RA, right atrium.

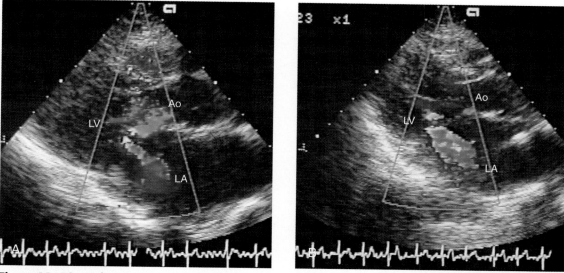

Figure 11•10 Color Doppler images of mitral regurgitation in parasternal long-axis views immediately before *(A)* and after *(B)* balloon mitral valvuloplasty. Little change in regurgitant severity is apparent in this patient. Ao, aorta; LA, left atrium; LV, left ventricle.

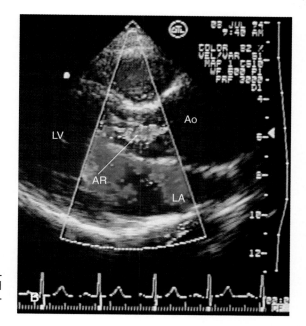

Figure 12 • 8 *B,* Central aortic regurgitation (AR), identified by color flow imaging, is caused by inadequate central coaptation of the stretched leaflets. Ao, aorta; LV, left ventricle; LA, left atrium.

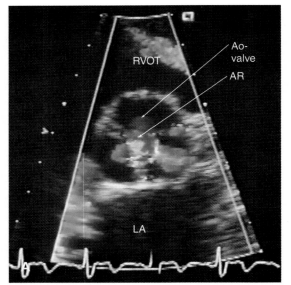

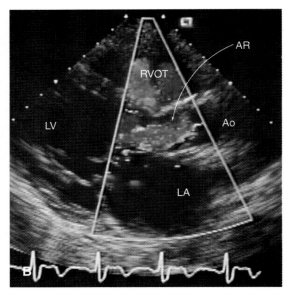

Figure 12•10   Parasternal short-axis *(A)* and long-axis *(B)* color flow images show aortic regurgitation (AR) in a patient with rheumatic valve disease. In short axis, the regurgitation jet is relatively small compared with the outflow tract, with the jet originating centrally and between the noncoronary and left coronary cusps of the aortic valve. In long axis, the narrow origin of the jet *(arrow)* can be appreciated even though the jet broadens as it extends into the left ventricular chamber. Ao, aorta; LA, left atrium; LV, left ventricle; RVOT, right ventricular outflow tract.

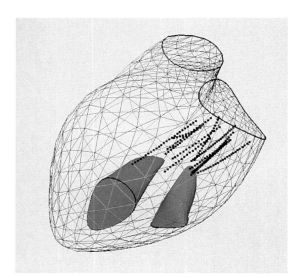

Figure 13•2   Three-dimensional reconstruction of the mitral valve apparatus. (Courtesy of Florence H. Sheehan, M.D.)

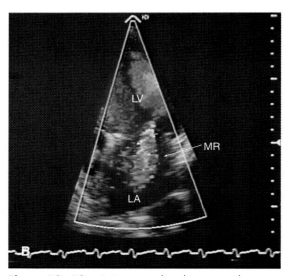

Figure 13•10   *B,* Patient with ischemic mitral regurgitation (MR). Notice the inadequate coaptation, or tenting, of the mitral leaflets in systole *(arrows)* and the centrally directed regurgitant jet. LA, left atrium; LV, left ventricle.

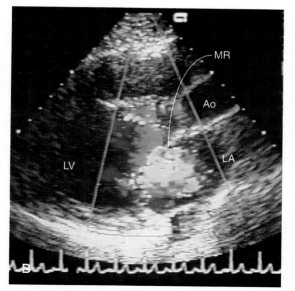

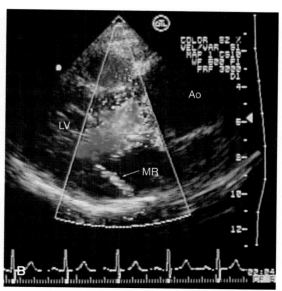

Figure 13•11 *B,* In systole, coaptation appears normal, but severe mitral regurgitation (MR) is caused by inadequate leaflet apposition and decreased leaflet flexibility. Ao, aorta; LA, left atrium; LV, left ventricle.

Figure 13•13 *B,* Color flow imaging showing only mild mitral regurgitation (MR). Ao, aorta; LV, left ventricle.

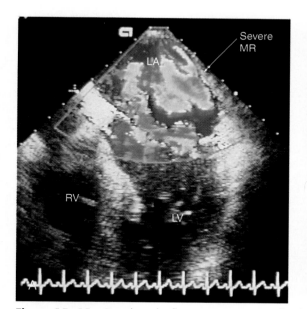

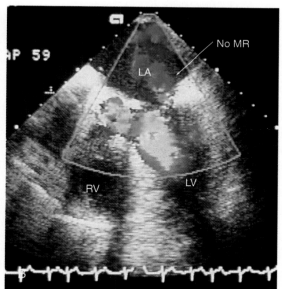

Figure 15•11 Doppler color flow images correspond to the two-dimensional images in Figure 15-10 and show severe mitral regurgitation (MR) with an anteriorly directed jet at baseline *(A)* and no significant regurgitation after mitral valve repair *(B).* The mean arterial pressure was similar during the preoperative and postoperative recordings. LA, left atrium; LV, left ventricle; RV, right ventricle.

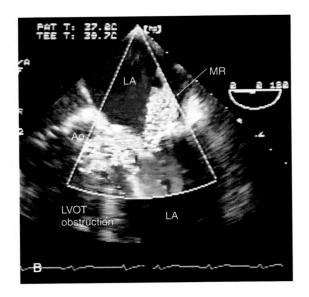

Figure 15•14   *B,* The resulting dynamic outflow tract obstruction and mitral regurgitation are seen on color flow imaging. After volume loading, mitral valve motion normalized, and no significant mitral regurgitation or outflow obstruction was evident. At the 6-month follow-up evaluation, the patient had no evidence of outflow obstruction or mitral regurgitation demonstrated by echocardiography. Ao, aorta; LA, left atrium; LVOT, left ventricular outflow tract.

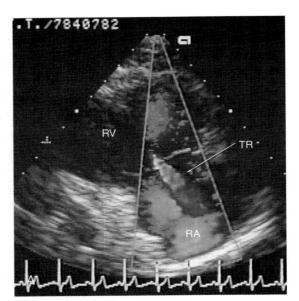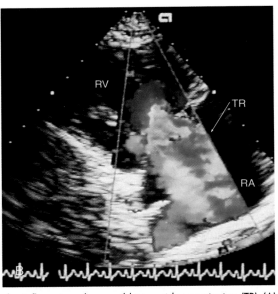

Figure 16•4   Color Doppler flow imaging in a right ventricular inflow view shows mild tricuspid regurgitation (TR) *(A)* and severe tricuspid regurgitation *(B)*. With severe regurgitation, a broad jet of turbulent flow extends to the distal wall of the atrium. RA, right atrium; RV, right ventricle.

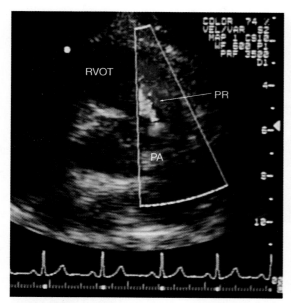

Figure 16•14 The color Doppler image shows mild pulmonic regurgitation in a patient with moderate pulmonic stenosis and mild pulmonic regurgitation (PR). The regurgitant jet is narrow as it crosses the valve plane. PA, pulmonary artery; RVOT, right ventricular outflow tract.

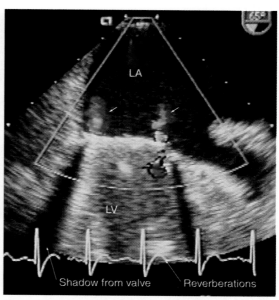

Figure 17•10 The transesophageal echocardiographic image of a St. Jude mitral valve shows the normal small regurgitant jets at valve closure. Notice the prominent reverberations *(arrows)* distal to the valve obscuring evaluation of structures in the far field of the image. LA, left atrium; LV, left ventricle.

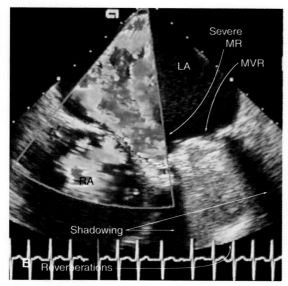

Figure 17•19 *B,* Color flow imaging documented severe paraprosthetic mitral regurgitation with a large color flow jet filling the entire enlarged left atrium and with systolic flow reversal in the pulmonary veins. LA, left atrium; RA, right atrium.

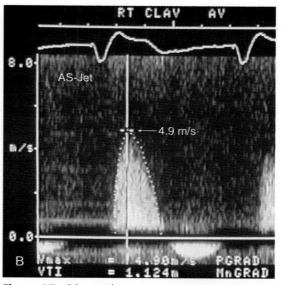

Figure 17•20 *B,* The continuous wave Doppler signal shows a velocity of 4.9 m/s, corresponding to a maximum gradient of 96 mm Hg and a mean gradient of 53 mm Hg across the valve.

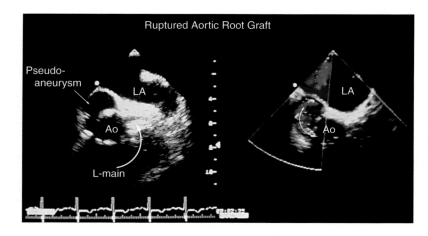

Figure 17·21 Transesophageal echocardiographic imaging in a patient with an ascending aortic graft demonstrates a pseudoaneurysm around the graft with color flow from the aorta into the pseudoaneurysm *(arrow)*. Ao, aorta; LA, left atrium; L-main, left main coronary artery.

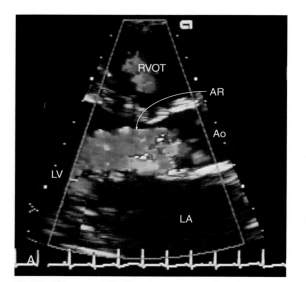

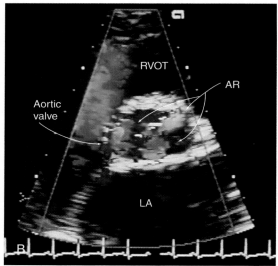

Figure 18·4 Color flow Doppler images in the same patient as in Figure 18-2 show severe aortic regurgitation (AR) due to valve destruction by infective endocarditis in long-axis *(A)* and short-axis *(B)* views. Ao, aorta; LA, left atrium; LV, left ventricle; RVOT, right ventricular outflow tract.

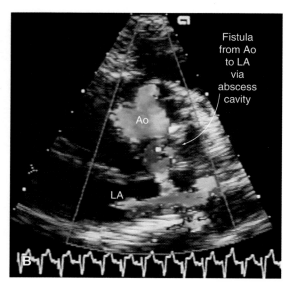

Figure 18·6 *B,* Color flow imaging shows a fistula from the aortic root into the left atrium *(arrow)*. Ao, aorta; LA, left atrium.

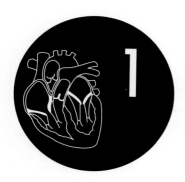

1 Etiology and Prevalence of Valvular Heart Disease

OVERALL PREVALENCE OF VALVULAR HEART DISEASE

During the past 50 years, there has been a dramatic shift in the causes of valvular heart disease in the United States, with a marked decline in the incidence of rheumatic valve disease and an increase in age-related degenerative valve disease.[1-3] However, although relatively uncommon in the United States, rheumatic heart disease remains a major case of mortality and morbidity worldwide.[4] The World Health Organization estimates that more than 12 million people are affected by rheumatic fever or rheumatic heart disease. Children and young adults mainly account for the more than 400,000 deaths annually. In many countries, more than 50% of patients with rheumatic heart disease are unaware of the condition and are therefore not receiving prophylaxis to prevent recurrent rheumatic fever. The primary episode of rheumatic fever and the long-term valvular sequelae produce substantial medical costs for this potentially preventable disease.[5] The incidence of acute rheumatic fever, the prevalence of rheumatic heart disease among school children, and the mortality associated with these conditions show wide geographic variations (Table 1–1). Most cases of rheumatic valve disease affect the mitral valve (mitral stenosis is the most common lesion), but aortic and tricuspid valve involvement also occur.

It is difficult to estimate the prevalence of specific types of nonrheumatic valvular disease, because the International Classification

	TABLE 1·1 WORLDWIDE IMPACT OF RHEUMATIC FEVER AND RHEUMATIC HEART DISEASE			
WHO Region	**Incidence of Acute RF in School Children (per 100,000)**	**Prevalence of RHD in School Children (per 1000)**	**Mortality (All Ages) for RF (per 100,000)**	**Mortality (All Ages) for RHD (per 100,000)**
Africa	3000	1.7–15.0	15	35
Americas	0.2–50.5	0.2–8.5	0–0.4	0.8–2.1
Eastern Mediterranean	51–100	1.6–10.5	7	81
Europe			0	1.0–5.3
Southeast Asia	30–54	1.3–5.0	2	4
Western Pacific	93–150	0.1–18.6	0–0.4	1.0–8.0

RF, rheumatic fever; RHD, rheumatic heart disease.
   From World Health Organization, October 28, 1996 (http://www.who.ch.programmes/ncd/cvd/cvd_epi.html).

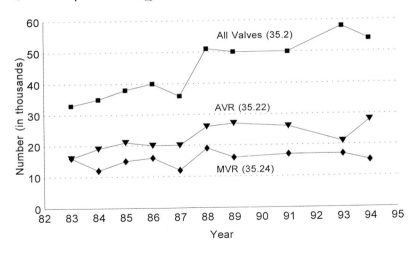

Figure 1·1 The number of heart valve surgery procedures performed in the United States between 1983 and 1994 is based on the procedure codes of the National Center for Health Statistics International Classification of Disease, version 9 (procedure code in parentheses).

of Disease, version 9 (ICD-9), discharge and procedure codes distinguish between aortic and mitral valve disease but not between valve stenosis and regurgitation. In the United States in 1994, there were about 54,000 surgical valve procedures, about two thirds of which were aortic valve replacements (Fig. 1–1). In the same period, there were 931,000 coronary artery bypass grafting procedures, making surgery for coronary artery disease 15 to 20 times more common than surgery for valve disease.[2] These statistics do not include nonsurgical valve procedures such as percutaneous balloon valvuloplasty.

Compared with the number of patients undergoing surgical procedures, far more persons are discharged with a diagnosis of valvular heart disease (Fig. 1–2). In 1994, a discharge diagnosis of nonrheumatic mitral valve disease was made for 422,000 patients and nonrheumatic aortic valve disease for 242,000 patients.

Many of these patients probably have valve disease of only mild to moderate severity, often resulting from other disease processes such as left ventricular systolic dysfunction or aortic root atherosclerosis, and most do not need surgical intervention. For comparison, there were 865,000 discharge diagnoses of acute myocardial infarction and 2.7 million cases of heart failure.

In the 1994 National Health Interview Study,[6] the reported incidence of a heart murmur was relatively high, particularly among younger adults, suggesting that patients often are aware of the possibility of valvular heart disease without needing hospitalization or valve surgery (Table 1–2). This perception emphasizes the importance of correctly diagnosing valvular heart disease, because the number of patients with a flow murmur or only mild valve disease greatly exceeds the number of patients with significant valve dysfunction. It is

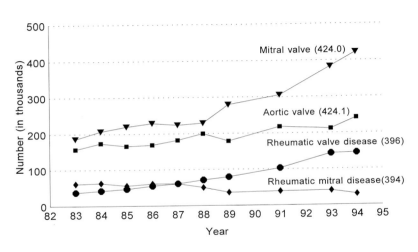

Figure 1·2 The number of patients discharged with diagnoses of valvular heart disease in the United States between 1983 and 1994 is based on the discharge code data of the National Center for Health Statistics International Classification of Disease, version 9 (diagnosis code in parentheses). The number of diagnoses of mitral valve disease appears to have increased, but this may reflect the expanded diagnostic use of echocardiography.

TABLE 1·2 REPORTED CASES OF CHRONIC CARDIAC CONDITIONS PER 1000 PERSONS IN THE UNITED STATES

Condition	Male			Female		
	<45 y	45–65 y	>65 y	<45 y	45–65 y	>65 y
Ischemic heart disease	3.8	81.9	191.8	—	32.5	123.3
Heart rhythm disorders	16.5	41.8	78.8	25.8	53.1	96.2
Hypertension	31.9	220.0	319.5	32.4	53.1	96.2
Heart murmurs	11.5	15.8	15.2	18.5	29.0	25.3

From Adams PF, Marano MA: Current estimate from the National Health Interview Survey, 1994. Vital Health Stat 1995;193:83–84.

a challenge for the primary care physician and the specialist to correctly identify which patients need further evaluation. Excessive use of diagnostic tests for patients with insignificant disease escalates medical costs, while failure to recognize progressive disease may result in unnecessary morbidity and mortality.

AORTIC VALVE DISEASE
Aortic Valve Stenosis
Prevalence

In adults, valvular aortic stenosis is caused by rheumatic disease, secondary calcification of a congenitally bicuspid valve, or fibrocalcific changes of a trileaflet valve.[7, 8] Children and young adults may have congenital aortic valve stenosis due to a unicuspid or severely deformed bicuspid valve. Valvular aortic stenosis must be differentiated from membranous or muscular subaortic stenosis and from supravalvular stenosis in younger patients. In older adults, the primary differential diagnosis is obstructive hypertrophic cardiomyopathy, although previously unrecognized subaortic ste-

nosis occasionally is identified in adult patients. In adults undergoing surgical intervention for aortic stenosis in the United States, calcific aortic stenosis is most common, accounting for 51% of cases, with a bicuspid valve accounting for 36% of cases and rheumatic disease accounting for only 9% of cases (Fig. 1–3).[1] The increased prevalence of calcific disease largely reflects aging of the population. Of the 28,000 aortic valve replacements performed in the United States in 1994, 61% were performed in patients older than 65 years of age.[2]

Rheumatic involvement of the aortic valve is characterized by fusion of the commissures between the aortic valve leaflets. Because rheumatic heart disease typically affects the mitral valve first, rheumatic disease of the aortic valve is invariably accompanied by rheumatic mitral valve disease.

The prevalence of a congenital bicuspid valve may be as high as 1% to 2% of the general population, with a threefold to fourfold male predominance.[9–11] Most patients with a congenital bicuspid valve develop superimposed calcific changes, eventually requiring

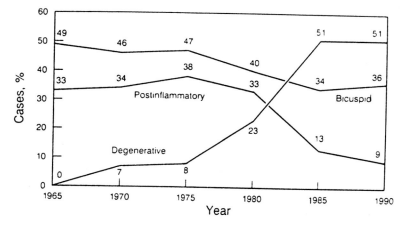

Figure 1·3 Among patients undergoing surgery for isolated aortic stenosis (637 cases total), the relative number of cases attributed to various causes changed from 1965 to 1990. (From Dare AJ, Veinot JP, Edwards WD, Tazelaar HD, Schaff HV: New observations on the etiology of aortic valve disease: a surgical pathologic study of 236 cases from 1990. Hum Pathol 1993; 24:1336.)

intervention for valve stenosis in the sixth or seventh decade of life. It is unusual for a congenital bicuspid valve to remain normal after age 70 years, although rare cases have been reported. The histologic changes in the stenotic bicuspid valve appear to be similar to those described for degenerative disease of a trileaflet valve. However, patients with a bicuspid valve present with significant obstruction about 2 decades earlier than patients with a trileaflet valve.[11] The abnormal stress-strain characteristics of the bicuspid valve probably account for the earlier onset of disease compared with disease onset in patients with a trileaflet valve.

Etiology

Until recently, "degenerative" calcific aortic stenosis was considered to be a nonspecific, age-related process. However, many elderly patients have relatively normal valve leaflets,[12, 13] although the prevalence of valvular aortic stenosis increases with age in men and women (Table 1–3). Aortic sclerosis, defined as irregular thickening of the aortic valve leaflets in the absence of significant obstruction, appears to represent a milder form of the same disease process. Although the prevalence of aortic sclerosis increases with age, other factors are important in determining whether a person develops clinically or echo-

cardiographically evident aortic valve disease. Studies on clinical factors associated with aortic valve disease and immunohistochemical studies of valve leaflets suggest that calcific aortic stenosis is caused by an active disease process.[14, 15]

In the Cardiovascular Health Study of 5201 persons older than 65 years of age, clinical factors associated with aortic sclerosis or stenosis identified by echocardiography were age, male sex, a history of hypertension, low-density lipoprotein cholesterol levels, lipoprotein (a) levels, height, and current smoking.[12] Smaller studies also support the association of these clinical factors with calcific aortic valve disease (Table 1–4).[16–21] Other studies indicate that radiation exposure and conditions that result in a high cardiac output state (eg, renal failure, Paget's disease) may be associated with aortic valve disease.[22–24]

At the histologic level, calcific aortic stenosis is characterized by lesions on the aortic side of the leaflet in areas of disruption of the normal subendothelial basement membrane and in association with displacement of the subendothelial elastic lamina (Fig. 1–4).[14, 15] These lesions consist of lipid, calcification, and proteoglycans,[25] along with macrophages and T lymphocytes. The active role of macrophages in lesion formation is demonstrated by the presence of foam cells and by a subset of lesion macrophages that produce osteopontin,

TABLE 1•3   ECHOCARDIOGRAPHIC PREVALENCE OF AORTIC VALVE ABNORMALITIES

Age Group	No Abnormality	Aortic Valve Abnormality*		Aortic Valve Calcification and Thickening*	
		Sclerosis	*Stenosis*	*Slight*	*Severe*
Cardiovascular Health Study† (n = 5201)					
All subjects	72%	26%	2%		
Women	76%	22%	1.5%		
Men	67%	31%	2%		
65–74 y	78%	20%	1.3%		
75–84 y	62%	35%	2.4%		
≥85 y	48%	48%	4%		
Helsinki Aging Study‡ (n = 651)					
55–71 y	72%			21%	7%
75–76 y	52%			39%	9%
80–81 y	45%			38%	17%
85–86 y	25%			56%	19%

*Percentages of patients in each age group with the observed valve abnormality.
†Stewart BF, Siscovick D, Lird BK, et al: Clinical factors associated with calcific aortic valve disease. J Am Coll Cardiol 1997;29:630–634.
‡Lindroos M, Kupari M, Heikkila J, Tilvis R: Prevalence of aortic valve abnormalities in the elderly: an echocardiographic study of a random population sample. J Am Coll Cardiol 1993;21:1220–1225.

TABLE 1·4 CLINICAL FACTORS ASSOCIATED WITH CALCIFIC AORTIC VALVE DISEASE

Clinical Factor*	P Value	Odds Ratio
Age	<0.001	2.18†
Male gender	<0.001	2.03
Lipoprotein (a)	<0.001	1.23‡
Height	0.001	0.84§
History of hypertension	0.002	1.23
Smoking (current)	0.006	1.35
Low-density lipoprotein cholesterol (mg/dL)	0.006	1.12‡

*Clinical factors are listed according to the Cardiovascular Health Study[12]; other studies also identified associated clinical factors of age,[17, 19] lipoprotein (a),[17] smoking,[16] gender,[16] cholesterol,[18,21] hypertension,[18] and diabetes.[18, 21]
†Ten-year increase.
‡Ten-unit increase.
§Comparison of 75th and 25th percentiles.

a protein involved in vascular calcification (see Chapter 2).[26] Sclerotic valves show similar, but less severe, histologic changes. Unlike atherosclerosis, smooth muscle cells are not present in the valvular lesions or in normal valvular tissue.

The identification of potential clinical risk factors for calcific aortic valve disease and the evidence that stenosis may be the end stage of an active disease process suggest that interventions to prevent or slow disease progression may be possible in the future.

Aortic Valve Regurgitation

Prevalence

The prevalence of significant aortic regurgitation is difficult to ascertain, because current diagnostic codes (ICD-9) classify valve disease as rheumatic and nonrheumatic, rather than as stenosis or regurgitation, and procedure codes list aortic valve operations as a single group, regardless of whether valve replacement was performed for stenosis or regurgitation. Moreover, many patients have mixed patterns of stenosis and regurgitation, ranging from severe stenosis with minimal regurgitation to severe regurgitation with minimal stenosis. Clinical decision making for patients with mixed moderate stenosis and moderate regurgitation is particularly difficult, because most of the published literature is limited to patients with predominant stenosis or regurgitation.

In surgical series of patients undergoing aortic valve surgery, isolated aortic regurgitation accounts for about 20% to 30% of cases, and

mixed stenosis and regurgitation accounts for an additional 12% to 30% of cases.[27, 28] Of patients older than 70 years, a lower percentage undergo aortic valve replacement for aortic regurgitation, and a higher percentage are treated for aortic stenosis.[27]

Patients undergoing surgical intervention for valvular regurgitation represent only the extreme of the disease spectrum. Less severe aortic regurgitation, which does not require surgical intervention, is much more common. Although accurate estimates of disease prevalence are not available, several echocardiographic studies have found an increasing prevalence of detectable aortic regurgitation with age,[29–31] with Doppler examinations demonstrating aortic regurgitation for as many as 11% of subjects older than 50 years[31] and 29% of subjects older than 75 years.[13] Most of these elderly patients do not have hemodynamically significant regurgitation, show no evidence of left ventricular dilation, and usually require no specific follow-up or treatment. The presumed cause of aortic regurgitation in the elderly is a combination of mild aortic root dilation[32] and mild fibrocalcific changes of the valve leaflets. Chronic hypertension is associated with mild aortic root dilation,[33] and although an increased prevalence of aortic regurgitation has not been documented in asymptomatic hypertensive patients, aortic regurgitation is a feature of end-stage hypertensive heart disease.[34]

For younger patients, the echocardiographic finding of more than trace aortic regurgitation elicits concern, especially if they do not have a history of hypertension. A careful clinical history and echocardiographic examination of the valve leaflets and aortic root is indicated to determine the mechanism and severity of regurgitation. Patients with moderate or severe regurgitation require close follow-up and treatment as discussed in Chapter 12. Even when aortic regurgitation is hemodynamically insignificant, appropriate endocarditis prophylaxis may be indicated. Whether the patient has trivial, nonprogressive aortic regurgitation or is at risk of progression to more severe regurgitation is often unclear. In these cases, a repeat examination at a later date may clarify the issue.

Etiology

The integrity of aortic valve closure depends on the anatomy of the valve leaflets and on the three-dimensional geometry of the aortic root and sinuses of Valsalva. Aortic regurgita-

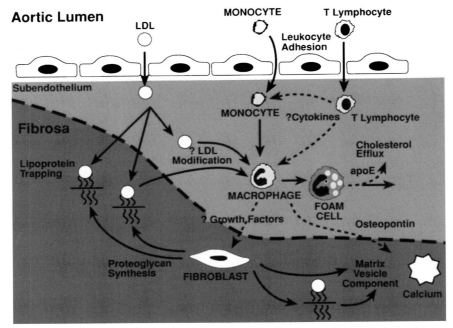

Figure 1·4 Potential roles of lipoproteins in the pathogenesis of aortic valvular lesions. Endothelial injury allows insudation of circulating lipoproteins into the subendothelial space. Sequestered in a microenvironment in which actively metabolizing cells (ie, resident fibroblasts and endothelial cells) consume antioxidants, these lipoproteins become minimally oxidized and possibly stimulate leukocyte adhesion. After more extensive oxidative modification, lipoproteins may be recognized and endocytosed by macrophage scavenger receptors, resulting in foam cell formation. Human leukocyte antigens and interleukin-2 receptors are present in lesions, suggesting the possibility of induction of cytokine and growth factor release by macrophages and fibroblasts. Lipid accumulation in macrophages leads to expression of apolipoprotein E (apoE). The cytokines released by macrophages and fibroblasts stimulate fibroblast production of proteoglycans. Low-density lipoprotein (LDL) and apoE then may be trapped by proteoglycans and lipoprotein(a) trapped by proteoglycans and fibrinogen, leading to lipoprotein accumulation and repetition of the cycle of events previously described. The presence of lipoproteins, release of calcification-mediating molecules such as osteopontin by inflammatory cells and possibly by fibroblasts, and participation of proteoglycans in matrix vesicle formation may facilitate calcium deposition. Features whose presence is inferred but not proved are indicated with question marks. (From O'Brien KD, Reichenbach DD, Marcovina SM, Kuusisto J, Alpers CE, Otto CM: Apolipoproteins B, (a), and E accumulate in the morphologically early lesion of "degenerative" valvular aortic stenosis. Arterioscler Thromb Vasc Biol 1996;16:523.)

tion can result from a variety of disease processes affecting the valve leaflets, commissures, aortic sinuses, and aortic root. For 50% of patients undergoing surgery for aortic regurgitation, the cause is root dilation, with leaflet abnormalities accounting for the remainder of the cases (Fig. 1–5).

LEAFLET ABNORMALITIES

Although most patients with congenitally bicuspid aortic valves present with stenosis later in life,[10, 11, 35] 15% to 20% have incomplete valve closure caused by distorted valve anatomy that leads to significant regurgitation. These patients typically present in the third or fourth decade of life with asymptomatic murmurs, cardiac enlargement identified by chest radiography, or symptoms resulting from aortic regurgitation.[3, 9, 36–38]

The finding of a bicuspid aortic valve prompts evaluation for associated abnormalities, including aortic coarctation[39–43] and aortic root dilation. Aortic root dilation in patients with a bicuspid aortic valve is unrelated to age or the hemodynamic severity of the valvular lesion.[44] In addition, patients with bicuspid valves are at increased risk for acute aortic dissection.[45, 46] Thus, a patient with baseline mild to moderate valve dysfunction may present emergently with severe aortic regurgitation caused by a superimposed aortic dissection. Other rare congenital causes of aortic regurgitation include congenital valve fenes-

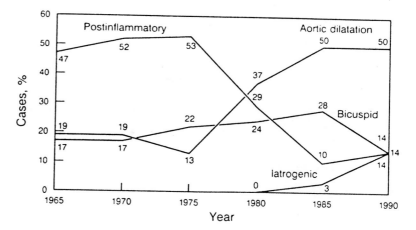

Figure 1·5 Among patients undergoing surgery for isolated aortic insufficiency (323 cases total), the relative number of cases attributed to various causes has changed over time. (From Dare AJ, Veinot JP, Edwards WD, Tazelaar HD, Schaff HV: New observations on the etiology of aortic valve disease: a surgical pathologic study of 236 cases from 1990. Hum Pathol 1993;24:1336.)

trations, unicommissural valves, and quadricuspid valves.[28]

Acquired diseases of the valve leaflets resulting in aortic regurgitation include rheumatic aortic valve disease, which is characterized by thickening and deformity along the valve commissures and which is invariably accompanied by rheumatic mitral valve disease. Infective endocarditis may result in acute regurgitation because of leaflet perforation or may result in chronic regurgitation caused by deformity of valve closure (see Chapter 18). Thickening and incomplete closure of the aortic valve leaflets can be caused by irradiation and by systemic diseases such as Fabry's disease, mucopolysaccharidosis, and Cogan's syndrome.[28] Degenerative valve disease may lead to mild aortic regurgitation but rarely causes a hemodynamically significant lesion unless concurrent aortic root dilation exists. Nonbacterial thrombotic endocarditis or other valve masses (eg, papillary fibroelastoma) rarely result in significant valve incompetence.

AORTIC ROOT DISEASE

Congenital or genetic abnormalities may be associated with aortic regurgitation because of abnormal geometry of the outflow tract, sinuses, or aortic root. Examples include a perimembranous ventricular septal defect with inadequate support of the base of the aortic annulus; conditions such as tetralogy of Fallot that are associated with an enlarged aortic root; congenital sinus of Valsalva aneurysms, which may lead to distortion of the normal supporting structures; and collagen-vascular diseases such as Ehlers-Danlos syndrome, pseudoxanthoma elasticum, and osteogenesis imperfecta, which result in aortic root dilation

because of the abnormal molecular components of the aortic wall. Marfan's syndrome, although rare, is important to recognize as a potential cause of aortic regurgitation, because diagnosis and appropriate surgical therapy for patients with this genetic disease can be lifesaving.

Acquired dilation of the aortic root or distortion of its normal anatomy leads to symmetric stretching of the annulus until the size of the stretched valve leaflets is inadequate to cover the cross-sectional area of the outflow tract, resulting in a central regurgitant jet. Inadequate support of the valve commissures results in a more eccentric jet origin and direction.

The most prevalent acquired abnormality of the aortic root is dilation due to hypertension, atherosclerotic changes of the aortic wall, or both conditions. Although some degree of aortic regurgitation is common in this situation, severe regurgitation that requires medical or surgical therapy is rare. Annuloaortic ectasia, also known as cystic medial necrosis, is more likely to lead to progressive root dilation and hemodynamically significant regurgitation, requiring surgical intervention.[47] Systemic diseases accompanied by aortic root dilation that may result in significant aortic regurgitation include rheumatoid arthritis,[48] psoriatic arthritis, ankylosing spondylitis,[49, 50] systemic lupus erythematosus, Reiter's syndrome,[51] relapsing polychondritis,[52] syphilitic aortitis, Kawasaki's disease, and Takayasu's aortitis.[28]

Acute aortic regurgitation, although much less common than chronic regurgitation, is a medical and surgical emergency. Acute aortic regurgitation may occur as a result of aortic dissection. The mechanisms of regurgitation include nonspecific aortic root enlargement, loss of normal commissural support, and extension of the dissection flap into a leaflet. Acute aortic regurgitation may result from leaflet perforation caused by endocarditis. Trauma also can lead to acute aortic regurgitation by means of iatrogenic damage to a valve leaflet from a catheter or other intravascular device or from leaflet prolapse after traumatic rupture of the ascending aorta.[53, 54]

MITRAL VALVE DISEASE
Mitral Stenosis
Prevalence

In Europe and North America, the prevalence of mitral stenosis due to rheumatic disease has decreased dramatically during the past 40 years. Mitral stenosis accounted for 43% of all valve disease cases at a European center in 1960, compared with 9% in 1985.[55]

Etiology

Rheumatic heart disease is by far the most common cause of mitral valve stenosis. Although only 75% of patients with mitral stenosis report a history consistent with rheumatic fever,[55, 56] surgical pathology series show rheumatic involvement in 99% of mitral valves excised because of stenosis.[57–60] About 38% of mitral stenosis cases have multivalve involvement. The aortic valve is affected most often (93%), with rheumatic tricuspid valve changes seen in 6% of patients with rheumatic mitral valve disease and involvement of all three valves in 1% of patients with rheumatic mitral valve disease.[58]

Severe mitral annular calcification with involvement of the mitral leaflets by the degenerative process is an unusual cause of hemodynamically significant mitral stenosis, accounting for less than 3% of mitral stenosis cases. These patients tend to be elderly and often have associated aortic valve calcification.[61] Rarer causes of mitral stenosis include carcinoid disease,[62] Fabry's disease,[63] mucopolysaccharidosis,[64] Whipple's disease,[65, 66] gout,[67] rheumatoid arthritis, or obstruction by a large valvular vegetation.[68, 69]

Congenital mitral stenosis accounts for less than 1% of mitral stenosis cases. Congenital abnormalities include shortened chordae and obliteration of interchordal spaces, a hypoplastic mitral valve associated with hypoplastic left heart syndrome, a supramitral ring, and a "parachute" mitral valve with insertion of all the chordae into a single papillary muscle. Congenital mitral stenosis often is associated with other congenital abnormalities and is rarely seen in adults, because the median age at death is only 2 months.[70]

Mitral Regurgitation

A variety of disease processes lead to mitral valve regurgitation. Mitral regurgitation may be caused by a primary disease of the valve apparatus, a secondary consequence of another cardiac disease, or a systemic or genetic disease that involves the mitral valve.

Prevalence

The relative prevalence of different causes of mitral regurgitation depends on whether only patients with severe regurgitation requiring surgical intervention or patients with milder degrees of regurgitation are included in the study. Estimates of disease prevalence are confounded by the observation that a small degree of physiologic mitral regurgitation can be detected on careful Doppler echocardiography in as many as 80% of normal, healthy persons.

Etiology

In patients undergoing surgical intervention for severe mitral regurgitation, the most common causes are mitral valve prolapse (20% to 70% of cases), ischemic mitral regurgitation (13% to 30%), rheumatic disease (3% to 40%), and endocarditis (10% to 12%).[57, 60, 68, 71–74] In patients followed medically for milder degrees of regurgitation, mitral valve prolapse and coronary artery disease also are common, but more patients are seen with mitral regurgitation resulting from dilated cardiomyopathy or as a component of a systemic disease. In many of these patients, therapy is directed to the underlying disease process rather than directly toward reduction of mitral regurgitation severity. In others, mitral regurgitation is an incidental finding that does not contribute to the disease process, does not progress to more severe regurgitation, and does not require surgical intervention. Surgical series of patients with mitral regurgitation represent only a small subset of the overall population of patients with this abnormality.

As might be expected from the complexity of the mitral valve apparatus, mitral regurgitation can have many other causes, including primary valve abnormalities, other cardiac diseases with mitral valvular involvement, systemic diseases that also affect the mitral valve, and external forces such as radiation therapy[75] or surgical trauma. In addition to myxomatous mitral valve disease (eg, mitral valve prolapse), primary disease of the valve leaflets includes endocarditis (see Chapter 18) with destruction of valve tissue leading to perforation, incomplete leaflet coaptation, chordal rupture, and consequent mitral regurgitation. Congenital abnormalities of the leaflets include a cleft anterior mitral leaflet and mitral valve fenestrations. A cleft anterior leaflet often accompanies defects of the atrioventricular septum but also may occur as an isolated defect.

An example of a primary cardiac disease that secondarily affects the mitral valve is hypertrophic cardiomyopathy. Although the systolic anterior motion of the mitral leaflets contributes to mitral regurgitation because of distortion of leaflet closure, the leaflets also are elongated and increased in size.[76, 77] Another example is Marfan's syndrome, in which the anterior mitral leaflet is long and redundant but minimally thickened, with systolic bowing into the left atrium and associated mitral regurgitation. Although sometimes classified as mitral valve prolapse, the echocardiographic appearance of the mitral valve in Marfan's syndrome is quite different from that of myxomatous mitral valve disease. Both show leaflet elongation and redundancy, but with Marfan's syndrome, there is little leaflet thickening, the anterior leaflet is most often affected, chordal rupture is rare, and mitral valve surgery is needed infrequently.[78-80] In contrast, mitral prolapse is characterized by marked leaflet thickening, predominant involvement of the posterior leaflet, and more frequent chordal rupture.[81, 82]

An example of systemic diseases that may affect the mitral valve is hypereosinophilic syndrome, in which fixation of the posterior leaflet by subannular thrombus leads to mitral regurgitation that, if severe, may require valve replacement.[83] Another example is systemic lupus erythematosus; about 50% of these patients have detectable valve disease on echocardiography, with significant valve regurgitation in approximately 25% that sometimes requires valve surgery.[84] Left-sided valve thickening and pathologic regurgitation have been associated with the use of fenfluramine-phentermine therapy used for appetite suppression. The pathologic changes seen with this therapy

mimic those seen in patients with carcinoid involvement of the tricuspid valve.[85]

Mitral regurgitation also is associated with mitral annular calcification. The presumed mechanism of regurgitation with mitral annular calcification is increased rigidity of the annulus, although calcification may involve the base of the posterior leaflet in some cases. Mitral annular calcification is most common in the elderly, particularly women, and is associated with hypertension, aortic stenosis, renal failure, and diabetes mellitus.[86-88] Typically, the degree of mitral regurgitation is only mild to moderate, and these patients rarely need intervention for mitral regurgitation.

TRICUSPID AND PULMONIC VALVE DISEASE

Primary involvement of the right-sided heart valves is uncommon in adults, but tricuspid regurgitation from pulmonary hypertension with secondary right ventricular enlargement and systolic dysfunction frequently accompanies significant mitral valve disease. Primary abnormalities of the tricuspid valve leading to regurgitation, although less common, include endocarditis, Ebstein's anomaly, and carcinoid syndrome. Tricuspid valve stenosis is a rare diagnosis, complicating rheumatic mitral disease in only 3% to 6% of cases.[58, 89, 90] Pulmonic valve disease most often is congenital and encountered in young adults with or without prior cardiac surgical procedures (see Chapter 16).

Minor degrees of tricuspid and pulmonic regurgitation can be detected in up to 80% of normal individuals and are not associated with progressive valve dysfunction or adverse clinical outcomes. Mild amounts of tricuspid and pulmonic regurgitation are considered to be normal.

ENDOCARDITIS

The estimated incidence of infective endocarditis is 3 to 6 cases per 100,000 inhabitants, based on data from a prospective Swedish study.[91] A population-based study in the United States also found an incidence of community-acquired native valve infective endocarditis of 4.5 cases per 100,000 persons. However, an additional 5 cases of infective endocarditis per 100,000 persons were associated with intravenous drug use.[92] It is estimated that infective endocarditis accounts for about 0.5 to 1.0% of hospital admissions in the United States. A discharge diagnosis of endocarditis (ICD-9 424.9) was recorded for 27,000 cases in 1994.

Before antibiotics were available, the mortality rate for infective endocarditis was nearly 100%. Although the use of high-dose, prolonged antibiotic therapy and surgical intervention in appropriate cases has dramatically improved survival rates, clinical outcome remains poor, with an overall mortality rate of 26% to 40%. Mortality is even higher for certain subgroups, depending on the specific organism and degree of intracardiac destruction from the infective process.[93, 94]

Concurrent with improved therapies for infective endocarditis is an increase in the age of affected individuals, with an estimated mean age of 30 years in the preantibiotic era compared with a mean age of 40 to 70 years in modern studies.[91, 95–98] The types of predisposing structural heart disease have shifted from chronic rheumatic disease in the past to predominantly degenerative valve disease and congenital heart disease in more recent series. The proportion of cases associated with intravenous drug use also has increased.

References

1. Dare AJ, Veinot JP, Edwards WD, Tazelaar HD, Schaff HV: New observations on the etiology of aortic valve disease: a surgical pathologic study of 236 cases from 1990. Hum Pathol 1993;24:1330–1338.
2. Vital and Health Statistics, Series 13. National Center for Health Statistics 1995;127.
3. Passik CS, Ackermann DM, Pluth JR, Edwards WD: Temporal changes in the causes of aortic stenosis: a surgical pathologic study of 646 cases. Mayo Clin Proc 1987;62:119–123.
4. World Health Organization: Bull World Health Organ 1995;73:583–587.
5. North DA, Heynes RA, Lennon DR, Neutze J: Analysis of costs of acute rheumatic fever and rheumatic heart disease in Auckland. N Z Med J 1993;106:400–403.
6. Adams PF, Marano MA: Current estimates from the National Health Interview Survey, 1994. Vital Health Stat 1995;10:83–84.
7. Roberts WC: Morphologic aspects of cardiac valve dysfunction. Am Heart J 1992;123:1610–1632.
8. Selzer A: Changing aspects of the natural history of valvular aortic stenosis. N Engl J Med 1987;317:91–98.
9. Roberts WC: Anatomically isolated aortic valvular disease: the case against its being of rheumatic etiology. Am J Med 1970;49:151–159.
10. Roberts WC: The congenitally bicuspid aortic valve: a study of 85 autopsy cases. Am J Cardiol 1970;26:72–83.
11. Beppu S, Suzuki S, Matsuda H, Ohmori F, Nagata S, Miyatake K: Rapidity of progression of aortic stenosis in patients with congenital bicuspid aortic valves. Am J Cardiol 1993;71:322–327.
12. Stewart BF, Siscovick D, Lind BK, Gardin JM, et al:

13. Lindroos M, Kupari M, Heikkila J, Tilvis R: Prevalence of aortic valve abnormalities in the elderly: an echocardiographic study of a random population sample. J Am Coll Cardiol 1993;21:1220–1225.
14. Otto CM, Kuusisto J, Reichenbach DD, Gown AM, O'Brien KD: Characterization of the early lesion of "degenerative" valvular aortic stenosis: histologic and immunohistochemical studies. Circulation 1994;90:844–853.
15. Olsson M, Dalsgaard CJ, Haegerstrand A, Rosenqvist M, Ryden L, Nilsson J: Accumulation of T lymphocytes and expression of interleukin-2 receptors in nonrheumatic stenotic aortic valves. J Am Coll Cardiol 1994;23:1162–1170.
16. Mohler ER, Sheridan MJ, Nichols R, Harvey WP, Waller BF: Development and progression of aortic valve stenosis: atherosclerosis risk factors—a causal relationship? A clinical morphologic study. Clin Cardiol 1991;14:995–999.
17. Gotoh T, Kuroda T, Yamasawa M, et al: Correlation between lipoprotein (a) and aortic valve sclerosis assessed by echocardiography (the JMS Cardiac Echo and Cohort Study). Am J Cardiol 1995;76:928–932.
18. Aronow WS, Schwartz KS, Koenigsberg M: Correlation of serum lipids, calcium, and phosphorus, diabetes mellitus and history of systemic hypertension with presence or absence of calcified or thickened aortic cusps or root in elderly patients. Am J Cardiol 1987;59:998–999.
19. Pomerance A, Darby AJ, Hodkinson HM: Valvular calcification in the elderly: possible pathogenic factors. J Gerontol 1978;33:672–675.
20. Hoagland PM, Cook EF, Flatley M, Walker C, Goldman L: Case-control analysis of risk factors for presence of aortic stenosis in adults (age 50 years or older). Am J Cardiol 1985;55:744–747.
21. Deutscher S, Rockette HE, Krishnaswami V: Diabetes and hypercholesterolemia among patients with calcific aortic stenosis. J Chron Dis 1984;37:407–415.
22. Strickberger SA, Schulman SP, Hutchins GM: Association of Paget's disease of bone with calcific aortic valve disease. Am J Med 1987;82:953–956.
23. Carlson RG, Mayfield WR, Normann S, Alexander JA: Radiation-associated valvular disease. Chest 1991;99:538–545.
24. Maher ER, Pazianas M, Curtis JR: Calcific aortic stenosis: a complication of chronic uraemia. Nephron 1987;47:119–122.
25. O'Brien KD, Reichenbach DD, Marcovina SM, Kuusisto J, Alpers CE, Otto CM: Apolipoproteins B, (a), and E accumulate in the morphologically early lesion of "degenerative" valvular aortic stenosis. Arterioscler Thromb Vasc Biol 1996;16:523–532.
26. O'Brien KD, Kuusisto J, Reichenbach DD, et al: Osteopontin is expressed in human aortic valvular lesions. Circulation 1995;92:2163–2168.
27. Fremes SE, Goldman BS, Ivanov J, Weisel RD, David TE, Salerno T: Valvular surgery in the elderly. Circulation 1989;80(suppl I):77–90.
28. Edwards WD: Surgical pathology of the aortic valve. *In* Waller BF, ed. Pathology of the heart and great vessels. New York: Churchill Livingstone, 1988:43–100.
29. Aronow WS, Kronzon I: Correlation of prevalence and severity of aortic regurgitation detected by pulsed Doppler echocardiography with the murmur of aortic regurgitation in elderly patients in a long-

term health care facility. Am J Cardiol 1989;63:128–129.

30. Akasaka T, Yoshikawa J, Yoshida K, et al: Age-related valvular regurgitation: a study by pulsed Doppler echocardiography. Circulation 1987;76:262–265.

31. Klein AL, Burstow DJ, Tajik AJ, et al: Age-related prevalence of valvular regurgitation in normal subjects: a comprehensive color flow examination of 118 volunteers. J Am Soc Echocardiogr 1990;3:54–63.

32. Seder JD, Burke JF, Pauletto FJ: Prevalence of aortic regurgitation by color flow Doppler in relation to aortic root size. J Am Soc Echocardiogr 1990;3:316–319.

33. Kim M, Roman MJ, Cavallini MC, Schwartz JE, Pickering TG, Devereux RB: Effect of hypertension on aortic root size and prevalence of aortic regurgitation. Hypertension 1996;28:47–52.

34. Waller BF, Zoltick JM, Rosen JH, et al: Severe aortic regurgitation from systemic hypertension (without aortic dissection) requiring aortic valve replacement: analysis of four patients. Am J Cardiol 1982;49:473–477.

35. Roberts WC: The structure of the aortic valve in clinically isolated aortic stenosis: an autopsy study of 162 patients over 15 years of age. Circulation 1970;42:91–97.

36. Subramanian R, Olson LJ, Edwards WD: Surgical pathology of pure aortic stenosis: a study of 374 cases. Mayo Clin Proc 1984;59:683–690.

37. Subramanian R, Olson LJ, Edwards WD: Surgical pathology of combined aortic stenosis and insufficiency: a study of 213 cases. Mayo Clin Proc 1985;60:247–254.

38. Olson LJ, Subramanian R, Edwards WD: Surgical pathology of pure aortic insufficiency: a study of 225 cases. Mayo Clin Proc 1984;59:835–841.

39. Elliott LP: Radiologic differentiation of the common anomalies. *In* Roberts WC, ed. Adult congenital heart disease. Philadelphia: FA Davis, 1987;191–220.

40. Becker AE, Becker MJ, Edwards JE: Anomalies associated with coarctation of aorta: particular reference to infancy. Circulation 1970;41:1067–1075.

41. Campbell M: Natural history of coarctation of the aorta. Br Heart J 1970;32:633–640.

42. Edwards JE: The congenital bicuspid aortic valve. Circulation 1961;23:485.

43. Tawes RL Jr, Berry CL, Aberdeen E: Congenital bicuspid aortic valves associated with coarctation of the aorta in children. Br Heart J 1969;31:127–128.

44. Hahn RT, Roman MJ, Mogtader AH, Devereux RB: Association of aortic dilation with regurgitant, stenotic and functionally normal bicuspid aortic valves. J Am Coll Cardiol 1992;19:283–288.

45. Larson EW, Edwards WD: Risk factors for aortic dissection: a necropsy study of 161 cases. Am J Cardiol 1984;53:849–855.

46. Edwards WD, Leaf DS, Edwards JE: Dissecting aortic aneurysm associated with congenital bicuspid aortic valve. Circulation 1978;57:1022–1025.

47. Carlson RG, Lillehei CW, Edwards JE: Cystic medial necrosis of the ascending aorta in relation to age and hypertension. Am J Cardiol 1970;25:411–415.

48. Robinowitz M, Virmani R, McAllister JHA: Rheumatoid heart disease: a clinical and morphologic analysis of 34 autopsy patients. Lab Invest 1980;42:145.

49. Bulkley BH, Roberts WC: Ankylosing spondylitis and aortic regurgitation: description of the characteristic cardiovascular lesion from study of eight necropsy patients. Circulation 1973;48:1014–1027.

50. Roberts WC, Hollingsworth JF, Bulkley BH, Jaffe RB, Epstein SE, Stinson EB: Combined mitral and aortic regurgitation in ankylosing spondylitis: angiographic and anatomic features. Am J Med 1974;56:237–243.

51. Paulus HE, Pearson CM, Pitts W Jr: Aortic insufficiency in five patients with Reiter's syndrome: a detailed clinical and pathologic study. Am J Med 1972;53:464–472.

52. Pearson CM, Kroening R, Verity MA, Getzen JH: Aortic insufficiency and aortic aneurysm in relapsing polychondritis. Trans Assoc Am Physicians 1967;80:71–90.

53. Obadia JF, Tatou E, David M: Aortic valve regurgitation caused by blunt chest injury. Br Heart J 1995;74:545–547.

54. German DS, Shapiro MJ, Willman VL: Acute aortic valvular incompetence following blunt thoracic deceleration injury: case report. J Trauma 1990;30:1411–1412.

55. Horstkotte D, Niehues R, Strauer BE: Pathomorphological aspects, aetiology and natural history of acquired mitral valve stenosis. Eur Heart J 1991;12(suppl):55–60.

56. Balloon Valvuloplasty Registry: Multicenter experience with balloon mitral commissurotomy: NHLBI Balloon Valvuloplasty Registry report on immediate and 30-day follow-up results: the National Heart, Lung, and Blood Institute Balloon Valvuloplasty Registry participants. Circulation 1992;85:448–461.

57. Olson LJ, Subramanian R, Ackerman DM, Orszulak T, Edwards WD: Surgical pathology of the mitral valve: a study of 712 cases spanning 21 years. Mayo Clin Proc 1987;62:22–34.

58. Waller BF: Morphological aspects of valvular heart disease: part II. Curr Probl Cardiol 1984;9:1–74.

59. Allen WB, Karp RB, Kouchoukos NT: Mitral valve replacement with Starr-Edwards cloth-covered composite-seat prosthesis. Arch Surg 1974;109:642–647.

60. Hanson TP, Edwards BS, Edwards JE: Pathology of surgically excised mitral valves. One hundred consecutive cases. Arch Pathol Lab Med 1985;109:823–828.

61. Hammer WJ, Roberts WC, deLeon AC: "Mitral stenosis" secondary to combined "massive" mitral anular calcific deposits and small, hypertrophied left ventricles: hemodynamic documentation in four patients. Am J Med 1978;64:371–376.

62. Pellikka PA, Tajik AJ, Khandheria BK, et al: Carcinoid heart disease. Clinical and echocardiographic spectrum in 74 patients. Circulation 1993;87:1188–1196.

63. Leder AA, Bosworth WC: Angiokeratoma corporis diffusum universale (Fabry's disease) with mitral stenosis. Am J Med 1965;38:814.

64. Roberts WC: Morphologic features of the normal and abnormal mitral valve. Am J Cardiol 1983;51:1005–1028.

65. McAllister HA Jr, Fenoglio JJ Jr: Cardiac involvement in Whipple's disease. Circulation 1975;52:152–156.

66. Rose AG: Mitral stenosis in Whipple's disease. Thorax 1978;33:500–503.

67. Scalapino JN, Edwards WD, Steckelberg JM, Wooten RS, Callahan JA, Ginsburg WW: Mitral stenosis associated with valvular tophi. Mayo Clin Proc 1984;59:509–512.

68. Waller BF, McManus BM, Roberts WC: Mitral valve stenosis produced by or worsened by active bacterial endocarditis. Chest 1982;82:498–500.

69. Matula G, Karpman LS, Frank S, Stinson E: Mitral obstruction from staphylococcal endocarditis, corrected surgically. JAMA 1975;233:58–59.

70. Ruckman RN, Van Praagh R: Anatomic types of congenital mitral stenosis: report of 49 autopsy cases with consideration of diagnosis and surgical implications. Am J Cardiol 1978;42:592–601.

71. Amlie JP, Langmark F, Storstein O: Pure mitral regurgitation: etiology, pathology and clinical patterns. Acta Med Scand 1976;200:201–208.

72. Falco A, Sante P, Renzulli A, et al: Etiology and incidence of pure mitral insufficiency: a morphological study of 926 native valves [translated]. Cardiologia 1990;35:327–330.

73. Turri M, Thiene G, Bortolotti U, Mazzucco A, Gallucci V: Surgical pathology of disease of the mitral valve, with special reference to lesions promoting valvar incompetence. Int J Cardiol 1989;22:213–219.

74. Rao V, Christakis GT, Weisel RD, et al: Changing pattern of valve surgery. Circulation 1996;94[Supp II]:113–120.

75. Jones RA, Hall RJ, Fraser AG: Severe mitral regurgitation caused by immobile posterior leaflet after radiotherapy. J Am Soc Echocardiogr 1995;8:207–210.

76. Klues HG, Roberts WC, Maron BJ: Morphological determinants of echocardiographic patterns of mitral valve systolic anterior motion in obstructive hypertrophic cardiomyopathy. Circulation 1993;87:1570–1579.

77. Klues HG, Proschan MA, Dollar AL, Spirito P, Roberts WC, Maron BJ: Echocardiographic assessment of mitral valve size in obstructive hypertrophic cardiomyopathy: anatomic validation from mitral valve specimen. Circulation 1993;88:548–555.

78. Marsalese DL, Moodie DS, Vacante M, et al: Marfan's syndrome: natural history and long-term follow-up of cardiovascular involvement. J Am Coll Cardiol 1989;14:422–428.

79. Pyeritz RE, McKusick VA: The Marfan syndrome: diagnosis and management. N Engl J Med 1979;300:772–777.

80. Legget ME, Unger TA, O'Sullivan CK, Zwink TR, Bennett RL, Byers PH, Otto CM: Aortic root complications in Marfan's syndrome: identification of a lower risk group. Heart 1996;75:389–395.

81. Perloff JK, Child JS, Edwards JE: New guidelines for the clinical diagnosis of mitral valve prolapse. Am J Cardiol 1986;57:1124–1129.

82. Devereux RB: Recent developments in the diagnosis and management of mitral valve prolapse. Curr Opin Cardiol 1995;10:107–116.

83. Boustany CW Jr, Murphy GW, Hicks GL Jr: Mitral valve replacement in idiopathic hypereosinophilic syndrome. Ann Thorac Surg 1991;51:1007–1009.

84. Roldan CA, Shively BK, Crawford MH: An echocardiographic study of valvular heart disease associated with systemic lupus erythematosus. N Engl J Med 1996;335:1424–1430.

85. Connolly HM, Crary JL, McGoon MD, et al: Valvular heart disease associated with fenfluramine-phentermine. N Engl J Med 1997;337:581–588.

86. Fenster MS, Feldman MD: Mitral regurgitation: an overview. Curr Probl Cardiol 1995;20:193–280.

87. Marzo KP, Herling IM: Valvular disease in the elderly. Cardiovasc Clin 1993;23:175–207.

88. Korn D, DeSanctis RW, Sell S: Massive calcification of the mitral annulus. N Engl J Med 1962;267:900.

89. Kitchin A, Turner R: Diagnosis and treatment of tricuspid stenosis. Br Heart J 1964;16:354.

90. Bousvaros GA, Stubington D: Some auscultatory and phonocardiographic features of tricuspid stenosis. Circulation 1964;29:26.

91. Hogevik H, Olaison L, Andersson R, Lindberg J, Alestig K: Epidemiologic aspects of infective endocarditis in an urban population: a 5-year prospective study. Medicine (Baltimore) 1995;74:324–339.

92. Berlin JA, Abrutyn E, Strom BL, et al: Incidence of infective endocarditis in the Delaware Valley, 1988–1990. Am J Cardiol 1995;76:933–936.

93. Mansur AJ, Grinberg M, da Luz PL, Bellotti G: The complications of infective endocarditis: a reappraisal in the 1980s. Arch Intern Med 1992;152:2428–2432.

94. Witchitz S, Reidiboym M, Bouvet E, et al: Role of transoesophageal echocardiography in the diagnosis and management of aortic root abscess. Br Heart J 1994;72:175–181.

95. Werner GS, Schulz R, Fuchs JB, et al: Infective endocarditis in the elderly in the era of transesophageal echocardiography: clinical features and prognosis compared with younger patients. Am J Med 1996;100:90–97.

96. Bayer AS, Ward JI, Ginzton LE, Shapiro SM: Evaluation of new clinical criteria for the diagnosis of infective endocarditis. Am J Med 1994;96:211–219.

97. Durack DT, Lukes AS, Bright DK: New criteria for diagnosis of infective endocarditis: utilization of specific echocardiographic findings: Duke Endocarditis Service. Am J Med 1994;96:200–209.

98. Jaffe WM, Morgan DE, Pearlman AS, Otto CM: Infective endocarditis, 1983–1988: echocardiographic findings and factors influencing morbidity and mortality. J Am Coll Cardiol 1990;15:1227–1233.

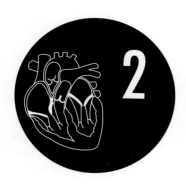

2 Pathology and Etiology of Heart Disease

Corinne L. Fligner and Dennis D. Reichenbach

Valvular heart disease is the diagnostic term used to describe cardiac dysfunction caused by structural or functional abnormalities in heart valves. In the past 30 years, the causes of valvular heart disease have changed in Western countries from primarily rheumatic to more degenerative and inherited conditions. In non-Western countries, rheumatic heart disease continues to account for the major proportion of valvular heart disease. The type of pathologic specimen received for evaluation also has changed, from hearts obtained at autopsy to valves excised at surgery; this change reflects the increasing number of valve replacement procedures performed and the decreasing number of autopsies performed, particularly in the United States.

The importance of careful pathologic examination of all valvular heart disease for definitive diagnosis and clinical correlation with imaging procedures cannot be overemphasized. In this chapter, we describe cardiac valvular pathology based on the primary disease processes involved and correlate disease states with functional abnormalities.

PATHOLOGIC EXAMINATION

In major cardiovascular surgical centers, most pathologic examination of cardiac valves is done in the surgical pathology laboratory, rather than by autopsy examination of intact hearts. The most important component of the evaluation of excised cardiac valves is the gross examination. According to Waller, "routine histologic sectioning of all cardiac valves will add little, if any, additional information beyond the morphologic evaluation, pertinent to the etiology or to therapy, except in two instances: infective endocarditis, and metabolic or inborn errors of metabolism."[1] In cases of endocarditis, histologic examination is required to characterize the vegetation as inflammatory or thrombotic and to detect pathologic organisms. For a patient with metabolic or enzymatic abnormalities, such as the mucopolysaccharidoses, Whipple's disease, or carcinoid syndrome, histologic evaluation can establish the cause. Although representative microscopy is appropriate in evaluating valvular heart disease, it cannot replace careful gross examination, which usually is more important in determining the cause.

Waller[1] recommends that the following 10 morphologic observations be made for each operatively excised valve:

1. Valve weight
2. Degree of fibrous thickening (mild to severe)
3. Degree (mild to severe) and extent (focal to diffuse) of calcification
4. Valve tissue deficiency (loss, perforation, or indentation) or excess
5. Absence or presence and degree of commissural fusion (mild to severe)
6. Vegetations
7. Status of chordae tendineae (fused, elongated, shortened, or ruptured)
8. Status of attached papillary muscles
9. Number of semilunar cusps
10. Measurement of "annular" circumference of atrioventricular valves (reconstructed)

Because of the importance of gross examination, photographs of resected valves are recommended. Radiographs may be helpful in evaluating the degree of calcification.

Structural and functional classification requires that the entire excised valve specimen be received, although culture of suspected vegetations should optimally be done in the operating room. In some instances, functional classification may necessitate obtaining catheterization data or information about other valvular structural or functional abnormalities. In Rose's survey of 100 consecutively excised surgical valves, etiologic classification was possible for 81% of cases for which the pathologist was given adequate information by the surgeon about the gross appearance of the intact valve before removal; when this information was not provided, an etiologic diagnosis could be made for only 35% of valves. For 62% of patients in this study, no clinical information was provided on the pathology request form, and for only 15% of patients did the request form and the operative note agree on the etiologic diagnosis.[2] Good communication between the clinician and pathologist is essential for obtaining clinically relevant, etiologically correct diagnoses. Preoperative completion of pathology information forms by knowledgeable parties and correlative conferences can facilitate optimal practice.

NORMAL VALVULAR ANATOMY AND HISTOLOGY

Aortic and Pulmonic Valves

The anatomic structures of the aortic and pulmonic valves are similar, except that the pulmonic valve structure is finer because of the lower pressures in the right than in the left heart systems. The anatomy is described for the aortic valve, which is more commonly seen because of disease. The valve has three semilunar cusps inserted into a fibrous connective tissue sleeve, which is attached to the aortic media above and below to the myocardium of the left ventricular outflow tract and to the anterior mitral leaflet (Figs. 2–1 and 2–2).

Each cusp is attached along its curved edge, and the cusps meet at three commissures, which are equally spaced along the circumference of the sleeve at the supraaortic ridge, a "bump" that marks the superior edge of the connective tissue sleeve. The sinuses of Valsalva are located between the valve sleeve and cusps. The left coronary, right coronary, and noncoronary cusps are named according to the location of the coronary ostia. During ventricular outflow, the cusps fold back toward the sinuses. Valve closure occurs when pressure in the aortic root exceeds ventricular pressure,

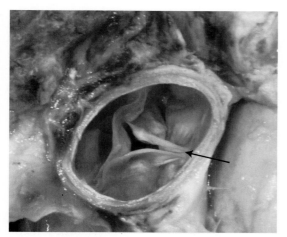

Figure 2·1 The normal trileaflet aortic valve is viewed from above in an intact aorta. Notice the flexible cusps and nonfused commissures *(arrow)*.

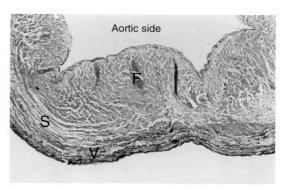

Figure 2·3 Microscopic appearance of a normal aortic valve, showing the fibrosa (F), spongiosa (S), and ventricularis (V). The spongiosa is relatively inapparent, and the ventricularis is marked by prominent elastic fibers (Verhoeff–van Gieson stain).

and the cusps oppose exactly. The line of opposition slants upward on each cusp from the commissures to the centrally located nodulus of Arantius. The area of the valve above the line of closure, the *lunula*, acts as a supporting strut and overlaps the adjacent cusps; fenestrations in this portion of the cusp are common and have no functional significance. The area of the valve is about 40% greater than the area of the aortic root. In the normal aortic valve, the cusps are symmetric, mobile, and free to the commissures, with equal overlap on closure.[3]

Microscopically, the valve consists of three layers, which are more robust in the aortic than in the pulmonic valve (Fig. 2–3). The dense collagen core, the *fibrosa*, is continuous

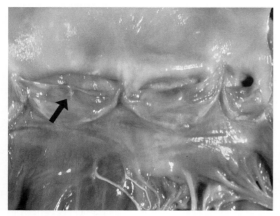

Figure 2·2 In the normal aortic valve in an opened heart, notice the thin cusps and relatively inapparent corpora Arantii *(arrow)*.

with the valve sleeve, extends to the free edge, and comprises the major structural support of the valve. It contains scattered fibroblasts and a few fine elastic fibers. The ventricularis on the ventricular or outflow surface of the valve also extends to the free edge; this layer is rich in elastic fibers and is continuous with the endocardium. Between these two layers is the spongiosa, which consists of loosely arranged collagen fibers, scattered fibroblasts, less-well-differentiated mesenchymal cells, and large amounts of proteoglycan. The spongiosa does not extend to the free edge; it is most prominent in the basal third of the valve. The normal valve is avascular and is surfaced by a single endothelial layer on the aortic and ventricular aspects.[3, 4]

Mitral and Tricuspid Valves

The atrioventricular valve apparatus consists of several components: the annulus, leaflets, chordae tendineae, and papillary muscles. The structure of the tricuspid valve is similar to that of the mitral valve, except that it is thinner because of the lower pressures to which it is subjected. When atrial pressure exceeds ventricular pressure, the valve leaflets open into the ventricle; the leaflets are lifted and meet and close when ventricular pressure rises. Function of the atrioventricular valves requires complex interaction of all components; the papillary muscles and chordae tendineae interact to prevent prolapse of the leaflets back into the atria during systole.

The mitral and tricuspid valve leaflets insert into a slender, fibrous ring called the *annulus*. The mitral valve is composed of the anterior leaflet, which has the greatest area and is semicircular in the open position, and the posterior leaflet, which is smaller and crescentic and more elongated than the anterior cusp (Fig. 2–4). The depth of the anterior leaflet from attachment to free edge is up to three times greater than that of the posterior leaflet, a feature particularly important in the evaluation of mild degrees of floppy mitral valve. In the closed position, the leaflets overlap by approximately 0.5 cm. The leaflets meet at the medial and lateral commissures, which can be identified by the fan-shaped commissural chordae. Normal hearts have no chordal fusion. The base of the anterior leaflet is continuous with the left coronary cusp of the aortic valve, and the anterior leaflet divides the left ventricular chamber into inflow and outflow portions. The chordae insert into the free edge of the valve or into the so-called rough zone on the ventricular aspect of the valve. The central portion of the anterior leaflet is relatively clear, because the chordae insert mainly medially and laterally. Some chordae contain smooth muscle and may contain blood vessels and collagen (ie, muscular chordae); these thicker chordae can be misinterpreted as showing pathologic postinflammatory changes.[3]

Tricuspid valvular anatomy is more variable than mitral anatomy, although the basic structures are the same. The three leaflets are the anterior, posterior, and septal, and the septal leaflet usually is quite small and rudimentary. The commissures can be identified by the presence of fan chordae. The anterior leaflet divides the right ventricular cavity in a fashion analogous to the anterior mitral leaflet on the left.

Microscopically, the atrioventricular valve consists of three layers. The dense collagenous fibrosa is continuous with the annulus and extends to the free edge of the leaflet and into the cores of the chordae tendineae, spreading out on the surface of the tips of the papillary muscles. On the ventricular aspect, the fibrosa is surfaced only by a single layer of endothelium. On the atrial aspect of the valve, the fibrosa is surfaced by the spongiosa, similar to that seen in the aortic and pulmonic valves, composed mainly of proteoglycan containing loosely arranged collagen and elastic fibers. In the mitral valve, the spongiosa may contain cardiac muscle bundles that extend from the left atrium into the proximal third (posterior leaflet) or middle third (anterior leaflet) of the leaflet. The spongiosa is surfaced on the atrial aspect by the atrialis layer, is continuous with the atrial endocardium, consists of prominent elastic fibers and smooth muscle cells similar in appearance to the ventricularis in the semilunar valves, and is surfaced by a single layer of endothelium. The normal valve is avascular. The chordae tendineae consist of a central, longitudinally arranged collagenous core that is continuous with the valve fibrosa surrounded by a looser layer of collagen, elastic fibers, and proteoglycan and surfaced by a single layer of endothelium. Histologic differences between the tricuspid and mitral valves include thinner layers and absence of atrial muscle extension into the leaflets in the tricuspid valve.[3, 4]

Age-Related Changes in Cardiac Valves

Age-related changes in all valves appear to be caused by "wear and tear" and primarily involve accentuation of the normal valvular architecture. The aortic valve shows enlargement of the corpora Arantii and increased prominence of the lines of closure; fibrous

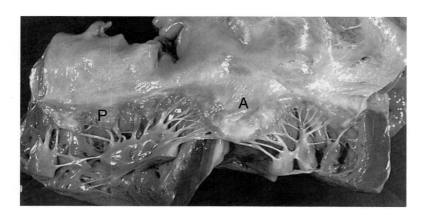

Figure 2·4 In this normal mitral valve, notice the difference in the sizes of the posterior (P) and anterior (A) leaflets from the annulus to the leaflet edge. The leaflets are thin and somewhat transparent, with fine, branching chordae.

thickening of the cusp body is associated with thinning and fenestration of the lunula (Fig. 2–5). Lipid deposits can occur in the cusps or sinuses, but they rarely calcify. Aortic sclerosis and stenosis, previously considered to be wear-related processes, may instead be active processes amenable to modulation.

In the mitral valve, age-related changes include fibrous thickening of the leaflets, causing them to be less translucent. The changes also may include deposition of lipid in the anterior leaflet, nodular thickening along the closure lines, and some hooding of the posterior leaflet, similar to that seen in floppy mitral valve. Other changes include isolated amyloid deposits, usually transthyretin, associated with other cardiac nodules of senile cardiac amyloidosis, and isolated myxomatous changes in the valve fibrosa.

Lambl's excrescences are tiny (1 to 4 mm long), solitary or multiple, whisker-like projections that are usually seen on the lines of closure or free margins of aortic and mitral valves, including the corpora Arantii.[3, 5] These should be differentiated from a papillary fibroelastoma, which consists of an endocardial sea anemone–like structure that is composed of multiple, endothelium-lined papillary fronds with avascular fibrous cores.[6]

RHEUMATIC OR POSTINFLAMMATORY VALVULAR DISEASE

Although the declining incidence of rheumatic fever in developed countries has resulted in a steadily decreasing incidence of rheumatic valvular disease, as seen in surgical and autopsy specimens, rheumatic valvular disease continues to predominate globally and to be a major cause of valvular dysfunction in

valves that are surgically removed in Western countries. The gross and microscopic features of rheumatic valvular disease are indistinguishable from those of other chronic postinflammatory valvular diseases, and many researchers use the more generic term, *postinflammatory,* recognizing that most of these cases are rheumatic in origin. These terms are used interchangeably in this discussion.

Rheumatic fever is an immunologic disease, with inflammatory manifestations involving the heart, joints, and skin; it occurs after a pharyngeal, not skin, infection with group A β-hemolytic streptococci. An autoimmune reaction is initiated by the streptococcal infection with an enhanced immune response to streptococcal antigens, evoking antibodies that cross-react with human tissue antigens. The factors determining which persons develop rheumatic fever after streptococcal pharyngitis are unknown, although they probably include immune-response genes. Although the sporadic attack rate is only 3%, susceptible individuals have a recurrence risk for acute rheumatic fever of 50%. The factors determining which individuals develop chronic rheumatic valvular disease after rheumatic fever also are unknown. The putative cross-reacting antigens are not definitively known, although possibilities include heart valve glycoproteins that cross-react with the hyaluronate capsule of the streptococcus, identical to human hyaluronate; myocardial and smooth muscle sarcolemma, cross-reactive with streptococcal membrane antigens; and cardiac myosin, which shares antigenic determinants with streptococcal M protein, the chief virulence factor of group A streptococcus.[7]

Rheumatic heart disease results from organization of the endocardial lesions of acute rheumatic fever. Rheumatic fever is a pancarditis. Acute endocardial and primarily left-sided valvular involvement takes the form of mild leaflet or cuspal thickening, with formation of small, relatively inapparent, warty vegetations or verrucae along the lines of valve closure, which may also be seen on the chordae tendineae, the endocardium lining the cardiac chambers, and the body of the leaflets or cusps (Fig. 2–6). Microscopically, the vegetations consist of fibrin-platelet thrombi that cover areas of focal fibrinoid necrosis, probably a result of fibrin deposition at sites of endocardial erosion occurring where the edematous leaflets come into contact during closure. Histologically, the leaflets are edematous with a pleomorphic inflammatory infiltrate. The in-

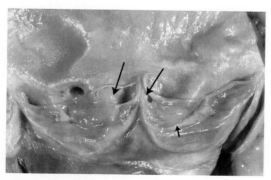

Figure 2·5 Age-related changes in an aortic valve. Notice the sagging of cusps, prominent fenestrations *(large arrows)*, and prominent contact zone *(small arrow)*. The fenestrations in the lunula are not functionally significant.

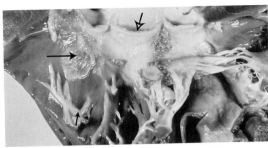

Figure 2·6 Chronic rheumatic aortic insufficiency with cuspal fibrosis, thickening, and retraction, with a jet lesion consisting of endocardial fibrosis *(large arrow)* and a "pocket" *(small arrow)* below the valve. Warty, small vegetations resulting from acute rheumatic fever are on the aortic valve edge, the aortic and mitral valve leaflets, and the chordae tendineae *(open arrow)*.

creased pressures on the left side of the heart compared with the right heart, with more forceful closure of inflamed valves, may explain the more severe involvement of left-sided valves in chronic rheumatic valvular disease.[8] Acute rheumatic fever is rarely seen today at autopsy in developed countries; in the past, death usually occurred as a result of the nonvalvular cardiac involvement.

Although the acute lesions do not cause significant functional abnormalities, scarring from the inflammatory process results in deformation of the valve. Hemodynamic alterations caused by valvular deformation probably result in recurrent endocardial damage, with fibrin-platelet deposition and organization resulting in progressive valvular damage. The pathologic lesion characteristic of rheumatic heart disease, the Aschoff body, is usually not seen in valves. It is more frequently

identified in the myocardium and becomes apparent about 5 weeks into the acute rheumatic episode. Because of the long interval between acute rheumatic fever and chronic valvular disease, Aschoff bodies are identified in only 4% to 21% of left atrial specimens from patients with mitral stenosis and in only 2% of autopsied patients with severe chronic valvular heart disease.[9, 10]

The macroscopic hallmark of post-rheumatic valvular disease in all valves is commissural fusion associated with leaflet fibrosis. Subsequent leaflet thickening, calcification, and retraction to some degree are often accompanied by chordal fusion in the atrioventricular valves. Microscopically, obliteration of the underlying architecture by fibrosis occurs, with increased collagen and variable cellularity, and neovascularization results in thick-walled blood vessels in the normally avascular valve (Fig. 2–7). Superimposed calcification, ulceration, and thrombosis may be present. In general, valves that are functionally stenotic show more fibrosis, calcification, and commissural fusion than valves that are functionally regurgitant, which tend to show retraction, shortening, and minimal calcification.

Although rheumatic heart disease often involves multiple valves, left-sided valve involvement is usually clinically and pathologically more severe. The mitral valve is virtually always involved in chronic rheumatic valvular disease. Isolated mitral valvular disease is most common, with combined mitral and aortic disease occurring frequently; the prevalence varies by whether the study involves clinical, pathologic, surgical, or autopsy material. Although clinical symptoms related to aortic valvular disease

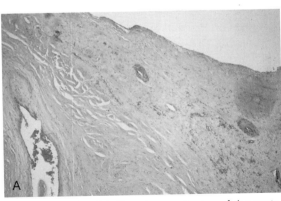
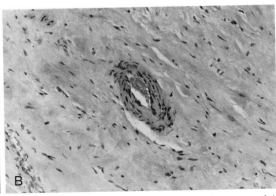

Figure 2·7 *A* and *B*, The microscopic view of rheumatic mitral valve disease shows fibrosis and vascularization of the leaflet. Notice the prominent large blood vessels and distortion of the valvular architecture compared with the normal valvular architecture of the aortic valve in Figure 2–4 and mitral valve in Figure 2–23C (hematoxylin and eosin stain; original magnification ×2 [*A*] and ×25 [*B*]).

may predominate, pathologic mitral involvement is typical when rheumatic aortic disease is present. Tricuspid valve involvement is less common, is always accompanied by mitral involvement, and is usually clinically insignificant. Pulmonic valvular involvement is rarely seen.[7]

Rheumatic valvular disease accounts for most cases of mitral stenosis, with only 1% of cases attributed to a cause other than postinflammatory.[11–16] The characteristic "button-hole" or "fish-mouth" appearance of mitral stenosis (Fig. 2–8) results from the marked bridging fibrosis of the commissures, producing a tiny orifice; variable calcification, sometimes nodular and often severe, can occur.[16] Ulceration of calcified areas can result in surface thrombosis. The degree of left atrial enlargement varies but may be severe in cases of mitral stenosis and incompetence; because the stenotic valve is also incompetent, endocardial fibrotic plaques that represent atrial jet lesions may be identified if the jet is directed toward the wall. Although mitral stenosis is the most frequent pathologic finding in patients with rheumatic mitral valvular disease, the valve may also be incompetent if the dominant pathology is leaflet and chordal retraction and shortening (Fig. 2–9).

Rheumatic aortic valvular disease most commonly causes aortic stenosis, characterized by commissural fusion and variable cusp fibrosis and calcification. Asymmetric fusion may

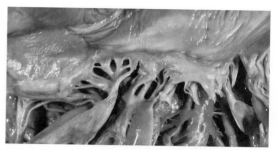

Figure 2·9 Rheumatic mitral valve disease is evident in this opened mitral valve with thickening and fibrosis of the leaflets and prominent fusion and shortening of the chordae tendineae. This valve probably was associated with predominantly regurgitant physiology.

mimic a bicuspid aortic valve, but close examination may show that two cusps are "stuck together." If necessary, histologic sectioning can show fibrous tissue between the two cusps at the commissures and preserved cusp architecture.[8] The classic appearance of rheumatic aortic stenosis is a valve with fusion of all three commissures, a central triangular orifice, and calcification that involves the edges of the cusps (Fig. 2–10). Central regurgitation typically occurs through the fixed orifice, which may not produce a jet lesion.[11] In degenerative aortic stenosis, the cusp edges usually are not calcified and the commissures not fused (Fig. 2–11).

In end-stage calcific aortic stenosis, advanced calcification with distortion can preclude determination of underlying valve anatomy. Because rheumatic aortic involvement is virtually always accompanied by mitral abnor-

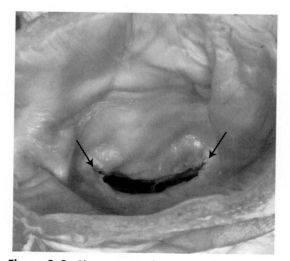

Figure 2·8 Rheumatic mitral stenosis with a fish-mouth configuration and mild calcification. Notice the commissural fusion *(arrows)* and cusp fibrosis. Although the defect is mainly stenotic, some degree of regurgitation would exist.

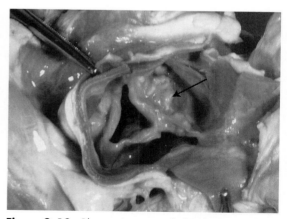

Figure 2·10 Rheumatic aortic valvular disease, with stenosis and central regurgitation. The trileaflet valve shows fusion of all three commissures with cuspal calcification *(arrow)*.

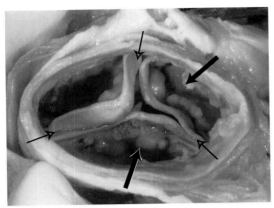

Figure 2·11 Degenerative type of calcific aortic stenosis. This intact aortic valve seen from the aortic aspect demonstrates nodules of calcium *(large arrows)* in the sinuses of Valsalva and an absence of commissural fusion *(open arrows)*.

malities, albeit sometimes mild, and limited to minimal fibrosis or commissural or chordal fusion, assessment of the mitral valve can be helpful in determining the cause of the aortic valvular pathology.

As with the mitral valve, variable retraction and scarring of the aortic valve can result in an incompetent valve, and the corresponding jet lesion may be identified as a fibrotic plaque or "pocket" on the upper left ventricular endocardium if the regurgitant blood is directed toward the chamber wall (see Fig. 2–6). Regurgitant aortic valves usually have minimal calcification.

Tricuspid stenosis in surgically excised valves usually is caused by rheumatic heart disease and accompanied by mitral stenosis. The anatomic features are similar to those seen in mitral disease, with diffuse fibrous thickening of the leaflets and fusion of two or usually three commissures. Chordal fusion and shortening are less severe than in the mitral valve. In contrast to left-sided valvular involvement, stenotic tricuspid valves have no significant calcification. Pulmonic valve involvement by rheumatic disease is uncommon and is always accompanied by involvement of other valves; the morphology is similar to that of tricuspid involvement, with fibrous thickening and commissural fusion and with minimal or no calcification.[17, 18]

DEGENERATIVE VALVULAR DISEASE
Isolated Calcific Aortic Stenosis of the Degenerative Type

In developed countries, the most common form of aortic stenosis is degenerative calcific aortic stenosis. The prevalence increases with increasing age, with aortic valve calcification found in more than 59% of subjects between the ages of 75 and 86 years.[19] Acquired calcific aortic stenosis manifests at different ages, depending on the underlying valve anatomy. The valve configuration can be predicted based on the age of presentation of aortic stenosis; in patients between 15 and 65 years of age, nearly 75% are bicuspid or unicuspid, and in patients older than 75 years of age, 90% of the stenotic aortic valves are tricuspid.[20]

Degenerative-type aortic stenosis is characterized by the accumulation of calcium in the cusps, which usually extends as nodules of calcium into the sinuses of Valsalva, preventing normal opening of the valve. The cusp edges typically are not involved, and the commissures are not fused (see Fig. 2–11). Nodules of dystrophic calcium are deposited in the valve fibrosa, but the underlying valvular architecture is preserved.

The early stage, designated aortic valve sclerosis, consists primarily of fibrosis and mild calcification. The end stage of the process shows extensive distortion by calcification and fibrotic thickening, which may make evaluation of the underlying valve anatomy difficult. Unlike rheumatic aortic stenosis, the mitral valve does not show postinflammatory changes. However, it may be involved by the changes of mitral annular calcification, or a bar of calcium can extend from the aortic valve onto the anterior mitral leaflet.[7]

Degenerative aortic stenosis was thought to be caused by wear and tear of a normal trileaflet aortic valve or a congenital unicuspid or bicuspid aortic valve. However, results of several studies have suggested that this may not be the case. Age, height, hypertension, smoking, and elevated levels of lipoprotein(a) and low-density lipoprotein cholesterol are clinical risk factors; although similar to those for atherosclerosis, other factors probably are important, because only 50% of patients with severe aortic stenosis also have significant coronary artery disease.[21] Several studies have indicated that degenerative calcific aortic stenosis is a histologically active process, with the early lesions having similarities (eg, lipoprotein accumulation, macrophage and T-cell infiltration, basement membrane disruption) and dissimilarities (eg, mineralization, small numbers of smooth muscle cells) to atherosclerosis.[22, 23] Osteopontin, a protein implicated in normal and dystrophic calcification, is actively synthesized in aortic tissue, suggesting that the calcification may be in part an actively regulated process.[24]

Mitral Annular Calcification

Calcification of the mitral annulus occurs when amorphous masses of calcium are deposited in the area of the mitral annulus. It is seen most prominently between the posterior leaflet of the mitral valve and the left ventricular endocardium (Fig. 2–12). This condition is most common in elderly women, and the incidence markedly increases after the age of 70 years; the prevalence is 43.5% among women older than 90 years.[25]

Although usually functionally insignificant, a murmur may be detected. The most common functional abnormality is mitral regurgitation, caused by interference with annular contraction during systole or by failure of leaflet coaptation because of fibrotic adherence between leaflets and calcific masses. More unusual is mitral stenosis caused by failure of annular relaxation during diastole or interference with leaflet retraction by the mass effect of the calcific nodules.[26] Large nodules can trap the chordae tendineae and may be

most easily visualized from the ventricular aspect. Although most commonly involving the posterior leaflet, the process can be circumferential and involve the anterior leaflet as well. The rock-hard masses are visualized well on specimen radiography, usually as a J-shaped or C-shaped area of calcification or less commonly as an O-shaped area.[27] Calcification may elicit a foreign body–type reaction. The calcific nodules can provide a nidus for thrombi or endocarditis; rarely, involvement of the conduction system by calcification results in complete heart block.[3, 7]

CONGENITAL VALVULAR DISEASE
Aortic Valve

The most frequent congenital abnormality of the aortic valve is the bicuspid aortic valve, which occurs in 1% to 2% of the population. At birth and in childhood, the bicuspid valve usually is asymptomatic and is neither stenotic nor regurgitant. However, degenerative fibrosis and calcification result in calcific aortic stenosis, which occurs at an earlier age than with a tricuspid aortic valve. Regurgitant physiology

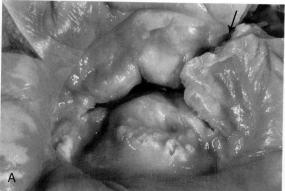

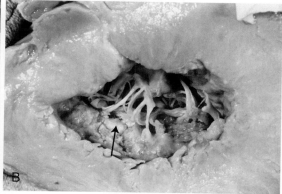

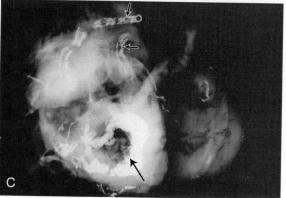

Figure 2·12 Mitral annular calcification with mitral stenosis. *A,* Atrial aspect of the mitral valve shows surface calcification, leaflet stenosis, and an artifactual cut at 2:00 o'clock *(arrow). B,* Ventricular aspect of the mitral valve shows nodules of calcium deposited at the annulus adherent to the valve leaflet and chordae *(arrow). C,* The postmortem radiograph shows nearly O-shaped mitral annular calcification *(large arrow)* and calcified coronary arteries *(small arrows).*

may occur but is less common. The frequency of bicuspid aortic valve is increased in certain congenital cardiac abnormalities, such as ventricular septal defect, coarctation of the aorta, and patent ductus arteriosus; patients with bicuspid aortic valves have an increased risk for aortic dissection.[28]

Congenital bicuspid aortic valve cusps are approximately equal in size. In about two thirds of cases, a raphe or ridge runs across one cusp, marking where the commissure should have formed (ie, false commissure).[29] The raphe usually ends before the free edge of the cusp but can sometimes extend to the free edge, mimicking acquired aortic stenosis. Rarely, the raphe may consist of a strand of tissue, which may rupture and cause prolapse of the cusp and aortic insufficiency.

The two main anatomic configurations of bicuspid valve occur approximately equally. In the anterior-posterior type, both coronary orifices open from the anterior sinus, which also contains the raphe, when present. In the right-left type, the coronary orifices are located in separate sinuses, and if a raphe is present, it is always located in the right cusp (Fig. 2–13).[1]

Gross inspection generally determines whether a bicuspid valve is congenital or acquired. In an acquired bicuspid valve, because the circumferential distances between each commissure of a tricuspid valve are equal, the cusp containing the fused commissure is approximately twice as long as the other cusp. Histologic inspection may assist in determining whether a raphe represents a congenital or acquired alteration. In acquired stenosis, the ventricularis of each leaflet may be seen in the raphe and is often associated with fibrous tissue between the cusps. Such assessment is difficult for a markedly calcified valve. The calcified and stenotic bicuspid aortic valve

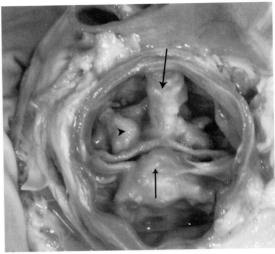

Figure 2·14 Congenital bicuspid aortic valve with calcific aortic stenosis. Notice the prominent calcification, with marked calcification of the raphe *(large arrow)*, nodules of calcium in the sinuses of Valsalva *(arrowhead)*, and more nodules at the edges of the valve *(small arrow)*. The commissures are not fused.

shows gross morphologic features similar to those of the degenerative-type calcific tricuspid valve, with the exception of the number of cusps (Fig. 2–14).

Less common is the unicuspid aortic valve, which has two main configurations. The dome-shaped valve has no lateral attachments and has a central stenotic orifice, similar in appearance to the dome-shaped valve of congenital pulmonic stenosis. The unicommissural valve has one lateral attachment and two raphes where the leaflets should have formed, resulting in an orifice with the shape of an exclamation mark. These valves typically become stenotic in adolescence or early adulthood.

Quadricuspid aortic valves are uncommon. They are more likely to be dysfunctional than quadricuspid pulmonic valves and may result in regurgitant or stenotic physiology.[30, 31]

Mitral Valve

Congenital abnormalities of the mitral valve are uncommon. In atrioventricular canal defects (ie, endocardial cushion), the anterior leaflet is abnormal. It usually has a central cleft and is associated with an ostium primum atrial septal defect. Associated with secundum-type atrial septal defects are several secondary mitral valvular anomalies, including floppy mitral valve, coexistent rheumatic mitral stenosis and atrial septal defect (Lutembacher's syn-

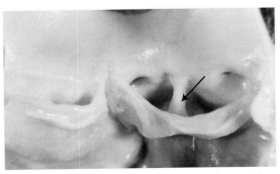

Figure 2·13 Congenital bicuspid aortic valve with flexible cusps in an opened aorta. The raphe *(arrow)* is located in the single cusp, which contains both coronary ostia.

drome), and thickening of the mitral leaflets adjacent to the medial commissure and under the atrial defect, without contraction or scarring, which is probably related to blood flow across the defect.[3]

Tricuspid Valve

In series of surgically excised adult valves, the tricuspid valve is more frequently affected by congenital abnormalities than the mitral valve. Most common is Ebstein's anomaly, which is usually purely regurgitant but which can produce stenosis. Ebstein's anomaly occurs when part of the line of attachment of the valve leaflets is shifted downward toward the ventricle. The anatomic abnormality varies in the degree of displacement and in the structure of the distal attachments, from a modest downward shift of relatively normal leaflets to markedly abnormal leaflets adherent to the ventricular endocardium. As a result of the displacement, part of the ventricle becomes atrialized; the most common functional abnormality is regurgitation. If the valve leaflets are fused, the valve may appear as a stenotic diaphragm with small peripheral openings, and tricuspid stenosis may occur, although this is rare.[3, 18, 32]

Isolated tricuspid valve stenosis is usually congenital and manifests during infancy. Congenitally abnormal valves may have poorly developed leaflets, shortened or absent chordae tendineae, abnormal sizes and numbers of papillary muscles, or a combination of defects.[18]

Pulmonic Valve

The most common underlying condition detected in operatively excised pulmonic valves is congenital heart disease. Although the frequency of stenosis (95%) as a functional category for the pulmonic valve is similar to that seen in aortic and mitral valves, the frequency of congenital causes for pulmonic valve dysfunction (95%) is much greater than that for left-sided valves (30% to 40%).[33, 34] Congenital pulmonic stenosis is most frequently a component of tetralogy of Fallot or an isolated entity (ie, isolated pulmonic stenosis). It can occur in conjunction with other malformations, including double-outlet right ventricle or complete atrioventricular canal. Valve morphology tends to vary with the type of congenital heart disease. In tetralogy of Fallot, pulmonic steno-

sis is most commonly associated with a bicuspid valve with a small annulus.

In isolated pulmonic stenosis, the valve is most commonly a dome-shaped, acommissural valve with a central opening (Fig. 2–15). It may also be a dysplastic pulmonic valve, with thickened cusps and a small annulus, but no commissural fusion. The dysplastic cusps contain increased amounts of acid mucopolysaccharide material and fibrous tissue. Gikonyo and colleagues reviewed the features of domed, unicuspid, bicuspid, tricuspid, and dysplastic types of congenital pulmonic valves and found that all forms had thickened cusps, without (domed, unicommissural, dysplastic) or with (bicuspid, tricuspid) commissural fusion.[35] Isolated pulmonic stenosis is one of the common congenital heart abnormalities in which adult survival is common. Noonan syndrome is pulmonic valvular stenosis, generally with a dysplastic valve, associated with other noncardiac defects.

Quadricuspid pulmonic valves are uncommon. They rarely result in functional abnormality significant enough to require surgical excision.[17, 30, 33]

INFECTIVE ENDOCARDITIS AND OTHER VEGETATIONS

Infective endocarditis occurs when microorganisms colonize and invade platelet-fibrin thrombi on valves, mural endocardium, or both. Endocarditis is clinically classified based on disease severity and time course as subacute

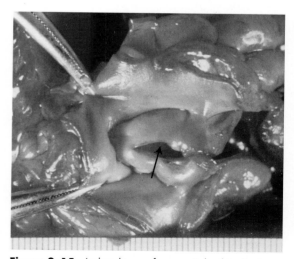

Figure 2·15 Isolated type of congenital pulmonic stenosis with a dome-shaped pulmonic valve containing a central aperture *(arrow)*.

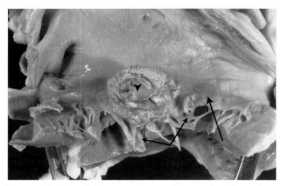

Figure 2·16 Subacute infective bacterial endocarditis, with a large vegetation *(arrowhead)* attached to the anterior leaflet of the mitral valve. The underlying mitral valve is abnormal, with a fused commissure *(large arrow)* and fusion of the chordae tendineae *(small arrows)*.

or acute; these terms are primarily related to organism virulence and the presence of underlying cardiac disease. Acute endocarditis is a rapidly progressive, destructive process that is caused by more virulent organisms (eg, staphylococci, fungi) and that usually involves anatomically normal valves, causing clinically severe illness and often causing death. Subacute endocarditis has a smoldering, longer clinical course, usually is caused by organisms of low virulence (eg, *Streptococcus viridans*), and involves previously damaged valves.

In the past, the most common underlying valvular pathology was healed rheumatic valvulitis; other abnormalities are more common today, such as mitral valve prolapse, calcific aortic stenosis, congenital heart disease with fibrotic mural jet lesions, prosthetic valves, and vascular grafts. This reflects the changing etiologic prevalence of valve disease. Immune compromise, which increases patient vulnerability to infection, occurs with human immunodeficiency virus infection, chemotherapy, therapeutic immunosuppression, and chronic alcoholism. Intravenous drug users have an increased risk of endocarditis; although left-sided endocarditis is more common among intravenous drug users, the prevalence of right-sided endocarditis has also increased. Other predisposing factors include indwelling catheters and instrumentation causing bacteremia, including dental therapy and gastrointestinal or genitourinary procedures.

Although many cases of subacute endocarditis continue to be caused by *S. viridans*, the prevalence of acute endocarditis caused by *Staphylococcus* organisms has increased. *Staphylococcus epidermidis* causes a significant propor-

tion of infections after cardiac surgery and in prosthetic valves, and *Staphylococcus aureus* causes most cases of endocarditis in intravenous drug users. Approximately 20% of endocarditis is culture negative because of antibiotic therapy or microbiologic technical difficulties or because the organism is found deep in the vegetation and does not readily seed the blood.

Infective vegetations are usually located on the "downstream" side of the valve or cardiac anatomic abnormality; typically, the vegetation is seen along the lines of closure, on the atrial aspect of the atrioventricular valves, and on the ventricular aspect of the semilunar valves. The vegetations of infective endocarditis are bulky and friable, are variable in size but measuring up to several centimeters, and are attached to single or multiple valves on either side of the heart (Fig. 2–16). Left-sided vegetations are most common, with the aortic valve most commonly involved, followed by mitral and combined aortic and mitral involvement. Fungal vegetations tend to be larger and more bulky than bacterial vegetations.

In subacute endocarditis, the underlying valve usually is abnormal, and there may be evidence of healing or organization of the vegetation. In acute endocarditis, the native valve usually is anatomically normal, but more tissue destruction, with ulceration and perforation, has occurred (Fig. 2–17). In both types, the vegetations consist of fibrin admixed with organisms and abundant leukocytes—neutrophils in the acute stage and more chronic inflammatory cells later. The organisms are often centrally located in the vegetation and can be difficult to demonstrate with time because of calcification or loss of Gram staining after antibiotic treatment. Healing can result in calcification of organisms and formation of

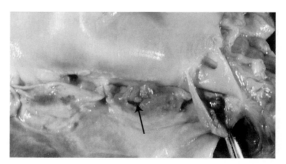

Figure 2·17 Acute bacterial endocarditis with perforation *(arrow)*. Notice the irregular vegetation at the superior margins of the perforation and vegetation on the adjacent transected cusp near the hemostat.

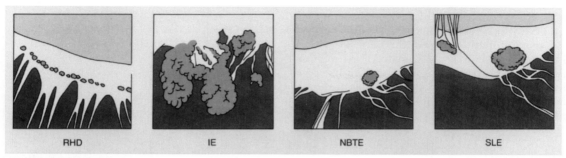

Figure 2·18 Comparison of the four major forms of vegetative endocarditis. The rheumatic fever phase of rheumatic heart disease (RHD) is marked by a row of warty, small vegetations along the lines of closure of the valve leaflets. In infective endocarditis (IE), large, irregular masses on the valve cusps can extend onto the chordae. Nonbacterial thrombotic endocarditis (NBTE) shows one or multiple, small, bland vegetations, usually at the line of valve closure. Libman-Sacks endocarditis of systemic lupus erythematosus (SLE) has small or medium-sized vegetations on either or both sides of the valve leaflets. (From Schoen FJ: The heart. *In* Cotran R, Kumar V, Robbins S, eds. Robbins Pathologic Basis of Disease, ed 5. Philadelphia: WB Saunders, 1994:543–557.)

fibrocalcific nodules on the surface of the valves.

Large and bulky vegetations can cause functional valvular stenosis; with healing, perforation or deformation usually results in a regurgitant valve. Local complications include extension into the myocardium as valve ring abscesses, formation of aneurysms in the sinuses of Valsalva, or extension into the pericardium as pericarditis. Septic embolization into the systemic circulation can also occur, producing cerebral, renal, and splenic infarcts.[7, 36] With right-sided valvular involvement, the presentation is often that of acute pneumonia because of septic pulmonary embolization.

The pathogenesis of infective endocarditis involves several factors. The valvular surface is altered by immune factors (in post-rheumatic disease) or damage related to turbulence or scarring. A fibrin-platelet thrombus forms on the damaged endocardium, resulting in a vegetation of the nonbacterial thrombotic endocarditis type (ie, NBTE lesion). Bacteremia leads to colonization of the thrombus, requiring bacterial adherence and cell receptors for specific bacteria. Bacterial proliferation then occurs, and interaction with the coagulation system results in the deposition of a fibrin-platelet mesh, which can enhance bacterial adhesion. The reason apparently anatomically normal valves become colonized and destroyed by acute endocarditis is related to the interaction of endocardial damage, thrombosis, and bacterial adhesion with host immune factors.[36, 37]

Not all vegetations represent infective endocarditis. Fig. 2–18 contrasts the morphologic characteristics of the four major forms of vegetations. Most common are those of NBTE, which consist of small thrombi-like vegetations found singly or in groups along the lines of closure of any valve without underlying tissue destruction (Fig. 2–19). Histologically, these are bland fibrin and platelet deposits, without organisms or significant numbers of leukocytes. This type of endocarditis is commonly found in debilitated or very ill patients, including those with cancer, sepsis, and multiorgan failure; right-sided vegetations are not uncom-

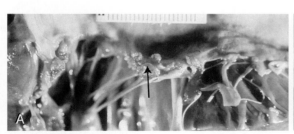
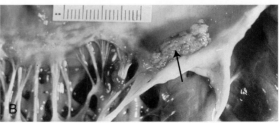

Figure 2·19 A, Nonbacterial thrombotic endocarditis of the mitral valve is evidenced by minute, bland vegetations attached at the line of closure (arrow). B, The vegetation on this valve is somewhat larger than in A, measuring approximately 1.5 cm in greatest dimension (arrow).

mon in patients with diffuse alveolar damage. The pathogenesis of NBTE is probably related to the combination of endothelial damage and loss and a hypercoagulable state. These vegetations may become superinfected and evolve into infective endocarditis. Systemic and pulmonary embolic phenomena are not uncommon, depending on the valves which are involved.

Other types of vegetations include the tiny wartlike vegetations of rheumatic fever (see Figs. 2–6 and 2–18) and the Libman-Sacks vegetation of systemic lupus erythematosus (SLE). In SLE, the small, bland thrombotic-type vegetations are characteristically seen on the undersurface of the valve, but they may be seen in many sites, including the chordae tendineae and mural endocardium. Notable is valvulitis underlying the vegetation, which can result in significant valve destruction and subsequent healing with anatomic and functional abnormalities.[7]

MITRAL VALVE PROLAPSE

Mitral valve prolapse, also called floppy mitral valve, is the most common cause of isolated mitral regurgitation in series of operatively excised valves. Many terms have been used to describe this entity, including myxomatous valve disease and floppy mitral valve syndrome. The descriptive terminology is confusing, and pathologic and clinical terminologies do not always agree. The terms *prolapse* and *floppy* imply functional regurgitation and some degree of bulging or billowing of variably enlarged leaflets into the left atrium (Fig. 2–20); the macroscopic and microscopic anatomic features do not always correlate well with the echocardiographic findings of prolapse. The

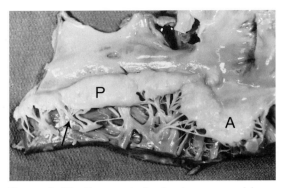

Figure 2·21 Floppy mitral valve in an opened heart. Notice the thickened, opaque leaflets with thickened chordae tendineae. The posterior (P) and anterior (A) leaflets are enlarged. An endocardial friction lesion probably is beneath the chordae tendineae of the posterior leaflet, near the cut edge *(arrow)*.

term *floppy mitral valve* is used here for the pathologic features that most commonly cause the clinical syndrome of mitral valve prolapse.

The floppy mitral valve, as classically described, has enlarged, thickened opaque leaflets, an increased leaflet area, and dilated annular circumference. The posterior leaflet often is most notably affected, with prominent elongation such that it is similar in size to the anterior leaflet (Figs. 2–21 and 2–22). The condition is characterized by interchordal hooding and hooding or doming of the leaflets toward the left atrium. The valve leaflets are soft, grayish white, and have a smooth surface. The apparent thickening of the spongiosa results from the deposition of acid mucopolysaccharide material; the spongiosa appears to extend into and replace the fibrosa (Fig. 2–23). The chordae tendineae are elongated and tortuous; they can show

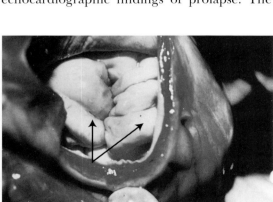

Figure 2·20 Mitral valve prolapse is viewed from the left atrial aspect. Enlarged leaflets have ballooned into the left atrium *(arrows)*.

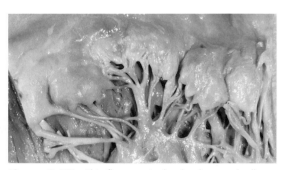

Figure 2·22 This floppy mitral valve has markedly enlarged, hooded leaflets. The anterior and posterior leaflets are nearly equal in size. The chordae are elongated and tortuous.

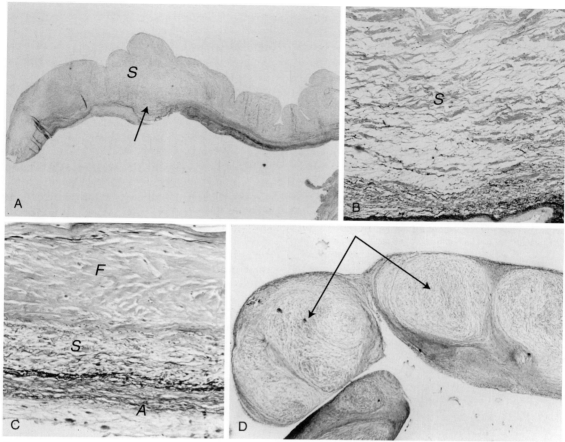

Figure 2·23 Microscopic section of a floppy mitral valve (Verhoeff–van Gieson stain). *A,* Low-power view of the mitral valve shows expansion of the spongiosa (S), virtual absence of the fibrosa, and focally absent elastic fibers in the atrialis *(arrow). B,* Higher-power view shows separation of fibers in the spongiosa (S). *C,* More normal mitral valve at a slightly higher power than in *B* shows the mildly thickened atrialis (A), fibrosa (F), and relatively inapparent spongiosa (S). *D,* The chordae tendineae show changes similar to those of the valve, with marked expansion of the spongiosa by acid mucopolysaccharide *(arrows).*

thinning or may appear thickened as a result of microscopic changes similar to those in the leaflets, with a mucopolysaccharide-rich spongiosa surfacing the central collagenous chordal core. Tortuosity is most prominent in the attachment of chordae to leaflets, and an important feature is the haphazard architecture of the chordal distribution and anchoring.[15] Secondary effects include endocardial friction lesions under the posterior leaflet or the chordae tendineae and left atrial enlargement (Figs. 2–24 and 2–25). Adherence of the leaflet to the friction lesions distorts the valve anatomy and increases the degree of regurgitation. Rupture of chordae tendineae can occur because of marked thinning (Fig. 2–26) and can result in a flail leaflet.[38, 39]

Most cases of floppy mitral valve are not associated with an underlying systemic disease.

However, patients with Marfan's syndrome or other inherited connective tissue diseases, such as Ehlers-Danlos syndrome, pseudoxanthoma elasticum, and osteogenesis imperfecta, have a high incidence of mitral valve prolapse. In autopsy and clinical series, 39% and 48%, respectively, of patients with Marfan's syndrome had mitral valve prolapse. A high incidence of mitral valve prolapse has also been associated with secundum-type atrial septal defect, hypertrophic cardiomyopathy, ventricular septal defect, patent ductus arteriosus, tetralogy of Fallot, and congenital heart disease in adults.[38]

Some patients with Marfan's syndrome have floppy aortic valves with expanded valve area, downward prolapse with resulting regurgitation, and histologic changes similar to those seen with mitral valve prolapse. An autopsy

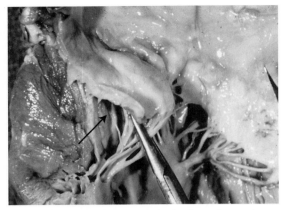

Figure 2·24   The floppy mitral valve has a friction lesion (ie, endocardial fibrosis) beneath the leaflet and chordae tendineae *(arrow)*. The leaflet is bound to the endocardium.

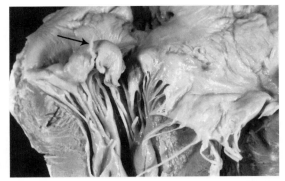

Figure 2·26   Floppy mitral valve with ruptured chordae tendineae *(arrow)*. The tortuous chordae tendineae are elongated and thickened.

study of 102 patients with floppy mitral valves who died at a community hospital showed a 2% incidence of floppy aortic valves, but none was associated with aortic valvular regurgitation.[40] Similarly, a floppy tricuspid valve can be associated with floppy mitral valve (Fig. 2–27). Autopsy studies have reported a prevalence of floppy tricuspid valve of 0.3% to 40%, with the higher percentage found in two autopsy series of patients with an antemortem diagnosis of floppy mitral valve or mitral valve prolapse.[40–42]

Davies reported that approximately one third of patients with floppy mitral valves had similar involvement of the tricuspid valve, although generally not clinically significant.[3] Floppy tricuspid valves are rarely seen as surgical pathology specimens, because the tricuspid regurgitation usually is not severe enough to require surgical treatment. The gross and microscopic changes are similar to those seen in

the mitral valve. In the autopsy series by Edwards and Lucas,[40] a thickened, floppy pulmonic valve was found in 11%, but none had signs of pulmonic regurgitation.

SYSTEMIC DISEASES THAT INVOLVE THE CARDIAC VALVES

Marfan's Syndrome and Other Connective Tissue Disorders

Marfan's syndrome is a disorder of the connective tissues caused by mutations in the fibrillin gene. Fibrillin is a glycoprotein that is secreted by fibroblasts and aggregates with other proteins to form a microfibrillar network in the extracellular matrix, serving as scaffolding for the deposition of elastin. Microfibrillar structures are particularly abundant in the aorta, in ligaments, and in the ciliary zonules that support the lens. Characteristic clinical abnormalities are skeletal, with long, slender

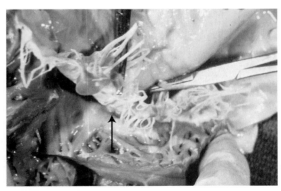

Figure 2·25   Endocardial fibrosis beneath the floppy mitral valve results in adherence of the chordae tendineae *(arrow)*.

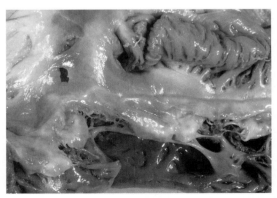

Figure 2·27   Floppy tricuspid valve with thickening and hooding of the leaflets that are less prominent than the changes seen with mitral valve prolapse.

extremities (including fingers and toes), tall stature, and lax ligaments; ocular, with subluxation of the lens of the eyes; and cardiovascular, most commonly dilatation of the ascending aorta caused by cystic medial degeneration and associated mitral valve prolapse.[43]

Cystic medial degeneration is also seen in patients who do not have Marfan's syndrome. It is characterized by fragmentation and loss of elastic fibers in the aortic media, accompanied by accumulation of acid mucopolysaccharide material (ie, extracellular matrix-type material or ground substance) in cleft-like cystic pools or spaces. Aortic dissection is a sequela of cystic medial degeneration and has an increased incidence among patients with Marfan's syndrome; however, aortic dissection can occur in the absence of histologic abnormalities of the aorta.[44]

As a result of the abnormal aortic wall, patients with Marfan's syndrome can develop aortic root or annular dilatation (ie, aortoannular ectasia), with resulting aortic insufficiency. Changes characteristic of aortic regurgitation due to annular dilatation include thickened, rolled edges of the aortic cusps and a "tadpole" appearance on microscopic examination (Figs. 2–28 and 2–29). The aortic valve may otherwise appear normal with thin cusps, or it may also show changes similar to those seen in the floppy mitral valve. Myxomatous change is not always seen histologically.

The prevalence of floppy mitral valve is increased among patients with Marfan's syndrome. Pure mitral regurgitation may also de-

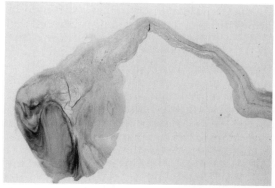

Figure 2·29 Microscopic section of the aortic valve cusps in Figure 2–28 show the tadpole appearance of the bulbous edge of the valve in cross section, which is characteristic of valvular aortic insufficiency due to aortic root dilatation (Verhoeff–van Gieson stain).

velop as a result of dilated mitral annulus with normal mitral valvular anatomy. Pure tricuspid regurgitation can occur because of floppy tricuspid valve or tricuspid annular dilatation with normal leaflets. Tricuspid dysfunction is always seen in conjunction with changes of the mitral or aortic valve or both.

Aortic and mitral alterations similar to those seen in Marfan's syndrome are associated with other inherited connective tissue disorders, principally Ehlers-Danlos syndrome and osteogenesis imperfecta. The changes, including floppy mitral valve, aortic dissection or rupture, and aortic valvular regurgitation, are more variable in these entities than in Marfan's syndrome.[45]

Aortic Root Dilatation

The most common cause of isolated aortic regurgitation is idiopathic aortic root dilatation. The characteristic features are a dilated aortic root and ascending aorta, without inflammation of the aorta and with negative serologic results characteristic of the inflammatory aortic processes. All patients with idiopathic aortic root dilatation have some degree of cystic medial degeneration, with variable destruction of the elastica. Aortic regurgitation occurs when the root dilates, because the degree of cusp overlap is reduced until one or more cusps prolapse. Regurgitant flow results in localized cusp fibrosis and a rolled edge with a characteristic tadpole shape. The aortic valve is otherwise anatomically normal. Idiopathic aortic root dilatation can be seen in Marfan's syndrome and other heritable connective tissue disorders.[3]

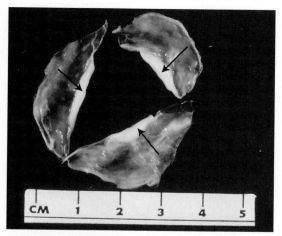

Figure 2·28 The surgically excised aortic valve shows changes of aortic insufficiency due to aortic root dilatation. Notice the thickened and rolled edges of the cusps (arrows). The patient had Marfan's syndrome, although these pathologic changes are not specific for that entity.

Aortic root dilatation can also be caused by various forms of aortitis: syphilis, giant cell and Takayasu's aortitis, rheumatoid arthritis, and ankylosing spondylitis. In syphilis, the aortic root is mildly dilated and has a wrinkled intima. Histologic inspection reveals a lymphoplasmacytic inflammatory infiltrate with destruction of smooth muscle and elastic tissue, resulting in formation of a medial scar. The valve has widened, separated commissures, without other valvular distortion. In ankylosing spondylitis, fibrosis distorts the aortic root and aortic valve and extends into the base of the mitral valve; the latter finding is considered characteristic of ankylosing spondylitis. The inflammatory process is similar to that of syphilis, and it can extend into the conduction system, with resultant heart block. In ankylosing spondylitis and syphilis, the appropriate serologic test results are positive.

Rheumatoid arthritis can be associated with an aortitis similar to that seen in ankylosing spondylitis. Cases in which there is inflammatory aortitis, with pathology similar to that seen in syphilis or ankylosing spondylitis but with negative serologic results or no clinical history of the associated disease's symptoms, are called nonspecific inflammatory aortitis. Idiopathic giant cell aortitis also has been described.[3] Other causes of aortic root dilatation include aortic dissection, with or without cystic medial degeneration, and systemic hypertension, in which the valve may be normal or show nonspecific myxoid degeneration.[46, 47]

Immune-Mediated Diseases

The prototypical immune disease is systemic lupus erythematosus (SLE). The characteristic acute lesion is Libman-Sacks endocarditis, which is a variant of nonbacterial thrombotic endocarditis (NBTE), in which tiny vegetations occur on both sides of the valve leaflets and are scattered on the mural endocardium and elsewhere. The vegetations are fibrin rich and may contain hematoxylin bodies. They often surface an area of valvulitis, characterized by fibrinoid necrosis and accompanied by a mixed inflammatory reaction. The acute vegetations can be differentiated from NBTE by their distribution, by the presence of hematoxylin bodies, and by their association with SLE. Healing has been associated with corticosteroid therapy and results in fibrous thickening, distortion, and calcification of the valve, similar to that seen in rheumatic valvular disease.

Clinically important valvular heart disease (acute and chronic) is a relatively common clinical problem in SLE, occurring in 18% of cases in one clinical study and mainly involving aortic and mitral valves with stenosis and regurgitation. The chronic valvular changes are often significant enough to require surgery.[5, 7, 48–50] High levels of anticardiolipin antibodies are associated with valvular abnormalities in SLE and other lupus-like diseases with antiphospholipid syndrome.[51]

In rheumatoid arthritis, diffusely or focally distributed rheumatoid granulomas can occur in the valve or annulus, causing valvular distortion and usually regurgitant physiology.[52]

Carcinoid Heart Disease and Drug-Related Valvular Abnormalities

Carcinoid heart disease occurs in the setting of the carcinoid syndrome, usually occurring with gastrointestinal carcinoid tumors that have metastasized to the liver or to regional lymph nodes. In the latter circumstance, the systemically drained venous blood bypasses the liver to reach the heart. The cardiovascular lesions mainly involve the right side of the heart, including the endocardium and the tricuspid and pulmonic valves, but may occur on the intima of the great veins, coronary sinus, and pulmonary trunk. Some cases have been reported with left-sided valvular involvement.[53]

The characteristic lesions consist of focal or diffuse, white, shiny, fibrous endocardial plaques (Fig. 2–30). The most extensive involvement is usually on the ventricular surface of the tricuspid valve leaflets and on the arterial aspect of the pulmonic valve. The tricuspid leaflets may adhere to the underlying ventricle, resulting in functional regurgitation. Stenosis is the most common abnormality of the pulmonic valve. The fibrous plaques also occur on the right atrial endocardium, resulting in a noncompliant chamber.

The carcinoid plaques are histologically distinctive. They consist of smooth muscle cells and sparse collagen embedded in abundant acid mucopolysaccharide matrix with no elastic fibers (Fig. 2–31). The plaques surface the endocardium and encase the valvular structures, causing no underlying destruction, and the subjacent structures appear unaltered.[7, 54]

The pathogenesis of these lesions is thought to be related to the chemical products of the carcinoid tumors, mainly serotonin but also bradykinin, histamine, and tachykinins. Plasma concentrations of these bioactive amines

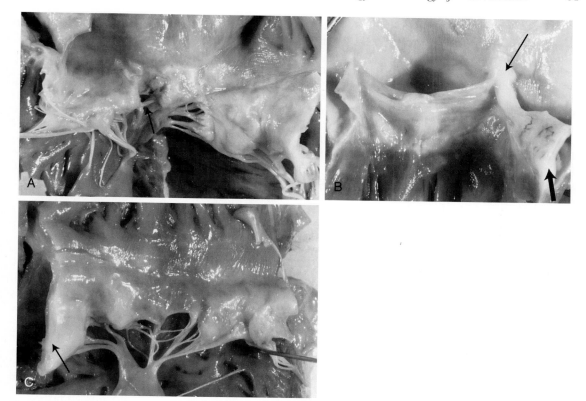

Figure 2·30 Carcinoid heart disease. The patient had histologically proved carcinoid tumor in the paraaortic lymph nodes but no hepatic metastases. Typical carcinoid-type changes involved all four valves but were more marked in the tricuspid and pulmonic valves. *A,* The tricuspid valve shows marked fibrous thickening and chordal fusion, with distortion of the valve caused by adherence of the leaflet to the ventricular endocardium *(arrow). B,* A thickened, white plaque encases the valve cusp *(large arrow)* on the cut section of the pulmonic valve and is seen adjacent to the commissure and on the pulmonary arterial wall *(small arrow). C,* The mitral valve is less involved than the tricuspid valve. The leaflet thickening is particularly well seen on cross section *(arrow).* These left-sided valvular changes can occur when drainage of metastases enters the systemic circulation and bypasses the liver, as in this case.

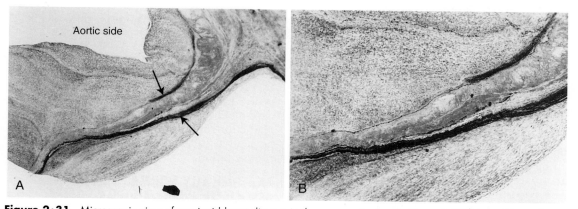

Figure 2·31 Microscopic view of carcinoid heart disease in the same patient as in Figure 2–30 (Verhoeff–van Gieson stain). *A,* Low-power view of an aortic valve with typical carcinoid plaque encasing the normal valve structure, which is relatively intact and bounded by the black-staining elastic tissue *(small arrows). B,* Higher power demonstrates that the plaque is composed of a cellular, fibrous connective tissue, with abundant matrix and no identifiable elastic tissue.

roughly correlate with the severity of the cardiac changes. The preponderance of right-sided changes is explained by inactivation of the bioactive amines by pulmonary monoamine oxidase. Because of hepatic inactivation of the amines, gastrointestinal carcinoid tumors without hepatic metastases do not produce cardiac lesions unless their venous drainage bypasses the liver. Left-sided cardiac lesions are thought to occur because of high levels of circulating amines, the presence of pulmonary tumors, or right-to-left cardiac shunts.[7, 55]

Changes microscopically identical to those seen in carcinoid syndrome have been reported in patients treated with methysergide and ergotamine for migraine headaches. The drug-related lesions demonstrate more left-sided involvement and more involvement of the chordae tendineae and the tips of the papillary muscles than carcinoid lesions.[56, 57] The similar chemical structures of serotonin, methysergide, and ergotamine may provide an explanation for the similarity in the pathologic changes.

Changes histologically identical to those of carcinoid valve disease have been described in patients treated with the appetite suppressants fenfluramine, dexfenfluramine, or the combination of fenfluramine and phentermine. These drugs, which had been known to cause pulmonary hypertension, have been reported to be associated with right-sided and left-sided valvular lesions (ie, mitral, tricuspid, aortic, and pulmonic abnormalities, in decreasing order of frequency), and multiple valve involvement has been common. It has been postulated that the changes seen with fenfluramine-phentermine therapy are related to changes in circulating concentrations of serotonin and other bioactive amines produced by the drugs.[58–61]

Miscellaneous Systemic Diseases and Alterations

Radiation-Induced Valvular Heart Disease

Valvular changes related to irradiation are uncommon and consist of focal fibrotic thickening of valve leaflets or cusps that may be associated with chordal fibrous thickening. The tricuspid and mitral valves are most frequently involved, followed by the aortic and pulmonic valves. Valvular changes are less frequent than other radiation-induced changes, including pericardial fibrous thickening, interstitial and perivascular myocardial fibrosis, and accelerated coronary atherosclerosis.[62]

Metabolic and Enzymatic Disorders

Inherited storage disease can result in accumulation of the storage product in cells in valves, resulting primarily in stenosis-type physiology. Accumulations are most commonly seen in the mitral and tricuspid valves. Most common of these uncommon diseases are the mucopolysaccharidoses. The histologic appearance of the valves is similar to the characteristic tissue involvement for each disease. In Fabry's disease, caused by deficiency of lysosomal galactosidase A and disrupted lipid metabolism, valvular lesions have been described functionally but not well characterized pathologically.[45] Young adults with type II hyperlipidemia can develop aortic stenosis as a result of marked lipid deposition, typically followed by calcification.[29] In Whipple's disease, periodic acid-Schiff–positive macrophages, which appear identical to those seen in intestinal biopsies, accumulate in the valve, most commonly in the mitral valve, followed by the tricuspid and aortic valves. The valves are thickened and generally stenotic.[62]

Amyloid

Amyloid may be present in valves of persons with systemic amyloidosis or senile cardiac amyloidosis. The mitral and tricuspid valves are primarily involved by the deposition of small nodules of amyloid, generally of no functional significance. However, the valve may be thickened enough to cause stenosis. Amyloid has been detected in areas of dense scarring in valves that have been surgically removed for valvular heart disease. This condition is called dystrophic amyloidosis.[63]

Endomyocardial Fibrosis

Endomyocardial fibrosis, also called hypereosinophilic syndrome, appears to be caused by elevated numbers of circulating eosinophils. The lesions consist of ventricular endocardial fibrosis, resulting in papillary muscle retraction, adherence of atrioventricular valvular leaflets to the ventricular wall, and valvular regurgitation.[25, 64]

ANATOMICALLY NORMAL VALVES ASSOCIATED WITH VALVULAR DYSFUNCTION

Aortic regurgitation can be caused by diseases that affect the aorta only but do not affect an anatomically normal valve (eg, Marfan's syndrome, idiopathic aortic root dilatation, and aortic dissection) and by diseases that do not compromise the anatomically normal aorta and valve (eg, systemic hypertension, ventricular septal defect). In all of these entities, there can be focal valvular thickening and the changes characteristic of aortic regurgitation caused by aortic annular dilatation (ie, thickening and rolling of the cusp edges), depending on the degree and duration of the hemodynamic alteration.[65]

Isolated mitral regurgitation may result from papillary muscle dysfunction, in which the valve leaflets are essentially normal. The underlying mechanism appears to be papillary muscle malalignment, without annular dilatation, particularly when it occurs with systemic hypertension, hypertrophic or dilated cardiomyopathy, or left ventricular dilatation. The most common cause of papillary muscle dysfunction in the mitral valve is atherosclerotic coronary artery disease. Acute papillary muscle rupture may occur in the setting of acute myocardial infarction; the severity of the mitral regurgitation depends on the degree of disruption of the chordae tendineae and papillary muscle (Fig. 2–32). Rupture of a papillary muscle head or trunk produces severe regurgitation and is often fatal. Chronic papillary muscle dysfunction occurs in the setting of remote myocardial infarction with scarring of the papillary muscle head and the adjacent left ventricle. Other infiltrative myocardial conditions can produce papillary muscle dysfunction, including sarcoidosis, amyloidosis, infection, neoplasm, and endomyocardial fibrosis.[39]

Dysfunction of the tricuspid papillary muscles can produce acute or chronic tricuspid regurgitation. However, the most common reason for tricuspid regurgitation with normal leaflets is tricuspid annular dilatation caused by right ventricular systolic or diastolic hypertension. Common causes include pulmonary hypertension of any origin, mitral or pulmonic valvular stenosis, right ventricular failure, or dilated cardiomyopathy. The mechanism for tricuspid regurgitation with an anatomically normal valve is related to annular dilatation and papillary muscle malalignment.[42] Other causes for tricuspid regurgitation with a normal valve are similar to those for the normal mitral valve, including necrosis (acute) or fibrosis (chronic) caused by atherosclerotic coronary artery disease with a posterior myocardial infarct involving the right ventricle;

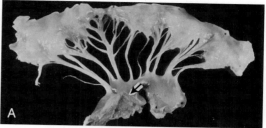

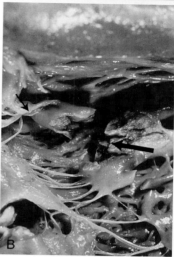

Figure 2·32 *A,* Mitral insufficiency was caused by rupture of the papillary muscle *(arrow).* The valve and chordae are normal in this surgically resected specimen. *B,* Close-up view of the ruptured papillary muscle *(large arrow)* that caused acute mitral regurgitation, a flail leaflet, and twisting of the chordae tendineae *(small arrow).*

myocarditis; infection with abscess formation; granuloma (as in sarcoidosis); amyloid; and endomyocardial fibrosis. Penetrating trauma of the right ventricle can disrupt the papillary muscle. Waller has proposed that leaflet appearance and annular circumference measurements can be used to establish the cause of pure tricuspid regurgitation.[66]

Pure pulmonic regurgitation with an anatomically normal pulmonary valve most commonly is caused by dilatation of the pulmonary trunk and annulus. This usually results from pulmonary arterial hypertension of any cause, but it also occurs in persons with Marfan's syndrome or with idiopathic pulmonary trunk dilatation.[17]

FUNCTIONAL CLASSIFICATION CORRELATED WITH ETIOLOGY

Tables 2–1 through 2–4 show the major causes of valvular dysfunction, classified func-

TABLE 2·1	CLASSIFICATION OF AORTIC VALVE DISORDERS AND FUNCTIONS

Stenosis
  Congenital conditions
    Bicuspid
    Unicuspid
    Acommissural
    Other (eg, tricuspid, quadricuspid)
  Degenerative conditions
  Rheumatic conditions
  Active infective endocarditis
  Other conditions
    Homozygous type II hyperlipoproteinemia
    Metabolic or enzymatic (eg, Fabry's disease)
    Systemic lupus erythematosus
Isolated regurgitation
  Abnormal valve
    Congenital bicuspid
    Rheumatic conditions
    Infective endocarditis (active or healed)
    Floppy aortic valve
    Systemic lupus erythematosus
    Rheumatoid arthritis
  Abnormal aorta and normal valve
    Idiopathic aortic root dilatation
    Marfan's syndrome
    Aortic dissection
  Normal aorta and normal valve
    Systemic hypertension
    Prolapse due to ventricular septal defect
  Abnormal aorta and abnormal valve
    Ankylosing spondylitis
    Marfan's syndrome
    Syphilis (ie, aortitis with commissural separation)

17). Both respond passively to changes in pressure and flow, and the bases of both types are surrounded by a fabric (usually Dacron) sewing ring, which is sutured to the surgically prepared host annulus (Fig. 2–33). This represents the primary site of host-prosthesis interaction, which is important in the pathogenesis of many of the complications of prosthetic valves, including thrombosis, infection, and tissue ingrowth. In most cases, organized thrombus or fibrous tissue from the endocardium, myocardium, or aorta surfaces the sewing ring (Fig. 2–34). Both types of valves can be placed in the atrioventricular or semilunar position, although there may be differences in the sewing rings for different sites.

Mechanical valves are composed of nonbiologic materials, and all consist of a valve base or body, which includes the sewing ring; a rigid, mobile occluder, also called a poppet; and a cagelike structure that restricts the pop-

tionally as stenosis or regurgitation. Most stenotic valves have some degree of regurgitation. By definition, isolated regurgitation has no stenotic component.

COMPLICATIONS OF PROSTHETIC VALVES

Pathologic evaluation of prosthetic valves is important in the management of patients and in the evaluation of safety and efficacy of particular prostheses in humans, specifically in the recognition of complications. The Federal Safe Medical Devices Act of 1990 (PL 101-629) requires that hospitals and health care personnel report all device-related deaths, injuries, or serious illness to the U.S. Food and Drug Administration; this necessitates initiation of reporting through the institution by the examining pathologist who discovers a malfunctioning prosthetic valve or other device.[67]

Types of Valve Prostheses

There are two types of heart valve prostheses in use: mechanical and tissue (see Chapter

TABLE 2·2	CLASSIFICATION OF MITRAL VALVE DISORDERS AND FUNCTIONS

Stenosis
  Rheumatic conditions (>95%)
  Other causes
    Active infective endocarditis, with obstruction by vegetation
    Mitral annular calcification
    Metabolic or enzymatic
      Whipple's disease, mucopolysaccharidosis, Fabry's disease
      Carcinoid
      Methysergide therapy
    Congenital conditions
Isolated regurgitation
  Abnormal valve
    Floppy mitral valve
    Rheumatic conditions
    Infective endocarditis, active or healed
    Marfan's syndrome and other heritable connective tissue disorders
    Mitral annular calcification
    Congenital (cleft or fenestration)
    Systemic lupus erythematosus
    Rheumatoid arthritis
    Radiation therapy
    Pharmacologic agents (eg, methysergide, fenfluramine-phentermine)
    Carcinoid syndrome
    Endomyocardial fibrosis
  Normal valve
    Papillary muscle dysfunction, including rupture
      Acute or remote myocardial infarct
      Infiltrative myocardial disease (eg, amyloid, sarcoid, infection)
    Hypertrophic and dilated cardiomyopathy
    Systemic hypertension
    Ventricular dilatation of any cause

TABLE 2·3 CLASSIFICATION OF TRICUSPID VALVE DISORDERS AND FUNCTIONS

Stenosis
  All stenosis
    Rheumatic conditions (>90%)
  Isolated stenosis
    Carcinoid syndrome
    Congenital conditions
  Other causes
    Active infective endocarditis with obstructing
      vegetation
    Metabolic or enzymatic disorders (eg, Whipple's
      disease, Fabry's disease)
    Pharmacologic agents (eg, methysergide,
      fenfluramine-phentermine)
    Giant blood cyst
Isolated regurgitation
  Normal valve
    Conditions producing annular dilatation and
      papillary muscle malalignment
    Pulmonary hypertension of any cause, with right
      ventricular dilatation
    Papillary muscle dysfunction
    Right ventricle trauma
    Acute or remote myocardial infarct
    Infiltrative myocardial disease (eg, amyloid,
      sarcoid)
  Abnormal valve
    Rheumatic conditions
    Congenital (mainly Ebstein's anomaly)
    Infective endocarditis, active or healed
    Carcinoid syndrome
    Floppy tricuspid valve

TABLE 2·4 CLASSIFICATION OF PULMONIC VALVE DISORDERS AND FUNCTIONS

Stenosis
  Congenital (>95%)
    Isolated
    With other abnormalities, especially tetralogy of
      Fallot
  Acquired
    Carcinoid syndrome
    Rheumatic conditions
    Infective endocarditis with obstructing vegetation
Isolated regurgitation
  Normal valve
    Dilatation of pulmonic trunk and annulus
      Pulmonary arterial hypertension of any cause
      Idiopathic pulmonary trunk dilatation
      Marfan's syndrome
  Abnormal valve
    Congenital
    Carcinoid syndrome
    Infective endocarditis, with perforation or retraction
    Catheter trauma (balloon)
    External blunt trauma
    Rheumatic conditions
    Rheumatoid arthritis and syphilis
    Pharmacologic agents (eg, fenfluramine-
      phentermine)

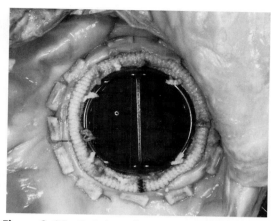

Figure 2·33 St. Jude mechanical valve recently inserted in the mitral position. The view from the atrial aspect shows pledgets around the sewing ring and no adherent thrombus.

pet motion. The most frequently used mechanical valve is the St. Jude Medical bileaflet tilting-disk valve prosthesis. It is composed of pyrolytic carbon, a thromboresistant material that is highly resistant to wear and fatigue, and it has bilateral and central flow patterns. Other previously widely used prostheses that may be encountered include the Starr-Edwards caged-ball valve, with a silicon ball; the Bjork-Shiley and Medtronic-Hall tilting-disk valves; and several types of caged-disk valves. Chronic anticoagulation, with its associated risk of hemorrhage, is required in patients with mechanical valves, because of the thrombogenicity of the nonbiologic materials and because of the tur-

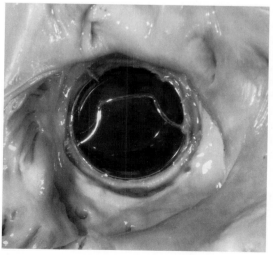

Figure 2·34 Bjork-Shiley mechanical valve with a well-healed sewing ring and no adherent thrombus.

bulence and stasis resulting from blood flow around the poppet.

Tissue valves have a more anatomic configuration; they are composed of three cusps of human or animal tissue. Heterograft or xenograft valves include porcine aortic or bovine pericardial prostheses. Homograft or allograft valves consist of human cadaveric aortic or pulmonic valves with or without attached aorta or pulmonary artery. Autograft valves consist of valves fashioned from the host fascia lata or pericardium or, more commonly, the patient's own pulmonic valve transplanted into the aortic position. The most commonly used tissue valve is the porcine aortic valve, consisting of a chemically preserved (cross-linked) pig aortic valve that is attached to a metal support structure or stent. The Hancock bioprosthesis is preserved in 0.2% glutaraldehyde, and the Carpentier-Edwards valve is preserved in 0.6% glutaraldehyde. The other commonly used tissue valve is the cryopreserved human aortic valve homograft, implanted into the host aortic valve without a stent.

The anatomic configuration of the tissue valves results in more physiologic central flow, increasing hemodynamic efficiency compared with mechanical valves. Because there is a relatively thromboresistant biologic blood surface contact, despite the absence of endothelial preservation, chronic anticoagulation is not required with homograft valves and most heterograft valves.[67]

Limitations of Prosthetic Valves

All prosthetic valves have limitations that significantly affect clinical function and survival of the patient. Pathologic complications of valve prostheses are major determinants of valve longevity and patient prognosis. Several studies have indicated that up to two thirds of deaths of patients with a prosthetic valve can be attributed to the prosthesis because of infective endocarditis, valve failure, and thromboembolic phenomena. Other causes of death include coincident coronary atherosclerosis and myocardial anatomic and functional abnormalities related to the valvular disease, such as significant cardiac left ventricular hypertrophy or congestive heart failure.[68–70]

Complications of valvular prostheses can be classified as follows:

1. Thromboembolism, including anticoagulant-related hemorrhage
2. Infection (such as endocarditis)

3. Structural degeneration or intrinsic failure (for mechanical valves: wear, fracture, or poppet escape; for bioprosthetic valves: cusp tear or calcification)
4. Nonstructural failure, such as paravalvular leak, tissue overgrowth or entrapment, suture entrapment, significant hemolysis, or audible valve clicks that disturb the patient

Studies have shown that these complications cause death or necessitate reoperation in as many as 50% to 60% of patients within 10 years of the first valve surgery.[7, 67, 71] Complications with mechanical valves are primarily related to thromboembolism and necessary anticoagulation, causing approximately 50% of deaths in one autopsy series mainly involving mechanical prostheses. A study of consecutive prostheses (45 mechanical, 112 bioprostheses) removed at surgery over a 5.5-year period demonstrated the following modes of failure: degenerative dysfunction (53%), endocarditis (16%), paravalvular leak (11%), thrombosis (9%), and tissue overgrowth (5%). However, the causes of failure were quite different for mechanical and bioprostheses. Bioprosthetic failure resulted from degenerative processes in 74% of the cases, compared with 10% of the mechanical prostheses; thrombosis-related complications caused failure in 18% of mechanical valves, compared with 4% of bioprostheses. Mechanical valves also had higher rates of complications from tissue overgrowth (18% versus 4%), sterile paravalvular leak (20% versus 8%), and endocarditis (16% versus 10%).[67, 72, 73]

Thromboembolism

Thromboembolic phenomena are related to obstruction of valve function, emboli to arterial beds, and anticoagulant-related hemorrhage. Complication rates are similar, at approximately 1% to 4% per year, for anticoagulated mechanical and nonanticoagulated bioprosthetic valves. Patients are at greatest risk for thromboembolic events when the valve is in the mitral position, when there is cardiac arrhythmia (eg, atrial fibrillation), and when anticoagulation is inadequate. Local thrombotic effects are predominantly seen with mechanical prostheses (Fig. 2–35), but they also occur with bioprostheses (Fig. 2–36). The thrombi can vary in appearance; erythrocyte-rich thrombi predominate (ie, red clots) in areas of stasis, and platelet-rich thrombi (ie, white clots) are related to the role of platelets

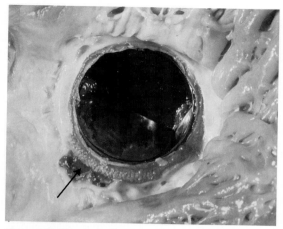

Figure 2·35 St. Jude mechanical valve in the mitral position with thrombus on the sewing ring, which is most prominent from 2 to 8 o'clock, and a small, sterile paravalvular leak at 8 o'clock *(arrow)*.

in initiating interaction with biomaterials in areas of high flow. Organization of thrombi is markedly altered from normal because of the absence of vascular ingrowth; this makes determining the age of such thrombi very difficult.

Endocarditis

Endocarditis can be an early or late complication (see Chapter 18). Early infection, defined as occurring within 60 days of valve placement, is usually related to normal skin flora, with *S. epidermidis* the predominant organism. Late infections are related to bacteremia. With mechanical valves, infection is localized to the sewing ring, and ring abscesses are common. Sequelae related to extension of the infection through tissue planes include suppurative pericarditis, aortitis, and pseudoaneurysm formation; valve dehiscence and septic paravalvular leak result from the local effects of the valve ring infection.

Infection of the cusps may occur with tissue valves, and organisms may be found deep in the cuspal connective tissue. Four stages of bioprosthetic valve infection are recognized: stage I, infection only in surface thrombi; stage II, invasion of superficial layers of the cusp; stage III, penetration of organisms into the central cusp (ie, spongiosa of porcine valves); and stage IV, cuspal perforation. Bacterial invasion of the spongiosa provides a path for sewing ring infection. Vegetations may calcify, making organisms difficult to identify.[74] Because of the presence of the foreign biomaterial and the lack of vascularity, these infections are very resistant to antibiotic therapy. The prevalence of staphylococcal infections in prosthetic valvular infections contrasts with the bacterial profile of native endocarditis (Fig. 2–37).

Nonstructural Abnormalities

Nonstructural abnormalities are a heterogeneous group of abnormalities related to the environment surrounding an otherwise normal-appearing and normal-functioning prosthetic valve. Exuberant fibrous tissue ingrowth extending from the sewing ring can cause valve obstruction, as can a loose suture in the sewing ring. Small, sterile paravalvular leaks usually result from tissue contraction during healing; the resulting leak may be clinically insignificant (see Fig. 2–35). Larger leaks may result from infection or from abnormality of the surgical annulus, as with mitral annular calcification, mitral valve prolapse, aortic valvular calcification, previous surgical procedure, or infection (eg, endocarditis with ring abscess). Significant hemolysis or congestive failure may occur. With sterile leaks, the prosthetic valve commonly appears normal. Although mild hemolysis generally occurs with mechanical valves as a result of turbulent blood flow, it is unusual for significant hemolysis to occur with modern mechanical prostheses or with bioprostheses. Development of significant hemolysis raises concerns about a paravalvular leak due to infection or a mechanical valve dysfunction.

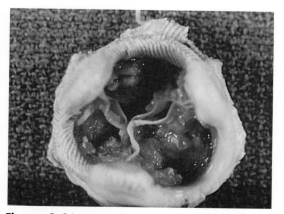

Figure 2·36 Hancock-type porcine heterograft bioprosthesis with extensive thrombus on the aortic aspect of the cusps (ie, sinuses of Valsalva).

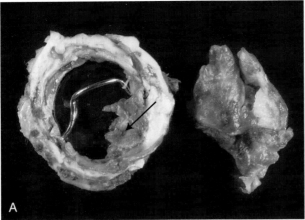

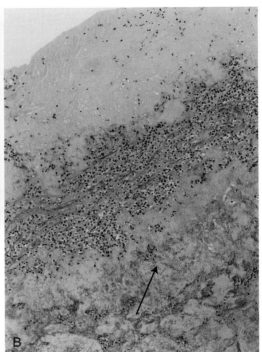

Figure 2·37 *A,* Bjork-Shiley mitral prosthesis with an adherent vegetation on the atrial aspect *(arrow).* The detached fragment of vegetation adjacent to the valve was attached on the ventricular aspect. *B,* Microscopic section of a vegetation shows abundant neutrophils and coccal-type organisms *(arrow)* admixed with fibrin and platelets. The blood culture was positive for *Staphylococcus aureus.*

Valve Degeneration

Bioprosthetic Valves

Intrinsic degeneration of the valve is the most common cause of bioprosthetic valve failure, generally occurring after 4 to 5 years of function and seen to greatest degree in heterograft valves (Fig. 2–38). More rapid progression is seen in children and youths; this increased risk for acceleration of primary valve failure extends to 35 years of age. The primary mechanism of failure is deposition of calcium phosphates, mainly in the form of hydroxyapatite, similar to the physiologic component of bone. Most of the calcium is deposited in the cusp bases and at the commissures; valves become stiff, and gray-white nodules of calcium can ulcerate through the cusp body, resulting in valvular insufficiency.

Because of the concentration of mineral at points of maximum flexion, the calcification appears to be related to but not dependent on mechanical stresses. The process does not seem to be immunologic or inflammatory in nature. It has been postulated that the nonviable cells in the prosthesis accumulate calcium based on the large concentration gradient that promotes transfer of calcium into cells, where it can react with membrane phosphorus. Calcification of collagen occurs later. It is likely that

tissue preservation is the primary determinant of valve failure, because pretreatment of tissue with an aldehyde cross-linking agent is a prerequisite for calcification. Microscopic and ultrastructural morphologic changes seen in glutaraldehyde-treated tissues include loss of endothelium, autolysis of connective tissue cells, collagen bundle loosening, and loss of ground substance. Postimplantation changes include plasma protein insudation, superficial fibrin deposition, inflammatory cell adherence with occasional penetration (mainly macrophages), generalized architectural homogenization, mineralization, and sometimes, amyloid deposition.[75] Treatment of the valve with a chemical surfactant (sodium dodecyl sulfate) may help mitigate leaflet calcification and extend durability.[76]

Cuspal tears can also occur in the absence of significant calcification by means of mechanical disruption of the collagen architecture (Fig. 2–39). Ishihara classified these cuspal lesions into four types. Type I lesions involve the free edges of the cusps and develop as a consequence of collagen breakdown at the free edges, usually near the commissures. Type II lesions consist of basal linear perforations parallel to the sewing ring and appear to be related to separation of collagen bundles. Type III lesions consist of centrally located,

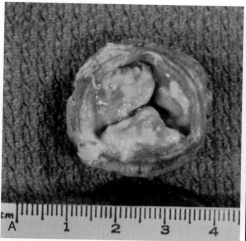
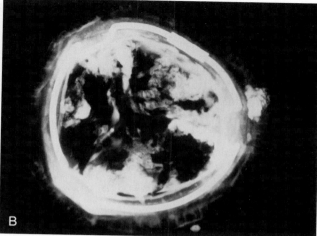

Figure 2·38 *A,* Porcine heterograft bioprosthesis with marked cuspal calcification resulting from primary valve failure. *B,* Radiograph of the valve shows extensive calcification of the cusps.

round to oval perforations that are associated with infection or severe degenerative changes with breakdown of collagen and calcification. Type IV lesions consist of multiple, pinhole-like perforations associated with calcific deposits.[74, 77]

Aortic Homografts

Aortic homograft or allograft valves are like heterograft valves in being hemodynamically efficient with minimal thromboembolic complications. They usually are cryopreserved in liquid nitrogen using dimethyl sulfoxide as a protective agent. As with porcine valves, they demonstrate late failure caused by progressive degeneration, including cusp rupture, perforation, or distortion and retraction, with vari-

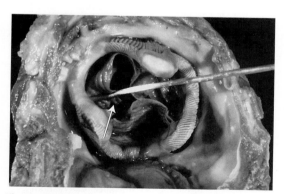

Figure 2·39 Porcine heterograft prosthesis with tears of all three cusps at the attachments. Notice the frayed edges of the tears *(arrow).* The valve had been in place in the mitral position for 17 years.

able calcification. The adjacent aortic wall shows variable calcification. These homografts are generally used in young patients with aortic valve disease or for those requiring pulmonic valve or pulmonary artery replacement for congenital heart disease. Stenosis can result from somatic growth of the recipient and lack of growth of the allograft.

Removed valves show relatively well-preserved connective tissue elements, with no surface endothelium, variably preserved and viable connective tissue cells in cusps and donor aorta, and mild, variable inflammatory cellularity. Immunologic rejection does not seem to play a role in the late failure of these grafts.[67]

Autograft Valves

Use of autograft valves has generally been confined to replacement of the aortic root with the autologous pulmonary valve and main pulmonary artery. In this procedure, the coronary arteries are implanted into the pulmonary artery, and the pulmonary valve and artery are replaced with cryopreserved pulmonary allograft. Advantages include excellent hemodynamic function without stenosis or progressive regurgitation, elimination of thromboembolic complications without anticoagulant therapy, and the potential for growth of these valves, making them particularly useful in young persons.[78]

Mechanical Valves

Contemporary mechanical valves (eg, St. Jude type) have good durability and structure, with minimal failure. A spectacular example of mechanical valve failure was seen in a group of Bjork-Shiley tilting-disk valves in which stress-induced strut fracture permitted disk escape, generally with a rapidly fatal result.[67, 70]

Approach to Pathologic Evaluation

The general approach to pathologic evaluation of prosthetic valves is similar to the evaluation of native valves, in that the gross examination of the valve provides the most useful information for diagnosis and clinical correlation.[67, 72, 79] The valve should be photographed at close range from inflow and outflow aspects and carefully examined for the presence of thrombi, vegetations, tissue overgrowth, structural defects, and wear. In autopsy specimens, complete evaluation of other cardiac structures is important, with attention to the presence of paravalvular leaks or annular (ring) abscesses. Removal of tissue for microbiologic culture is optimally performed in the operating room, although it may be done by the pathologist, and should be done at autopsy early in the cardiac examination. Some pathologists have advised that the prosthetic valve examined at autopsy must be completely removed from the intact heart to facilitate evaluation for possible ring abscess.

The specific type and model of the prosthesis can be identified using existing radiographic and morphologic keys; hidden under the sewing ring is the manufacturer's identification number.[67, 80–83] In addition to assistance in identification of the type of mechanical or bioprosthesis, radiography allows assessment of calcification of bioprosthetic valves. Semiquantitative radiographic grading of calcification correlates well with chemically determined mineral content.[84] The location of the calcification should be described (ie, free edge, commissures, cuspal base, or cuspal bodies).

Mechanical prostheses are assessed for intact function, including poppet excursion and disk mobility; structural integrity, including asymmetry, abnormal wear, strut abrasion or fracture, and poppet distortion or wear; and presence of even minute amounts of thrombus or vegetation. Attention is focused on the sewing ring and the attached tissue. Bioprosthetic valves are examined and palpated to assess cusp flexibility and mobility and to document calcification, ulceration, fenestrations, hematomas, and tears. Struts are evaluated for distortion. Histologic examination is directed toward the tissue-prosthesis junction, morphology of thrombi and vegetations, degenerative changes in cusps, and morphologic appearance and location of calcification. For calcified specimens, embedding in glycolmethacrylate allows optimal histologic examination of undecalcified specimens. Judicious use of special stains for organisms and calcium phosphate (ie, von Kossa's method) may be indicated.[67, 79]

Careful pathologic examination of valves removed at surgery and autopsy can provide information important for individual patient treatment and useful in further elucidating the causes of valvular heart disease. Application of newer technologies to understanding pathogenetic mechanisms may provide insights into common entities, such as floppy mitral valve syndrome, calcific aortic stenosis, and aortic root dilatation, and may assist in the development of improved valve prostheses.

ACKNOWLEDGMENT

Janet Miller provided excellent photographic assistance.

References

1. Waller B: Evaluation of operatively excised cardiac valves. *In* Waller B, ed. Contemporary Issues in Cardiovascular Pathology, vol 18. Philadelphia: FA Davis, 1988:203–247.
2. Rose A: Etiology of acquired valvular heart disease in adults: a survey of 18,132 autopsies and 100 consecutive valve-replacement operations. Arch Pathol Lab Med 1986;110:385–388.
3. Davies M: Pathology of Cardiac Valves. London: Butterworths, 1980.
4. Billingham M: Normal heart. *In* Sternberg S, ed. Histology for Pathologists. New York: Raven Press, 1992:215–231.
5. Silver M: Acquired disease of the valves and endocardium. *In* Bloom S, Lie J, Silver M, eds. Diagnostic Criteria for Cardiovascular Pathology: Acquired Diseases. Philadelphia: Lippincott-Raven, 1997:97–148.
6. Burke A: Tumors of the pericardium, myocardium, and blood vessels. *In* Bloom S, ed. Diagnostic Criteria for Cardiovascular Pathology: Acquired Diseases. Philadelphia: Lippincott-Raven, 1997:241–275.
7. Schoen FJ: The heart. *In* Cotran R, Kumar V, Robbins S, eds. Robbins Pathologic Basis of Disease, ed 5. Philadelphia: WB Saunders, 1994:543–557.
8. Becker A, Anderson R: Cardiac Pathology: An Integrated Text and Colour Atlas. New York: Raven Press, 1983.
9. Virmani R, Roberts W: Aschoff bodies in operatively excised atrial appendages and in papillary muscles: frequency and clinical significance. Circulation 1977;55:559–563.
10. Roberts W, Virmani R: Aschoff bodies at necropsy in valvular heart disease: evidence from an analysis of 543 patients over 14 years of age that rheumatic

heart disease, at least anatomically, is a disease of the mitral valve. Circulation 1978;57:803–807.

11. Tazelaar H: Surgical pathology of the heart, endomyocardial biopsy, valvular heart disease, and cardiac tumors. *In* Schoen F, Gimbrone M, eds. Cardiovascular Pathology: Clinicopathologic Correlations and Pathogenetic Mechanisms. Philadelphia: Williams & Wilkins, 1995:81–107.

12. Dare A, Harrity P, Tazelaar H, Edwards W, Mullany C: Evaluation of surgically excised mitral valves: revised recommendations based on changing operative procedures in the 1990's. Hum Pathol 1993;24:1286–1293.

13. Olson L, Subramanian R, Ackermann D, Orszulak T, Edwards W: Surgical pathology of the mitral valve: a study of 712 cases spanning 21 years. Mayo Clin Proc 1987;62:22–34.

14. Agozzino L, Falco A, de Vivo F, et al: Surgical pathology of the mitral valve: gross and histological study of 1288 surgically excised valves. Int J Cardiol 1992;37:79–89.

15. van der Bel-Kahn J, Becker A: The surgical pathology of rheumatic and floppy mitral valves: distinctive morphologic features upon gross examination. Am J Surg Pathol 1986;10:282–292.

16. Waller B, Howard J, Fess S: Pathology of mitral valve stenosis and pure mitral regurgitation—part I. Clin Cardiol 1994;17:330–336.

17. Waller B, Howard J, Fess S: Pathology of pulmonic valve stenosis and pure regurgitation. Clin Cardiol 1995;18:45–50.

18. Waller B, Howard J, Fess S: Pathology of tricuspid valve stenosis and pure tricuspid regurgitation—part I. Clin Cardiol 1995;18:97–102.

19. Lindroos M, Kupari M, Heikkila J: Prevalence of aortic valve abnormalities in the elderly: an echocardiographic study of a random population sample. J Am Coll Cardiol 1993;21:1220–1225.

20. Waller B, Howard J, Fess S: Pathology of aortic valve stenosis and pure aortic regurgitation: a clinical morphologic assessment—part I. Clin Cardiol 1994;17:85–92.

21. Stewart B, Siscovick D, Lind B, et al: Clinical factors associated with calcific aortic valve disease. J Am Coll Cardiol 1997;29:630–634.

22. Otto C, Kuusisto J, Reichenbach D, Gown A, O'Brien K: Characterization of the early lesion of "degenerative" valvular aortic stenosis: histological and immunohistochemical studies. Circulation 1994;90:844–853.

23. O'Brien K, Reichenbach D, Marcovina S, Kuusisto J, Alpers C, Otto C: Apolipoproteins B, (a), and E accumulate in the morphologically early lesions of "degenerative" valvular aortic stenosis. Arterioscler Thromb Vasc Biol 1996;16:523–532.

24. O'Brien K, Kuusisto J, Reichenbach D, et al: Osteopontin is expressed in human aortic valvular lesions. Circulation 1995;92:2163–2168.

25. Edwards J: Pathology of mitral incompetence. *In* Silver M, ed. Cardiovascular Pathology, ed 2. New York: Churchill Livingstone, 1991:961–984.

26. Osterberger L, Goldstein S, Khaja F, Lakier J: Functional mitral stenosis in patients with massive mitral annular calcification. Circulation 1981;64:472–476.

27. Roberts W, Waller B: Mitral valve "anular" calcium forming a compete circle or "O" configuration: clinical and necropsy observations. Am Heart J 1981;101:619–621.

28. Schoen F, St. John Sutton M: Contemporary patho-

logic considerations in valvular heart disease. *In* Virmani R, Atkinson J, Fenoglio J, eds. Cardiovascular Pathology. Philadelphia: WB Saunders, 1991:334–353.

29. Silver M: Blood flow obstruction related to the aortic valve. *In* Silver M, ed. Cardiovascular Pathology, ed 2. New York: Churchill Livingstone, 1991:985–1012.

30. Hurwitz L, Roberts W: Quadricuspid semilunar valve. Am J Cardiol 1973;31:623–626.

31. Moore G, Hutchins G, Brito J, Kang H: Congenital malformations of the semilunar valves. Hum Pathol 1980;11:367–372.

32. Zuberbuhler J, Allwork S, Anderson R: The spectrum of Ebstein's anomaly of the tricuspid valve. J Thorac Cardiovasc Surg 1979;77:202–211.

33. Altrichter P, Olson L, Edwards W, Puga F, Danielson G: Surgical pathology of the pulmonary valve: a study of 116 cases spanning 15 years. Mayo Clin Proc 1989;64:1352–1360.

34. Waller B: The operatively excised pulmonic valve—a forgotten entity. Mayo Clin Proc 1989;64:1452–1454.

35. Gikonyo B, Lucas R, Edwards J: Anatomic features of congenital pulmonary valvar stenosis. Pediatr Cardiol 1987;8:109–116.

36. Atkinson J, Virmani R: Infective endocarditis: changing trends and general approach for examination. *In* Virmani R, Atkinson J, Fenoglio J, eds. Cardiovascular Pathology. Philadelphia: WB Saunders, 1991:435–450.

37. Bansal R: Infective endocarditis. Med Clin North Am 1995;79:1205–1240.

38. Virmani R, Atkinson J, Forman M, Robinowitz M: Mitral valve prolapse. *In* Virmani R, Atkinson J, Fenoglio J, eds. Cardiovascular Pathology. Major Problems in Pathology, vol 23. Philadelphia: WB Saunders, 1991:419–434.

39. Waller B, Howard J, Fess S: Pathology of mitral valve stenosis and pure mitral regurgitation—part II. Clin Cardiol 1994;17:395–402.

40. Edwards J: Floppy mitral valve syndrome. *In* Waller B, ed. Contemporary Issues in Cardiovascular Pathology. Cardiovascular Clinics Series, vol 18. Philadelphia: FA Davis, 1988:249–271.

41. van Son J, Miles C, Starr A: Tricuspid valve prolapse associated with myxomatous degeneration. Ann Thorac Surg 1995;59:1237–1239.

42. Waller B, Howard J, Fess S: Pathology of tricuspid valve stenosis and pure tricuspid regurgitation—part II. Clin Cardiol 1995;18:167–174.

43. Genetic disorders. *In* Cotran R, Kumar V, Robbins S, eds. Robbins Pathologic Basis of Disease, ed 5. Philadelphia: WB Saunders, 1994:123–170.

44. Schoen F: Blood vessels. *In* Cotran R, Kumar V, Robbins S, eds. Robbins Pathologic Basis of Disease, ed 5. Philadelphia: WB Saunders, 1994:467–516.

45. Ferrans V: Metabolic and familial diseases. *In* Silver M, ed. Cardiovascular Pathology, ed 2. New York: Churchill Livingstone, 1991:1073–1149.

46. Olson L, Subramanian R, Edwards W: Surgical pathology of pure aortic insufficiency: a study of 225 cases. Mayo Clin Proc 1984;59:835–841.

47. Allen W, Matloff J, Fishbein M: Myxoid degeneration of the aortic valve and isolated severe aortic regurgitation. Am J Cardiol 1985;55:439–444.

48. Bulkley B: Systemic lupus erythematosus as a cause of severe mitral regurgitation: new problem in an old disease. Am J Cardiol 1975;35:305–308.

49. Bulkley B, Roberts W: The heart in systemic lupus erythematosus and the changes induced in it by corticosteroid therapy: a study of 36 necropsy patients. Am J Med 1975;58:243–263.

50. Galve E, Candell-Riera J, Pigrau C, Permanyer-Mira-lda G, Garcia-Del-Castillo H, Soler-Soler J: Prevalence, morphologic types, and evolution of cardiac valvular disease in systemic lupus erythematosus. N Engl J Med 1988;319:817–823.

51. Ducceschi V, Sarubbi B, Iacono I: Primary antiphospholipid syndrome and cardiovascular disease. Eur Heart J 1995;16:441–445.

52. Roberts W, Kehoe J, Carpenter D, Golden A: Cardiac valvular lesions in rheumatoid arthritis. Arch Intern Med 1968;22:141–146.

53. Materazzo C, Meazza R, Stefanelli M, Biasi S: Left valvular involvement in carcinoid: description of a case. G Ital Cardiol 1994;24:429–433.

54. Ferrans V, Roberts W: The carcinoid endocardial plaque: an ultrastructural study. Hum Pathol 1976;4:387–409.

55. McAllister H Jr: Endocrine diseases and the cardiovascular system. In Silver M, ed. Cardiovascular Pathology, ed 2. New York: Churchill Livingstone, 1991:1181–1203.

56. Hendrikx M, Van Dorpe J, Flameng W, Daenen W: Aortic and mitral valve disease induced by ergotamine therapy for migraine: a case report and review of the literature. J Heart Valve Dis 1996;5:235–237.

57. Hauck A, Edwards W, Danielson G, Mullany C, Bresnahan D: Mitral and aortic valve disease associated with ergotamine therapy for migraine: report of two cases and review of literature. Arch Pathol Lab Med 1990;114:62–64.

58. Connolly H, Crary J, McGoon M, et al: Valvular heart disease associated with fenfluramine-phentermine. N Engl J Med 1997;337:581–588.

59. Department of Health and Human Services: Cardiac valvulopathy associated with exposure to fenfluramine or dexfenfluramine: US Department of Health and Human Services Interim Public Health Recommendations. JAMA 1997;278:1729–1731.

60. Graham D, Green L: Further cases of valvular heart disease associated with fenfluramine-phentermine. N Engl J Med 1997;337:635.

61. Cannistra L, Davis S, Bauman A: Valvular heart disease associated with dexfenfluramine. N Engl J Med 1991;337:636.

62. McAllister H Jr: Collagen vascular diseases and the cardiovascular system. In Silver M, ed. Cardiovascular Pathology, ed 2. New York: Churchill Livingstone, 1991:1151–1179.

63. Goffin Y: Microscopic amyloid deposits in the heart valves: a common local complication of chronic damage and scarring. J Clin Pathol 1980;33:262–268.

64. Boudoulas H, Vavuranakis M, Wolley C: In response to valvular heart disease: the influence of changing etiology on nosology. J Heart Valve Dis 1994;3:692–693.

65. Waller B, Howard J, Fess S: Pathology of aortic valve stenosis and pure aortic regurgitation: a clinical morphologic assessment—part II. Clin Cardiol 1994;17:150–156.

66. Waller B, Howard J, Fess S: Pathology of tricuspid valve stenosis and pure tricuspid regurgitation—part III. Clin Cardiol 1995;18:225–230.

67. Schoen F: Pathologic considerations in replacement heart valves and other cardiovascular prosthetic devices. In Schoen F, Gimbrone M, eds. Cardiovascular Pathology: Clinicopathologic Correlations and Pathogenetic Mechanisms. Philadelphia: Williams & Wilkins, 1995:194–222.

68. Schoen F, Titus J, Lawrie G: Autopsy-determined causes of death after cardiac valve replacement. JAMA 1983;249:899–902.

69. Rose A: Autopsy-determined causes of death following heart valve replacement. Am J Cardiovasc Pathol 1987;1:39–46.

70. Zeien L, Klatt E: Cardiac valve prostheses at autopsy. Arch Pathol Lab Med 1990;114:933–937.

71. Hammermeister K, Sethi G, Henderson W, Oprian C, Kim T, Rahimtoola S: A comparison of outcomes in men 11 years after heart valve replacement with mechanical valve or bioprosthesis. N Engl J Med 1993;328:1289–1296.

72. Schoen F: Surgical pathology of removed natural and prosthetic heart valves. Hum Pathol 1987;18:558–567.

73. Schoen F, Hobson C: Anatomic analysis of removed prosthetic heart valves: causes of failure of 33 mechanical valves and 58 bioprostheses, 1980–1983. Hum Pathol 1985;16:549–559.

74. Ferrans V, Hilbert S, Fujita S, Jones M, Roberts W: Morphologic abnormalities in explanted bioprosthetic heart valves. In Virmani R, Atkinson J, Fenoglio J, eds. Cardiovascular Pathology. Philadelphia: WB Saunders, 1991:373–398.

75. Fishbein M, Gissen S, Collins J: Pathologic findings after cardiac valve replacement with glutaraldehyde-fixed porcine valves. Am J Cardiol 1977;40:331–337.

76. Bortolotti U, Milano A, Mossuto E, Mazzaro E, Thiene G, Casarotto D: Porcine valve durability: a comparison between Hancock standard and Hancock II bioprostheses. Ann Thorac Surg 1995;60(suppl 5):S216–S220.

77. Ishihara T, Ferrans V, Boyce S, Jones M, Roberts W: Structure and classification of cuspal tears and perforations in porcine bioprosthetic cardiac valves implanted in patients. Am J Cardiol 1981;48:665–677.

78. Kouchoukos N, Davila-Roman V, Spray T, Murphy S, Perrillo J: Replacement of the aortic root with a pulmonary autograft in children and young adults with aortic-valve disease. N Engl J Med 1994;330:1–6.

79. Schoen F: Evaluation of surgically removed natural and prosthetic heart valves. In Virmani R, Atkinson J, Fenoglio J, eds. Cardiovascular Pathology. Philadelphia: WB Saunders, 1991:399–418.

80. Mehlman D: A guide to the radiographic identification of prosthetic heart valves: an addendum. Circulation 1984;69:102–105.

81. Schoen F: Pathology of bioprostheses and other tissue heart valve replacements. In Silver M, ed. Cardiovascular Pathology, ed 2. New York: Churchill Livingstone, 1991:1547–1605.

82. Silver M, Wilson G: Pathology of mechanical heart valve prostheses and vascular grafts made of artificial materials. In Silver M, ed. Cardiovascular Pathology, ed 2. New York: Churchill Livingstone, 1991:1487–1545.

83. Mehlman D: A pictorial and radiographic guide for identification of prosthetic heart valve devices. Prog Cardiovasc Dis 1988;30:441–464.

84. Schoen F, Kujovich J, Webb C, Levy R: Chemically determined mineral content of explanted porcine aortic valve bioprostheses: correlation with radiographic assessment of calcification and clinical data. Circulation 1987;76:1061–1066.

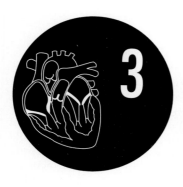

3 Echocardiographic Evaluation of Valvular Heart Disease

Echocardiography provides detailed, noninvasive information about valve anatomy, the cause of valve disease, the severity of valve stenosis or regurgitation, the impact of the valvular lesion on left ventricular (LV) size and function, and any associated cardiac abnormalities. Echocardiographic evaluation is the standard diagnostic approach to the patient with suspected or known valvular heart disease. This chapter provides an overview of the echocardiographic evaluation of the patient with valvular heart disease; more detailed discussions are available in standard echocardiography texts.[1–4]

ANATOMIC IMAGING

The first step in evaluation of the patient with valvular heart disease is assessment of valvular anatomy with two-dimensional (2D) imaging (Table 3–1). Although in many cases the specific valve involved is known from previous evaluation or based on clinical history and physical examination, in other cases, the exact diagnosis may be unknown or may have been incorrectly inferred from clinical data. A careful examination of all four valves and screening for other lesions that could be mistaken for valvular disease are important aspects of the examination. For example, in a patient with a systolic murmur referred for suspected valvular aortic stenosis, other diagnostic possibilities that could account for the systolic murmur include a subaortic membrane, mitral regurgitation, ventricular septal defect, or hypertrophic obstructive cardiomyopathy. An appropriate examination includes exclusion or

TABLE 3·1 CLINICAL ECHOCARDIOGRAPHIC EVALUATION OF THE PATIENT WITH VALVULAR HEART DISEASE

Two-Dimensional Imaging

Valve anatomy and cause of disease
Two-dimensional echocardiographic valve area (in mitral
    stenosis)
Qualitative evaluation of global and regional left
    ventricular (LV) function
Quantitative LV dimensions, volumes, ejection fraction
    and mass
Associated chamber enlargement (eg, left atrium)
Right heart structure and function
Complications of valve disease (ie, left atrial thrombus)

Doppler Evaluation of Severity of Valve Disease

Valve stenosis
    Velocity data
    Maximum and mean pressure gradients
    Valve area (continuity equation and/or pressure
        half-time)
    Other measures of stenosis severity, if needed
Valve regurgitation
    Color flow mapping
    Calculation of regurgitant fraction in selected cases
    Flow reversals
    Continuous wave velocity curve
    Other approaches in selected cases

Other Doppler Echocardiographic Data

LV diastolic function
Pulmonary pressures

---

confirmation of each differential diagnosis
and evaluation of the aortic valve.

Echocardiographic Valve Anatomy and Cause of Disease

Two-dimensional imaging allows identification of the involved valve and often allows
precise definition of the cause of the valvular
lesion on the basis of the typical anatomic
features of each disease process. Mitral stenosis
most often is caused by rheumatic valvular disease with pathognomonic features of commissural fusion, thickening of the leaflet tips, and
chordal thickening, fusion, and shortening
(Fig. 3–1), all of which are easily recognized
on 2D imaging.[5–7] In contrast, the occasional
elderly patient with functional mitral stenosis
caused by extension of mitral annular calcification onto the valve leaflets has thin, mobile
leaflet tips, with calcification and thickening
at the leaflet bases. The specific anatomic features of the rheumatic mitral valve apparatus,
as seen on 2D imaging, are important factors
in predicting prognosis and in clinical decision
making, particularly with regard to mitral commissurotomy (see Chapter 11).

Whereas aortic valve stenosis of any cause is
characterized by thickened, stiff leaflets with
reduced systolic opening, calcific aortic stenosis (most commonly seen) is typified by increased echogenicity and thickness of the
leaflet bodies without evidence of commissural
fusion, resulting in a stellate orifice in systole
(Fig. 3–2).[8, 9] It may be difficult to separate
calcific changes superimposed on a bicuspid
aortic valve from calcification of a trileaflet
valve by 2D imaging alone. However, the different age distribution of symptom onset in patients with stenosis due to a bicuspid (50 to 60
years) compared with that for a trileaflet valve
(70 to 90 years) allows a reasonable guess
about the cause of disease.[10] Rheumatic aortic
valve disease is characterized by commissural
fusion with increased thickening and echogenicity along the leaflet closure lines and invariably is associated with rheumatic mitral valve
disease.[11] Congenital aortic stenosis, seen in
young adults, is characterized by a deformed
(often unicuspid) valve that "domes" in systole with a restrictive orifice.

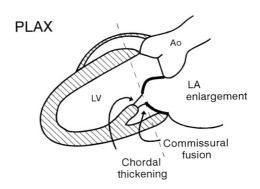

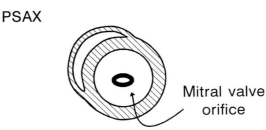

Figure 3·1 Schematic diagram of the two-dimensional
echo findings in mitral stenosis. The parasternal long-axis
view (PLAX) shows commissural fusion with diastolic doming of the mitral leaflets, chordal thickening, and fusion. In
a parasternal short-axis view (PSAX) at the mitral valve
orifice, the area of opening can be planimetered. The
plane of the short-axis view is indicated by a *dashed line*
on the long-axis image. Ao, aorta; LA, left atrium; LV, left
ventricle. (From Otto CM, Pearlman AS: The Textbook of
Clinical Echocardiography. Philadelphia: WB Saunders,
1995:228.)

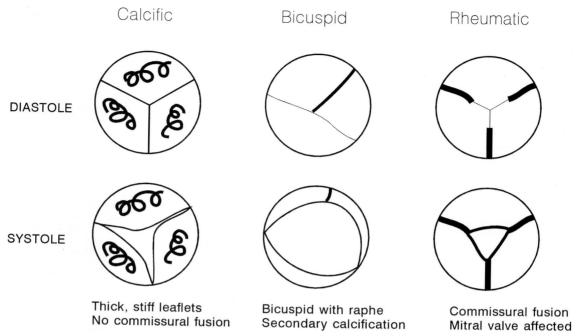

Figure 3·2 Schematic diagram of the three most common causes of valvular aortic stenosis. Calcific aortic stenosis is characterized by fibrocalcific masses on the aortic side of the leaflet that result in increased leaflet stiffness without commissural fusion. A congenital bicuspid valve undergoes secondary degenerative changes. The diagnostic features of rheumatic stenosis are commissural fusion and mitral valve involvement. (From Otto CM, Pearlman AS: The Textbook of Clinical Echocardiography. Philadelphia: WB Saunders, 1995:213.)

Evaluation of the cause of a regurgitant lesion by echocardiography is challenging because of the wide range of abnormalities that can lead to valvular incompetence. Mitral regurgitation may be caused by abnormalities of the mitral annulus, leaflets, subvalvular apparatus, or papillary muscle, or it may result from regional or global LV dysfunction (Figs. 3–3 and 3–4). Echocardiographic imaging allows assessment of each of these components of the valve apparatus, and the cause of the regurgitant lesion can be discerned in many cases (see Chapter 13). This evaluation is critical is selecting patients for mitral valve repair procedures (see Chapter 15). However, multiple abnormalities of the valve apparatus may make determination of the mechanism of regurgitation difficult. For example, in a patient with a dilated, hypokinetic left ventricle and irregular thickening of the valve leaflets, it may be unclear whether mitral regurgitation is caused by the abnormal leaflets, annular dilation, malalignment or dysfunction of the papillary muscles, or a combination of these factors. In the future, three-dimensional (3D) reconstruction of echocardiographic images in combination with computer modeling of nor-

mal valve anatomy and function may provide more precise definition of the mechanism of regurgitation.[12, 13]

Aortic regurgitation may result from abnormalities of the valve leaflets (eg, bicuspid valve, endocarditis), inadequate support of the valve structures (eg, subaortic ventricular septal defect), or from aortic root dilation (eg, Marfan's syndrome, annuloaortic ectasia) (Fig. 3–5).[14, 15] Echocardiographic imaging provides accurate measurements of aortic root dimensions and allows detailed evaluation of valve anatomy and dynamics. A bicuspid valve is diagnosed on the basis of the typical appearance in *systole* of two open leaflets; the closed valve in diastole may mimic a trileaflet valve if there is a raphe in one leaflet. Other recognized abnormalities of the valve leaflets that correspond to a specific cause include valvular vegetations in endocarditis, redundant leaflets in myxomatous disease, and commissural thickening and mitral valve involvement in rheumatic disease, all of which can be recognized on 2D imaging.

With aortic root disease, the specific pattern of root dilation and associated features may indicate a specific cause, such as the "water

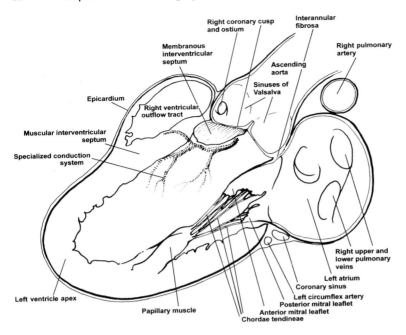

Figure 3·3 Anatomic drawing in a long-axis orientation illustrates the close relationship between the aortic root and anterior mitral valve leaflet. The mitral valve apparatus includes the left atrial wall, the annulus, the anterior and posterior mitral leaflets, the mitral chordae, and the papillary muscles. (Drawing by Starr Kaplan.)

balloon" appearance of the root in Marfan's syndrome, with a loss of the normal tapering at the sinotubular junction and associated mitral valve abnormalities.[16, 17] In other cases, the

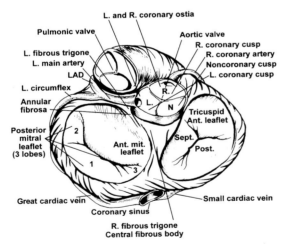

Figure 3·4 Anatomic view of the cardiac valves from the perspective of the base of the heart with the left and right atrium "cut away" and the great vessels transected. Notice the close anatomic relationships of all four cardiac valves. In particular, the aortic valve is adjacent to the mitral valve along the middle segment of the anterior mitral valve leaflet. The pulmonic valve is slightly superior to the aortic valve, and the aortic and pulmonic valve planes are nearly perpendicular to each other. Ant., anterior; LAD, left anterior descending artery; L., left; mit., mitral; Post., posterior; R., right; Sept., septum. (Drawing by Starr Kaplan.)

pattern of root dilation is nonspecific, and other clinical information is needed to determine the cause of disease. For example, aortic root dilation in a patient with a systemic immune-mediated process (eg, rheumatoid arthritis) probably results from this systemic disease.[18] In contrast, dilation of the ascending aorta in a patient with aortic valve stenosis can be attributed to "post-stenotic" dilation, which is thought to be caused by the effect of blood flow turbulence on restructuring of the vascular wall.[19]

Right-sided valve abnormalities in adults usually are caused by residual congenital heart disease (eg, congenital pulmonic stenosis, Ebstein's anomaly of the tricuspid valve) or result from left-sided heart disease (eg, tricuspid annular dilation due to pulmonary hypertension in a patient with mitral stenosis). Two-dimensional imaging usually allows determination of the valve anatomy and cause of the valvular lesion, particularly when other aspects of the examination and clinical features are incorporated in the echocardiographic interpretation.

Transthoracic Versus Transesophageal Imaging

Transthoracic imaging provides diagnostic images for most patients with valvular heart disease and is the standard approach for initial

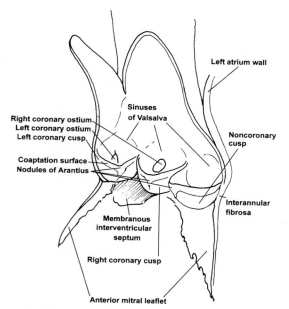

Figure 3·5 Detailed view of the aortic valve with the aorta opened to show the valve leaflets and the anterior mitral leaflet bisected. The aortic valve consists of three leaflets and associated sinuses of Valsalva, with each leaflet-sinus pair forming a cup-shaped unit when the valve is closed. The load-bearing section of the leaflet appears linear when viewed in the long axis (see Fig. 3·3) but curved in cross section, consistent with a hemicylindrical shape. The coaptation surfaces of the leaflets thicken toward the center of each leaflet; areas of prominent thickening are called the nodes of Arantius. Lambl's excrescences, filamentous attachments on the ventricular side of the nodules of Arantius, are common in older subjects. (Drawing by Starr Kaplan.)

evaluation and for follow-up studies. Transesophageal imaging is used when transthoracic images are nondiagnostic or when higher-resolution images are needed for clinical decision making. With trained and experienced sonographers, diagnostic images can be obtained by transthoracic imaging for most patients; exceptions include patients with poor ultrasound access because of body habitus, hyperexpanded lungs, or poor postoperative status. For these patients, transesophageal imaging may be necessary. The improved image quality, particularly of posterior structures such as the mitral valve, may provide critical anatomic information in specific clinical situations, such as determining the likelihood of mitral valve repair in a patient with myxomatous mitral valve disease or excluding left atrial thrombus in a candidate for mitral balloon commissurotomy.

Other indications for transesophageal echocardiography in patients with valvular disease include assessment of regurgitant severity when transthoracic images are nondiagnostic or when a prosthetic mitral valve is present, intraoperative monitoring of valve repair procedures, and determining the exact level of obstruction in a patient with a differential diagnosis of valvular or subvalvular obstruction. Rarely, transesophageal imaging is needed to evaluate the severity of stenosis when the transthoracic data are not diagnostic.

EVALUATION OF LEFT VENTRICULAR SYSTOLIC FUNCTION

Evaluation of the LV response to pressure or volume overload is a critical step in echocardiographic examination of the patient with left-sided valvular heart disease. The degree of LV dilation and evidence of impaired contractility is particularly important in patients with chronic valvular regurgitation (see Chapters 12 and 15).

Left Ventricular Volumes and Ejection Fraction

Two-dimensional echocardiography allows qualitative and quantitative evaluation of LV size and systolic function.[20, 21] Tomographic images are acquired in several image planes, and mental integration of the data provides an overall view of ventricular size, shape, and function. As 3D imaging protocols become more widely available, the integration of tomographic images may be performed by computer with 3D display of the resultant images.[22] Because mental reconstruction can only be "seen" by the echocardiographer, computer display of the 3D images will facilitate communication with referring physicians and surgeons.

Images of the left ventricle are acquired from the parasternal window in a long-axis view and in sequential short-axis views at the basal, midventricular, and when possible, apical levels. From an apical approach, images are acquired in four-chamber, two-chamber, and long-axis views. Additional subcostal views in four-chamber and short-axis orientations can be used to supplement the parasternal and apical windows, particularly if image quality is suboptimal.

Qualitative Evaluation

Qualitative evaluation of the left ventricle includes descriptors of LV hypertrophy, chamber dilation, shape, overall systolic function, and regional wall motion abnormalities. Visual estimates of the degree of LV hypertrophy or dilation can be made by comparing wall thickness with chamber dimensions and by comparing LV size with other normal cardiac structures, such as the aortic root. However, qualitative assessment of LV size is limited. The structures used for comparison may be abnormal, and considerable observer variability is likely. Although qualitative evaluation of LV size and hypertrophy by an experienced echocardiographer may be reliable, quantitative measures of LV size and hypertrophy are preferable.

In contrast, qualitative evaluation of global and regional systolic function by an experienced observer has great clinical utility. Classification of overall LV systolic function as normal or as mildly, moderately, or severely reduced is of prognostic value for patients with valvular heart disease, such as those with symptomatic aortic stenosis.[23] Evaluation of overall

systolic function by an experienced observer correlates well with quantitative measures of systolic function. Individual echocardiographers should "calibrate" themselves and improve the accuracy of qualitative assessment by ongoing comparison with other measures of LV function.

Regional wall motion is assessed as normal, hypokinetic, akinetic, or dyskinetic for each region of the left ventricle using one of several segmental schemes.[24] In the most widely used scheme, the ventricle is divided into thirds from base to apex (ie, basal, middle, apex) with evaluation (clockwise in a short-axis view) of anterior septum, anterior wall, lateral wall, posterior wall, inferior wall, and inferior septum at the basal and midventricular levels, with three segments (ie, anterior, posterolateral, and inferior) at the apical level (Fig. 3–6).[25] Although regional wall motion abnormalities are not considered features of valvular heart disease, their presence may alert the

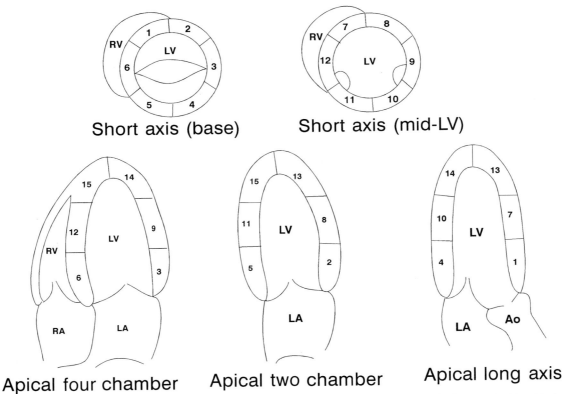

Figure 3·6 Echocardiographic views for wall motion evaluation. In the short-axis view at the base and midventricular levels, the left ventricle (LV) is divided into the anterior septum (1, 7) and free wall (2, 8); lateral (3, 9), posterior (4, 10), and inferior free wall (5, 11); and inferior septal (6, 12) segments. These same wall segments are seen in the apical views along with the anterior (13), inferior (15), and posterolateral (14) apical segments. Ao, aorta; LA, left atrium; RA, right atrium; RV, right ventricle. (From Otto CM, Pearlman AS: The Textbook of Clinical Echocardiography. Philadelphia: WB Saunders, 1995:140.)

clinician to the probability of coexisting coronary artery disease. Because wall motion may be normal at rest even when significant coronary disease is present, stress echocardiography or coronary angiography may be indicated if coronary disease is suspected clinically.[26–32]

Quantitative Measures

The simplest quantitative measures of LV size and wall thickness are 2D-guided M-mode recordings at the midventricular level (Table 3–2). Typical measurements include LV end-diastolic (EDD) and end-systolic dimensions (ESD), septal and posterior wall thickness at end-diastole, and calculation of the percentage of fractional shortening (FS):

$$\%FS = [(EDD - ESD)/EDD] \times 100\%$$

Using long- and short-axis views from a parasternal window, the 2D image is used to ensure that the M-mode beam is centered in the LV chamber and is perpendicular to the long-axis of the left ventricle. The advantages of M-mode measurements are that they are based on the axial resolution of the ultrasound system (rather than the less accurate lateral resolution) and that they are reasonably reproducible when performed by experienced laboratories using careful recording and measurement techniques. The value of changes seen on serial studies is higher if side-by-side comparisons of the data are made to ensure consistency in recording and measurement techniques between the two examinations.

The disadvantages of M-mode data are that an oblique orientation of the M-mode beam or incorrect identification of endocardial borders leads to measurement errors. End-diastolic dimensions change with changes in preload caused by volume status or medications. Although end-systolic dimensions depend less on preload, they may be affected by afterload. However, the major disadvantage of M-mode data is that a single linear measurement assumes a symmetric pattern of LV dilation, hypertrophy, and systolic function. Although this assumption may be valid in patients with isolated valvular disease, concurrent coronary disease results in asymmetric LV abnormalities in others. Even in the absence of coronary disease, LV shape changes associated with valvular disease (eg, increased sphericity of the left ventricle with chronic aortic regurgitation) make M-mode data less useful.

Quantitative 2D measurements of LV size and function include LV end-diastolic (EDV) and end-systolic volumes (ESV) with calculation of ejection fraction (EF):

$$EF = (EDV - ESV)/EDV$$

Several methods for the calculation of LV volumes from tomographic 2D images have been described,[33–36] some of which are shown in Figure 3–7. The consensus of the American Society of Echocardiography is that the preferred method is the apical biplane approach[21]:

$$V = (\pi/4) \sum_{I=1}^{20} a_i b_i \times (L/20)$$

In this equation, a and b represent the minor axis dimensions in two image planes at each of 20 intervals perpendicular to the long axis of the ventricle, from apex to the base, with a length, L. For the apical biplane method, images of the left ventricle are acquired in apical four-chamber and two-chamber views for tracing of endocardial borders at end-diastole and end-systole.

Accurate LV volume measurements on 2D imaging depend on correct image plane orientation and inclusion of the true long axis of the ventricle in the image (Table 3–3). Use of a cutout in the bed to allow positioning the transducer on the apex with the patient in a steep left lateral decubitus position helps avoid inadvertent foreshortening of the apex. Accuracy also depends on accurate identification of endocardial borders. Manual tracing of borders by an experienced observer remains the most accurate method for calculation of volumes from 2D images. Approaches to automated border detection remain experimental and require further validation. During image acquisition, care is taken to optimize endocardial definition based on patient positioning, transducer frequency and focusing, subtle adjustments in transducer position and orientation, preprocessing and postprocessing curves, gray scale, and gain settings. The addition of harmonic imaging to the ultrasound system markedly improves endocardial definition in many patients.

The quality of image acquisition is improved if the LV borders are traced by the sonographer performing the examination. Systems that allow evaluation of the motion of the endocardium during the tracing process (ie, using a cine-loop feature) facilitate correct border identification. The views most suited to quantitative measurement (ie, apical views)

TABLE 3·2   SELECTED NORMAL ECHOCARDIOGRAPHIC DIMENSIONS IN ADULTS

Site	Range	Range Indexed to BSA	Upper Limit of Normal
Aorta			
Annulus diameter (cm)	1.4–2.6	$1.3 + 0.1$ cm/m^2	<1.6 cm/m^2
Diameter at leaflet tips (cm)	2.2–3.6	$1.7 + 0.2$ cm/m^2	<2.1 cm/m^2
Ascending aorta diameter (cm)	2.1–3.4	$1.5 + 0.2$ cm/m^2	
Arch diameter (cm)	2.0–3.6		
Left ventricle			
Short-axis dimension (cm)			
Diastole	3.5–6.0	2.3–3.1 cm/m^2	
Systole	2.1–4.0	1.4–2.1 cm/m^2	
Long-axis dimension (cm)			
Diastole	6.3–10.3	4.1–5.7 cm/m^2	
Systole	4.6–8.4		
End-diastolic volume (mL)			
Men	96–157	67 ± 9 mL/m^2	
Women	59–138	61 ± 13 mL/m^2	
End-systolic volume (mL)			
Men	33–68	27 ± 5 mL/m^2	
Women	18–65	26 ± 7 mL/m^2	
Ejection fraction			
Men	0.59 ± 0.06		
Women	0.58 ± 0.07		
LV wall thickness (cm) (end-diastole)	0.6–1.1		
Men			<1.2 cm
Women			<1.1 cm
LV mass (g)			
Men	<294 g	109 ± 20 g/m^2	<150 g/m^2
Women	<198 g	89 ± 15 g/m^2	<120 g/m^2
Left atrium			
Anterior-posterior dimension (cm) (PLAX)	2.3–4.5	1.6–2.4 cm/m^2	
Medial-lateral dimension (cm) (A4C)	2.5–4.5	1.6–2.4 cm/m^2	
Superior-inferior dimension (cm) (A4C)	3.4–6.1	2.3–3.5 cm/m^2	
Mitral annulus			
End-diastole (cm)	2.7–0.4		
End-systole (cm)	2.9–0.3		
Right ventricle			
Wall thickness (cm)	0.2–0.5	0.2 ± 0.05 cm/m^2	
Minor dimension (cm)	2.2–4.4	1.0–2.8 cm/m^2	
Length, diastole (cm)	5.5–9.5	3.8–5.3 cm/m^2	
Length, systole (cm)	4.2–8.1		
Pulmonary artery			
Annulus diameter (cm)	1.0–2.2		
Main PA (cm)	0.9–2.9		
Inferior vena cava diameters (at RA junction) (cm)	1.2–2.3		

A4C, apical four-chamber view; BSA, body surface area; LV, left ventricular; PA, pulmonary artery; PLAX, parasternal long-axis view; RA, right atrium.

Data from Erbel: Dtsch Med Wochenschr 1982;107:107; Levy et al: AJC 1987;59:956; Hahn et al: Z Kardiol 1982;71:445; Pearlman et al: J Am Coll Cardiol 1988;12:1432; Pini et al: Circulation 1989;80:915; Roman et al: Am J Cardiol 1989;64:507; Schnittger et al: J Am Coll Cardiol 1983;2:934; Truiulzi et al: Echocardiography 1984;1:403.

From Otto CM, Pearlman AS: The Textbook of Clinical Echocardiography. Philadelphia: WB Saunders, 1995.

Biplane apical

 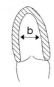 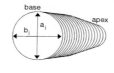

Single-plane ellipsoid

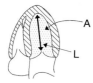 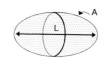

Hemisphere-cylinder

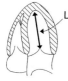 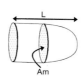

Figure 3·7 Examples of three formulas for left ventricular volume calculations show the two-dimensional echocardiographic views and measurements on the left and the geometric model on the right. For the biplane apical method, endocardial borders are traced in apical four-chamber and two-chamber views, which are used to define a series of orthogonal diameters (a and b). A Simpson's rule assumption based on stacked disks is used to calculate the volume. The single-plane ellipsoid method uses the two-dimensional area (A) and length (L) in a single (usually apical four-chamber) view. The hemisphere-cylinder method uses a short-axis endocardial area at the midventricular level (Am) and a long-axis length (L). For each method, end-diastolic and end-systolic measurements are needed for calculation of end-diastolic and end-systolic volumes, respectively, and for ejection fraction determinations. (From Otto CM, Pearlman AS: The Textbook of Clinical Echocardiography. Philadelphia: WB Saunders, 1995:91.)

use the lateral (rather than axial) resolution of the ultrasound system, limiting the overall precision with which the endocardial border can be identified.

In an experienced laboratory, the accuracy and reproducibility of 2D echocardiographic LV volumes and ejection fractions is high, with 95% confidence intervals for LV end-diastolic volume of $\pm 15\%$, for end-systolic volume of $\pm 25\%$, and for ejection fraction of $\pm 10\%$.[37] These values are similar to reported variability for ventricular volumes or ejection fractions determined by contrast or radionuclide ventriculography.[38] Because many of the factors leading to measurement variability are con-

stant in an individual patient, when serial studies are evaluated, a change in end-systolic volume of more than 5% and a change in the ejection fraction of more than 2% is clinically significant.[37]

LV mass can be determined by 2D echocardiography using a mean end-diastolic wall thickness, calculated from traced endocardial and epicardial borders in a parasternal short-axis view at the midventricular level.[39, 40] The mean wall thickness allows calculation of the volume of myocardium as the difference between the epicardial (V_{epi}) and endocardial (V_{endo}) volume, which then is multiplied by the mass density of myocardium to yield LV mass:

$$LV \text{ mass} = 1.05 \, (V_{epi} - V_{endo})$$

Three-Dimensional Echocardiography

Substantial research data suggest that quantitative 3D echocardiographic measurements of LV volume, ejection fraction, and mass are more accurate and more reproducible than 2D measurements (Table 3–4).[22, 38, 41, 42] Potential advantages of 3D measurements are the absence of geometric assumptions, little dependence on image orientation, and the use of axial resolution for endocardial definition. Disadvantages include the need for manual tracing of endocardial borders in multiple views, respiratory and electrocardiographic gating during image acquisition, an accurate system for locating the position and orientation of each 2D image in 3D space, and the consequent time required for analysis. As these technical problems are resolved and 3D capability becomes more widely available, it is likely that 3D quantitative assessment of LV volume, ejection fraction, and mass will become the clinical standard.

Left Ventricular Wall Stress

LV wall stress can be calculated from 2D echocardiographic data in combination with measurement of ventricular systolic pressure. Wall stress calculations provide a relatively load-independent measure of LV systolic function. Meridional wall stress (σ_m) is calculated as the ratio of ventricular cavity area (Ac) to total myocardial area (Am) in a short-axis view at the midventricular level, multiplied by LV pressure (P):[43–45]

$$\sigma_m = 1.33P \, (Ac/Am) \times 10^3 \text{ dyne/cm}^2$$

TABLE 3·3   SELECTED STUDIES VALIDATING TWO-DIMENSIONAL ECHOCARDIOGRAPHIC LEFT VENTRICULAR VOLUME MEASUREMENTS

Study/Year	Volume/Method	n	r	Regression Equation	SEE	Standard of Reference
Teicholz/74	Ejection fraction $V = [7.0/(2.4 + D)] \times D^3$	25	0.87	Echo = 0.61 angio + 0.01 mL		Biplane LV-angio
Schiller/79	Modified Simpson's rule	30				Biplane angio
	Diastolic volume		0.80	Echo = 0.7 angio − 1 mL	15 mL	
	Systolic volume		0.90	Echo = 0.7 angio − 2 mL	8.5 mL	
	Ejection fraction		0.87	Echo = angio + 5	7.6%	
Folland/79	Modified Simpson's rule	35				
	Ejection fraction		0.78	Angio = 1.01 echo + 0.04	9.7%	Single-plane angio
	Ejection fraction		0.75	Radionuclide = 0.75 echo + 0.07	8.7%	Radionuclide Single-plane angio
Parisi/79	Modified Simpson's rule	50				
	Diastolic volume		0.82	Angio = 1.08 echo + 30 mL	39 mL	
	Systolic volume		0.90		29 mL	
	Ejection fraction		0.80		9%	
Gueret/80	Modified Simpson's rule	11				Cineangiography in closed-chest dogs
	Diastolic volume		0.89	Cine = 0.88 echo + 22 mL	10 mL	
	Systolic volume		0.86	Cine = 0.95 echo + 11 mL	9 mL	1 h S/P LAD occlusion
	Ejection fraction		0.92	Cine = 1.13 echo − 7.5%	5%	
Silverman/80	Biplane area-length	20				Biplane angio
	Diastolic volume		0.96	Echo = 1.05 angio − 3.64		
	Systolic volume		0.91	Echo = 1.37 angio − 1.37		
	Ejection fraction		0.82	Echo = 9.87 angio + 0		
Wyatt/80	Modified Simpson's rule	21	0.98	Echo = 1.0x − 0.7 mL	6.6 mL	Directly measured fluid volume in fixed hearts
	⅔ area-length		0.97	Echo = 1.0x − 8.9 mL	8.6 mL	
	Area-length (cylinder)		0.97	Echo = 1.49x − 13.4 mL	12.8 mL	
	Hemiellipsoid (bullet)		0.97	Echo = 1.25x − 11.1 mL	10.9 mL	
Starling/81	Simpson's rule	70				Single or biplane (n = 30) LV angio
	Diastolic volume		0.80	Echo = 0.66 angio + 42 mL	34 mL	
	Systolic volume		0.88	Echo = 0.72 angio + 18 mL	27 mL	
	Ejection fraction		0.90	Echo = 0.76 angio + 12%	7%	
Quinones/81	Simplified method	55				Radionuclide
	Ejection fraction		0.93		6.7%	Angio
			0.91		7.4%	Single-plane angio
Tortoledo/83	Simplified method	52				
	Diastolic volume		0.88	Angio = 1.07 echo − 7.3 mL	28 mL	
	Systolic volume		0.94	Angio = 1.0 echo + 1.3 mL	19 mL	
	Ejection fraction		0.92	Angio = 0.93 echo + 3.5 mL	7%	
Weiss/83	Modified Simpson's rule (15–19 "slices")	52	0.97		6.6% (mean % error)	Direct volume measurement in isolated ejecting dog hearts
Erbel/85	Simpson's rule	46				Single-plane LV-angio
	Diastolic volume		0.91	Echo = 0.66 angio + 0.8 mL	26 mL	
	Systolic volume		0.94	Echo = 0.57 angio + 18 mL	19 mL	
	Ejection fraction		0.80	Echo = 0.61 angio + 13%	9%	
Zoghbi/90	Echo-tilt method	24				Biplane angio
	Diastolic volume		0.92	Angio = 0.80 echo + 37 mL	23 mL	
	Systolic volume		0.96	Angio = 0.97 echo − 1 mL	16 mL	
	Ejection fraction		0.82	Angio = 1.17 echo − 4	10%	
Smith/92	TEE Simpson's rule	36				LV angio (single plane)
	Diastolic volume		0.85	Echo = 0.75 angio + 0.2 mL	42 mL	
	Systolic volume		0.94	Echo = 0.78 angio − 3.5 mL	22 mL	
	Ejection fraction		0.85	Echo = 0.82 angio + 9.0 mL	8%	
Zile/92	Prolate ellipsoid using constant long-axis/short-axis ratio	25				LV angio in dog model
	Diastolic volume		0.96	Echo = 1.0 angio − 1.8 mL		
	Systolic volume		0.95	Echo = 0.98 angio − 0.65 mL		

Angio, angiography; cine, cineangiography; echo, echocardiography; LV, left ventricular; SEE, standard error of the estimate; TEE, transesophageal echocardiography.

Data from Teicholz LE et al: N Engl J Med 1974;291:1220; Schiller NB et al: Circulation 1979;60:547; Folland AD et al: Circulation 1979;60:760; Parisi AF et al: Clin Cardiol 1979;2:257; Gueret P et al: Circulation 1980;62:1308; Silverman NH et al: Circulation 1980;62:548; Wyatt HL et al: Circulation 1980;61:1119; Kan G et al: Eur Heart J 1981;2:337; Starling MR et al: Circulation 1981;63:1075; Quinones MA et al: Circulation 1981;64:7444; Tortoledo FA et al: Circulation 1983;67:579; Weiss JL et al: Circulation 1983;67:889; Erbel R et al: Circulation 1983;67:205; Zoghbi WA et al: J Am Coll Cardiol 1990;15:610; Smith MD et al: J Am Coll Cardiol 1992;19:1213; Zile MR et al: J Am Coll Cardiol 1992;20:986.

From Otto CM, Pearlman AS: The Textbook of Clinical Echocardiography. Philadelphia: WB Saunders, 1995.

TABLE 3·4	SELECTED STUDIES VALIDATING THREE-DIMENSIONAL ECHOCARDIOGRAPHIC LEFT VENTRICULAR VOLUME MEASUREMENTS						
Study/Year	**Method**	*n*	*r*	**Regression Equation**	**SEE**	**Standard of Reference**
Nessly/91	Dog model, 3D reconstruction	33	0.86	Echo = 0.83 RN + 4 mL	6 mL	RN
Kuroda/91	Balloons in water bath					True volume by weight
	Pull-back reconstruction		0.99	Echo = 1.1x − 10 mL	5.8 mL	
	Rotational reconstruction		0.99	Echo = 1.0x − 7 mL	6.5 mL	
Handschumacher/93	Ventricular phantoms and gel-filled		0.99	Echo = 0.96x + 2.2 mL	2.7 mL	Direct volumes
	excised ventricles		0.99	Echo = 0.99x + 0.11 mL	5.9 mL	
Gopal/93	Normal adults, 6–8 nonparallel nonintersecting short-axis planes	15				MRI
	End-diastolic volume		0.92	Echo = 0.84 MRI + 22 mL	7 mL	
Sui/93	End-systolic volume		0.81	Echo = 0.51 MRI + 18 mL	4 mL	
	Canine model, spark-gap 3D location	84	0.98	Echo = 1.0x − 0.8 mL	3.6 mL	Direct volumes
		19	0.94	Echo = 0.96x + 1.3 mL	4.3 mL	Doppler stroke volume
Sapin/93	Excised porcine hearts	25	0.99	y = 1.02 Echo + 3.7 mL	7.1 mL	Direct volume

Echo, echocardiography; MRI, magnetic resonance imaging; Rn, radionuclide; 3D, three dimensional.
Data from Nessley ML et al: Cardiothorac Vasc Anesth 1991;5:40; Kuroda T et al: Echocardiography 1991;4:475; Handschumacher MD et al: J Am Coll Cardiol 1993;21:743; Gopal AS et al: J Am Coll Cardiol 1993;22:258; Sui et al: Circ 88(1):1715, 1993; Sapin et al: JACC 1993;22:1530.
From Otto CM, Pearlman AS: The Textbook of Clinical Echocardiography. Philadelphia, WB Saunders, 1995.

Circumferential stress (σ_c) requires a measurement of ventricular length (L) from an apical four-chamber view in addition to the above variables.[44, 46, 47]

$$\sigma_c = \frac{(1.33)\,\text{P}\,\sqrt{\text{Ac}}}{\sqrt{\text{Am}+\text{Ac}}-\sqrt{\text{Ac}}} \times \left(1 - \frac{4\text{Ac}\sqrt{\text{Ac}}/\pi\text{L}^2}{\sqrt{\text{Am}+\text{Ac}}+\sqrt{\text{Ac}}}\right)\,\text{kdyn/cm}^2$$

Wall stress can be calculated at any point in the cardiac cycle at which these measurements can be made, but end-systolic wall stress provides the most useful clinical information.

Cardiac Output

Another clinically useful measure of LV systolic function is stroke volume or cardiac output. Stroke volume (SV) can be measured using 2D and Doppler echocardiography at any intracardiac site where flow is undisturbed by multiplying the cross-sectional area (CSA) of flow by flow velocity (v) and by the duration of flow (t):

$$\text{SV (cm}^3) = \text{CSA (cm}^2) \times \text{v(cm/sec)} \times \text{t (sec)}$$

Because the Doppler spectral output displays the instantaneous velocity on the *y* axis versus time on the *x* axis, the velocity-time integral (VTI, in centimeters) represents the mean velocity during the period of flow (Fig. 3–8) so that:

$$\text{SV} = \text{CSA} \times \text{VTI}$$

Cardiac output (CO) is the stroke volume times the heart rate (HR):

$$\text{CO} = \text{SV} \times \text{HR}$$

The cross-sectional area typically is calculated from a 2D echocardiographic measurement of the diameter (d) as the area of a circle, with the assumption that flow fills the anatomic cross-sectional area:

$$\text{CSA} = \pi(\text{d}/2)^2$$

Several other assumptions underlie this equation. First, flow velocity and cross-sectional area must be measured at the *same* anatomic

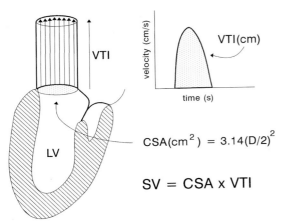

$$CSA(cm^2) = 3.14(D/2)^2$$

$$SV = CSA \times VTI$$

Figure 3·8 Doppler stroke volume calculation. The cross-sectional area (CSA) of flow is calculated as a circle based on a two-dimensional echo diameter (D) measurement. The length of the cylinder of blood ejected through this cross-sectional area on a single beat is the velocity-time integral (VTI) of the Doppler curve. Stroke volume (SV) is calculated as CSA × VTI. LV, left ventricle. (From Otto CM, Pearlman AS: The Textbook of Clinical Echocardiography. Philadelphia: WB Saunders, 1995:98.)

site; this factor becomes important when diameter and flow are measured nonsimultaneously in different views. Second, the pattern of flow is assumed to be laminar; flow occurs in an undisturbed pattern in parallel streamlines at uniform velocities. The measurement of a centerline velocity assumes that the spatial flow profile is "flat," specifically that velocity is the same at the edges and center of the flow stream. The ultrasound beam is assumed to be oriented parallel to the direction of flow for accurate velocity measurement.

Despite potential theoretical concerns about whether these assumptions are strictly met, numerous studies have demonstrated the accuracy and reproducibility of Doppler stroke volume measurements in the absence of valvular disease and in both animal studies and patients with valvular disease (Table 3–5).[48–51] The most useful sites for stroke volume measurement in patients with valvular disease are the LV outflow tract (LVOT) proximal to the aortic valve, the mitral annulus, and the pulmonary artery (Table 3–6). In normal individuals, volume flow rates are equal at these sites; however, when valvular regurgitation is present, differences in volume flow rates can be used to quantify regurgitant severity. In addition, accurate quantitation of stenosis severity depends on measurement of the antegrade volume flow rate across the affected valve.

For the LVOT, diameter is averaged from three to five measurements in mid-systole adjacent to the aortic valve leaflet insertions, from the endocardium of the septum to the leading edge of the anterior mitral valve leaflet (Fig. 3–9). A parasternal long-axis image is used to facilitate identification of the correct site of measurement and to utilize the axial resolution of the ultrasound system. The flow velocity curve is recorded from an apical approach (anteriorly angulated four-chamber or long-axis view), with the sample volume (5 to 10 mm long) positioned on the ventricular side of the aortic valve. A parallel intercept angle between the direction of flow and the ultrasound beam is obtained by careful patient positioning and transducer angulation. The region of flow acceleration proximal to the jet (recognized by spectral broadening in mid-systole) must be avoided while maintaining a position immediately adjacent to the valve for correspondence with the site of diameter measurement. Optimal sample volume positioning results in a smooth velocity curve with a well-defined peak velocity and an aortic valve closing click. Wall filters are adjusted to a low setting, and the sweep speed of the recording device is maximized to allow precise identification of the onset and end of flow. Transaortic stroke volume (SV_{Ao}) then is calculated:

$$SV_{Ao} = CSA_{LVOT} \times VTI_{LVOT}$$

This approach results in an accurate calculation of transaortic stroke volume even when stroke volume across the aortic valve is increased (as with aortic regurgitation) or when there is downstream flow obstruction (as with aortic stenosis), because the upstream flow pattern remains laminar[50, 52] and flow in the outflow tract continues to equal transaortic flow, even when aortic stenosis or regurgitation is present.

Transmitral stroke volume (SV_{MV}) is calculated as the product of the annular cross-sectional area (CSA_{MA}) and the velocity-time integral of flow at the mitral annulus (VTI_{MA}):

$$SV_{MV} = CSA_{MA} \times VTI_{MA}$$

Although measurement of transmitral flow at the leaflet tip level has been described,[53] this method is more difficult because of the complex motion of the leaflets in diastole. Measurement of stroke volume at the annulus assumes that flow is laminar at this site with a spatially flat velocity profile; these assumptions are likely to be valid for patients with a normal mitral valve or with mitral regurgitation but

TABLE 3·5 SELECTED STUDIES VALIDATING DOPPLER VOLUME FLOW MEASUREMENT

Study/Year	Volume Flow Site/Method	n	r	Regression Equation	SEE	Standard of Reference
Huntsman/83	Ascending aorta	100	0.94	DOP = 0.95x + 0.38	0.58 L/min	TD-CO
Fisher/83	Mitral leaflets	52	0.97	DOP = 0.98x + 0.02	0.23 L/min	Roller pump
Meijboom/83	Mitral leaflets	26	0.99	DOP = 0.97x + 0.07	0.13 L/min	EM flow and roller pump
	RVOT	26	0.99	DOP = 0.96x + 0.11	0.16 L/min	Roller pump
Lewis/84	Mitral annulus	35	0.96	TD = 0.91x + 5.1	5.9 mL	TD-SV
	LVOT	39	0.95	TD = 0.91x + 7.8	6.4 mL	TD-SV
Stewart/85	Mitral leaflets	29	0.97	DOP = 0.98x + 0.3	0.3 L/min	Roller pump
	Aortic annulus	33	0.98	DOP = 1.06x + 0.2	0.3 L/min	Roller pump
	Pulmonary annulus	30	0.93	DOP = 0.89x + 0.4	0.5 L/min	Roller pump
Bouchard/87	Aortic leaflets	41	0.95	DOP = 0.97x + 1.7	7 mL	TD-SV
Dittmann/87	Mitral annulus	40	0.86	DOP = 0.88 + 1.75	0.80 L/min	TD-CO
	LVOT (M-mode)	40	0.93	DOP = 0.94x + 0.44	0.59 L/min	TD-CO
DeZuttere/88	Mitral orifice (instantaneous)	30	0.91	DOP = 0.92x + 0.35	0.53 L/min	TD-CO
Hoit/88	Mitral leaflets	48	0.93	DOP = 1.1x − 0.45	0.36 L/min	TD-CO
Otto/88	LVOT (proximal to stenotic aortic valve)	52	0.91	DOP = 1.0x + 0.03	0.25 L/min	EM flow and timed collection
Burwash/93	LVOT (proximal to aortic stenosis)	75	0.86	CO = 0.92 DOP + 0.26	0.50 L/min	Transit-time flow probe

CO, cardiac output; DOP, Doppler; EM flow, volume flow rate measured by electromagnetic flowmeter; LVOT, left ventricular outflow tract; RVOT right ventricular outflow tract; SV, stroke volume; TD, thermodilution.

Data from Huntsman et al: Circulation 1983;67:593; Fisher et al: Circulation 1983;67:872; Meijboom et al: Circulation 1983;68:437, Lewis et al: Circulation 1984;70:425; Stewart et al: J Am Coll Cardiol 1985;6:653; Bouchard et al: J Am Coll Cardiol 1987;9:75; Dittmann et al: J Am Coll Cardiol 1987;10:818; DeZuttere et al: J Am Coll Cardiol 1988;11:343; Hoit et al: Am J Cardiol 1988;62:131; Otto et al: Circulation 1988;78:435; Burwash et al: Am J Physiol 1993;265:1734.

From Otto CM, Pearlman AS: The Textbook of Clinical Echocardiography. Philadelphia: WB Saunders, 1995.

may not be appropriate for patients with mitral stenosis given proximal flow acceleration on the left atrial side of the stenotic valve in diastole.

Mitral annular cross-sectional area is best described as the area of an ellipse, with the major axis measured from the four-chamber view and the minor axis measured from an apical or parasternal long-axis view. However, a simplified approach using a single-diameter measurement with calculation of a circular cross-sectional area provides acceptable results. Transmitral flow velocity is recorded from an apical approach with the sample volume positioned at the level of the mitral annulus in diastole. A sample volume length of 5 to 10 mm with low wall filters and a fast sweep speed on the spectral display is used to improve the accuracy of tracing the velocity-time integral. The major potential source of error in calculating stroke volume across the mitral annulus is measurement of annulus diameter, because the annulus is at a substantial depth in the image from the apical view, resulting in beam width artifact superimposed on the lateral resolution of the imaging system.

Stroke volume in the pulmonary artery is calculated from 2D measurement of the pulmonary artery diameter in a parasternal short-axis or right ventricular outflow view, assuming a circular cross-sectional area (CSA_{PA}) and the velocity time integral of flow at that site (VTI_{PA}):

$$SV_{PA} = CSA_{PA} \times VTI_{PA}$$

TABLE 3•6 NORMAL ANTEGRADE DOPPLER FLOW VELOCITIES	
Site	**Normal Range (m/s)**
Ascending aorta	1.0–1.7
LV outflow tract	0.7–1.1
LV inflow	
E-velocity	0.6–1.3 (0.72 ± 0.14)
Deceleration slope	5.0 ± 1.4 m/s
A-velocity	0.2–0.7 (0.47 ± 0.4)
Pulmonary artery	0.5–1.3
RV inflow	
E-velocity	0.3–0.7
RA filling (SVC, HV)	
Systole	0.32–0.69 (0.46 ± 0.08)
Diastole	0.06–0.45 (0.27 ± 0.08)
LA filling (pulmonary vein)	
Systole	0.56 ± 0.13
Diastole	0.44 ± 0.16
Atrial reversal	0.32 ± 0.07

LA, left atrial; LV, left ventricular; RA, right atrial; RV, right ventricular; HV, hepatic vein; SVC, superior vena cava.

Data from Appleton et al: J Am Coll Cardiol 1987;10:1032; Jaffe et al: Am J Cardiol 1991;68:550; Van Dam et al: Eur Heart J 1987;8:1221; Van Dam et al Eur Heart J 1988;9:165; Wilson et al: Br Heart J 1985;53:451; Hattle & Angelsen: Doppler Ultrasound in Cardiology, ed 2. Philadelphia: Lea & Febiger, 1985.

From Otto CM, Pearlman AS: The Textbook of Clinical Echocardiography. Philadelphia: WB Saunders, 1995.

As for the mitral annulus approach, the major potential source of error, particularly in adults, is accurate diameter measurement because it often is difficult to clearly define the lateral wall of the pulmonary artery. Alternatively, diameter and flow can be measured in the right ventricular outflow tract, just proximal to the pulmonary valve, although it may be difficult to obtain a parallel intercept angle between the Doppler beam and flow direction at this site.

EVALUATION OF STENOSIS SEVERITY
Velocity Data and Pressure Gradients

The fluid dynamics of a stenotic valve are characterized by a high-velocity jet in the narrowed orifice; laminar, normal velocity flow proximal to the stenosis; and a flow disturbance distal to the obstruction (Fig. 3–10).[54] The pressure gradient across the valve (ΔP) is related to the high velocity jet (V_2) in the stenosis, the proximal velocity (V_1), and the mass density of blood (ρ), as stated in the Bernoulli equation, which includes terms for conversion of potential to kinetic energy (convective acceleration), the effects of local acceleration, and viscous (v) losses:

$$\Delta P = 1/2\, \rho (V_2^2 - V_1^2) + \rho\left(\frac{dv}{dt}\right) dx + R\,(v)$$

$$\underbrace{}_{\substack{\text{Convective} \\ \text{acceleration}}} \quad \underbrace{\phantom{\rho\left(\frac{dv}{dt}\right)dx}}_{\substack{\text{Local} \\ \text{acceleration}}} \quad \underbrace{}_{\substack{\text{Viscous} \\ \text{losses}}}$$

In clinical practice, the terms for acceleration and viscous losses are ignored, so that a shorter form of the equation can be used:

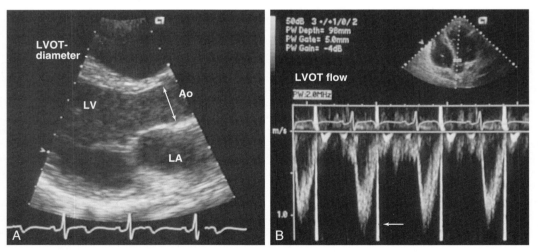

Figure 3•9 This example shows the data needed to calculate stroke volume in the left ventricular outflow tract (LVOT). *A,* Outflow tract diameter *(arrow)* is measured in a parasternal long-axis view to take advantage of the axial resolution of the ultrasound system. *B,* The flow velocity curve at this site is measured from an apical approach using pulsed Doppler echocardiography with a sample volume length of 5 to 10 mm. Care is taken to ensure the velocity and diameter data are from the same anatomic site by including the aortic valve closing click *(arrow)* in the Doppler recording. Ao, aorta; LA, left atrium; LV, left ventricle.

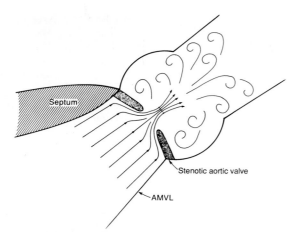

Figure 3·10 Fluid dynamics of the stenotic aortic valve in systole. The left ventricular outflow tract (LVOT) is bounded by the septum and anterior mitral valve leaflet (AMVL). As LVOT flow accelerates and converges, a relatively flat velocity profile occurs proximal to the stenotic valve *(arrows)*. Flow accelerates in a spatially small zone adjacent to the valve as blood enters the narrowed orifice. In the stenotic orifice, a high-velocity laminar jet is formed with the narrowest flow stream, called the vena contracta *(dots)*, occurring downstream from the orifice. Beyond the jet, flow is disturbed, with blood cells moving in multiple directions and velocities. (From Judge KW, Otto CM: Doppler echocardiographic evaluation of aortic stenosis. Cardiol Clin 1990;8:203.)

$$\Delta P = 4 (V_2^2 - V_1^2)$$

In this equation, the constant 4 accounts for the mass density of blood and conversion factors for measurement of pressure in units of millimeters of mercury and velocity in units of meters per second. When the proximal velocity is low (<1.5 m/s) and the jet velocity is high ($V_1^2 << V_2^2$), this equation[55, 56] can be further simplified:

$$\Delta P = 4 V_2^2$$

Maximum instantaneous gradient is calculated from the maximum transvalvular velocity, and the mean gradient is calculated by averaging the instantaneous gradients over the flow period (Fig. 3–11).

The accuracy of the simplified Bernoulli equation in measuring transvalvular pressure gradients has been shown in in vitro studies, animal models, and clinical studies of patients with valvular disease (Table 3–7).[55, 57–61] However, accuracy depends on optimal data acquisition as detailed in textbooks of echocardiography.[1, 4] Specifically, care is needed to obtain a parallel intercept angle between the continu-

ous wave Doppler beam and direction of blood flow to avoid underestimation of the velocity and therefore pressure gradient across the valve. The high velocities encountered in aortic and pulmonic stenosis mandate the use of continuous wave Doppler to avoid signal aliasing. Pulsed or high-pulse-repetition-frequency Doppler can be used for evaluation of the lower velocities seen in mitral and tricuspid stenosis, with the advantage of a better signal-to-noise ratio and clearer definition of

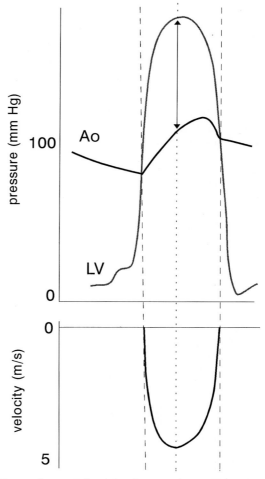

Figure 3·11 Relationship between the transaortic pressure gradient *(top)* and the Doppler velocity curve *(bottom)* in valvular aortic stenosis. The maximum instantaneous pressure gradient *(arrow)* corresponds to the maximum instantaneous velocity across the valve *(dotted line)*. Mean transaortic gradients are calculated by integrating the instantaneous gradients over the systolic ejection period using invasive pressure data or noninvasive Doppler data. Because the peak left ventricular (LV) and peak aortic (Ao) pressures are not simultaneous, the difference between these two pressures does not correspond to any point on the Doppler velocity curve.

TABLE 3·7   SELECTED STUDIES VALIDATING DOPPLER PRESSURE GRADIENTS IN VALVULAR STENOSIS (IN VIVO SIMULTANEOUS DATA)

Study/Year	n	Study Group/Model	r	Range (mm Hg)	SEE (mm Hg)
Callahan/1985	120	Supravalvular constriction (canines)	0.99 (ΔP_{max})	7–179	5.2
			0.98 (ΔP_{mean})	N/A	4.3
Smith/1985	88	Supravalvular constriction (canines)	0.98 (ΔP_{max})	5–166	5.3
			0.98 (ΔP_{mean})	5–116	3.3
Currie/1985	100	Adults with valvular aortic stenosis	0.92 (ΔP_{max})	2–180	15
			0.92 (ΔP_{mean})	0–112	10
Smith/1986	33	Adults with valvular aortic stenosis	0.85 (ΔP_{max})	27–138	N/A
Simpson/1985	24	Adults with valvular aortic stenosis	0.98 (ΔP_{max})	0–120	N/A
Burwash/1993	98	Chronic valvular aortic stenosis (canines)	0.95 (ΔP_{max})	10–128	8.4
			0.91 (ΔP_{mean})	5–77	5.3

N/A, not available; ΔP_{mean}, mean pressure gradient; ΔP_{max}, maximum pressure gradient; SEE, standard error of the estimate.

   Data from Callahan MJ et al: Am J Cardiol 1985;56:989; Smith MD et al: J Am Coll Cardiol 1985;6:1306; Currie PJ et al: Circulation 1985;71:1162; Smith MD et al: Am Heart J 1986;11:245; Simpson IA et al: Br Heart J 1985;53:636; Burwash IG et al: Am J Physiol 1993;265:H1734.

   From Otto CM, Pearlman AS: The Textbook of Clinical Echocardiography. Philadelphia: WB Saunders, 1995.

the diastolic deceleration slope than with continuous wave Doppler. Other potential technical sources of error in measuring transvalvular velocities include poor acoustic access with an inadequate flow signal, incorrect identification of the flow signal (eg, mistaking the mitral regurgitation signal for aortic stenosis), respiratory motion, and measurement variability. Physiologic sources of error include beat-to-beat variability with irregular rhythms and interim changes in volume flow rates leading to changes in the velocity and pressure gradient.

In many clinical situations, the velocity itself across the stenotic valve provides important diagnostic and prognostic information (see Chapter 9). As stated in the Bernoulli equation, a consistent relationship exists between maximum velocity and the maximum pressure gradient. Because of the consistent relationship between maximum velocity and *mean* gradient in native aortic valve stenosis, the maximum velocity, maximum gradient, and mean gradient all convey the same information about the degree of valve narrowing. Increasingly, clinicians rely on velocity data alone in clinical decision making, without the intermediate step of converting velocities to pressure gradients.

Valve Area Concept and Measurement

Pressure gradients and velocities depend on the volume flow rate across the valve and on the degree of valve narrowing. In theory and in practice, valve area (or the 2D size of the stenotic orifice) is a robust measure of stenosis severity that more closely reflects valve anatomy independently of the flow rate across the valve. Valve area can be calculated from invasive data (see Chapter 4) or noninvasively from 2D and Doppler data as described here.

Although the concept of valve area is simple, the actual valve area in a patient with valvular disease is more elusive (Table 3–8). The fluid dynamics of a stenotic valve are complex, and there may be no simple descriptor of stenosis severity that is constant for a given valve anatomy. Moreover, the difference between anatomic and functional valve area is related to the coefficients of orifice contraction and velocity, which depend on the specific shape and eccentricity of the valve orifice and on the geometry and tapering of proximal flow.[62, 63] Several studies have demonstrated that valve area is flow dependent to some extent, at least in valvular aortic stenosis (see Chapter 9).[64–71] Despite these concerns, valve area determination remains a standard clinical approach for evaluation of patients with valvular disease.

Two-Dimensional Imaging

The valve orifice in rheumatic mitral stenosis is a relatively planar structure with a constant shape and size throughout diastole (Fig. 3–12). From a parasternal short-axis view, the orifice can be imaged, taking care to identify the minimum orifice area by scanning from the apex toward the base, using low-gain settings and tracing the inner border of the black-white interface. Measurement of the 2D mitral valve area has been well validated compared with direct measurement at surgery[5, 72]

TABLE 3·8 POTENTIAL SOURCES OF ERROR IN ECHOCARDIOGRAPHIC VALVE AREA CALCULATIONS

Two-Dimensional Valve Area

Tomographic plane not a minimum valve orifice
Image plane oblique
Image quality
Gain settings
Measurement error
Complex, nonplanar valve anatomy
Shadowing and reverberations

Continuity Equation Valve Area

Proximal flow diameter measurement
Position of proximal sample volume
Proximal spatial flow profile
Intercept angle between proximal flow and ultrasound
 beam
Identification of orifice jet velocity
Intercept angle between stenotic jet and ultrasound
 beam
Measurement and calculation error

Pressure Half-Time Valve Area

Definition of maximum early diastolic velocity
Definition of early diastolic deceleration slope
Nonlinear diastolic deceleration slope
Use of empiric constant for prosthetic valves
Short early diastolic filling period (rapid heart rate,
 prolonged PR in sinus rhythm)
Changing left ventricular and left atrial compliances

and compared with invasive valve area calculations.[72] Mitral valve area determinations by 2D echocardiography is a standard part of the clinical examination.

The anatomy of valvular aortic stenosis is variable and more complex than mitral stenosis. A congenitally unicuspid valve may have a relatively symmetric orifice that can be imaged in a single tomographic plane. Although the opening of a bicuspid valve often is clearly seen early in the disease course, superimposed calcific changes result in shadowing and reverberations, making planimetry of the stenotic valve orifice problematic. The orifice of a calcified trileaflet valve may be complex, with a nonplanar stellate shape further complicating direct planimetry of valve area. Some of these limitations are minimized on transesophageal imaging, and accurate measurement of aortic valve area has been reported using this approach compared with continuity equation valve area and invasive valve area calculations.[73–76] However, this approach is rarely needed, because the aortic valve area can be calculated on transthoracic echocardiography using the continuity equation for most patients.[50, 58, 77, 78]

Continuity Equation

Valve area is calculated using the continuity equation based on the principle of conservation of mass, specifically that the stroke volume proximal to and in the stenotic orifice are equal:

$$SV_{Proximal} = SV_{Stenotic\ orifice}$$

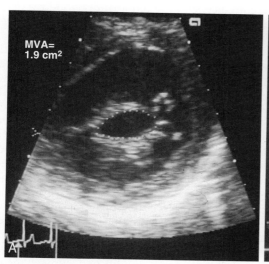
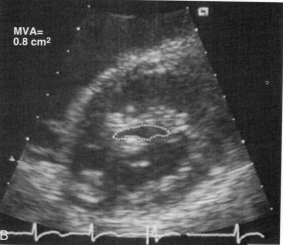

Figure 3·12 Two-dimensional echocardiographic short-axis views at the level of the mitral valve orifice in mid-diastole in a patient with moderate mitral stenosis *(A)* and in a patient with severe mitral stenosis *(B)*. Minimal orifice area is identified by scanning slowing from the apex toward the base, with the valve area (MVA) calculated directly by planimetry of the white-black interface. More severe commissural fusion is evident in the patient with severe stenosis.

Because stroke volume is the product of cross-sectional area and velocity-time integral of flow,

$$CSA_{Proximal} \times VTI_{Proximal} = Area_{Stenotic\ orifice} \times VTI_{Stenotic\ orifice}$$

This equation then is solved for stenotic orifice area:

$$Area_{Stenotic\ orifice} = (CSA_{Proximal} \times VTI_{Proximal})/VTI_{Stenotic\ orifice}$$

The continuity equation is used routinely for evaluation of aortic stenosis severity.[79-81] For calculation of aortic valve area, transaortic stroke volume is measured in the LV outflow tract just proximal to the stenotic valve, as described previously. The high-velocity aortic jet signal is recorded with continuous wave Doppler from the window that yields the highest velocity signal.

Continuity equation valve area calculations depend on accurate measurement of transaortic stroke volume and on optimal recording of the high velocity flow in the stenotic orifice (Fig. 3–13). The underlying assumptions of these methods and potential sources of error are described in the previous sections on cardiac output and velocity measurement. Continuity equation valve area calculations have been validated in comparison with invasive measures of valve area in animal models and clinical studies, and the utility of this measurement in patient management is clear (Table 3–9).[50, 77] In an experienced laboratory, with meticulous attention to technical details, the reproducibility of continuity equation valve area measurements is 5% to 8%, such that an interim change of more than 0.15 cm² is clinically significant.

Pressure Half-Time

In contrast to stenosis of a semilunar valve, where ventricular ejection drives blood across the narrowed orifice and results in the characteristic ejection type velocity curve, the time course of the decline in velocity (or pressure gradient) across a narrowed atrioventricular valve is a passive process, largely dependent on the area of the stenotic valve. This rate of pressure decline across the stenotic valve is independent of heart rate and volume flow rate and is inversely related to valve area.[82]

The rate of pressure decline typically is measured as the pressure half-time (T½) de-fined as the time interval between the maximum initial gradient and the point where this gradient has declined to one half of the initial value (Fig. 3–14). Although this method was initially described using invasive pressure measurement,[82] it now is used noninvasively with the pressure half-time measured from the Doppler velocity curve as the time from maximum velocity to the maximum velocity divided by the square root of 2 (given the quadratic relationship between velocity and pressure).[56, 83-85] A normal pressure half-time is 40 to 60 ms, with progressively longer half-times indicating more severe stenosis (Table 3–10). For the stenotic native mitral valve, an empiric constant of 220 is used to convert the half-time (in milliseconds) to mitral valve area (MVA, in centimeters squared):

$$MVA = 220/T\frac{1}{2}$$

The pressure half-time concept also can be applied to the stenotic tricuspid valve and to prosthetic valves, although it is preferable to report only the half-time itself, because the empiric constant has not been as well validated in these situations.

A major assumption of the pressure half-time method is that valve area is the predominant factor affecting ventricular diastolic filling. Although this assumption is appropriate for clinically stable patients with severe mitral stenosis, caution is needed in other clinical situations. For example, when mitral stenosis is not severe, the time course of the pressure decline between the left atrium and left ventricle in diastole is determined by the diastolic compliance of the two chambers, the initial (or opening) gradient across the valve, and atrial contractile function in addition to the effect of the restrictive mitral orifice. Similarly, in the patient undergoing percutaneous mitral commissurotomy, changing ventricular and atrial compliances in the immediate postprocedure period can lead to inaccuracies.[86, 87] Another potential concern is coexisting aortic regurgitation, because LV diastolic filling results from antegrade transmitral and retrograde transaortic flow, although this theoretical concern does not appear to significantly impact the accuracy of the pressure half-time in the clinical setting.[88]

Despite these limitations, the mitral pressure half-time is an established clinical technique that provides accurate results, particularly in patients with evidence for significant mitral stenosis on 2D echocardiography. As

TABLE 3•9 SELECTED STUDIES OF AORTIC VALVE AREA DETERMINATION

Study/Year	Comparison	n	Study Group	r	Range (cm²)	SEE (cm²)
Hakki/1981	Simplified vs original Gorlin formula	60	Aortic stenosis	0.96	0.2–2.0	0.10
Skjaerpe/1985	Cont eq vs Gorlin	30	Aortic stenosis	0.89	0.4–2.4	0.12
Zoghbi/1986	Cont eq vs Gorlin	39	Aortic stenosis	0.95	0.4–2.0	0.15
Otto/1988	Cont eq vs Gorlin	103	Aortic stenosis	0.87	0.2–3.7	0.34
Teirstein/1986	Cont eq vs Gorlin	30	Aortic stenosis	0.88	0.3–1.6	0.17
Oh/1988	Cont eq vs Gorlin	100	Aortic stenosis	0.83	0.2–1.8	0.19
Danielson/1989	Cont eq vs Gorlin	100	Aortic stenosis	0.96	0.4–2.0	
Cannon/1985	Gorlin vs videotape of valve opening	42	Porcine valves in pulsatile flow model	0.87	0.6–2.5	0.28
	New formula vs actual orifice area	42	Porcine valves in pulsatile flow model	0.98	0.6–2.5	0.11
Segal/1987	Cont eq vs actual valve area		In vitro pulsatile flow with orifice plates	0.99	0.05–0.5	0.016
	Gorlin formula vs actual valve area			0.87		0.047
Cannon/1988	Gorlin vs known valve area	135	Prosthetic aortic valves	0.39	0.6–2.3	
Come/1987	Gorlin vs Gorlin	28	Aortic stenosis	0.42	0.3–1.1	
	Cont eq vs Gorlin	40	Pre-BAV	0.71	0.2–1.1	
			Post-BAV	0.85	0.5–2.6	
Nishimura/1988	Cont eq vs Gorlin	55	Pre-BAV	0.72	0.2–0.9	0.10
			Post-BAV	0.61	0.5–1.3	0.17
Desnoyers/1988	Cont eq vs Gorlin	42	Pre-BAV	0.74	0.3–1.3	
Stoddard/1989	Cont eq vs Gorlin	41	Pre-BAV	0.84	0.2–0.8	0.08
			Post-BAV	0.87	0.3–1.2	0.10

BAV, balloon aortic valvuloplasty; Cont eq, continuity equation; Gorlin, Gorlin formula for valve area; SEE, standard error of the estimate.

Data from Hakki et al: Circulation 1981;63:1050; Skjaerpe et al: Circulation 1985;72:810; Zoghbi et al: Circulation 1986;73:452; Otto et al: Arch Intern Med 1988;148:2553; Teirstein et al: J Am Coll Cardiol 1986;8:1059; Oh et al: J Am Coll Cardiol 1988;11:1227; Danielson et al: Am J Cardiol 1989;63:1107; Cannon et al: Circulation 1985;71:1170; Segal et al: J Am Coll Cardiol 1987;9:1294; Cannon et al: Am J Cardiol 1988;62:113; Come et al: J Am Coll Cardiol 1987;10:115; Nishimura et al: Circulation 1988;78:791; Desnoyers et al: Am J Cardiol 1988;62:1078; Stoddard et al: J Am Coll Cardiol 1989;14:1218.

From Otto CM, et al: Am J Cardiol 1992;69:1607.

for other methods of evaluation of stenosis severity, careful attention to technical details and an awareness of potential pitfalls are essential to the accuracy of the technique.[88]

Other Measures of Stenosis Severity

Although maximum velocity, pressure gradient, and valve area calculations usually provide sufficient diagnostic data for clinical decision making, in some situations other measures are needed. Examples include discrepancies between the clinical presentation and diagnostic test results, discrepancies between different measure of stenosis severity, or because it is unclear whether the primary disease process is valvular or ventricular. In some patients, measurement of stenosis severity at two different flow rates (eg, with exercise, with pharmacologic stress agents) may be helpful clinically. In other situations, alternate measures of stenosis severity are needed.

Velocity Ratios

The velocity ratio is the dimensionless ratio of the maximum velocity proximal to a stenosis to the high-velocity jet in the orifice:

Velocity ratio = Proximal velocity/Jet velocity

A normal velocity ratio is slightly less than 1, with smaller ratios indicating more severe stenosis. For example, a velocity ratio of 0.25 implies that valve opening is reduced to one

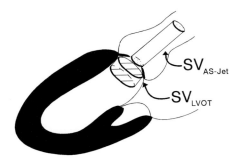

$$SV_{LVOT} = SV_{AS\text{-}Jet}$$

$$CSA_{LVOT} \times VTI_{LVOT} = AVA \times VTI_{AS\text{-}Jet}$$

$$AVA = (VTI_{LVOT} \times CSA_{LVOT})/VTI_{AS\text{-}Jet}$$

Figure 3·13 Continuity equation. Stroke volume (SV) in the left ventricular outflow tract (LVOT) and in the stenotic orifice must be equal. Because stroke volume at each site equals the cross-sectional area of flow (CSA) times the velocity-time integral (VTI), the aortic valve area (AVA) can be calculated as shown. AS-Jet, aortic stenosis jet.

fourth of its normal size. In one sense, the velocity ratio is a simplification of the continuity equation, with elimination of the term for cross-sectional area of the proximal flow stream. In another sense, the velocity ratio is a more robust descriptor of stenosis severity. Normal valve area is a function of body size, and stenotic valve areas need to be interpreted in the context of patient size, specifically by indexing valve area to body surface area. The velocity ratio has the advantage of being already "indexed" to body size. Normal intracardiac velocities are similar in people of all ages and sizes; differences in stroke volume are related to differences in the cross-sectional area of flow rather than to flow velocities. By looking at velocities alone, the velocity ratio assumes that the proximal cross-sectional area is normal for that patient and the resulting descriptor of stenosis severity is already indexed for body size. The velocity ratio has proven to be most useful for patients with native aortic stenosis when outflow tract diameter is difficult to visualize and for patients with prosthetic valves in the aortic and pulmonic positions.[89, 90]

Valve Resistance

Valve resistance (VR), calculated as the ratio of mean pressure gradient (ΔP_{mean}) to mean flow rate (Q_{mean}) across the stenotic valve, has been proposed[91–94] as a measure of stenosis severity:

$$VR = (\Delta P_{mean}/Q_{mean}) \times 1333$$

In this equation, ΔP_{mean} is measured in millimeters of mercury, Q_{mean} in milliliters per second, and valvular resistance in dynes-seconds per centimeters to the fifth power.

As the mathematics indicate, valve resistance is inversely related to valve area in a curvilinear fashion, with small valve areas corresponding to a large resistance. Initially, it was postulated that valve resistance might be flow independent, but subsequent data have shown that valve area and valve resistance change with changes in flow rate across the valve, probably because of an increase in the degree of opening of the valve leaflets at increased flow rates.[64, 65, 95] In addition, valve resistance assumes that the relationship between pressure and flow across a stenotic valve is linear, not quadratic as is assumed in the Bernoulli equation. Most theoretical and experimental data support a quadratic pressure-flow relationship in the ranges encountered clinically,[96] raising questions about the validity of the concept of valve resistance. For these reasons, valve resistance has not gained wide acceptance as a measure of stenosis severity, although it continues to be evaluated in ongoing research studies.

QUALITATIVE AND QUANTITATIVE ASSESSMENT OF VALVULAR REGURGITATION

Echocardiographic assessment of valvular regurgitation includes integration of data from 2D imaging of the valve and ventricle as well as Doppler measures of regurgitant severity. No single Doppler method provides a definitive measure of regurgitant severity, nor can the Doppler findings be interpreted in the absence of qualitative and quantitative imaging data. The specific Doppler parameters that are measured in an individual patient depend on the clinical situation, but the standard examination of a patient with valvular disease includes color flow imaging, pulsed Doppler transvalvular velocities, downstream flow reversals, and continuous wave Doppler measures of regurgitant severity (Table 3–11).

Color Flow Mapping

Color flow imaging provides a 2D display of blood flow direction and velocity superim-

TABLE 3·10 SELECTED STUDIES OF MITRAL VALVE AREA DETERMINATION

Study/Year	Comparison	n	Study Group	r	Range (cm²)	SEE (cm²)
Gorlin/1951	MVA by Gorlin formula vs direct autopsy or surgery	11	Mitral stenosis	0.89	0.5–1.5	0.15
Hakki/1981	MVA by original vs simplified Gorlin formula	40	Mitral stenosis	0.94	0.4–2.6	0.19
Libanoff/1968	T½ at rest vs exercise	20	Mitral valve disease	0.98	20–340 ms	21 ms
Henry/1975	2D echo vs direct measurement at surgery	20	MS pts undergoing surgery	0.92	0.5–3.5	
Holen/1977	MVA by Doppler vs Gorlin	10	Mitral stenosis	0.98	0.6–3.4	0.18
Hatle/1979	T½ vs Gorlin MVA	32	Mitral stenosis	−0.74	0.4–3.5	
Smith/1986	2D echo vs Gorlin	37	MS alone	0.83	0.4–2.3	0.26
		35	Prior commissurotomy	0.58		0.28
	T½ MVA vs Gorlin	(37)	MS alone	0.85		0.22
		(35)	Prior commissurotomy	0.90		0.14
Reid/1987	T½ MVA vs Gorlin	12	Pre-CBV	0.80	0.6–3.6	0.4
			Post-CBV	0.30		0.3
	2D echo vs Gorlin		Pre- and post-CBV	0.80		
Come/1988	T½ MVA vs Gorlin	37	Pre-CBV	0.51	0.6–1.3	
			Post-CBV	0.47	1.2–3.8	
	Gorlin vs Gorlin		Repeat-cath	0.74	0.4–1.4	
Thomas/1988	Predicted vs actual T½	18	Pre-CBV	0.93–0.96		
			Post-CBV	0.52–0.66		
Abascal/1988	2D echo vs Gorlin	17	Pre-CBV	0.81		
			Post-CBV	0.75		
			Pre- and post-CBV	0.88	0.5–3.0	
	T½ MVA vs Gorlin	17	Pre-CBV	0.75		
			Immediately post-CBV	0.46		
			Follow-up	0.78	0.8–3.0	
Chen/1989	T½ MVA vs Gorlin	18	Pre-CBV	0.81	0.4–1.2	0.11
			Immediately post-CBV	0.84	1.3–2.6	0.20
			24–48 h post-CBV	0.72	1.3–2.6	0.49

CBV, catheter balloon valvuloplasty; 2D, two dimensional; echo, echocardiography; MS, mitral stenosis; MVA, mitral valve area; pts, patients; SEE, standard error of the estimate; T½, pressure half-time.

Data from Gorlin et al: Am Heart J 1951;41:1; Hakki et al: Circulation 1981;63:1050; Libanoff et al: Circulation 1968;38:144; Henry et al: Circulation 1975;51:827; Holen et al: Acta Med Scand 1977;201:83; Hatle et al: Circulation 1979;60:1096; Smith et al: Circulation 1986;73:100; Reid et al: Circulation 1987;76:628; Come et al: Am J Cardiol 1988;61:817; Thomas et al: Circulation 1988;78:980; Abascal et al: J Am Coll Cardiol 1988;12:606; Chen et al: J Am Coll Cardiol 1989;13:1309.

From Otto CM, et al: Am J Cardiol 1992;69:1607.

posed on the 2D image. Although the physics of color Doppler are complex and numerous factors affect the final display, the color flow image provides an intuitive and appealing real-time display of blood flow patterns in the heart.[97-100] Color flow Doppler has a high sensitivity (nearly 100%) and specificity (nearly 100%) for identification of valvular regurgitation based on identification of the flow disturbance in the receiving chamber, exceeding the detection rates for auscultation or angiography.[101] With a meticulous examination, a small degree of valvular regurgitation is seen in many normal individuals; tricuspid regurgitation is detectable in 80% to 90% of normal individuals, pulmonic regurgitation in 70% to 80%, mitral regurgitation in 70% to 80%, and aortic regurgitation in 5% to 10%, with an increasing frequency of detectable regurgitation with age.[102]

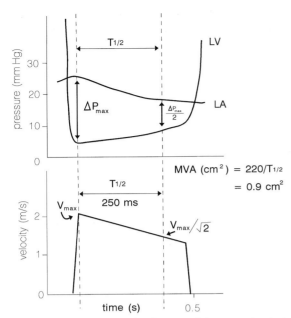

Figure 3·14 Relationship between left ventricular (LV) and left atrial (LA) pressures *(top)* and the transmitral velocity curve *(bottom)* recorded with Doppler ultrasound. The shape of the pressure gradient is reflected in the Doppler velocity curve. The pressure half-time (T½) is the same whether measured from the pressure data or from the velocity data. Mitral valve area (MVA) is calculated using an empiric constant as 220/T½; the valve area is in square centimeters (cm²), and T½ is in milliseconds (ms). (From Otto CM, Pearlman AS: The Textbook of Clinical Echocardiography. Philadelphia: WB Saunders, 1995:231.)

Physiologic or "normal" regurgitation is characterized by a small volume of backflow, with only a small area of flow disturbance seen on color flow and a weak continuous wave Doppler signal. Pathologic regurgitation is associated with a larger area of flow disturbance on color flow imaging, with the size of the flow disturbance corresponding roughly with the severity of regurgitation.

Color flow regurgitant severity is graded on a 0 to 4+ scale as follows:

0 = none (no flow disturbance in the receiving chamber)

1+ = mild (disturbed flow localized to the region immediately adjacent to valve closure, may not be seen on every beat, consistent with normal or physiologic regurgitation)

2+ = mild to moderate (disturbed flow filling up to one third of the cross-sectional area of the receiving chamber, seen on every beat)

3+ = moderate to severe (disturbed flow filling up to two thirds of the cross-sectional area of the receiving chamber, seen on every beat)

4+ = severe (disturbed flow almost filling the cross-sectional area of the receiving chamber, distal flow reversal also present)

The assigned grade is based on examination from at least two orthogonal image planes and integration of the extent of the flow disturbance in both views (Figs. 3–15 and 3–16).[101, 103, 104] For the atrioventricular valves, severe regurgitation is associated with systolic flow reversal in the veins filling the atrium. Severe semilunar valve regurgitation is associated with downstream flow reversal in the great vessels.

Color flow evaluation of regurgitant severity has become a standard clinical technique and is valid for differentiating minimal from moderate or severe regurgitation. However, more precise quantitation of regurgitant severity from color flow images is problematic because, in addition to regurgitant severity, the color flow display depends on technical and physiologic factors.[97–100] For example, the size of the aortic regurgitant jet often is overestimated in the apical views because of beam width artifact and depth of interrogation from this window. Perhaps the most useful view for routine clinical assessment of aortic regurgitation is the parasternal short-axis view just on the ventricular side of the aortic valve.[104–106] This provides a cross-sectional image of regurgitant jet area relative to the area of the outflow tract. Even with this view, attention is needed to optimize gain and other instrument settings and to position the image plane immediately adjacent to the valve.

For mitral regurgitation, signal attenuation from the transthoracic apical views may lead to underestimation of regurgitant severity, a problem that is exacerbated by the presence of a prosthetic mitral valve due to acoustic shadowing and reverberations. Transesophageal imaging allows optimization of the mitral regurgitant color flow image; however, the clinician needs to be aware of the effects of depth, pulse repetition frequency, carrier frequency, and other factors that lead to differences in jet size on transesophageal compared with transthoracic echocardiography.[107] In addition, eccentric jets may have smaller jet areas than central jets with the same regurgitant volume because of differences in entrainment of blood in the receiving chamber and adherence of the regurgitant jet to adjacent surfaces.[108–110]

TABLE 3•11 SELECTED STUDIES VALIDATING QUANTITATIVE EVALUATION OF REGURGITANT SEVERITY USING DOPPLER ECHOCARDIOGRAPHY

Study/Year	Method	Standard of Reference	n	r	SEE
Downstream Flow Reversal					
Boughner/1975	Diastolic flow reversal in descending Ao	Angio LV, Fick CO	15 AR pts	0.91 (RF)	
Touché/1985	Diastolic flow reversal in descending Ao	Angio LV, TD-CO	30 AR pts	0.92 (RF)	8.8%
Volume Flow at Two Sites					
Ascah/1985	Transmitral vs transaortic SV	EM flow	30 flow rates in canine model	0.83 (RF)	
Kitabatake/1985	Transaortic vs transpulmonic SV	Angio LV, TD-CO	20 AR pts	0.94 (RF)	
Rokey/1986	Transmitral vs transaortic SV	Angio LV, TD-CO	19 MR and 6 AR pts	0.91 (RF)	7%
Continuous Wave Doppler					
Teague/1986	AR half-time	Angio LV, Fick CO	32 AR pts	−0.88 (RF)	11%
Masuyama/1986	AR half-time	Angio LV, ID-CO	20 AR pts	−0.89 (RF)	
Jenni/1989	CW Doppler Amplitude weighted velocity	Angio LV, Fick CO	25 MR pts	0.96 (RF)	6.1%
Color Flow Imaging (Regurgitant Jet)					
Spain/1989	Color jet area	Angio LV, TD-CO	15 MR pts	0.62 (RF)	
Tribouilloy/1992	Regurgitant jet width at origin	Angio LV, TD-CO	31 MR pts	0.85 (RSV)	
Enriquez-Sarano/1993	Color jet area	Doppler SV at two sites	80 MR pts	0.69 (RF)	4.4 cm²
Proximal Acceleration (Color Flow)					
Recusani/1991	PISA (hemispherical)	Rotometer	In vitro, constant flow	0.94–0.99 (flow rate)	1–1.6 L/min
Utsunomiya/1991	PISA (hemispherical)	Actual flow rate, stopwatch and cylinder	In vitro, pulsatile flow	0.99 (flow rate)	0.53 L/min
Vandervoort/1993	PISA	Actual flow rate	In vitro, steady flow	0.98–0.99 (flow rate)	
Giesler/1993	PISA	LV angio, Fick CO	16 MR pts	0.88 (RSV)	17 mL
Chen/1993	PISA	Doppler SV at two sites	46 MR pts	0.94 (RSV)	18 mL
Jet Momentum					
Cape/1989	Conservation of momentum	EM flow	In vitro, constant flow	0.98	0.18 L/min

Ao, aortic; AR, aortic regurgitation; CO, cardiac output; EM flow, volume flow rate measured by electromagnetic flowmeter; ID, indicator dilation; LV, left ventricle; MR, mitral regurgitation; PISA, proximal isovelocity surface area method; RF, regurgitant fraction; RSV, regurgitant stroke volume; SV, stroke volume; TD, thermodilution.

Data from Boughner et al: Circulation 1975;52:874; Touché et al: Circulation 1985;72:819; Ascah et al: Circulation 1985;72:377; Kitabatake et al: Circulation 1985;72:523; Rokey et al: J Am Coll Cardiol 1986;7:1273; Teague et al: J Am Coll Cardiol 1986;8:592; Masuyama et al: Circulation 1986;73:460; Jenni et al: Circulation 1989;79:1294; Spain et al: J Am Coll Cardiol 1989;13:585; Tribouilloy et al: Circulation 1992;85:1248; Enriquez-Sarano et al: J Am Coll Cardiol 1993;21:1211; Rescusani et al: Circulation 1991;83:594; Utsunomiya et al: J Am Soc Echocardiogr 1991;4:338; Vandervoort et al: J Am Coll Cardiol 1993;22:535; Giesler et al: Am J Cardiol 1993;71:217; Chen et al: J Am Coll Cardiol 1993;121:374; Cape et al: Circulation 1989;79:1343.

From Otto CM, Pearlman AS: The Textbook of Clinical Echocardiography. Philadelphia: WB Saunders, 1995.

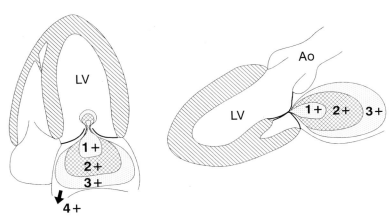

Apical four chamber   Parasternal long axis

Figure 3·15 Mitral regurgitation semiquantitative flow mapping. Multiple views are used during the examination, and jet geometry is considered in conjunction with the jet area in grading the degree of regurgitation. Severe (4+) mitral regurgitation is associated with systolic reversal in the pulmonary veins. Ao, aorta; LV, left ventricle. (From Otto CM, Pearlman AS: The Textbook of Clinical Echocardiography. Philadelphia: WB Saunders, 1995;248.)

Despite these limitations, qualitative color flow mapping is the most widely used noninvasive approach for assessment of regurgitant severity and has proven its clinical utility in patient management. In the clinical setting, color flow information must be interpreted in conjunction with 2D images of the valve and left ventricle and with other Doppler measures of regurgitant severity. The potential limitations of this technique also must be recognized.

Calculation of Regurgitant Fraction With Two-Dimensional and Pulsed Doppler Echocardiography

The amount of backflow across the regurgitant valve is expressed as the regurgitant stroke volume (per beat) or regurgitant volume (per minute). Regurgitant stroke volume (RSV) can be determined using 2D and pulsed Doppler echocardiography by calculation of the total stroke volume (TSV) antegrade across the regurgitant valve minus the forward stroke volume (the amount of blood delivered to the body) across a normal valve (Fig. 3–17). For aortic regurgitation (AR), total stoke volume is measured in the LVOT and forward stroke volume across the mitral or pulmonic (PA) valve:

$$RSV_{AR} = (CSA_{LVOT} \times VTI_{LVOT}) - (CSA_{PA} \times VTI_{PA})$$

For mitral regurgitation (MR), total stroke volume is measured across the mitral annulus (MA) and forward stroke volume across the LVOT or pulmonic valve:

$$RSV_{MR} = (CSA_{MA} \times VTI_{MA}) - (CSA_{LVOT} \times VTI_{LVOT})$$

The regurgitant fraction (RF) is the ratio of regurgitant stroke volume to total stroke volume:

$$RF = RSV/TSV$$

The validity of this method has been demon-

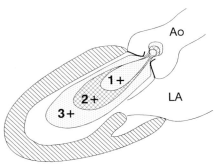

Long axis

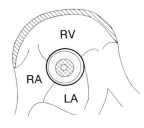

Short axis just below aortic valve

Figure 3·16 Semiquantitation of aortic regurgitant severity using color flow mapping in parasternal long-axis and short-axis views. The depicted jet areas are only rough guides. In the clinical setting, multiple views are used, and jets often are eccentric and asymmetric. Ao, aorta; LA, left atrium; RA, right atrium; RV, right ventricle. (From Otto CM, Pearlman AS: The Textbook of Clinical Echocardiography. Philadelphia: WB Saunders, 1995;248.)

Figure 3·17 The aortic regurgitant stroke volume (SV) is calculated by measurement of the transvalvular volume flow rate at two intracardiac sites. Transaortic flow, representing the total stroke volume, is calculated from the cross-sectional area (CSA) and velocity-time integral (VTI) of the left ventricular outflow tract (LVOT). Transmitral flow, representing the forward stroke volume, is calculated from the CSA and VTI of LV inflow (LVI) across the mitral annulus. Regurgitant stroke volume is the difference between the total and forward stroke volumes. (From Otto CM, Pearlman AS: The Textbook of Clinical Echocardiography. Philadelphia: WB Saunders, 1995: 252.)

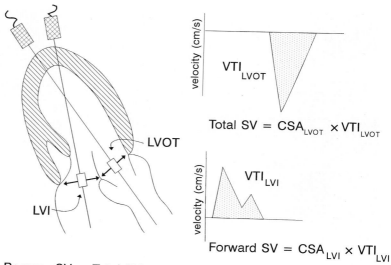

$$\text{Total SV} = \text{CSA}_{LVOT} \times \text{VTI}_{LVOT}$$

$$\text{Forward SV} = \text{CSA}_{LVI} \times \text{VTI}_{LVI}$$

$$\text{Regurg. SV} = \text{Total SV} - \text{Forward SV}$$

strated in animal and clinical studies of valvular regurgitation.[111–113] However, the accuracy of this method for calculation of regurgitant fraction depends on the caveats described earlier for measurement of cardiac output by Doppler echocardiography. Given the potential error of this approach, particularly if there are errors in diameter measurement, and the complexity of data acquisition and measurement, most laboratories perform these calculations only in selected cases.

Flow Reversals

When atrioventricular valve regurgitation is severe, the backflow across the valve fills the atrium and extends into the veins, resulting in reversal of the normal flow pattern in systole. Severe tricuspid regurgitation results in systolic flow reversal in the inferior vena cava and hepatic veins, which can be demonstrated from the subcostal view using pulsed Doppler recordings (Fig. 3–18). Severe mitral regurgitation results in systolic flow reversal in the pulmonary veins (Fig. 3–19). On transthoracic echocardiography, the flow pattern in the right inferior pulmonary vein can be recorded from the apical four-chamber view in most patients, although the signal-to-noise ratio may be suboptimal at this depth in some adult patients. On transesophageal echocardiography, the flow pattern in the pulmonary veins

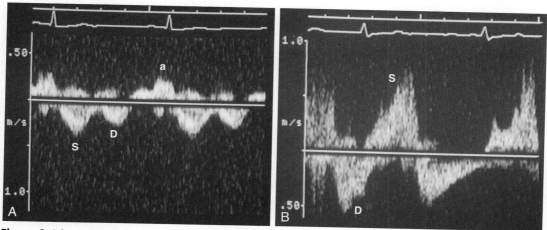

Figure 3·18 *A,* Normal hepatic vein flow shows systolic (S) and diastolic (D) atrial filling, with a small flow reversal after atrial contraction (a). *B,* With severe tricuspid regurgitation, systolic flow reversal is observed.

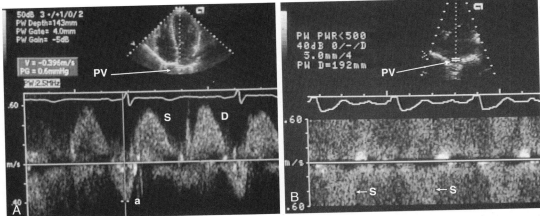

Figure 3·19 *A*, Pulmonary vein (PV) flow recorded from a transthoracic apical four-chamber view shows normal systolic (S) and diastolic (D) atrial filling, with reversal of flow after atrial contraction (a). *B*, With severe mitral regurgitation, systolic flow reversal *(arrows)* is observed, even though the signal strength is suboptimal.

can be recorded at high resolution. Examination of all four pulmonary veins is especially helpful with an eccentric regurgitant jet, because the pattern of systolic flow reversal may not be uniform.

Other physiologic factors affect the atrial inflow patterns, including respiratory phase, cardiac rhythm, atrial and venous compliance, ventricular diastolic filling, and age.[114–118] Although the presence and severity of venous systolic flow reversal is a useful adjunct in the evaluation of atrioventricular valve regurgitant severity, it is not a pathognomonic finding.

For the semilunar valves (aortic and pulmonic), severe regurgitation results in diastolic flow reversal in the associated great vessels as blood flows back into the ventricular chamber across the incompetent valve. A quantitative aortic regurgitant fraction can be derived from the extent of diastolic flow reversal in the descending aorta when systolic and diastolic aortic diameters and velocity time integrals are used to calculated antegrade compared with retrograde volume flow rates (Fig. 3–20).[119, 120] Because the distance that holodiastolic flow reversal extends down the aorta correlates with regurgitant severity, the presence of holodiastolic flow reversal in the proximal abdominal aorta provides a simple indicator of severe aortic regurgitation (see Fig. 3–20).[121] Holodiastolic flow reversal in the descending thoracic aorta is a more sensitive but less specific indicator of significant regurgitant, because patients with severe or with moderate aortic regurgitation are detected.

When performed carefully, with an adequate signal-to-noise ratio and low wall filters,

this approach is a simple and reliable method for qualitative evaluation of regurgitant severity. False-negative results result from poor examination technique or limited acoustic access. False-positive results result from other sources of diastolic run-off in the aorta, such as a patent ductus arteriosus.

Continuous Wave Doppler Data

Two types of data are inherent in the continuous wave Doppler spectral recording of a regurgitant jet velocity curve. First, the signal strength, especially relative to antegrade flow, is directly related to the volume of regurgitation.[122] Although acoustic attenuation and in-

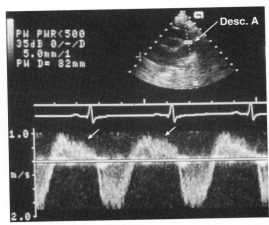

Figure 3·20 From a suprasternal notch window, holodiastolic flow reversal *(arrows)* is seen in the descending thoracic aorta (Desc. A) in a patient with severe aortic regurgitation.

strumentation variability make quantitation of signal strength problematic, qualitative assessment is a simple and useful clinical measure. Second, the time-velocity curve reflects the time course of the instantaneous pressure difference across the regurgitant valve. For each instantaneous velocity, the pressure difference across the valve is $4V^2$ (as stated in the Bernoulli equation), such that inferences about intracardiac pressures and the time course of pressure changes can be derived from the Doppler data.

For aortic regurgitation, the rate of pressure decline between the aorta and left ventricle in diastole is related to chronicity of disease and LV compensation (Fig. 3–21).[88, 123–125] The end-diastolic velocity across the regurgitant aortic valve corresponds to the end-diastolic pressure gradient, which, when subtracted from the cuff diastolic blood pressure, provides an approximation of LV end-diastolic pressure, although wide measurement variability limits the clinical utility of this estimate.[126]

The mitral regurgitant signal is characterized by a high maximum velocity, reflecting the high LV systolic pressure and low left atrial pressure in compensated disease. Typically, this high velocity persists through most of systole. However, when left atrial pressure rises in late systole (eg, a v wave) due to severe or acute mitral regurgitation, the velocity curve shows a steep decline in velocity in late systole, termed the Doppler "v wave" (Fig. 3–22). In addition, the rate of pressure rise in the left ventricle during early systole correlates with the rate of increase in velocity in the regurgitant jet. Thus, the LV dP/dt can be calculated from the Doppler mitral regurgitant jet as the

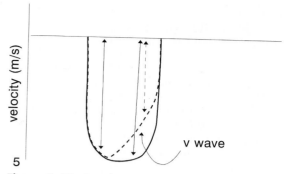

Figure 3·22 Doppler velocity curve for chronic *(solid line)* and acute *(dashed line)* mitral regurgitation. The rise in left atrial pressure in late systole in patients with acute regurgitation is associated with a more rapid decline in velocity in late systole, often called a v wave.

time interval (in milliseconds) between the points on the curve corresponding to 1 and 3 m/s, divided by the pressure difference between these two points:

$$dP/dt = time/[4(3)^2 - 4(1)^2] = time/32 \text{ mm Hg}$$

A value of less than 1000 indicates significant contractile dysfunction of the left ventricle.[127–129] Similarly, the rate of decline in the mitral regurgitant jet velocity corresponds to LV diastolic relaxation.[128]

On the right side of the heart, the tricuspid regurgitant jet velocity corresponds to the right ventricular to right atrial pressure difference in systole, so that right ventricular (and pulmonary systolic pressures) can be calculated from the maximum tricuspid regurgitant jet by using the Bernoulli equation. As for mitral regurgitation, severe or acute tricuspid regurgitation may result in a right atrial v wave, seen as a late systolic rapid decline in the velocity curve.

The pulmonic regurgitant jet velocity is related to the diastolic pressure difference between the pulmonary artery and right ventricle and, given that the normal pressure difference is low, typically is low in velocity. With pulmonary hypertension, pulmonic regurgitant velocities are increased, and the end-diastolic velocity, in combination with an estimate of right ventricular diastolic pressure, allows calculation of diastolic pulmonary pressure.

Other Quantitative Approaches to Evaluation of Regurgitant Severity

Several new quantitative approaches for evaluation of regurgitant severity have been

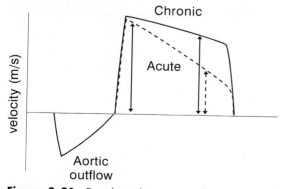

Figure 3·21 Doppler velocity curve for chronic and acute aortic regurgitation. The slope is steeper for acute regurgitation because of a more rapid equalization of aortic and left ventricular pressures in diastole as the regurgitant volume fills a noncompliant left ventricle.

proposed.[130] These include momentum quantification in the regurgitant jet, calculation of flow rates from the proximal convergence zone (also known as the proximal isovelocity surface area or PISA method), and calculation of regurgitant orifice area.

Momentum is defined as the product of velocity and volume flow rate. Because instantaneous volume flow rate is the product of flow area (A) and velocity, momentum is approximated at any time point in the cardiac cycle as the area of the jet multiplied by the velocity squared. Momentum is conserved in the regurgitant jet; momentum for any cross-sectional plane equals momentum at any other site. Theoretically, conservation of momentum allows calculation of regurgitant orifice area (ROA) from the area of the jet and velocity (V_{jet}) at any downstream site in conjunction with the velocity in the regurgitant orifice ($V_{orifice}$)[131]:

$$ROA = (\text{area of jet} \times V^2_{jet})/V^2_{orifice}$$

Clinical application of this approach has been problematic because of non-axisymmetric and turbulent jets, the need for accurate velocity resolution, the assumptions of this simplified approach, and the technical difficulties in implementing the technique.

The proximal isovelocity surface area approach is based on the concept that flow accelerates on the upstream side of a regurgitant valve, resulting in successively higher velocities as flow approaches the regurgitant orifice (see Fig. 13–3).[132–136] For any given velocity (v) an isovelocity surface area can be visualized as the aliasing velocity on a color flow image. By definition, the volume flow rate (Q) at this site is the area of flow multiplied by velocity. The area of flow can be calculated as the area of a hemisphere or hemiellipse (with radius r):

$$Q = \pi r^2 v$$

The regurgitant orifice area then can be calculated[137] from the maximal continuous wave Doppler velocity (V):

$$ROA = Q/V$$

In the clinical setting, this approach has proven most useful for evaluation of mitral regurgitation, as imaging of proximal acceleration is more difficult for aortic regurgitation. In addition, methodologic problems, such as integration of the flow rate over diastole, have not been fully worked out. Qualitatively, visualization of the proximal flow convergence region is helpful in determining the site of regurgitation, particularly with complex valve lesions.

OTHER ECHOCARDIOGRAPHIC DATA

Echocardiographic evaluation of the patient with valvular heart disease also includes assessment of other parameters, depending on the specific valve involved and the severity of valve disease. For example, in a patient with mitral stenosis, measurement of left atrial size and estimation of pulmonary pressures are important components of the examination. In a patient with severe aortic stenosis and heart failure symptoms despite normal LV systolic function, evaluation of diastolic ventricular function may be needed.

Left Ventricular Diastolic Function

LV diastolic function is reflected in the Doppler velocity patterns of ventricular inflow and atrial filling (Table 3–12).[109, 138–141] LV diastolic inflow is recorded from the transthoracic approach in the apical four-chamber view with the sample volume positioned at the mitral leaflet tips in diastole. The normal pattern of LV diastolic filling in young, healthy individuals is a short isovolumic relaxation time, a high early diastolic filling velocity (E-velocity), a steep early diastolic deceleration slope, and a smaller late diastolic filling velocity after atrial contraction (A-velocity), with a high ratio of early to late diastolic filling velocities (E/A ratio) (Fig. 3–23).

TABLE 3·12   PARAMETERS OF LEFT VENTRICULAR DIASTOLIC FUNCTION

Parameter	Echocardiographic Measurement
Ventricular relaxation	Isovolumic relaxation time (aortic closure to mitral opening)
	$-dP/dt$ (from mitral regurgitant jet)
Rapid filling rate	Early diastolic velocity (E-velocity) or velocity time integral
Atrial filling rate	Late diastolic velocity (A-velocity) or velocity time integral
Ventricular compliance (dV/dP)	E/A ratio
	Diastolic deceleration slope
Left ventricular end-diastolic pressure	Calculate from aortic regurgitant velocity curve minus diastolic blood pressure
	Estimate from pattern of pulmonary vein flow

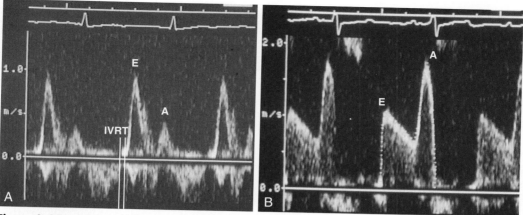

Figure 3·23 *A,* Normal left ventricular diastolic filling is characterized by rapid early diastolic filling (E), with a steep deceleration slope and a small atrial contribution to ventricular filling (A). The isovolumic relaxation time (IVRT) is measured as the interval from aortic valve closure to mitral valve opening. *B,* With impaired ventricular relaxation, as is seen in patients with concentric hypertrophy, the early diastolic filling velocity is diminished, the deceleration slope is prolonged, and the atrial contribution to filling is more prominent.

Pulmonary vein flow is recorded from the apical four-chamber view on transthoracic echocardiography with the sample volume positioned in the right inferior pulmonary vein, using color Doppler to aid in positioning the Doppler beam. Higher-quality pulmonary vein flow signals can be obtained from the transesophageal approach with the sample volume positioned in the left superior pulmonary vein. Normal pulmonary vein flow patterns show systolic and diastolic flow into the atrium, with diastolic flow (D) exceeding systolic flow (S) in young, normal individuals. A small flow reversal after atrial contraction (a-reversal) also is seen.

With diastolic dysfunction from impaired LV relaxation, the LV inflow pattern shows a reduced E-velocity and increased A-velocity, resulting in a low E/A ratio. The isovolumic relaxation time is prolonged, and the deceleration slope is reduced. Pulmonary vein flow shows a reduced diastolic filling velocity, prominent systolic filling velocity, and increased atrial reversal.

With diastolic dysfunction from decreased compliance of the left ventricle, the pattern of LV diastolic filling is characterized by an increased E-velocity, reduced A-velocity resulting in a high E/A ratio in conjunction with a reduced isovolumic relaxation time, and an increased early diastolic deceleration slope. A reduced systolic filling and increased diastolic filling curve is seen on the pulmonary venous flow curve with an increase in the velocity and duration of the atrial reversal velocity curve.

Between these two extremes, diastolic dysfunction may manifest a "pseudonormal" pattern in which the LV filling curve appears normal, but the pulmonary vein flow pattern shows reduced diastolic filling and an increased atrial reversal velocity.

Unfortunately, although the Doppler velocity curves accurately portray LV diastolic filling, evaluation of LV diastolic *function* by echocardiography is limited by the numerous technical and physiologic factors other than the diastolic properties of the ventricle that affect diastolic *filling.* LV diastolic filling is affected by technical factors such as sample volume position and intercept angle; normal physiologic variation, including respiration, heart rate, age, and PR interval; and other physiologic variables, such as preload, coexisting mitral regurgitation, LV systolic function, and atrial contractile function.[115, 116, 142-145] Pulmonary vein flow is affected by age, left atrial size, left atrial pressure, atrial contractile function, and cardiac rhythm, in addition to LV and left atrial compliance, LV diastolic relaxation, and the gradient from the pulmonary veins to the left ventricle.

Evaluation of diastolic function in a patient must take into consideration whether technical or physiologic factors affect the findings. With a knowledge of these potential limitations, clinically useful information about LV diastolic function can be derived from the Doppler patterns of LV inflow and pulmonary vein flow in patients with valvular heart disease.

Left Atrial Enlargement and Thrombus Formation

Left atrial size can be assessed on 2D transthoracic imaging from parasternal, apical, and subcostal views. Although methods for calculation of left atrial volume based on planimetry of atrial area in two views have been validated and provide a quantitative measure of atrial size, a single anterior-posterior diameter, in conjunction with 2D visual estimates of atrial size, provides adequate information for patient management in most clinical situations.

The specificity of identification of a left atrial thrombus on transthoracic imaging is high (95% to 99%), but sensitivity is low (about 60%) because of poor image quality at the depth of the left atrium and difficulty in visualizing the atrial appendage.[146–148] Transesophageal imaging provides high-quality images of the left atrium and atrial appendage, resulting in a very high sensitivity (nearly 100%) and specificity (nearly 100%) for detection of atrial thrombus.[149, 150] When atrial thrombus is suspected clinically, transesophageal imaging is necessary for reliable exclusion of this potential diagnosis.

Determination of Pulmonary Pressures

Several noninvasive methods for estimation of pulmonary artery pressures have been proposed.[100, 151–154] The most accurate and widely used method is based on measurement of tricuspid regurgitant jet velocity in combination with an estimate of right atrial pressure.[58, 155, 156] A small degree of tricuspid regurgitation is present in most healthy persons, and the prevalence is higher among patients with valvular disease. Because the velocity of the regurgitant jet is related to the pressure difference across the valve, not to the volume of regurgitation, this degree of tricuspid regurgitation, although not hemodynamically significant, allows recording of jet velocity and calculation of pulmonary pressures.

The velocity in the tricuspid regurgitant jet (TR_{jet}) reflects the right ventricular to right atrial systolic pressure difference, as stated in the Bernoulli equation. Addition of right atrial pressure (RAP) to this pressure difference yields right ventricular systolic pressure, which, in the absence of pulmonic stenosis, equals pulmonary artery systolic pressure ($PA_{systolic}$) (Table 3–13):

$$PA_{systolic} = 4(TR_{jet})^2 + RAP$$

TABLE 3·13   SELECTED STUDIES VALIDATING NONINVASIVE PULMONARY ARTERY PRESSURE MEASUREMENT

Study/Year	Method	n	r	Regression Equation	SEE (mm Hg)
Kitabatake/83	Time to peak flow (RVOT)	33	−0.88	Log (mean PAP) = 0.0068 (AcT) + 2.1 mm Hg	
Stevenson/84	IVRT (Burstin method, in sedated patients)	95	0.97	Doppler mean PAP = 0.97 (cath) + 1.7 mm Hg	6.4
Isobe/86	PEP/AcT	45	0.89	PEP/AcT = 0.023 mean PAP + 0.48 mm Hg	
Stevenson/89	TR-jet	50	0.96		6.9
	Time to peak flow (PA)		0.63		16.4
	IVRT		0.97		5.4
	Pulmonic regurgitation		0.96		4.5
Yock/84	TR-jet	62	0.95	Doppler RV-RA ΔP = 1.03 ΔP + 0.71 mm Hg	7
Berger/85	TR-jet	69	0.97	Systolic PAP = 1.23 (Doppler ΔP) − 0.09 mm Hg	4.9
Currie/85	TR-jet	127	0.96	Doppler RV-RA ΔP = 0.88 ΔP + 2.2 mm Hg	7
Lee/89	Pulmonic regurgitation	29	0.94	Diastolic PAP (echo) = 0.95 (cath) − 1.0 mm Hg	Mean diff: 3.3 ± 2.2

AcT, acceleration time; IVRT, isovolumic relaxation time; ΔP, pressure gradient; PAP, pulmonary artery pressure; PEP, pre-ejection period; RA, right atrial; RV, right ventricular; RVOT, right ventricular outflow tract; SEE, standard error of the estimate; TR-jet, tricuspid regurgitant jet.

Data from Kitabatake A et al: Circulation 1983;68:302; Stevenson JG et al: J Am Coll Cardiol 1984;4:1021; Isobe M et al: Am J Cardiol 1986;57:316; Stevenson JG et al: J Am Soc Echocardiogr 1989;2:157; Yock PG, Popp RL: Circulation 1984;70:657; Berger M et al: J Am Coll Cardiol 1985;6:359; Currie PJ et al: J Am Coll Cardiol 1985;6:750; Lee RT et al: Am J Cardiol 1989;64:1366.

From Otto CM, Pearlman AS: The Textbook of Clinical Echocardiography. Philadelphia: WB Saunders, 1995.

Right atrial pressure is estimated from the appearance of the inferior vena cava at its entrance into the right atrium, as imaged from a subcostal view during normal respiration (Table 3–14).[157, 158] Because this method depends on normal intrathoracic pressure changes with respiration, right atrial pressure cannot be estimated by this method in mechanically ventilated patients.

Examination of the tricuspid regurgitant jet from parasternal and apical windows with careful transducer angulation to record the highest velocity signal is essential to avoid underestimation of jet velocity and pulmonary artery pressures. When a clear maximum regurgitant jet velocity cannot be identified or only an incomplete waveform is obtained, pulmonary pressures cannot be reliably determined from the regurgitant jet. Instead, indirect evidence for pulmonary hypertension (eg, mid-systolic notching and short time to peak velocity in the pulmonary artery velocity wave, abnormal septal motion) or other methods for evaluation of pulmonary pressures should be used.

Right Heart Structure and Function

Qualitative evaluation of right ventricular size and systolic function on 2D echocardiography is an important component of the examination in patients with valvular heart disease. The right ventricle is imaged in the parasternal short-axis and right ventricular inflow views and in the apical and subcostal four-chamber views. Right ventricular size is described as normal or as mildly, moderately, or severely enlarged based on integration of data from these views. Similarly, right ventricular systolic function is graded on a scale of normal to severely reduced. The pattern of ventricular

septal motion also is helpful in the diagnosis of right ventricular pressure or volume overload. Although quantitative evaluation of right ventricular size and function has been described using 3D echocardiography, these techniques are complex and have not been widely used clinically.

THE UTILITY OF STRESS ECHOCARDIOGRAPHY

Stress echocardiography may be useful in assessing coexisting coronary disease in patients with valvular heart disease. Evaluation of the severity of valvular disease (stenosis or regurgitation) at two volume flow rates, changes in pulmonary pressures, and the overall response of the left ventricle to stress provide important diagnostic and prognostic information.

Valvular Stenosis

Because clinical measures of stenosis severity are flow dependent, there has been increasing interest in using the degree of change in stenosis severity relative to a change in volume flow rate as an index of disease severity. This concept has been applied predominantly to valvular aortic stenosis in an effort to differentiate patients with a small valve area due to LV systolic dysfunction from those with severe aortic stenosis resulting in LV dysfunction (see Chapter 9).

In patients with mitral stenosis, assessment of the rise in pulmonary pressures with exercise provides insight into the relationship between hemodynamic severity and clinical symptoms. Exercise Doppler data also may be useful in determining the optimal timing of intervention in patients with mitral stenosis to prevent the development of irreversible pulmonary hypertension (see Chapter 10).

Valvular Regurgitation

The volume of retrograde flow across a regurgitant valve depends on heart rate and the driving pressure across the valve, as well as the size of the regurgitant orifice. Evaluation of the change in regurgitant severity with stress may be helpful in identifying patients with exertional symptoms from valvular regurgitation or those with intermittent regurgitation (eg, mitral prolapse, ischemia) that is precipitated by stress.

In patients with chronic valvular regurgita-

TABLE 3·14	ESTIMATION OF RIGHT ATRIAL PRESSURE	
Size of the IVC at IVC-RA Junction	Respiratory Change	RA Pressure (mm Hg)
Small (<1.5 cm)	Collapse	0–5
Normal (1.5–2.5 cm)	Decrease by >50%	5–10
Normal	Decrease by <50%	10–15
Dilated (>2.5 cm)	Decrease by <50%	15–20
Dilated with dilated hepatic veins	No change	>20

IVC, inferior vena cava; RA, right atrial.
From Otto CM, Pearlman AS: The Textbook of Clinical Echocardiography. Philadelphia: WB Saunders, 1995.

tion, the response of the left ventricle to stress, using radionuclide techniques, has been proposed as an indicator of disease severity. The ejection fraction can be measured at rest and after exercise by using 2D echocardiography providing similar information (see Chapters 12 and 13).

References

1. Otto CM, AS Pearlman: Textbook of Clinical Echocardiography. Philadelphia: WB Saunders, 1995.
2. Weyman AE: Principles and Practice of Echocardiography. Philadelphia: Lea & Febiger, 1994.
3. Feigenbaum H: Echocardiography. Philadelphia: Lea & Febiger, 1994.
4. Otto CM: The Practice of Clinical Echocardiography. Philadelphia: WB Saunders, 1997.
5. Henry WL, Griffith JM, Michaelis LL, McIntosh CL, Morrow AG, Epstein SE: Measurement of mitral orifice area in patients with mitral valve disease by real-time, two-dimensional echocardiography. Circulation 1975;51:827–831.
6. Abascal VM, Wilkins GT, Choong CY, et al: Echocardiographic evaluation of mitral valve structure and function in patients followed for at least 6 months after percutaneous balloon mitral valvuloplasty. J Am Coll Cardiol 1988;12:606–615.
7. Reid CL, Otto CM, Davis KB, Labovitz A, Kisslo KB, McKay CR: Influence of mitral valve morphology on mitral balloon commissurotomy: immediate and six-month results from the NHLBI Balloon Valvuloplasty Registry. Am Heart J 1992;124:657–665.
8. Roberts WC: Morphologic aspects of cardiac valve dysfunction. Am Heart J 1992;123:1610–1632.
9. Selzer A: Changing aspects of the natural history of valvular aortic stenosis. N Engl J Med 1987;317:91–98.
10. Beppu S, Suzuki S, Matsuda H, Ohmori F, Nagata S, Miyatake K: Rapidity of progression of aortic stenosis in patients with congenital bicuspid aortic valves. Am J Cardiol 1993;71:322–327.
11. Roberts WC: Anatomically isolated aortic valvular disease: the case against its being of rheumatic etiology. Am J Med 1970;49:151–159.
12. He S, Fontaine AA, Schwammenthal E, Yoganathan AP, Levine RA: Integrated mechanism for functional mitral regurgitation—leaflet restriction versus coapting force: in vitro studies. Circulation 1997;96:1826–1834.
13. Otsuji Y, Handschumacher MD, Schwammenthal E, et al: Insights from three-dimensional echocardiography into the mechanism of functional mitral regurgitation: direct in vivo demonstration of altered leaflet tethering geometry. Circulation 1997;96:1999–2008.
14. Subramanian R, Olson LJ, Edwards WD: Surgical pathology of combined aortic stenosis and insufficiency: a study of 213 cases. Mayo Clin Proc 1985;60:247–254.
15. Olson LJ, Subramanian R, Edwards WD: Surgical pathology of pure aortic insufficiency: a study of 225 cases. Mayo Clin Proc 1984;59:835–841.
16. Pyeritz RE, McKusick VA: The Marfan syndrome: diagnosis and management. N Engl J Med 1979;300:772–777.
17. Marsalese DL, Moodie DS, Vacante M, et al: Marfan's syndrome: natural history and long-term follow-up of cardiovascular involvement. J Am Coll Cardiol 1989;14:422–428.
18. Roldan CA, Shively BK: Echocardiographic findings in systemic diseases characterized by immune-mediated injury. In Otto CM, ed. The Practice of Clinical Echocardiography. Philadelphia: WB Saunders, 1997:585–601.
19. Hahn RT, Roman MJ, Mogtader AH, Devereux RB: Association of aortic dilation with regurgitant, stenotic and functionally normal bicuspid aortic valves. J Am Coll Cardiol 1992;19:283–288.
20. Otto CM, Pearlman AS: Echocardiographic evaluation of left and right ventricular systolic function. In Otto CM, Pearlman AS, eds. Textbook of Clinical Echocardiography. Philadelphia: WB Saunders, 1995:85–116.
21. American Society of Echocardiography: American Society of Echocardiography Committee on Standards, Subcommittee on Quantitation of Two-Dimensional Echocardiograms: recommendation for quantitation of the left ventricle by two-dimensional echocardiography. J Am Soc Echocardiogr 1989;2:361–367.
22. Gopal AS, King DL: Three-dimensional echocardiography. In Otto CM, ed. The Practice of Clinical Echocardiography. Philadelphia: WB Saunders, 1997:131–166.
23. Otto CM, Mickel MC, Kennedy JW, et al: Three-year outcome after balloon aortic valvuloplasty: insights into prognosis of valvular aortic stenosis. Circulation 1994;89:642–650.
24. Kaul S: Echocardiography in coronary artery disease. Curr Probl Cardiol 1990;15:239–298.
25. American Society of Echocardiography: Report of the American Society of Echocardiography Committee on Nomenclature and Standards: Identification of Myocardial Wall Segments. Durham, NC: American Society of Echocardiography, 1982.
26. Marwick T, Willemart B, D'Hondt AM, et al: Selection of the optimal nonexercise stress for the evaluation of ischemic regional myocardial dysfunction and malperfusion. Circulation 1993;87:345–354.
27. Marcovitz PA, Armstrong WF: Accuracy of dobutamine stress echocardiography in detecting coronary artery disease. Am J Cardiol 1992;69:1269–1273.
28. Segar DS, Brown SE, Sawada SG, Ryan T, Feigenbaum H: Dobutamine stress echocardiography: correlation with coronary lesion severity as determined by quantitative angiography. J Am Coll Cardiol 1992;19:1197–1202.
29. Mertes H, Sawada SG, Ryan T, et al: Symptoms, adverse effects, and complications associated with dobutamine stress echocardiography: experience in 1118 patients. Circulation 1993;88:15–19.
30. Armstrong WF: Stress echocardiography for detection of coronary artery disease. Circulation 1991;84:43–49.
31. Quinones MA, Verani MS, Haichin RM, Mahmarian JJ, Suarez J, Zoghbi WA: Exercise echocardiography versus 201 TI single-photon emission computed tomography in evaluation of coronary artery disease: analysis of 292 patients. Circulation 1992;85:1026–1031.
32. Marwick TH, Nemec JJ, Pashkow FJ, Stewart WJ, Salcedo EE: Accuracy and limitations of exercise echocardiography in a routine clinical setting. J Am Coll Cardiol 1992;19:74–81.
33. Folland ED, Parisi AF, Moynihan PF, Jones DR, Feld-

man CL, Tow DE: Assessment of left ventricular ejection fraction and volumes by real-time two-dimensional echocardiography: a comparison of cineangiographic and radionuclide techniques. Circulation 1979;60:760–766.

34. Zile MR, Tanaka R, Lindrith JR, Spinale F, Carabello BA, Mirsky I: Left ventricular volume determined echocardiographically by assuming a constant left ventricular epicardial long-axis/short-axis dimension ratio throughout the cardiac cycle. J Am Coll Cardiol 1992;20:986–993.

35. Zoghbi WA, Buckey JC, Massey MA, Blomqvist CG: Determination of left ventricular volumes with use of a new nongeometric echocardiographic method: clinical validation and potential application. J Am Coll Cardiol 1990;15:610–617.

36. Smith MD, MacPhail B, Harrison MR, Lenhoff SJ, DeMaria AN: Value and limitations of transesophageal echocardiography in determination of left ventricular volumes and ejection fraction. J Am Coll Cardiol 1992;19:1213–1222.

37. Gordon EP, Schnittger I, Fitzgerald PJ, Williams P, Popp RI: Reproducibility of left ventricular volumes by two-dimensional echocardiography. J Am Coll Cardiol 1983;2:506–513.

38. Nessly ML, Bashein G, Detmer PR, Graham MM, Kao R, Martin RW: Left ventricular ejection fraction: single-plane and multiplanar transesophageal echocardiography versus equilibrium gated-pool scintigraphy. J Cardiothorac Vasc Anesth 1991;5:40–45.

39. Schiller NB, Maurer G, Ritter SB, et al: Transesophageal echocardiography. J Am Soc Echocardiogr 1989;2:354–357.

40. Reichek N, Helak J, Plappert T, Sutton MS, Weber KT: Anatomic validation of left ventricular mass estimates from clinical two-dimensional echocardiography: initial results. Circulation 1983;67:348–352.

41. Handschumacher MD, Lethor J-P, Siu SC, et al: A new integrated system for three-dimensional echocardiographic reconstruction: development and validation for ventricular volume with application in human subjects. J Am Coll Cardiol 1993;21:743–753.

42. Gopal AS, Keller AM, Rigling R, King DLJ, King DL: Left ventricular volume and endocardial surface area by three-dimensional echocardiography: comparison with two-dimensional echocardiography and nuclear magnetic resonance imaging in normal subjects. J Am Coll Cardiol 1993;22:258–270.

43. Mirsky I, Cohn PF, Levine JA, Gorlin R, Herman MV, Kreulen TH, Sonnenblick EH: Assessment of left ventricular stiffness in primary myocardial disease and coronary artery disease. Circulation 1974;50:128–136.

44. Gaasch WH, Zile MR, Hoshino PK, Apstein CS, Blaustein AS: Stress-shortening relations and myocardial blood flow in compensated and failing canine hearts with pressure-overload hypertrophy. Circulation 1989;79:872–883.

45. Reichek N, Wilson J, St-John SM, Plappert TA, Goldberg S, Hirshfeld JW: Noninvasive determination of left ventricular end-systolic stress: validation of the method and initial application. Circulation 1982;65:99–108.

46. Douglas PS, Reichek N, Plappert T, Muhammad A, St. John-Sutton MG: Comparison of echocardiographic methods for assessment of left ventricular shortening and wall stress. J Am Coll Cardiol 1987;9:945–951.

47. St. John-Sutton MG, Plappert TA, Hirshfeld JW, Reichek N: Assessment of left ventricular mechanics in patients with asymptomatic aortic regurgitation: a two-dimensional echocardiographic study. Circulation 1984;69:259–268.

48. Lewis JF, Kuo LC, Nelson JG, Limacher MC, Quinones MA: Pulsed Doppler echocardiographic determination of stroke volume and cardiac output: clinical validation of two methods using the apical window. Circulation 1984;70:425–431.

49. Bouchard A, Blumlein S, Schiller NB, et al: Measurement of left ventricular stroke volume using continuous wave Doppler echocardiography of the ascending aorta and M-mode echocardiography of the aortic valve. J Am Coll Cardiol 1987;9:75–83.

50. Otto CM, Pearlman AS, Gardner CL, et al: Experimental validation of Doppler echocardiographic measurement of volume flow through the stenotic aortic valve. Circulation 1988;78:435–441.

51. Burwash IG, Otto CM, Pearlman AS: Use of Doppler-derived left ventricular time intervals for noninvasive assessment of systolic function. Am J Cardiol 1993;72:1331–1333.

52. Sjoberg BJ, Ask P, Loyd D, Wranne B: Subaortic flow profiles in aortic valve disease: a two-dimensional color Doppler study. J Am Soc Echocardiogr 1994;7:276–285.

53. Fisher DC, Sahn DJ, Friedman MJ, Larson D, et al: The mitral valve orifice method for noninvasive two-dimensional echo Doppler determinations of cardiac output. Circulation 1983;67:872–877.

54. Yoganathan AP: Fluid mechanics of aortic stenosis. Eur Heart J 1988;9:13–17.

55. Holen J, Aaslid R, Landmark K, Simonsen S: Determination of pressure gradient in mitral stenosis with a non-invasive ultrasound Doppler technique. Acta Med Scand 1976;199:455–460.

56. Hatle L, Angelsen B, Tromsdal A: Noninvasive assessment of atrioventricular pressure half-time by Doppler ultrasound. Circulation 1979;60:1096–1104.

57. Hatle L, Angelsen A, Tromsdal A: Noninvasive assessment of aortic stenosis by Doppler ultrasound. Br Heart J 1980;43:284–292.

58. Currie PJ, Seward JB, Reeder GS, et al: Continuous-wave Doppler echocardiographic assessment of severity of calcific aortic stenosis: a simultaneous Doppler-catheter correlative study in 100 adult patients. Circulation 1985;71:1162–1169.

59. Smith MD, Dawson PL, Elion JL, et al: Correlation of continuous wave Doppler velocities with cardiac catheterization gradients: an experimental model of aortic stenosis. J Am Coll Cardiol 1985;6:1306–1314.

60. Nishimura RA, Tajik AJ: Quantitative hemodynamics by Doppler echocardiography: a noninvasive alternative to cardiac catheterization. Prog Cardiovasc Dis 1994;36:309–342.

61. Callahan MJ, Tajik AJ, SuFan Q, Bove AA: Validation of instantaneous pressure gradients measured by continuous wave Doppler in experimentally induced aortic stenosis. Am J Cardiol 1985; 56:989–993.

62. Flachskampf FA, Weyman AE, Guerrero JL, Thomas JD: Influence of orifice geometry and flow rate on effective valve area: an in vitro study. J Am Coll Cardiol 1990;15:1173–1180.

63. Segal J, Lerner DJ, Miller DC, Mitchell RS, Alderman EA, Popp RL: When should Doppler-determined valve area be better than the Gorlin formula? Variation in hydraulic constants in low flow states. J Am Coll Cardiol 1987;9:1294–1305.

64. Burwash IG, Thomas DD, Sadahiro M, et al: Dependence of Gorlin formula and continuity equation valve areas on transvalvular volume flow rate in valvular aortic stenosis. Circulation 1994;89:827–835.

65. Burwash IG, Pearlman AS, Kraft CD, Miyake-Hull C, Healy NL, Otto CM: Flow dependence of measures of aortic stenosis severity during exercise. J Am Coll Cardiol 1994;24:1342–1350.

66. Casale PN, Palacios IF, Abascal VM, et al: Effects of dobutamine on Gorlin and continuity equation valve areas and valve resistance in valvular aortic stenosis. Am J Cardiol 1992;70:1175–1179.

67. Cochrane T, Kenyon CJ, Lawford PV, Black MM, Chambers JB, Sprigings DC: Validation of the orifice formula for estimating effective heart valve opening area. Clin Phys Physiol Meas 1991;12:21–37.

68. Montarello JK, Perakis AC, Rosenthal E, et al: Normal and stenotic human aortic valve opening: in vitro assessment of orifice area changes with flow. Eur Heart J 1990;11:484–491.

69. Tardif JC, Rodrigues AG, Hardy JF, et al: Simultaneous determination of aortic valve area by the Gorlin formula and by transesophageal echocardiography under different transvalvular flow conditions: evidence that anatomic aortic valve area does not change with variations in flow in aortic stenosis. J Am Coll Cardiol 1997;29:1296–1302.

70. Badano L, Cassottano P, Bertoli D, Carratino L, Lucatti A, Spirito P: Changes in effective aortic valve area during ejection in adults with aortic stenosis. Am J Cardiol 1996;78:1023–1028.

71. Bermejo J, Garcia Fernandez MA, Torrecilla EG, et al: Effects of dobutamine on Doppler echocardiographic indexes of aortic stenosis. J Am Coll Cardiol 1996;28:1206–1213.

72. Smith MD, Kwan OL, DeMaria AN: Value and limitations of continuous-wave Doppler echocardiography in estimating severity of valvular stenosis. JAMA 1986;255:3145–3151.

73. Kim KS, Maxted W, Nanda NC, et al: Comparison of multiplane and biplane transesophageal echocardiography in the assessment of aortic stenosis. Am J Cardiol 1997;79:436–441.

74. Cormier B, Iung B, Porte JM, Barbant S, Vahanian A: Value of multiplane transesophageal echocardiography in determining aortic valve area in aortic stenosis. Am J Cardiol 1996;77:882–885.

75. Tribouilloy C, Shen WF, Peltier M, Mirode A, Rey JL, Lesbre JP: Quantitation of aortic valve area in aortic stenosis with multiplane transesophageal echocardiography: comparison with monoplane transesophageal approach. Am Heart J 1994;128:526–532.

76. Stoddard MF, Hammons RT, Longaker RA: Doppler transesophageal echocardiographic determination of aortic valve area in adults with aortic stenosis. Am Heart J 1996;132:337–342.

77. Galan A, Zoghbi WA, Quinones MA: Determination of severity of valvular aortic stenosis by Doppler echocardiography and relation of findings to clinical outcome and agreement with hemodynamic measurements determined at cardiac catheterization. Am J Cardiol 1991;67:1007–1012.

78. Otto CM, Nishimura RA, Davis KB, Kisslo KB, Bashore TM: Balloon Valvuloplasty Registry Echocardiographers: Doppler echocardiographic findings in adults with severe symptomatic valvular aortic stenosis. Am J Cardiol 1991;68:1477–1484.

79. Otto CM, Pearlman AS, Gardner CL: Hemodynamic progression of aortic stenosis in adults assessed by Doppler echocardiography. J Am Coll Cardiol 1989;13:545–550.

80. Roger VL, Tajik AJ, Bailey KR, Oh JK, Taylor CL, Seward JB: Progression of aortic stenosis in adults: new appraisal using Doppler echocardiography. Am Heart J 1990;119:331–338.

81. Oh JK, Taliercio CP, Holmes DRJ, et al: Prediction of the severity of aortic stenosis by Doppler aortic valve area determination: prospective Doppler-catheterization correlation in 100 patients. J Am Coll Cardiol 1988;11:1227–1234.

82. Libanoff AJ, Rodbard S: Atrioventricular pressure half-time: measure of mitral valve orifice area. Circulation 1968;38:144–150.

83. Thomas JD, Weyman AE: Doppler mitral pressure half-time: a clinical tool in search of theoretical justification. J Am Coll Cardiol 1987;10:923–929.

84. Holen J, Aaslid R, Landmark K, Simonsen S, Ostrem T: Determination of effective orifice area in mitral stenosis from non-invasive ultrasound Doppler data and mitral flow rate. Acta Med Scand 1977;201:83–88.

85. Knutsen KM, Bae EA, Sivertssen E, Grendahl H: Doppler ultrasound in mitral stenosis: assessment of pressure gradient and atrioventricular pressure half-time. Acta Med Scand 1982;211:433–436.

86. Thomas JD, Wilkins GT, Choong CY, et al: Inaccuracy of mitral pressure half-time immediately after percutaneous mitral valvotomy: dependence on transmitral gradient and left atrial and ventricular compliance. Circulation 1988;78:980–993.

87. Braverman AC, Thomas JD, Lee RT: Doppler echocardiographic estimation of mitral valve area during changing hemodynamic conditions. Am J Cardiol 1991;68:1485–1490.

88. Grayburn PA, Handshoe R, Smith MD, Harrison MR, DeMaria AN: Quantitative assessment of the hemodynamic consequences of aortic regurgitation by means of continuous wave Doppler recordings. J Am Coll Cardiol 1987;10:135–135.

89. Otto CM, Pearlman AS, Gardner CL, Kraft CD, Fujioka MC: Simplification of the Doppler continuity equation for calculating stenotic aortic valve area. J Am Soc Echocardiogr 1988;1:155–157.

90. Zoghbi WA, Galan A, Quinones MA: Accurate assessment of aortic stenosis severity by Doppler echocardiography independent of aortic jet velocity. Am Heart J 1988;116:855–863.

91. Ford LE, Feldman T, Carroll JD: Valve resistance. Circulation 1994;89:893–895.

92. Ford LE, Feldman T, Chiu YC, Carroll JD: Hemodynamic resistance as a measure of functional impairment in aortic valvular stenosis. Circ Res 1990;66:1–7.

93. Cannon JDJ, Zile MR, Crawford FAJ, Carabello BA: Aortic valve resistance as an adjunct to the Gorlin formula in assessing the severity of aortic stenosis in symptomatic patients. J Am Coll Cardiol 1992;20:1517–1523.

94. Beyer RW, Olmos A, Bermudez RF, Noll HE: Mitral valve resistance as a hemodynamic indicator in mitral stenosis. Am J Cardiol 1992;69:775–779.

95. Voelker W, Berner A, Regele B, et al: Effect of exercise on valvular resistance in patients with mitral stenosis. J Am Coll Cardiol 1993;22:777–782.

96. Laskey WK, Kussmaul WG, Noordergraaf A: Valvular and systemic arterial hemodynamics in aortic

valve stenosis: a model-based approach. Circulation 1995;92:1473–1478.

97. Bolger AF, Eigler NL, Pfaff JM, Resser KJ, Maurer G: Computer analysis of Doppler color flow mapping images for quantitative assessment of in vitro fluid jets. J Am Coll Cardiol 1988;12:450–457.

98. Krabill KA, Sung HW, Tamura T, Chung KJ, Yoganathan AP, Sahn DJ: Factors influencing the structure and shape of stenotic and regurgitant jets: an in vitro investigation using Doppler color flow mapping and optical flow visualization. J Am Coll Cardiol 1989;13:1672–1681.

99. Simpson IA, Valdes-Cruz LM, Sahn DJ, Murillo A, Tamura T, Chung KJ: Doppler color flow mapping of simulated in vitro regurgitant jets: evaluation of the effects of orifice size and hemodynamic variables. J Am Coll Cardiol 1989;13:1195–1207.

100. Stevenson JG: Comparison of several noninvasive methods for estimation of pulmonary artery pressure. J Am Soc Echocardiogr 1989;2:157–171.

101. Spain MG, Smith MD, Grayburn PA, Harlamert EA, DeMaria AN: Quantitative assessment of mitral regurgitation by Doppler color flow imaging: angiographic and hemodynamic correlations. J Am Coll Cardiol 1989;13:585–590.

102. Klein AL, Burstow DJ, Tajik AJ, et al: Age-related prevalence of valvular regurgitation in normal subjects: a comprehensive color flow examination of 118 volunteers. J Am Soc Echocardiogr 1990;3:54–63.

103. Tribouilloy C, Shen WF, Qu Rey JL, Choquet D, Dufoss, Lesbre JP: Assessment of severity of mitral regurgitation by measuring regurgitant jet width at its origin with transesophageal Doppler color flow imaging. Circulation 1992;85:1248–1253.

104. Enriquez-Sarano M, Tajik AJ, Bailey KR, Seward JB: Color flow imaging compared with quantitative Doppler assessment of severity of mitral regurgitation: influence of eccentricity of jet and mechanism of regurgitation. J Am Coll Cardiol 1993;21:1211–1219 [published erratum appears in J Am Coll Cardiol 1993;22:342].

105. Taylor AL, Eichhorn EJ, Brickner ME, Eberhart RC, Grayburn PA: Aortic valve morphology: an important in vitro determinant of proximal regurgitant jet width by Doppler color flow mapping. J Am Coll Cardiol 1990;16:405–412.

106. Veyrat C, Lessana A, Abitbol G, Ameur A, Benaim R, Kalmanson D: New indexes for assessing aortic regurgitation with two-dimensional Doppler echocardiographic measurement of the regurgitant aortic valvular area. Circulation 1983;68:998–1005.

107. Smith MD, Harrison MR, Pinton R, Kandil H, Kwan OL, DeMaria AN: Regurgitant jet size by transesophageal compared with transthoracic Doppler color flow imaging. Circulation 1991;83:79–86.

108. Chen C, Rodriguez L, Guerrero JL, et al: Noninvasive estimation of the instantaneous first derivative of left ventricular pressure using continuous-wave Doppler echocardiography. Circulation 1991;83:2101–2110.

109. Thomas JD, Weyman AE: Echocardiographic Doppler evaluation of left ventricular diastolic function: physics and physiology. Circulation 1991;84:977–990.

110. Cape EG, Yoganathan AP, Weyman AE, Levine RA: Adjacent solid boundaries alter the size of regurgitant jets on Doppler color flow maps. J Am Coll Cardiol 1991;17:1094–1102.

111. Rokey R, Sterling LL, Zoghbi WA, et al: Determination of regurgitant fraction in isolated mitral or aortic regurgitation by pulsed Doppler two-dimensional echocardiography. J Am Coll Cardiol 1986;7:1273–1278.

112. Ascah KJ, Stewart WJ, Jiang L, et al: A Doppler-two-dimensional echocardiographic method for quantitation of mitral regurgitation. Circulation 1985;72:377–383.

113. Kitabatake A, Ito H, Inoue M, et al: A new approach to noninvasive evaluation of aortic regurgitant fraction by two-dimensional Doppler echocardiography. Circulation 1985;72:523–529.

114. Gardin JM, Drayer JI, Weber M, et al: Doppler echocardiographic assessment of left ventricular systolic and diastolic function in mild hypertension. Hypertension 1987;9:6.

115. Harrison MR, Clifton GD, Pennell AT, DeMaria AN: Effect of heart rate on left ventricular diastolic transmitral flow velocity patterns assessed by Doppler echocardiography in normal subjects. Am J Cardiol 1991;67:622–627.

116. Berk MR, Xie G, Kwan OL, et al: Reduction of left ventricular preload by lower body negative pressure alters Doppler transmitral filling patterns. J Am Coll Cardiol 1990;16:1387–1392.

117. Choong CY, Abascal VM, Thomas JD, et al: Combined influence of ventricular loading and relaxation on the transmitral flow velocity profile in dogs measured by Doppler echocardiography. Circulation 1988;78:672–683.

118. Dabestani A, Takenaka K, Allen B, et al: Effects of spontaneous respiration on diastolic left ventricular filling assessed by pulsed Doppler echocardiography. Am J Cardiol 1988;61:1356–1358.

119. Touche T, Prasquier R, Nitenberg A, de Zuttere D, Gourgon R: Assessment and follow-up of patients with aortic regurgitation by an updated Doppler echocardiographic measurement of the regurgitant fraction in the aortic arch. Circulation 1985;72:819–824.

120. Boughner DR: Assessment of aortic insufficiency by transcutaneous Doppler ultrasound. Circulation 1975;52:874–879.

121. Takenaka K, Dabestani A, Gardin JM, Russell D, Clark S, Allfie A, Henry WL: A simple Doppler echocardiographic method for estimating severity of aortic regurgitation. Am J Cardiol 1986;57:1340–1343.

122. Jenni R, Ritter M, Eberli F, Grimm J, Krayenbuehl HP: Quantification of mitral regurgitation with amplitude-weighted mean velocity from continuous wave Doppler spectra. Circulation 1989;79:1294–1299.

123. Labovitz AJ, Ferrara RP, Kern MJ, Bryg RJ, Mrosek DG, Williams GA: Quantitative evaluation of aortic insufficiency by continuous wave Doppler echocardiography. J Am Coll Cardiol 1986;8:1341–1347.

124. Teague SM, Heinsimer JA, Anderson JL, et al: Quantification of aortic regurgitation utilizing continuous wave Doppler ultrasound. J Am Coll Cardiol 1986;8:592–599.

125. Masuyama T, Kodama K, Kitabatake A, et al: Noninvasive evaluation of aortic regurgitation by continuous-wave Doppler echocardiography. Circulation 1986;73:460–466.

126. Mulvagh S, Quinones MA, Kleiman NS, Cheirif J, Zoghbi WA: Estimation of left ventricular end-diastolic pressure from Doppler transmitral flow veloc-

ity in cardiac patients independent of systolic performance. J Am Coll Cardiol 1992;20:112–119.

127. Pai RG, Bansal RC, Shah PM: Doppler-derived rate of left ventricular pressure rise: its correlation with the postoperative left ventricular function in mitral regurgitation. Circulation 1990;82:514–520.

128. Chen C, Rodriguez L, Lethor JP, et al: Continuous wave Doppler echocardiography for non-invasive assessment of left ventricular dP/dt and relaxation time constant from mitral regurgitant spectra in patients. J Am Coll Cardiol 1994;23:970–976.

129. Chen C, Rodriguez L, Levine RA, Weyman AE, Thomas JD: Noninvasive measurement of the time constant of left ventricular relaxation using the continuous-wave Doppler velocity profile of mitral regurgitation. Circulation 1992;86:272–278.

130. Vandervoort P, Thomas JD: New approaches to quantitation of valvular regurgitation. *In* Otto CM, ed. The Practice of Clinical Echocardiography. Philadelphia: WB Saunders, 1997:307–326.

131. Cape EG, Skoufis EG, Weyman AE, Yoganathan AP, Levine RA: A new method for noninvasive quantification of valvular regurgitation based on conservation of momentum: in vitro validation. Circulation 1989;79:1343–1353.

132. Recusani F, Bargiggia GS, Yoganathan AP, et al: A new method for quantification of regurgitant flow rate using color Doppler flow imaging of the flow convergence region proximal to a discrete orifice: an in vitro study. Circulation 1991;83:594–604.

133. Utsunomiya T, Ogawa T, Doshi R, et al: Doppler color flow "proximal isovelocity surface area" method for estimating volume flow rate: effects of orifice shape and machine factors. J Am Coll Cardiol 1991;17:1103–1111 [published erratum appears in J Am Coll Cardiol 1993;21:1537].

134. Vandervoort PM, Rivera JM, Mele D, et al: Application of color Doppler flow mapping to calculate effective regurgitant orifice area: an in vitro study and initial clinical observations. Circulation 1993;88:1150–1156.

135. Giesler M, Grossmann G, Schmidt A, et al: Color Doppler echocardiographic determination of mitral regurgitant flow from the proximal velocity profile of the flow convergence region. Am J Cardiol 1993;71:217–224.

136. Chen C, Koschyk D, Brockhoff C, et al: Noninvasive estimation of regurgitant flow rate and volume in patients with mitral regurgitation by Doppler color mapping of accelerating flow field. J Am Coll Cardiol 1993;21:374–383.

137. Reimold SC, Byrne JG, Caguioa ES, et al: Load dependence of the effective regurgitant orifice area in a sheep model of aortic regurgitation. J Am Coll Cardiol 1991;18:1085–1090.

138. Nishimura RA, Abel MD, Hatle LK, Tajik AJ: Assessment of diastolic function of the heart: background and current applications of Doppler echocardiography. Part II: clinical studies. Mayo Clin Proc 1989;64:181–204.

139. Spirito P, Maron BJ, Bonow RO: Noninvasive assessment of left ventricular diastolic function: comparative analysis of Doppler echocardiographic and radionuclide angiographic techniques. J Am Coll Cardiol 1986;7:518–526.

140. Friedman BJ, Drinkovic N, Miles H, Shih W-J, Mazzoleni A, DeMaria AN: Assessment of left ventricular diastolic function: comparison of Doppler echocardiography and gated blood pool scintigraphy. J Am Coll Cardiol 1986;8:1348–1354.

141. Rokey R, Kuo LC, Zoghbi WA, Limacher MC, Quinones MA: Determination of parameters of left ventricular diastolic filling with pulsed Doppler echocardiography: comparison with cineangiography. Circulation 1985;71:543–550.

142. Stoddard MF, Pearson AC, Kern MJ, Ratcliff J, Mrosek DG, Labovitz AJ: Influence of alteration in preload on the pattern of left ventricular diastolic filling as assessed by Doppler echocardiography in humans. Circulation 1989;79:1226–1236.

143. Thomas JD, Choong CYP, Flachskampf FA, Weyman AE: Analysis of the early transmitral Doppler velocity curve: effect of primary physiologic changes and compensatory preload adjustment. J Am Coll Cardiol 1990;16:644–655.

144. Appleton CP: Influence of incremental changes in heart rate on mitral flow velocity: assessment in lightly sedated, conscious dogs. J Am Coll Cardiol 1991;17:227–236.

145. Zoghbi WA, Bolli R: The increasing complexity of assessing diastolic function from ventricular filling dynamics. J Am Coll Cardiol 1991;17:238–248.

146. Shrestha NK, Moreno FL, Narciso FV, Torres L, Calleja HB: Two-dimensional echocardiographic diagnosis of left-atrial thrombus in rheumatic heart disease: a clinicopathologic study. Circulation 1983;67:341–347.

147. Chiang CW, Pang SC, Lin FC, Fang BR, Kuo CT, Lee YS, Chang CH: Diagnostic accuracy of two-dimensional echocardiography for detection of left atrial thrombus in patients with mitral stenosis. J Ultrasound Med 1987;6:525–529.

148. Bansal RC, Heywood JT, Applegate PM, Jutzy KR: Detection of left atrial thrombi by two-dimensional echocardiography and surgical correlation in 148 patients with mitral valve disease. Am J Cardiol 1989;64:243–246.

149. Aschenberg W, Schluter M, Kremer P, Schroder E, Siglow V, Bleifeld W: Transesophageal two-dimensional echocardiography for the detection of left atrial appendage thrombus. J Am Coll Cardiol 1986;7:163–166.

150. Olson JD, Goldenberg IF, Pedersen W, et al: Exclusion of atrial thrombus by transesophageal echocardiography. J Am Soc Echocardiogr 1992; 5:52–56.

151. Kitabatake A, Inoue M, Asao M, et al: Noninvasive evaluation of pulmonary hypertension by a pulsed Doppler technique. Circulation 1983;58:302–309.

152. Stevenson JG, Kawabori I, Guntheroth WG: Noninvasive estimation of peak pulmonary artery pressure by M-mode echocardiography. J Am Coll Cardiol 1984;4:1021–1027.

153. Isobe M, Yazaki Y, Takaku F, et al: Prediction of pulmonary arterial pressure in adults by pulsed Doppler echocardiography. Am J Cardiol 1986;57:316–321.

154. Lee RT, Lord CP, Plappert T, St John Sutton M: Prospective Doppler echocardiographic evaluation of pulmonary artery diastolic pressure in the medical intensive care unit. Am J Cardiol 1989;64:1366–1370.

155. Yock PG, Popp RL: Noninvasive estimation of right ventricular systolic pressure by Doppler ultrasound in patients with tricuspid regurgitation. Circulation 1984;70:657–662.

156. Berger M, Haimowitz A, Van TA, Berdoff RL, Goldberg E: Quantitative assessment of pulmonary hypertension in patients with tricuspid regurgitation

using continuous wave Doppler ultrasound. J Am Coll Cardiol 1985;6:359–365.

157. Simonson JS, Schiller NB: Sonospirometry: a new method for noninvasive estimation of mean right atrial pressure based on two-dimensional echocardiographic measurements of the inferior vena cava during measured inspiration. J Am Coll Cardiol 1988;11:557–564.

158. Kircher BJ, Himelman RB, Schiller NB: Noninvasive estimation of right atrial pressure from the inspiratory collapse of the inferior vena cava. Am J Cardiol 1990;66:493–496.

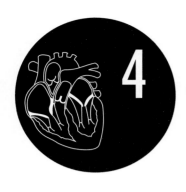

4 Cardiac Catheterization and Angiography for Evaluation of Valvular Disease

For most patients with valvular heart disease, information derived from the history, physical examination, and echocardiographic assessment is adequate for clinical decision making, including referral for valvular surgery.[1-4] However, cardiac catheterization continues to play an important diagnostic role for selected patients with valvular disease. First, in some cases, some additional information can only be acquired by cardiac catheterization. For example, coronary angiography may be needed for evaluation of concurrent coronary disease in the patient undergoing aortic valve replacement. Second, complex disease may best be evaluated by integration of data from echocar-

diography and cardiac catheterization. For the patient with multivalve disease, Doppler echocardiography often provides adequate evaluation of regurgitant severity, but catheterization is needed for calculation of pulmonary vascular resistance. Third, the quality of echocardiographic data depends on ultrasound tissue penetration, which is limited in some patients because of body habitus or coexisting lung disease and which can result in suboptimal data or nondiagnostic study results. Although transesophageal imaging offers improved image quality, quantitation of disease severity may be limited by difficulties in parallel alignment of the Doppler beam. Fourth, cardiac catheterization may help resolve significant discrepancies between the clinical assessment and echocardiographic data or be useful when disease severity is uncertain (Table 4–1).

As with any diagnostic technique, the accuracy of data obtained at cardiac catheterization depends on careful attention to methodology and technical details and on an understanding of the physiologic variables that may affect the recorded data. When echocardiographic and catheterization data diverge, the clinician should examine the original data from both studies, including the quality of the recorded data, the accuracy of measurements and calculations, and the interpretation of the findings (Table 4–2).[5] Apparent discrepancies between these two techniques often disappear when suboptimal data are disregarded and errors in measurement or interpretation are eliminated.

EVALUATION OF LEFT VENTRICULAR SYSTOLIC FUNCTION

Evaluation of left ventricular (LV) systolic function typically includes ventriculography, calculation of cardiac output, and measurement of LV pressures throughout the cardiac cycle. Although LV systolic function is best

TABLE 4·2 POTENTIAL SOURCES OF ERROR IN EVALUATION OF VALVULAR HEART DISEASE AT CATHETERIZATION

Pressure Data

Frequency response
Side-hole vs end-hole catheters
Catheter whip and impact artifacts
Signal damping
Calibration and zero
Recorder sweep speed and scale
Peripheral amplification

Cardiac Output

Fick
   Measurement of O_2 consumption
   Timing of arterial and venous O_2 samples
   Site of arterial and venous sampling
Thermodilution
   Uneven mixing of injectate within right atrium
    (tricuspid regurgitation)
   Poor accuracy at low outputs (extrapolation of curve)

Angiography

Geometric assumptions
Endocardial border identification
Catheter positioning
Cardiac rhythm

Valve Area Calculations

Transvalvular volume flow rate
Pressure measurements
Empiric constant

TABLE 4·1 PROTOCOL FOR EVALUATION OF VALVULAR HEART DISEASE AT CARDIAC CATHETERIZATION

Pressure Measurements

Right heart
Left ventricle
Left atrium (for mitral stenosis evaluation)
Aorta
Transvalvular gradients—simultaneous pressure recordings on both sides of stenotic valve

Cardiac Output

Thermodilution or Fick method (simultaneous with transvalvular gradient)

Angiography

Left ventricle—EDV, ESV, SV, ejection fraction
Aortic root—for evaluation of AR
Coronary—for assessment of coexisting coronary artery disease

Calculated Values

Valve areas—Gorlin and Gorlin formula; use transvalvular volume flow rate
Pulmonary vascular resistance
Systemic vascular resistance
Regurgitant volume and fraction

EDV, end diastolic volume; ESV, end-systolic volume; SV, stroke volume; AR, aortic regurgitation.

described in terms of contractility, defined as the intrinsic ability of the myocardium to shorten independent of loading conditions, measurement of contractility in the clinical setting is problematic. Most conventional measures of LV systolic function depend on ventricular preload and afterload and on myocardial contractility. Increased preload, defined as LV end-diastolic volume or pressure, increases myocardial shortening as described by the Frank-Starling relationship. Afterload, defined as the resistance or impedance to LV ejection, is inversely related to myocardial shortening. Loading conditions frequently are altered in patients with valvular disease (eg, increased afterload with aortic stenosis, increased preload with aortic regurgitation), complicating evaluation of LV systolic function.

Angiographic Volumes and Ejection Fraction

LV end-diastolic volumes (EDV) and end-systolic volumes (ESV) can be calculated by tracing the respective endocardial boundaries on angiographic images and applying a validated geometric formula for volume calculation (Figs. 4–1 and 4–2, Table 4–3). Stroke volume (SV) is calculated as

$$SV = EDV - ESV$$

and ejection fraction (EF) as

$$EF = \frac{SV}{EDV}$$

The stroke volume (or cardiac output when multiplied by heart rate) calculated by angiography represents the total amount of blood ejected by the ventricle, whether that blood is ejected forward into the aorta or backward into the left atrium across an incompetent mitral valve. Angiographic stroke volume often is called *total stroke volume.*

The geometric formulas for angiographic calculation of volume (V) typically assume a prolate ellipsoid shape of the left ventricle. Endocardial border tracings from two orthogonal views of the ventricle (ie, right and left anterior oblique projections) are used to measure the area (A) and length (L) of the ventricle, with the minor axis diameter (D) calculated for each view as

$$D = \left(\frac{4A}{\pi L}\right)$$

Calculated ventricular volume (V_c) is derived as follows:

$$V_c = \left(\frac{\pi}{6}\right)(L \times D_a \times D_b)$$

In the equation, D_a and D_b are the minor axis dimensions in the two orthogonal views.

In the clinical setting, a single plane right anterior oblique angiogram using the modified formula of Dodge and Sandler[6] also provides acceptable results:

$$V_c = \frac{(8A^2)}{(3\pi L)} \ or \ V_c = \left(\frac{\pi}{6}\right)(LD^2)$$

Although angiography and echocardiography depend on manual border tracing by an experienced observer, a slight but consistent overestimation of LV volumes by angiography is caused by contrast filling the ventricular trabeculations so that the traced endocardial border represents the outer edge of the myocardial trabeculations.[7–9] The volume occupied by the papillary muscles (which are excluded from the endocardial border tracing) also should be taken into account. Regression equations have been derived[6, 7, 9–11] to correct for the overestimation of volume on angiography resulting from these two factors:

$$V = 0.81 \ V_c + 1.9$$

In this equation, V_c is the calculated volume and V is the corrected volume. In contrast, on echocardiography, ultrasound is reflected from the inner edge of the myocardial trabeculations so that volume tends to be underestimated slightly.

With careful angiographic technique, tracing of endocardial borders by an experienced observer, and use of appropriate correction factors, ventricular volumes derived from angi-

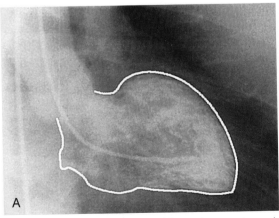
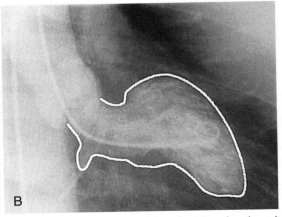

Figure 4·1 In a right anterior oblique view, angiography of the left ventricle shows end-diastolic *(A)* and end-systolic volumes *(B)*. The endocardial borders are traced for calculation of the left ventricular volumes.

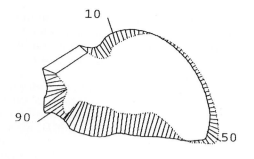

Measure	Value	Value/BSA
EDV (cc)	133.63	74.48
ESV (cc)	74.20	41.35
SV (cc)	59.43	33.12
CO (L/min)	5.94	3.31
Mass (g)	0.00	0.00
RRI (sec)	0.60	
HR (bpm)	100.00	
EF	0.44	
BSA (m^2)	1.79	
LV Vol = (RAO VOL)*0.81+1.9		

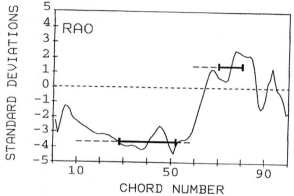

Region of interest (ROI):
                    L territory
  No. of vessels diseased: 3

  Hypokinesis in ROI, SD: −3.66
  Hyperkin. opposite ROI: 1.47

Percent of chords in LV contour
  with hypokinesis <−1 SD: 68
  with hyperkinesis >1 SD: 15
  with akinesis/dyskinesis: 37

Figure 4·2 Method for calculating the left ventricular volume and ejection fraction from a single-plane right anterior oblique left ventricular angiogram. BSA, body surface area; CO, cardiac output; EDV, end-diastolic volume; EF, ejection fraction; ESV, end-systolic volume, HR, heart rate; LV, left ventricle; RRI, R-R interval; SD, standard deviation; SV, stroke volume. (Courtesy of Florence Sheehan, M.D., University of Washington, Seattle, WA.)

ography correlate well with directly measured volumes and with echocardiographic volumes (Fig. 4–3).[8, 10, 12, 13] A biplane imaging approach[7, 9] using borders traced from right and left anterior oblique radiographic projections provides accurate results with a mean difference for measurement variability of 6 to 10 mL for end-systolic and 7 to 20 mL for end-diastolic volumes,[14–16] although the intertest variability is higher.[17]

Technical factors important in performing ventricular angiography include the need for complete opacification of the ventricle and clear definition of the endocardial borders at end-diastole and end-systole.[17, 18] This requires use of a 6, 7, or 8 French side-hole pigtail catheter and a power contrast injector using an injection rate and volume appropriate to the type of catheter, ventricular size, and hemodynamics. A nonionic contrast agent is optimal in patients with valvular disease to avoid

myocardial depression or hemodynamic changes. Correct positioning of the catheter in the middle of the ventricle is needed for complete opacification of the chamber to prevent movement of the catheter during the contrast injection and to minimize the risk of arrhythmias. Optimal catheter positioning also avoids artifactual mitral regurgitation caused by entrapment of the catheter in the mitral apparatus. A correction factor for the effect of magnification must be used for accurate volume determination. One method films a calibrated grid at the estimated level of the ventricle. Other factors that affect the accuracy and reproducibility of angiographic volumes include image quality, the experience of the individual tracing the endocardial borders, cardiac rhythm, and the potential cardiodepressant effect of the contrast agent.

LV mass can be determined angiographically based on the thickness (h) of the anterior

TABLE 4·3   NORMAL VALUES AT CARDIAC CATHETERIZATION FOR SUPINE, RESTING ADULTS

Angiographic Left Ventricular Volumes[17]	Mean ± 1 SD
End-diastolic volume	70 ± 20 mL/m²
End-systolic volume	24 ± 10 mL/m²
Ejection fraction	0.67 ± 0.08
LV mass	92 ± 16 g/m²

Cardiac Output[78]	Mean ± 1 SD
Rest	
Age 30–39	4.48 ± 0.31 L/min/m²
Age 60–69	3.51 ± 0.61 L/min/m²
Exercise	
Age 30–39	7.61 ± 0.35 L/min/m²
Age 60–69	6.64 ± 0.49 L/min/m²
O₂ consumption (resting)[32]	126 ± 26 mL/min/m²
Arterial O₂–saturation	$97 \pm 2\%$
Venous O₂–saturation	$73 \pm 4\%$

Pressures (mm Hg)[78]	Systolic/Diastolic	Mean
Right atrium	a3–6, v1–4	1–5
Right ventricle	20–30/2–7	
Pulmonary artery	16–30/4–13	9–18
Pulmonary wedge		5–12
Left atrial	a4–14, v6–16	6–11
Left ventricular	90–140/6–12	
Aorta	90–140/70–90	70–110

Vascular Resistance[78]	Mean ± 1 SD	Indexed to Body Surface Area
Pulmonary resistance	67 ± 30	123 ± 54 dynes-sec-cm^{-5}/m²
Wood units (mm Hg-L^{-1}-min)	$0.8–1.1 \pm 0.3–0.5$	
Systemic resistance	1170 ± 270	2130 ± 450

Valve Areas (cm²)[81]	Overall	Male	Female
Aortic	4.6 ± 1.1	4.8 ± 1.3	3.7 ± 1.0
Mitral	7.8 ± 1.9	8.3 ± 2.0	6.7 ± 1.3
Tricuspid	10.6 ± 2.6	11.5 ± 2.5	8.8 ± 1.7
Pulmonic	4.7 ± 1.2	4.9 ± 1.3	4.3 ± 1.0

wall (assuming a symmetric thickness around the ventricle), ventricular diameter in anterior-posterior (D_{AP}) and lateral views (D_{lat}), long-axis length (L), and ventricular volume (V):

$$\text{LV mass (g)} = \left(\frac{4}{3}\pi \left[\frac{D_{AP}}{2} + h\right]\left[\frac{D_{lat}}{2} + h\right]\left[\frac{L}{2} + h\right] - V\right) \times 1.05$$

However, ventricular mass calculations are limited by the inaccuracy in measuring LV wall thickness from the angiographic image[19, 20] and are not widely used clinically. Similarly, although LV wall stress can be calculated on the basis of angiographic measurement of LV

dimensions and wall thickness in combination with pressure data[21, 22] analogous to the method described for echocardiography (see Chapter 3), this method is rarely used in the clinical setting.

LV angiography allows qualitative and quantitative assessment of wall motion in valvular heart disease patients with concurrent coronary artery disease.[23, 24] The differences between echocardiographic and angiographic methods should be recognized. Angiography is a silhouette technique (ie, only abnormalities at the edge of the silhouette can be identified), and echocardiography is tomographic (ie, wall motion and thickening can be evaluated for each segment). Quantitative methods for evaluation of regional ventricular function by angiography are well validated and widely used, while echocardiographic evaluation remains largely qualitative or semiquantitative. Both techniques suffer from the problems inherent in evaluation of wall motion related to translation and rotation of the heart during the cardiac cycle.

Cardiac Output Measurement

Cardiac output can be calculated at cardiac catheterization by the dilution of a known concentration of an indicator (eg, dye, oxygen,

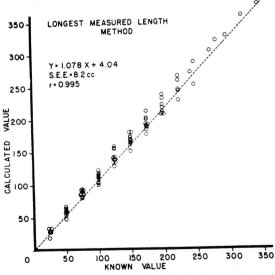

Figure 4·3 The area-length method of measuring left ventricular chamber volume was validated by comparing the volume calculated from angiograms of barium filled heart casts with the true volume of these hearts. (From Dodge HT, Sandler H, Ballew DW, Lord J Jr: The use of biplane angiocardiography for the measurement of left ventricular volume in man. Am Heart J 1960;60:752.)

cold saline) as it passes through the vascular bed. The injection of a known volume and concentration of dye (typically indocyanine green) into the venous circulation illustrates this concept. From the rate at which this dye appears in the arterial circulation, the volume of blood the dye was diluted in (ie, cardiac output) can be calculated. Although indicator dilution dye curves provide accurate cardiac output data, this method is cumbersome and depends on meticulous technique, and other methods are used in most laboratories.

Fick Technique

Oxygen serves as the indicator for cardiac output calculations in the Fick method. The Fick principle states that the uptake or release of oxygen by a tissue is the product of the amount of oxygen delivered to the tissue times the difference in oxygen content between the blood entering and leaving the tissue.[25] For the uptake of oxygen by the lungs,

$$\text{Oxygen uptake} = \text{Pulmonary blood flow} \times (O_2 \text{ content}_{PV} - O_2 \text{ content}_{PA})$$

If the amount of oxygen consumed by the patient (oxygen uptake) and the oxygen content of pulmonary arterial (PA) and pulmonary venous (PV) blood are measured, this equation can be solved for pulmonary blood flow:

$$\text{Pulmonary blood flow} = \frac{O_2 \text{ consumption}}{(O_2 \text{ content}_{PV} - O_2 \text{ content}_{PA})}$$

In the absence of an intracardiac shunt, pulmonary and systemic blood flow are equal, so that this method provides a measure of systemic (or forward) cardiac output that can be calculated as follows:

$$\text{Cardiac output} = \frac{O_2 \text{ consumption}}{[(O_2 \text{ content})_{arterial} - (O_2 \text{ content})_{venous}]}$$

In the equation, oxygen consumption is measured in milliliters of O_2 per minute and oxygen content as milliliters of O_2 per 100 mL of blood (often referred to as volume percent).

To ensure the sample of venous blood represents total venous return and that there is adequate mixing of the sample, a pulmonary artery blood sample is used for mixed systemic venous oxygen content in this equation, unless the patient has an intracardiac shunt. Although pulmonary venous blood provides the most accurate sample of oxygenated blood, the arterial sample typically is obtained from a systemic artery or the left ventricle. When the patient has an intracardiac shunt, separate calculations for systemic and pulmonary blood flow (using the appropriate arterial and venous oxygen contents) allow determination of the shunt ratio.

Oxygen consumption is measured by the polarographic O_2 method, by the breath-by-breath method using a metabolic cart, or by the Douglas bag method. The polarographic method uses a hood or face mask, with the rate of air flow through the servo unit controlled by an oxygen sensor cell to maintain a constant fractional content of oxygen. Oxygen consumption (VO_2) then is calculated from the fractional content of oxygen and flow rates of air entering and exiting the patient's mask. Although some laboratories have found this method to be accurate when performed carefully,[26] others have shown inaccuracies compared with the Douglas bag method.[27]

Oxygen consumption by the standard Douglas bag technique is based on analysis of oxygen content of room air and a timed collection of the patient's expired air. Oxygen consumption is calculated on the basis of the volume of expired air, the collection time, the oxygen content of inspired and expired air, and barometric pressure. Although this technique can be accurate, potential sources of error include incomplete air collection (leakage around the nose clip or through a perforated ear drum), failure to allow a period of equilibration to clear the dead space in the valve and tubing, and diffusion of air out of the collection bag because of an excessive delay before analysis. Both techniques for measurement of oxygen consumption assume the patient is at a steady state, specifically that there is no change in the residual volume of air in the lungs or in the patient's metabolic rate during the measurement period.

The arteriovenous oxygen difference is calculated from measurement of oxygen content in simultaneously drawn samples of arterial and mixed venous blood collected midway during the oxygen consumption measurement. Oxygen content typically is calculated as oxygen saturation times the theoretical oxygen capacity, which is estimated from the patient's hemoglobin (Hgb) level:

$$O_2 \text{ content} = \text{Hgb(g/dL)} \times 1.36 \text{ (mL } O_2/\text{g of Hgb)} \times 10 \times \% \text{ saturation}$$

For accurate cardiac output calculations, the arterial and venous oxygen samples must be collected from the correct sites with prompt processing of the samples, and oxygen consumption and content measurements are made simultaneously. Even with careful technique, the average error in measuring oxygen consumption is approximately 6%,[28] and the error in measurement of the arteriovenous oxygen difference is approximately 5%,[29, 30] resulting in an error in cardiac output measurement of about 10% by the Fick method.[31] Measurements are more inaccurate if physiologic changes that affect cardiac output, such as changes in heart rate or loading conditions, occur during the analysis period. Use of an assumed, rather than measured, oxygen consumption also leads to significant error because of the wide variation in the normal rate of oxygen consumption in adults.[32, 33] Fick cardiac outputs tend to be more accurate for low outputs, and thermodilution outputs are more accurate at high flow rates.

Thermodilution

Measurement of cardiac output by the thermodilution method is widely used in the evaluation of patients with valvular heart disease in the cardiac catheterization laboratory for quantitation of the severity of valvular disease

and in the intensive care unit for optimal hemodynamic management of the decompensated patient. With the thermodilution method, a fluid bolus of known volume and temperature is injected into the right atrium while a thermistor in the pulmonary artery continuously records temperature (Fig. 4–4). Cardiac output then is calculated from the known temperature (T) and volume (V) of the injectate and the integral of temperature over time ($\Delta T/dt$) in the pulmonary artery.[34, 35]

$$\text{Cardiac output} = \text{Constant} \left[\frac{V_{injectate} \times (T_{blood} - T_{injectate})}{(\Delta T/dt)} \right]$$

In the equation, the constant incorporates factors for the specific gravity and specific heat of blood and the injectate (1.08 if the injectate is 5% dextrose). An empiric correction factor (multiplication by 0.825) for the effect of warming of the injectate as it passes through the catheter also is needed.[36, 37]

As with the Fick technique, the thermodilution method measures the forward cardiac output, specifically the output of the right heart. Advantages of the thermodilution method include ease and repeatability, allowing multiple measurements over short time intervals with a reasonable accuracy (reproducibility of about 5% to 10% with proper technique).[36, 37] Disadvantages include relatively poor accuracy at low cardiac outputs[38, 39] and dependence on careful attention to technique, particularly avoidance of warming the injectate. Because this method depends on

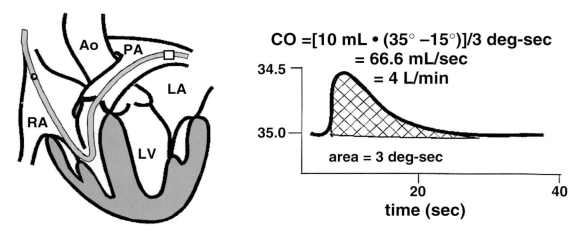

Figure 4·4 Thermodilution method for measuring cardiac output (CO). Ao, aorta; LA, left atrium; LV, left ventricle; RA, right atrium; PA, pulmonary artery.

even mixing of the injectate with the right atrial blood, thermodilution output measurements may be inaccurate when the patient has tricuspid regurgitation.

Pressures

Direct measurement of LV pressures throughout the cardiac cycle provide valuable data on LV systolic function, although the effect of concurrent valvular disease must also be taken into account (see Table 4–3). The rate of rise of LV pressure (dP/dt) during isovolumic contraction provides a relatively load-independent measure of LV systolic function, which is particularly useful for patients with altered loading conditions caused by valvular disease.

Pressure-Volume Loops

The relationship between LV pressure and volume throughout the cardiac cycle can be examined in detail by graphing instantaneous pressure (on the vertical axis) versus volume (on the horizontal axis). LV stroke volume is the distance on the horizontal axis between end-diastole and end-systole, and LV stroke work (the integral of pressure times volume over the cardiac cycle) is the area enclosed by the pressure-volume loop. When pressure-volume loops are recorded under different loading conditions, the slope of the end-systolic pressure-volume relationship, called elastance or E_{max}, provides a load-independent measure of LV systolic function. [40–46]

Valvular heart disease characterized by pressure overload of the left ventricle results in a taller pressure-volume loop that is shifted upward (see Chapter 7), reflecting the higher ventricular systolic pressures and greater LV stroke work. Volume overload of the ventricle also increases stroke work, producing a larger loop that is shifted upward and to the right. However, despite these shifts in the pressure-volume loop, the slope of the end-systolic pressure-volume relationship remains normal in patients with valvular disease and compensated ventricular systolic function. A reduced slope indicates impaired contractility superimposed on the pressure or volume overload state.

In practice, measurement of pressure-volume loops is technically demanding. Ventricular pressures must be recorded with high-fidelity catheters, and volumes must be determined at multiple points in the cardiac cycle with the use of contrast or radionuclide

angiography or experimental approaches such as a conductance catheter.[47] Although this approach provides insight into the pathophysiology of disease and provides key data in patient-based research studies, it rarely is used in the routine clinical management of patients with valvular heart disease.

EVALUATION OF STENOSIS SEVERITY
Normal and Abnormal Transvalvular Pressure-Flow Relationships
Semilunar Valves

The aortic and pulmonic valves each connect a ventricular chamber to a great vessel. Valve motion is related to characteristics of the valve leaflets and to the driving force of blood as it is ejected from the ventricular chamber. The following discussion focuses on the aortic valve, but the physiology of the pulmonic valve is similar, although with lower systolic pressures when valve function is normal.

With LV contraction, LV pressure rises rapidly during isovolumic contraction. When the LV pressure exceeds the aortic pressure, the aortic valve opens. Motion of normal cardiac valves is essentially a passive process, with the open leaflets assuming an orientation parallel to the flow stream and with valve closure caused by the adverse pressure field induced by flow deceleration.[48] Even with normal thin flexible valve leaflets, LV pressure continues to exceed aortic pressure by a slight amount in early systole as blood accelerates across the valve. The maximum pressure gradient in early systole corresponds to the maximum rate of rise in flow rate (dQ/dt) and to the maximum acceleration (steepest slope) of the Doppler velocity curve. With a normal aortic valve, the point in early systole where LV pressure falls below aortic pressure corresponds to the maximum flow rate (Q_{max}) and to the maximum Doppler velocity. Although aortic pressure is slightly higher than LV pressure in the later part of systole, blood flow continues to flow antegrade across the valve but at decreasing velocities (deceleration phase), with aortic valve closure occurring when the flow velocity falls to zero, corresponding to the dicrotic notch on the aortic pressure waveform (Fig. 4–5). Thus, normal transaortic pressure gradient and volume flow curves are asymmetric with respect to time (ie, peak early in systole) and are "out of phase" in that the maximum pressure gradient and the maximum flow rate do not occur simultaneously.[49, 50]

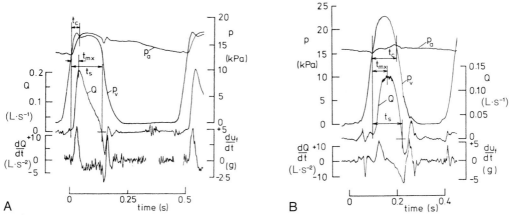

Figure 4·5 Pressures and flows measured in open-chest dogs with normal, healthy conditions *(A)* and with a moderately severe stenosis *(B)*. Acceleration (du_f/dt) was measured at the level of the flowmeter cuff. The times to maximum flow (t_{mx}) and to reversal of the pressure difference (t_c) are shown with the ejection time (t_s). The data have not been corrected for instrumentation phase shifts. Q, flow; Pa, aortic pressure; Pv, ventricular pressure. The conversion factor is 1 kPa = 7.52 mm Hg. (From Clark C: Relation between pressure difference across the aortic valve and left ventricular outflow. Cardiovasc Res 1978;12:276.)

When aortic valve stenosis is present, aortic valve opening still corresponds to the point where LV pressure first exceeds aortic pressure and, despite a reduction in total leaflet excursion, the timing and rate of aortic valve opening appear relatively normal as assessed by M-mode echocardiography. In contrast to the LV and aortic pressures seen with a normal valve, LV pressure remains higher than aortic pressure throughout systole, reflecting the additional force needed to keep the stiffened aortic valve leaflets open during the ejection period (for calcific stenosis) or to eject blood through a narrow fixed orifice (with congenital stenosis). LV and aortic pressures rise more slowly than normal, and maximum LV pressure, maximum aortic pressure, maximum transvalvular velocity, and the maximum volume flow rate (Q_{max}) all occur later in systole with a relatively symmetric ejection curve. With valvular obstruction, the pressure gradient and volume flow rate are in phase; specifically the maximum gradient and maximum flow rate occur simultaneously. During the deceleration phase of ventricular ejection, LV pressure (while declining) remains higher than aortic pressure, and aortic valve closure corresponds to the point where LV pressure falls just below aortic pressure. The magnitude of the pressure difference between the left ventricle and aorta in systole (ie, transvalvular gradient) is related to the severity of obstruction at the valvular level.

Atrioventricular Valves

The physiology of the right-sided and left-sided atrioventricular valves is similar. Because mitral stenosis is much more common than tricuspid stenosis, the following discussion focuses on the mitral valve, but the same concepts apply to the tricuspid valve.

Mitral valve opening occurs when LV pressure falls below left atrial pressure. As for the semilunar valves, valve opening appears to be a passive process, with the leaflets assuming a position parallel to the flow stream. When the mitral valve is normal, a slight pressure gradient exists between the left atrium and the left ventricle during early diastole, with equalization of pressures in mid-diastole (ie, diastasis). In mid-diastole, the leaflets move toward each other and may undulate as the flow rate decreases, but they typically do not completely close even though left atrial and LV pressures are equal and little flow occurs across the valve. After atrial contraction, atrial pressure again rises, and blood flows from the atrium to the ventricle, with a corresponding increase in the degree of leaflet separation. Valve closure occurs at the onset of LV contraction as LV pressure abruptly rises to exceed left atrial pressure, with valve closure related to the adverse pressure gradient resulting from flow deceleration.[48]

With mitral stenosis, left atrial pressure remains higher than LV pressure throughout diastole (Fig. 4–6). An increase in the trans-

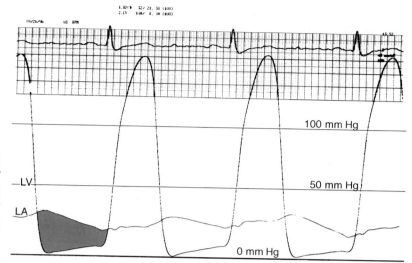

Figure 4·6 Left ventricular (LV) and left atrial (LA) pressure tracings in a 68-year-old man with symptomatic mitral stenosis. The mean transmitral pressure gradient is 19 mm Hg. The mitral valve area calculated by the Gorlin formula is 0.74 cm² and the pulmonary artery pressures are 98/40 mm Hg.

mitral pressure gradient in late diastole is seen when sinus rhythm is present because of the increase in atrial pressure after atrial contraction. As in stenosis of the semilunar valves, the magnitude of the mean diastolic pressure difference between the left atrium and left ventricle is an indicator of the degree of valvular stenosis. However, the absolute value of the pressure difference is much less than seen with semilunar valve stenosis because of the lower diastolic (compared with systolic) intracardiac pressures. As with any stenotic valve, transvalvular pressure gradients are flow dependent, increasing and decreasing as the volume flow rate across the valve increases or decreases. This effect is of particular importance for the atrioventricular valves, for which mild to moderate degrees of stenosis may be underestimated because of the difficulty in measuring the small diastolic pressure gradient. This problem can be avoided by recording the pressure gradient after increasing the transvalvular volume flow rate (ie, with exercise or pharmacologic therapy).

In evaluation of patients with mitral stenosis, venous pressure measured using a catheter occluding (or wedged in) a branch pulmonary artery often is substituted for left atrial pressure. Although this approach can provide a reasonable approximation of left atrial pressure in many cases, several technical and physiologic factors can affect the relationship between the measured "wedge pressure" and actual left atrial pressure. If an accurate measurement of the transmitral gradient is needed in a patient with mitral stenosis, direct mea-

surement of left atrial pressure by the transseptal technique is preferable.[51] If pulmonary wedge pressure is used, correct positioning of the catheter should be verified by fluoroscopy, the pressure waveform, and oxygen saturation measurements.

For the atrioventricular valves, the time course of the decline in pressure difference across the valve during the passive early diastolic phase is closely related to the severity of stenosis. The more severe the stenosis, the longer is the time interval for the initial pressure gradient to fall to one half of its initial value. Although this approach is rarely used for invasive data gathering, this concept is the basis of noninvasive evaluation of mitral valve stenosis using the pressure half-time method (see Chapter 3).[52–54]

Transvalvular Pressure Gradients
Reporting Pressure Gradients

Transvalvular pressure differences are best reported as the mean gradient averaged over the period of flow. Doppler and catheterization transvalvular mean gradients correlate well with each other if recorded simultaneously. Nonsimultaneous data also correlate closely if loading conditions and cardiac output are similar at the time of both recordings. Mean gradients are measured by averaging (by planimetry or digitally by computer) the instantaneous gradients over the flow period using meticulously recorded and correctly aligned tracings of the pressure curves on both sides of the valve (Fig. 4–7).

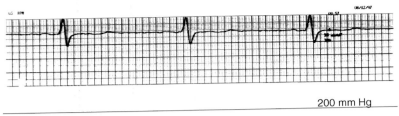

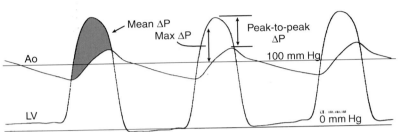

Figure 4·7 Left ventricular (LV) and aortic (Ao) pressures in a 70-year-old man with symptomatic valvular aortic stenosis. The peak-to-peak transvalvular gradient pressure is 50 mm Hg, with a mean gradient of 47 mm Hg. The aortic valve area is 0.91 cm² by the Gorlin formula, with an aortic valve index of 0.39 cm²/m².

For aortic stenosis, although the transvalvular gradient can be quickly estimated as the difference between the peak LV and peak aortic pressures, this peak-to-peak gradient may not accurately indicate stenosis severity, because these two peaks do not occur simultaneously and the pressure difference does not represent an actual gradient at any instant in time across the valve. Particularly with low gradients, the peak-to-peak gradient may underestimate the mean transvalvular gradient.

The maximum gradient (and maximum velocity) recorded by Doppler corresponds to the maximum instantaneous pressure gradient across the valve. The maximum instantaneous gradient is higher than the peak-to-peak or the mean gradient, as shown in Figure 4–7 for semilunar valves. For the atrioventricular valves, the maximum gradient at valve opening also may significantly overestimate the severity of stenosis, particularly with prosthetic valves. When pressure gradients are reported, it is important to specify the type of gradient measured (eg, mean, maximum, peak to peak) and to report mean gradient whenever possible.

Technical Factors

Technical and physiologic factors can significantly affect the accuracy of the reported transvalvular gradients. For example, the frequency response of the pressure measurement system significantly influences the recorded pressure waveform. Although micromanometer-tipped catheters have an optimal frequency response (at least 20 Hz) for intracardiac pressure recording, these catheters are expensive, and their use requires meticulous technique. In the clinical setting, fluid-filled catheters and strain-gauge external transducers are used more commonly with a frequency response of the system of only 10 to 20 Hz. The frequency response can be optimized by the use of stiff wide-bore catheters, short connecting tubing, and a low-density liquid. Simple side-hole catheters may provide more accurate data than end-hole catheters in some cases, because of the kinetic and pressure energy imparted to the fluid-filled column in an end-hole catheter. However, catheters with multiple side holes can lead to erroneous results if the position of the openings straddles the stenotic valve.

External pressure transducers are subject to a phenomenon called "ring-down" resulting from the conversion of pressure energy to an electrical signal, similar to the sound resulting from striking a bell. The use of a fluid-filled catheter between the chamber of interest and the transducer amplifies this phenomenon, leading to apparent fluctuations in the recorded pressure signal. This phenomenon, called underdamping, is characterized by a waveform consisting of diminishing harmonic oscillations of the underlying pressure signal (Fig. 4–8). To counter this effect, the recording system is damped just enough to avoid excessive oscillations while maintaining the frequency response of the system. Overdamping also must be avoided to prevent underestimation of pressure gradients. Damping typically can be optimized by using short, stiff tubing to connect the catheter to the pressure transducer, minimizing the number of connec-

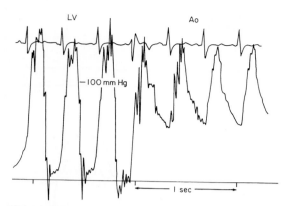

Figure 4·8 Pressure measurements recorded during a pullback of the catheter from the left ventricle (LV) to the aorta (Ao). The tracings are markedly underdamped, with rapid oscillations in the pressure tracing seen in diastole and in systole. These obscure the actual pressure measurements. Notice the harmonic oscillation caused by underdamping in the second left ventricular beat.

tions in the system, and using contrast (instead of saline) to fill the catheter.

Pressure recording systems must be zeroed and calibrated before and after data collection in each patient. The zero position is adjusted with the system open to room air. Calibration is optimally performed using a known input pressure, such as with a mercury manometer, but many systems include an electronic calibration that is adequate in most cases. With either type of calibration, both zero and the reference standard need to be rechecked periodically during and at completion of the study to avoid erroneous data interpretation. When two catheters are used to measure pressures simultaneously on both sides of a stenotic valve, the calibrations are checked together and, if possible, data are recorded again after switching the transducers to the other catheters to avoid any systematic bias.

Pressures are recorded at a fast sweep speed to allow accurate time measurements and to display the waveform in enough detail to allow analysis of the degree of damping and the subtleties of the pressure waveform. The vertical axis is adjusted, depending on the pressures being recorded, to use the full height of the recording while including the pressure waveforms of interest on the scale. For example, left atrial and LV pressures across a stenotic mitral valve may be recorded on a scale of 0 to 25 mm Hg, whereas severe aortic stenosis may require a scale of 0 to 200 mm Hg.

Physiologic Factors

The exact location of the pressures recorded on the upstream and downstream sides of a stenotic or regurgitant valve can significantly affect the measured transvalvular gradient for several reasons. First, the *timing* of the pressure waveform is different closer to the valve than at a greater distance, so that realignment of the waveforms may be needed for accurate gradient calculations. For example, the femoral artery pressure upstroke is delayed slightly compared with central aortic pressure, as predicted by the velocity of pressure propagation between these two sites. If a femoral artery waveform is used in place of central aortic pressure for calculating the aortic transvalvular gradient, this timing difference must be taken into account. Similarly, if the diastolic pressure curve for a catheter occluding a branch pulmonary artery (ie, pulmonary wedge pressure) is used in place of directly measured left atrial pressure in a patient with mitral stenosis, failure to consider timing differences may lead to erroneous mitral gradient calculations.

Second, the *shape* of the waveform adjacent to the valve compared with that more distally may affect the apparent transvalvular gradient. This difference is most evident when comparing central aortic and peripheral arterial (eg, femoral artery) pressures. Because of summation of the transmitted and reflected pressure waveforms, the femoral artery pressure curve is narrower and has a higher peak than the central aortic pressure, a phenomenon known as peripheral amplification. While simultaneously measured central aortic and LV pressures are used whenever possible for calculation of transaortic pressure gradients, if only a femoral pressure is available, realignment of timing and correction for peripheral amplification is needed (Fig. 4–9). Optimal mean gradient results are obtained by averaging aligned and unaligned LV and femoral artery pressure tracings when compared with gradients calculated using LV and central aortic pressure data.[55]

The third physiologic effect that may influence the measured transvalvular gradient is the phenomenon of *pressure recovery* distal to a stenosis, particularly in the case of aortic valve obstruction.[56–60] As the high-velocity jet of flow through the stenotic orifice decelerates and expands distal to the valve, the associated turbulence increases the aortic pressure (ie, pressure recovery) such that the pressure difference between the left ventricle and the distal

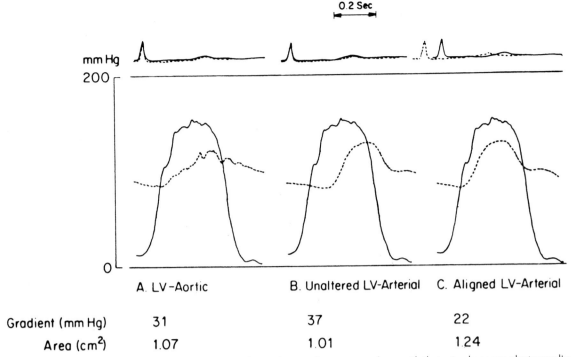

Figure 4·9 Methods for alignment of left ventricular and arterial pressures, along with their simultaneous electrocardiograms in patients with valvular aortic stenosis. A, The "true" aortic valve gradient measured by simultaneous left ventricular and ascending aortic recordings or by sequential left ventricular and ascending aortic recordings superimposed by lining up the electrocardiographic R waves. B, Unaltered left ventricular–femoral artery gradient obtained from simultaneous or sequential tracings synchronized on the R wave. C, Aligned left ventricular–femoral artery gradient obtained by temporally realigning the femoral artery tracing so that its upstroke matches that of the left ventricle. Although displayed here separately, ascending aortic and femoral artery pressures are measured simultaneously. Aortic valve gradients are most accurate when data from aligned and unaligned tracings are averaged. (From Folland ED, Parisi AF, Carbone C: Is peripheral arterial pressure a satisfactory substitute for ascending aortic pressure when measuring aortic valve gradients? J Am Coll Cardiol 1984;4:1207.)

ascending aorta is less than the difference between the left ventricle and the pressure in the stenotic orifice itself (Fig. 4–10). Although pressure recovery may account for some of the observed discrepancies between Doppler and catheter data and may lead to apparent underestimation of stenosis severity, the magnitude of this effect in the clinical setting appears to be small (on the order of 5 to 10 mm Hg) and is unlikely to affect clinical decision making. Pressure recovery is greatest when stenosis severity is mild and the aortic root dimension is small and is least with severe stenosis and poststenotic dilation. Potential underestimation of stenosis severity due to pressure recovery can be avoided by recording pressures immediately adjacent to the valve on the downstream side of the stenosis.

Several other factors may affect recorded pressure gradients. The transaortic pressure gradient may be affected by the presence of the catheter in the stenotic orifice. The catheter may increase the transvalvular pressure gradient by further decreasing the cross-sectional flow area or by inducing aortic regurgitation.[51, 61] Other physiologic variables that may affect recorded pressure data include the effect of atrial contraction, cardiac arrhythmias, and the compliance of the receiving chamber when regurgitation is present. The effect of atrial contraction is exemplified in the case of mitral stenosis, in which effective atrial contraction due to sinus rhythm increases the late-diastolic and mean transmitral gradient compared to when atrial fibrillation is present. Irregular heart rhythms affect measured pressure gradients in valvular stenosis because of the varying volume flow rates across the valve, necessitating averaging of several beats for clinical interpretation.

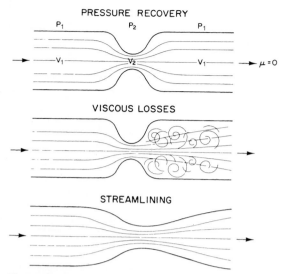

PRESSURE RECOVERY

VISCOUS LOSSES

STREAMLINING

Figure 4·10 Pressure recovery. *A,* Complete recovery of pressure (P) for inviscid flow (μ = 0) when velocity (V) increases and then decreases to its original value distal to the stenosis. *B,* In the real case, pressure recovery is limited by turbulence distal to the stenosis, created by flow separation from the chamber walls and viscous interactions between the jet and adjacent fluid. *C,* Streamlining the stenosis to minimize flow separation increases pressure recovery. (From Levine RA, Jimoh A, Cape EG, McMillan S, Yoganathan AP, Weyman AE: Pressure recovery distal to a stenosis: potential cause of gradient "overestimation" by Doppler echocardiography. Reproduced by permission from the American College of Cardiology, J Am Coll Cardiol 1989;13:706.)

Subvalvular Gradients in Valvular Aortic Stenosis

In valvular aortic stenosis, even in the absence of fixed or dynamic subvalvular obstruction, significant subvalvular pressure gradients can be seen due to the effect of a nonuniform (eg, tapering) flow field on convective acceleration (Fig. 4–11).[49, 62, 63] Although this phenomenon rarely is of sufficient magnitude to affect clinical measurements of pressure gradient, when present both the subvalvular and transvalvular gradients should be measured and reported. Overinterpretation of an apparent subvalvular gradient should be avoided; if subaortic stenosis or dynamic obstruction due to hypertrophic cardiomyopathy is suspected, pressure data should be confirmed by direct imaging of the site of obstruction using echocardiography or fluoroscopy.

Dynamic outflow obstruction also can be differentiated from fixed valvular aortic stenosis based on the effect of a premature ventricu-lar contraction (PVC) on the gradient recorded on the next beat. With both lesions, the LV to aortic pressure gradient is higher on the post-PVC beat, but with hypertrophic cardiomyopathy, the pulse pressure is narrower than on the normal beat preceding the premature beat (ie, Brockenbrough's sign).

Valve Areas

As with velocity and pressure gradient data recorded noninvasively with Doppler techniques, invasive measurement of intracardiac pressures and transvalvular pressure gradients provides valuable information for clinical decision making for individual patients. However, regardless of measurement technique, transvalvular gradients vary with transvalvular volume flow rates. A patient with aortic stenosis and a high cardiac output or mixed aortic stenosis and regurgitation may have a high transvalvular gradient despite only moderate disease. Conversely, a patient with severe valvular obstruction may have only a modest gradient because of coexisting LV systolic dysfunction or mitral regurgitation resulting in a low transaortic volume flow rate. Even in the same individual, the magnitude of the transvalvular gradient varies with transvalvular volume flow rate, such as with exercise, anxiety, volume depletion, or pharmacologic therapy.

In 1951, Gorlin and Gorlin proposed a hydraulic formula for calculation of cardiac valve areas. The concept underlying this approach is that valve area should be closely related to the actual valve anatomy and should be constant for any specific valve, regardless of volume flow rate. The proposed formula was derived from two accepted principles.[64, 65] The first principle is that the volume flow (F) through an orifice is the product of cross-sectional area (A), velocity (V), and the coefficient of orifice contraction (C_c):

$$F = AVC_c$$

In this equation, C_c corrects for the difference between the geometric cross-sectional area and the area of the flow stream.

The second principle is the relationship between pressure gradient (ΔP) and velocity (the Bernoulli equation), retaining the separate constants for acceleration due to gravity (*g*) and the coefficient of velocity (C_v), which relates to the conversion of potential to kinetic

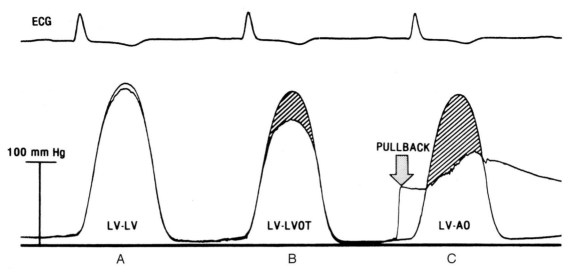

Figure 4·11 Intraventricular deep *(A)*, subvalvular *(B)*, and transvalvular *(C)* ejection gradients in aortic stenosis. AO, aortic root; LV, deep left ventricle; LVOT, left ventricular outflow tract at or immediately upstream from the aortic orifice. (From Pasipoularides A: Clinical assessment of ventricular ejection dynamics with and without outflow obstruction. J Am Coll Cardiol 1990;15:859.)

energy), to allow measurement of pressure, rather than velocity, in the equation:

$$V^2 = C_v^2 [2g\,(\Delta P_{mean})]\ or\ V = C_v \sqrt{2g\,(\Delta P_{mean})}$$

Combining these two equations,

$$F = A\,[C_v \sqrt{2gh\,(\Delta P_{mean})}]C_c$$

and solving for area,

$$A = F/[C_c C_v \sqrt{2gh(\Delta P_{mean})}]$$

In this equation, the volume flow rate (V in mL/s) is the stroke volume divided by the period of flow, and the mean transvalvular pressure gradient is measured in millimeters of mercury. Combining the $\sqrt{2g}$ and empiric estimates for C_v and C_c into a single constant[66] yields the following equations for aortic and mitral valves:

$$Aortic\ valve\ area = [SV/SEP]/[44.3 \sqrt{\Delta P_{mean}}]$$

and

$$Mitral\ valve\ area = [SV/DFP]/[37.7 \sqrt{\Delta P_{mean}}]$$

In these equations, SEP is the systolic ejection period, and DFP is the diastolic filling period (Fig. 4–12).

For calculation of valve area in the clinical setting, the mean transvalvular gradient is re-corded and averaged from several beats, as discussed previously. Stroke volume is measured by angiographic, Fick, or thermodilution techniques, taking care to use a cardiac output measurement that reflects the flow rate across the affected valve. For example, if aortic stenosis and regurgitation exist, an angiographic stroke volume represents transaortic flow rate, but Fick and thermodilution outputs do not. Similarly, if mitral regurgitation and stenosis exist, only the angiographic output reflects transmitral flow. Use of a forward cardiac output in these settings results in calculations that overestimate stenosis severity (eg, result in a smaller calculated valve area).

The invasive approach for calculation of valve area is based on the same basic principles underlying the Doppler approaches: calculation of volume flow rate as area times velocity and the Bernoulli relationship between velocity and pressure gradient. Significant differences between the invasive and noninvasive approaches include measurement of pressure rather than velocity and an attempt to calculate anatomic instead of physiologic orifice area. The constant in the Gorlin formula has been empirically derived and includes factors for the conversion of units of measure and factors for the coefficients of velocity and contraction in order to calculate an anatomic area. With the Doppler continuity equation, no constant is needed, because units of measure are congruent and the goal is to calculate

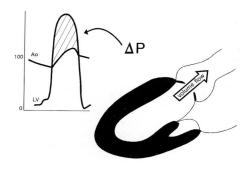

$$Flow = AVA \times V \times C_c$$

$$V^2 = (C_v)^2 \times 2g \times \Delta P$$

$$V = C_v \times \sqrt{2g\ \Delta P}$$

$$AVA = Flow/(44.3 \times C_c \times C_v \sqrt{\Delta P})$$

Figure 4·12 Schematic diagram of the Gorlin and Gorlin method for calculation of valve area. Ao, aorta; AVA, aortic valve area; V, velocity; C_c, coefficient of orifice contraction; C_v, coefficient of velocity; LV, left ventricle; ΔP, pressure gradient;

physiologic orifice area. In addition to potential inaccuracy in the empiric derivation of the Gorlin constant, results of in vitro and in vivo studies suggest that this "constant" varies with volume flow rate, orifice shape, and stenosis severity.[67-71] While less flow dependent than pressure gradients, invasive determinations of valve areas may vary with flow rate because of changes in the Gorlin constant. In addition, the degree of valve opening may vary with different flow rates, as also occurs with Doppler continuity equation valve areas (see Chapters 3 and 9).

Despite these concerns and although the initial evaluation of the accuracy of the formula of Gorlin and Gorlin was limited,[64, 72] the clinical utility of this measurement is well established. Gorlin and Gorlin valve areas have been used appropriately for clinical decision making for more than 40 years. Pragmatically, both Doppler and invasive techniques depend on careful and accurate data acquisition by experienced laboratory staff, so that while differences between invasively and noninvasively derived valve areas may be related to the different underlying assumptions of these two techniques, in the clinical setting the effect of data quality tends to predominate. Apparent discrepancies most often are caused by suboptimal technique with one or both approaches.

If discrepancies are seen even with optimal technique, the difference may provide useful information about the physiology of valvular obstruction, because the invasive formula estimates anatomic valve area, and the noninvasive formula measures physiologic orifice area.[65, 73]

ASSESSMENT OF VALVULAR REGURGITATION

Valvular regurgitation can be evaluated by cardiac catheterization with direct measurement of intracardiac pressures, semiquantitative evaluation of regurgitant severity by angiography, and calculation of regurgitant fraction on the basis of the difference between angiographic (total) stroke volume and forward stroke volume (by Fick or thermodilution methods).

Pressure Waveform Analysis

Evaluation of the pressure waveforms on both sides of the regurgitant valve allows inferences about the severity and chronicity of the regurgitant lesion and LV systolic function.

Aortic regurgitation may be associated with a systolic pressure gradient across the aortic valve, even in the absence of coexisting stenosis, because of the high-volume flow rate across the valve. This pressure gradient occurs predominantly in early systole and corresponds to an increased antegrade flow velocity with an early peaking of the Doppler velocity curve. Although the magnitude of the systolic pressure gradient is related to volume flow rate, pressure gradients for isolated severe aortic regurgitation are small, with mean pressure gradients ranging from 5 to 20 mm Hg, corresponding to Doppler maximum velocities of 1.5 to 2.5 m/s. Larger pressure gradients indicate associated outflow obstruction.

In diastole, central aortic pressure falls more rapidly than normal because of the diastolic run-off into the left ventricle, producing an end-diastolic aortic pressure that is lower than normal (Fig. 4–13). Conversely, LV diastolic pressure rises more rapidly than normal because of rapid ventricular filling retrograde across the incompetent aortic valve as well as antegrade across the mitral valve. With acute severe aortic regurgitation, this fall in aortic and rise in ventricular diastolic pressures results in equalization of aortic and ventricular pressures at end-diastole. Thus, the rate of equalization of aortic and LV diastolic pres-

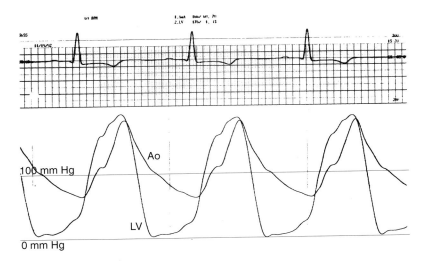

Figure 4·13 Left ventricular (LV) and aortic (Ao) pressures recorded in a 46-year-old man with severe prosthetic aortic regurgitation. Notice the mild gradient in systole because of the increased antegrade volume flow rate and the rapid rate of decrease in aortic pressure during diastole, resulting in near equalization of aortic and left ventricular end-diastolic pressures. His calculated regurgitant fraction from angiographic and forward cardiac outputs was 59%.

sures is related to regurgitant severity. This concept serves as the basis for using the diastolic slope of the Doppler velocity curve (see Chapter 3) as a measure of regurgitant severity. The limitation of this approach, whether invasive or noninvasive data are used, is that chronic regurgitation results in compensatory changes in LV diastolic compliance such that LV end-diastolic pressure may remain low, even with severe regurgitation. Therefore, interpretation of the pressure curves must take into account disease chronicity and severity.

This combination of systolic and diastolic pressure abnormalities leads to the most characteristic hemodynamic feature of chronic aortic regurgitation: an increased pulse pressure. Since systolic pressure is increased and end-diastolic pressure is decreased, the pulse pressure measured invasively or by blood pressure cuff is increased. Although the magnitude of increase is only modestly correlated with regurgitant severity,[74] this simple measure of regurgitant severity should be integrated with other imaging and pressure data in patient evaluation.

Mitral regurgitation results in an increase in left atrial pressure that peaks in late systole, called the *v wave* (Fig. 4–14). To some extent, the height of the v wave is related to regurgitant severity, although other factors, such as left atrial size and compliance, may modulate this effect. The left atrial pressure curve is transmitted variably to the pulmonary wedge tracing, again related to the modulating effects of the size and compliance of the pulmonary vascular bed.

For example, a patient with a prosthetic mitral valve with a small degree of regurgitation may show a prominent v wave due to a noncompliant pulmonary vascular bed, whereas the patient with chronic severe mitral regurgitation may demonstrate no v wave because of compensatory changes in the left atrium and pulmonary vasculature. Thus, while a v wave often is considered a hallmark of mitral regurgitation, this finding is not sensitive for the diagnosis of mitral regurgitation, nor is its absolute value a reliable predictor of regurgitant severity.[75, 76] However, except when a prosthetic mitral valve is present, the finding of a v wave is reasonably specific for the diagnosis of mitral regurgitation, and directional changes in its magnitude may be helpful in management of an individual patient.

The rate of rise of LV pressure during "isovolumic" contraction (dP/dt) provides a measure of LV systolic function in patients with mitral regurgitation. Normally, dP/dt is more than 1000 mm Hg/s, with diminished values reflecting progressively more severe impairment of contractility. Peak LV systolic pressure typically is normal in patients with mitral regurgitation, although severe regurgitation associated with decreased forward cardiac output may lead to decreased LV systolic pressures and clinical hypotension.

Analysis of pressure waveforms for *right-sided regurgitant lesions* is similar to that for left-sided valvular disease. Pulmonic regurgitation results in diminished diastolic pulmonary artery and increased diastolic right ventricular pressures, and the rate of pressure equalization is

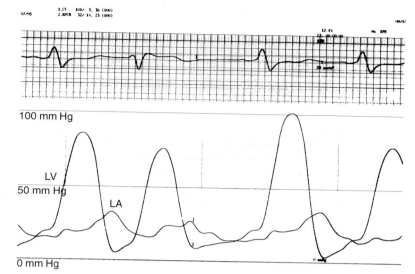

Figure 4·14 Left ventricular and pulmonary artery wedge tracings in a 53-year-old man with dilated cardiomyopathy, an ejection fraction of 31%, and moderately severe mitral regurgitation. The left atrial pressure tracing shows a prominent v wave. The mild early diastolic pressure gradient results from the increased antegrade flow rate across the mitral valve.

related to the severity and chronicity of disease. Acute severe tricuspid regurgitation results in a right atrial v wave.

Angiography

Angiographic evaluation of regurgitant severity is based on injection of contrast into the chamber downstream to the affected valve with imaging of reflux of contrast into the chamber receiving the regurgitant volume. For aortic regurgitation, contrast is injected into the aortic root; for mitral regurgitation, contrast is injected into the left ventricle. Regurgitation is graded on a semiquantitative scale of 0 to 4+, as shown in Table 4–4.

Although angiographic grading provides a useful clinical estimate of regurgitant severity that is conceptually similar to Doppler color flow mapping, this approach has several limitations. First, interobserver variability in grading regurgitant severity can be considerable unless the observers adhere strictly to accepted definitions. Although mild regurgitation is clearly distinct from severe regurgitation, intermediate grades may not be reliably estimated.

Second, technical factors may lead to an erroneous interpretation. The volume and rate of contrast injection must provide complete opacification of the upstream chamber; care is needed in positioning the catheter such that it is close to the valve but does not interfere with valve closing (eg, LV catheter entrapment in the mitral chordal apparatus or the aortic root catheter impinging on the closed aortic valve), and the data should be recorded

from an angle and with an image size that includes the upstream and downstream chambers fully without overlapping radiopaque structures. For aortic regurgitation, a 45-degree left anterior oblique view with 10% to 15% of cranial angulation tends to result in a

TABLE 4·4 ANGIOGRAPHIC GRADING OF REGURGITANT SEVERITY

Grade	Aortic Regurgitation	Mitral Regurgitation
1+	Contrast refluxes from the aortic root into the LV but clears on each beat.	Contrast refluxes into the left atrium but clears on each beat.
2+	Contrast refluxes into the LV with a gradually increasing density of contrast in the LV that never equals contrast intensity in the aortic root.	Left atrial contrast density gradually increases but never equals LV density.
3+	Contrast refluxes into the LV with a gradually increasing density such that LV and aortic root density are equal after several beats.	The density of contrast in the atrium and ventricle equalize after several beats.
4+	Contrast fills the LV rapidly, resulting in an equivalent radiographic density in the LV and aortic root on the first beat.	The left atrium becomes as dense as the LV on the first beat, and contrast is seen refluxing into the pulmonary veins.

LV, left ventricle.

image perpendicular to the valve plane, allowing assessment of the degree of reflux from the aortic root into the left ventricle. For mitral regurgitation, a 30-degree right anterior oblique view offers separation of the left ventricle and left atrium in a plane perpendicular to the mitral annulus. Caution is needed, because the descending aortic shadow is superimposed on the left atrium in this view, and contrast in the descending aorta may be mistaken for mitral regurgitation.

Third, physiologic factors, including heart rate, cardiac rhythm, preload, and afterload, affect the severity of regurgitation, so that images recorded under conditions disparate from the patient's baseline hemodynamic state may not accurately reflect disease severity.

Despite these potential limitations, evaluation of valvular regurgitation by angiography may be helpful in selected cases, particularly when clinical and noninvasive imaging data are discordant (Figs. 4–15 and 4–16). If the patient is undergoing cardiac catheterization for other indications, performing angiography adds relatively little risk or cost to the procedure. Angiographic images are familiar to most cardiologists and cardiac surgeons, with an apparent ease of interpretation that has led to widespread clinical acceptance.

Calculation of Regurgitant Volume and Fraction

For aortic and mitral insufficiency, regurgitant volume and fraction can be calculated at cardiac catheterization based on measurement of the amount of blood ejected by the left ventricle (total stroke volume) and the amount of blood delivered to the body (forward stroke volume) (Fig. 4–17). Total stroke volume is calculated from the LV angiogram, and forward stroke volume is measured by Fick or thermodilution techniques:

$$\text{Regurgitant SV} = \text{Total SV} - \text{Forward SV}$$

A regurgitation fraction of less than 20% indicates mild, 20% to 40% indicates moderate, 40% to 60% indicates moderately severe, and more than 60% indicates severe regurgitation.[76] The accuracy of this approach depends on the accuracy and potential limitations of cardiac output measurements by these two techniques. Given the normal range of variability for these measurements, meticulous attention to details and averaging of several determinations are needed for reliable results. Another limitation of this approach is that, when both aortic and mitral valves are regurgitant (often in adult patients), only a rough estimate can be made of the portion of the regurgitant fraction due to each valve.

Thus, while this method has the potential to provide a quantitative measure of regurgitant severity, now that reliable noninvasive measures of regurgitant severity are available, invasive data are most useful in patients with complex valve disease or when discrepancies exist between the clinical data and other imaging techniques. Calculation of regurgitant fractions for right heart valves is problematic because of the difficulties in calculating right ventricular volumes from angiographic data.

Although Gorlin and Gorlin's original hydraulic formula was proposed for calculation for regurgitant (as well as stenotic) orifice areas, this approach is rarely used clinically.[64, 72]

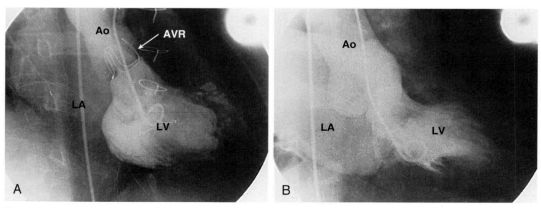

Figure 4·15 Examples of mild *(A)* and severe *(B)* mitral regurgitation are demonstrated on left ventricular angiography in a right anterior oblique projection. LV, left ventricle; Ao, aorta; AVR, aortic valve replacement; LA, left atrium; LV, left ventricle.

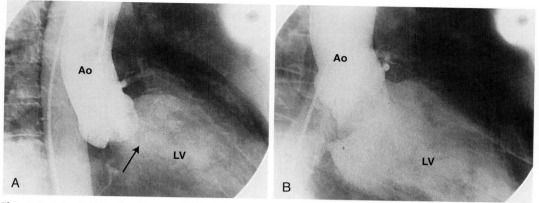

Figure 4·16 *A,* Example of mild aortic regurgitation. Contrast entering the left ventricle *(arrow)* did not completely opacify the chamber and cleared on each beat. *B,* Severe aortic regurgitation is shown by dense opacification of the left ventricle on the first beat. *Ao,* aorta; *LV,* left ventricle.

OTHER CATHETERIZATION DATA

In addition to direct measure of valvular and ventricular function, cardiac catheterization provides unique data that allow calculation of pulmonary and systemic vascular resistance, calculations that cannot be made using noninvasive approaches. Cardiac catheterization also allows direct measurement of LV end-diastolic pressure (or pulmonary capillary wedge pressure as a surrogate), data that may be essential for management of the decompensated patient.

Pulmonary Artery Pressures and Resistance

Direct measurement of pulmonary artery pressures at catheterization is needed when

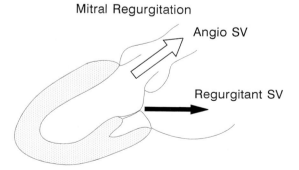

Regurgitant SV = Angio SV - Fick SV

Figure 4·17 Diagram of the method for calculation of the regurgitant fraction from the left ventricular angiographic output and the forward cardiac output in a patient with mitral regurgitation. *SV,* stroke volume.

noninvasively acquired data are nondiagnostic or are discordant with other clinical data. Pulmonary pressures should be measured before crossing the aortic valve in aortic stenosis patients, because an average increase in mean pulmonary pressure of 4 mm Hg (ranging up to 19 mm Hg) has been reported after the aortic valve is crossed.[77] Normal pulmonary pressures slightly increase with maximal exercise in young adults, from a resting pulmonary systolic pressure of 15 to 20 mm Hg at rest to a maximum of 25 to 35 mm Hg. Although resting pulmonary pressures increase minimally with age, the exercise increase becomes exaggerated, with an exercise systolic pulmonary pressure as high as 45 to 50 mm Hg in normal 60- to 70-year-old subjects.[78]

Pulmonary artery pressure depends not only on the resistance to flow imposed by pulmonary vascular bed but also on volume flow rate and the pulmonary venous (or left atrial) pressure. The rise in pulmonary pressure that occurs "passively" in response to an elevated left atrial pressure (eg, in mitral stenosis) reverses when left atrial pressure is lowered. Similarly, high pulmonary pressures caused by a high-volume flow rate revert toward normal with a reduction in the flow rate. Thus, it is important to calculate pulmonary vascular resistance (PVR), which takes volume flow rate and the pressure drop across the circuit into account:

$$PVR = \frac{(PA_{mean} - LA_{mean})}{Pulmonary\ blood\ flow}$$

When pressures are measured in millimeters of mercury (mm Hg) and blood flow in liters per minute (L/min), this equation results in Wood units of resistance, which can be converted to dynes-seconds per centimeter to the fifth power (dyne-s-cm⁻⁵) by multiplying by 80. In practice, pulmonary wedge pressure commonly is substituted for left atrial pressure in this calculation.

Even though pulmonary vascular resistance describes the component of pulmonary hypertension caused by the pulmonary vasculature, some of the increase in vascular resistance may be reversible after relief of the initiating cause, and some may represent an irreversible increase in pulmonary vascular resistance. The degree of reversibility of an elevated pulmonary vascular resistance often is difficult to predict in patients with valvular heart disease.

Systemic Vascular Resistance

Systemic vascular resistance (in dyne-s-cm⁻⁵) can be calculated at catheterization:

Systemic vascular resistance =

$$\left[\frac{(Ao_{mean} - RA_{mean})}{Cardiac\ output} \right] \times 80$$

In patients with valvular regurgitation, an elevated systemic vascular resistance may contribute to the total load imposed on the ventricle and can lead to increased LV wall stress and clinical symptoms.

Left Ventricular Diastolic Function

The most widely used clinical measure of LV diastolic function is the LV end-diastolic pressure, which is measured directly at catheterization. When repeat measurements are needed, an indwelling pulmonary artery catheter is used, with the assumption that the pulmonary artery wedge pressure reflects the pressure in the left atrium.

Although end-diastolic pressure typically is normal at rest in patients with chronic, mild to moderate valvular disease, significant elevations can occur with severe aortic stenosis, acute aortic or mitral regurgitation, or in the decompensated patient. For example, in the patient with acute aortic regurgitation, severe elevation of the LV end-diastolic pressure results from acute volume overload of the left ventricle that has not had time to dilate. Similarly, a superimposed systemic disease (eg, fever, anemia, sepsis) in a patient with LV dia-

stolic dysfunction (eg, patient with compensatory hypertrophy resulting from aortic valve stenosis) may result in acute decompensation with significant elevations in LV diastolic pressure. Other measures of diastolic function, such as the time constant of relaxation, also can be measured at catheterization but require special recording and analysis of data and are rarely performed in the clinical setting.

Coronary Angiography

Coronary angiography often is needed in patients with valvular heart disease as part of the preoperative evaluation or to evaluate other potential causes of clinical symptoms. Other texts should be consulted for details of coronary angiographic image acquisition and interpretation.[18, 79–81]

References

1. Cheitlin MD: Valvular heart disease: management and intervention. Clinical overview and discussion. Circulation 1991;84(suppl I):259–264.
2. Leitch JW, Mitchell AS, Harris PJ, Fletcher PJ, Bailey BP: The effect of cardiac catheterization upon management of advanced aortic and mitral valve disease. Eur Heart J 1991;12:602–607.
3. van den Brink RB, Verheul HA, Hoedemaker G, et al: The value of Doppler echocardiography in the management of patients with valvular heart disease: analysis of one year of clinical practice. J Am Soc Echocardiogr 1991;4:109–120.
4. Slater J, Gindea AJ, Freedberg RS, et al: Comparison of cardiac catheterization and Doppler echocardiography in the decision to operate in aortic and mitral valve disease. J Am Coll Cardiol 1991;17:1026–1036.
5. Cujec B, Welsh R, Aboguddah A, Reeder B: Comparison of Doppler echocardiography and cardiac catheterization in patients requiring valve surgery: search for a "gold standard." Can J Cardiol 1992;8:829–838.
6. Sandler H, Dodge HT: The use of single plane angiocardiograms for the calculation of left ventricular volume in man. Am Heart J 1968;75:325–334.
7. Dodge HT, Sandler H, Ballew DW, Lord JD Jr: The use of biplane angiocardiography for the measurement of left ventricular volume in man. Am Heart J 1960;70:752–762.
8. Greene DG, Carlisle R, Grant C, Bunnell IL: Estimation of left ventricular volume by one-plane cineangiography. Circulation 1967;35:61–69.
9. Wynne J, Green LH, Mann T, Levin D, Grossman W: Estimation of left ventricular volumes in man from biplane cineangiograms filmed in oblique projections. Am J Cardiol 1978;41:726–732.
10. Kennedy JW, Trenholme SE, Kasser IS: Left ventricular volume and mass from single-plane cineangiocardiogram: a comparison of anteroposterior and right anterior oblique methods. Am Heart J 1970;80:343–352.
11. Graham TP Jr, Jarmakani JM, Canent RV Jr, Morrow MN: Left heart volume estimation in infancy and childhood: reevaluation of methodology and normal values. Circulation 1971;43:895–904.

12. Kasser IS, Kennedy JW: Measurement of left ventricular volumes in man by single-plane cineangiocardiography. Invest Radiol 1969;4:83–90.

13. Sheehan FH, Mitten Lewis S: Factors influencing accuracy in left ventricular volume determination. Am J Cardiol 1989;64:661–664.

14. Cohn PF, Levine JA, Bergeron GA, Gorlin R: Reproducibility of the angiographic left ventricular ejection fraction in patients with coronary artery disease. Am Heart J 1974;88:713–720.

15. Chaitman BR, DeMots H, Bristow JD, Rosch J, Rahimtoola SH: Objective and subjective analysis of left ventricular angiograms. Circulation 1975;52:420–425.

16. Rogers WJ, Smith LR, Hood WP Jr, Mantle JA, Rackley CE, Russell RO Jr: Effect of filming projection and interobserver variability on angiographic biplane left ventricular volume determination. Circulation 1979;59:96–104.

17. Sheehan FH: Cardiac angiography. *In* Braunwald E, Marcus M, Skorton DJ, Schelbert HR, Wolf GL, Brundage BH, eds. Marcus Cardiac Imaging: A Companion to Braunwald's Heart Disease. Philadelphia: WB Saunders, 1996.

18. Baim DS, Grossman W: Cardiac Catheterization, Angiography, and Intervention, 5th Edition. Baltimore: Williams & Wilkins, 1996.

19. Rackley CE, Dodge HT, Coble YD Jr, Hay RE: A method for determining left ventricular mass in man. Circulation 1964;29:666.

20. Kennedy JW, Reichenbach DD, Baxley WA, Dodge HT: Left ventricular mass: a comparison of angiocardiographic measurements with autopsy weight. Am J Cardiol 1967;19:221–223.

21. Grossman W, Jones D, McLaurin LP: Wall stress and patterns of hypertrophy in the human left ventricle. J Clin Invest 1975;56:56–64.

22. Yin FC: Ventricular wall stress. Circ Res 1981;49:829–842.

23. Sheehan FH, Bolson EL, Dodge HT, Mathey DG, Schofer J, Woo HW: Advantages and applications of the centerline method for characterizing regional ventricular function. Circulation 1986;74:293–305.

24. Sheehan FH, Schofer J, Mathey DG, et al: Measurement of regional wall motion from biplane contrast ventriculograms: a comparison of the 30 degree right anterior oblique and 60 degree left anterior oblique projections in patients with acute myocardial infarction. Circulation 1986;74:796–804.

25. Fick A: Uber die messung des Blutquantums in den Herzventrikeln. Sitz der Physik-Med ges Wurtzberg 1870:16.

26. Grossman AR: Hemodynamic principles. *In* Baim DS, Grossman W, eds. Cardiac Catheterization, Angiography, and Intervention. Baltimore: Williams & Wilkins, 1996:109–182.

27. Lange RA, Dehmer GJ, Wells PJ, et al: Limitations of the metabolic rate meter for measuring oxygen consumption and cardiac output. Am J Cardiol 1989;64:783–786.

28. Barratt Boyes BG, Wood EH: The oxygen saturation of blood in the venae cavae, right heart chambers and pulmonary vessels of healthy subjects. J Lab Clin Med 1957;50:93.

29. Selzer A, Sudrann RB: Reliability of the determination of cardiac output in man by means of the Fick principle. Circ Res 1958;6:485.

30. Thomassen B: Cardiac output in normal subjects under standard conditions: the repeatability of measurements by the Fick method. Scand J Clin Lab Invest 1957;9:365.

31. Visscher MB, Johnson JA: The Fick principle: analysis of potential errors in its conventional applications. J Appl Physiol 1953;5:635.

32. Dehmer GJ, Firth BG, Hillis LD: Oxygen consumption in adult patients during cardiac catheterization. Clin Cardiol 1982;5:436–440.

33. Kendrick AH, West J, Papouchado M, Rozkovec A: Direct Fick cardiac output: are assumed values of oxygen consumption acceptable? Eur Heart J 1988;9:337–342.

34. Branthwaite MA, Bradley RD: Measurement of cardiac output by thermal dilution in man. J Appl Physiol 1968;24:434–438.

35. Ganz W, Donoso R, Marcus HS, Forrester JS, Swan HJ: A new technique for measurement of cardiac output by thermodilution in man. Am J Cardiol 1971;27:392–396.

36. Forrester JS, Ganz W, Diamond G, McHugh T, Chonette DW, Swan HJ: Thermodilution cardiac output determination with a single flow-directed catheter. Am Heart J 1972;83:306–311.

37. Weisel RD, Berger RL, Hechtman HB: Current concepts measurement of cardiac output by thermodilution. N Engl J Med 1975;292:682–684.

38. van Grondelle A, Ditchey RV, Groves BM, Wagner WW Jr, Reeves JT: Thermodilution method overestimates low cardiac output in humans. Am J Physiol 1983;245:H690–692.

39. Milnor WR: Cardiac dynamics. *In* Milnor WR, ed. Hemodynamics. Baltimore: Williams & Wilkins, 1982:244–272.

40. Mirsky I, Tajimi T, Peterson KL: The development of the entire end-systolic pressure-volume and ejection fraction-afterload relations: a new concept of systolic myocardial stiffness. Circulation 1987;76:343–356.

41. Wisenbaugh T, Yu G, Evans J: The superiority of maximum fiber elastance over maximum stress-volume ratio as an index of contractile state. Circulation 1985;72:648–653.

42. Sagawa K, Suga H, Shoukas AA, Bakalar KM: End-systolic pressure/volume ratio: a new index of ventricular contractility. Am J Cardiol 1977;40:748–753.

43. Grossman W, Braunwald E, Mann T, McLaurin LP, Green LH: Contractile state of the left ventricle in man as evaluated from end-systolic pressure-volume relations. Circulation 1977;56:845–852.

44. McKay RG, Aroesty JM, Heller GV, Royal HD, Warren SE, Grossman W: Assessment of the end-systolic pressure-volume relationship in human beings with the use of a time-varying elastance model. Circulation 1986;74:97–104.

45. Starling MR, Walsh RA, Dell'Italia LJ, Mancini GB, Lasher JC, Lancaster JL: The relationship of various measures of end-systole to left ventricular maximum time-varying elastance in man. Circulation 1987;76:32–43.

46. Borow KM, Neumann A, Wynne J: Sensitivity of end-systolic pressure-dimension and pressure-volume relations to the inotropic state in humans. Circulation 1982;65:988–997.

47. Kass DA, Midei M, Graves W, Brinker JA, Maughan WL: Use of a conductance (volume) catheter and transient inferior vena caval occlusion for rapid determination of pressure-volume relationships in man. Cathet Cardiovasc Diagn 1988;15:192–202.

48. Lee CS, Talbot TL: A fluid-mechanical study of the closure of heart valves. J Fluid Mechanics 1979;91:41–63.

49. Pasipoularides A: Clinical assessment of ventricular

ejection dynamics with and without outflow obstruction. J Am Coll Cardiol 1990;15:859–882.

50. Clark C: Relation between pressure difference across the aortic valve and left ventricular outflow. Cardiovasc Res 1978;12:276–287.

51. Carabello BA: Advances in the hemodynamic assessment of stenotic cardiac valves. J Am Coll Cardiol 1987;10:912–919.

52. Libanoff AJ, Rodbard S: Atrioventricular pressure half-time: measure of mitral valve orifice area. Circulation 1968;38:144–150.

53. Hatle L, Angelsen B, Tromsdal A: Noninvasive assessment of atrioventricular pressure half-time by Doppler ultrasound. Circulation 1979;60:1096–1104.

54. Holen J, Aaslid R, Landmark K, Simonsen S, Ostrem T: Determination of effective orifice area in mitral stenosis from non-invasive ultrasound Doppler data and mitral flow rate. Acta Med Scand 1977;201:83–88.

55. Folland ED, Parisi AF, Carbone C: Is peripheral arterial pressure a satisfactory substitute for ascending aortic pressure when measuring aortic valve gradients? J Am Coll Cardiol 1984;4:1207–1212.

56. Levine RA, Cape EG, Yoganathan AP: Pressure recovery distal to stenoses: expanding clinical applications of engineering principles. J Am Coll Cardiol 1993;21:1026–1028.

57. Voelker W, Reul H, Stelzer T, Schmidt A, Karsch KR: Pressure recovery in aortic stenosis: an in vitro study in a pulsatile flow model. J Am Coll Cardiol 1992;20:1585–1593.

58. Baumgartner H, Schima H, Tulzer G, Kuhn P: Effect of stenosis geometry on the Doppler-catheter gradient relation in vitro: a manifestation of pressure recovery. J Am Coll Cardiol 1993;21:1018–1025.

59. Laskey WK, Kussmaul WG: Pressure recovery in aortic valve stenosis. Circulation 1994;89:116–121.

60. Levine RA, Jimoh A, Cape EG, McMillan S, Yoganathan AP, Weyman AE: Pressure recovery distal to a stenosis: potential cause of gradient "overestimation" by Doppler echocardiography. J Am Coll Cardiol 1989;13:706–715.

61. Carabello BA, Barry WH, Grossman W: Changes in arterial pressure during left heart pullback in patients with aortic stenosis: a sign of severe aortic stenosis. Am J Cardiol 1979;44:424–427.

62. Pasipoularides A, Murgo JP, Bird JJ, Craig WE: Fluid dynamics of aortic stenosis: mechanisms for the presence of subvalvular pressure gradients. Am J Physiol 1984;246:H542–550.

63. Bird JJ, Murgo JP, Pasipoularides A: Fluid dynamics of aortic stenosis: subvalvular gradients without subvalvular obstruction. Circulation 1982;66:835–840.

64. Gorlin R, Gorlin SG: Hydraulic formula for calculation of the area of the stenotic mitral valve, other cardiac valves, and central circulatory shunts. Am Heart J 1951;41:1–29.

65. Gorlin R, Gorlin WB: Further reconciliation between pathoanatomy and pathophysiology of stenotic cardiac valves. J Am Coll Cardiol 1990;15:1181–1182.

66. Cohen MV, Gorlin R: Modified orifice equation for the calculation of mitral valve area. Am Heart J 1972;84:839–840.

67. Cannon SR, Richards KL, Crawford MH, et al: Inadequacy of the Gorlin formula for predicting prosthetic valve area. Am J Cardiol 1988;62:113–116.

68. Cannon SR, Richards KL, Crawford MH: Hydraulic estimation of stenotic orifice area: a correction of the Gorlin formula. Circulation 1985;71:1170–1178.

69. Richards KL, Cannon SR, Miller JF, Crawford MH: Calculation of aortic valve area by Doppler echocardiography: a direct application of the continuity equation. Circulation 1986;73:964–969.

70. Segal J, Lerner DJ, Miller DC, Mitchell RS, Alderman EA, Popp RL: When should Doppler-determined valve area be better than the Gorlin formula?: Variation in hydraulic constants in low flow states. J Am Coll Cardiol 1987;9:1294–1305.

71. Flachskampf FA, Weyman AE, Guerrero JL, Thomas JD: Influence of orifice geometry and flow rate on effective valve area: an in vitro study. J Am Coll Cardiol 1990;15:1173–1180.

72. Gorlin R, McMillan IKR, Medd WE, Matthews MB, Daley R: Dynamics of the circulation in aortic valvular disease. Am J Med 1955;18:855–870.

73. Dumesnil JG, Yoganathan AP: Theoretical and practical differences between the Gorlin formula and the continuity equation for calculating aortic and mitral valve areas. Am J Cardiol 1991;67:1268–1272.

74. Judge TP, Kennedy JW: Estimation of aortic regurgitation by diastolic pulse wave analysis. Circulation 1970;41:659–665.

75. Snyder RW, Glamann DB, Lange RA, et al: Predictive value of prominent pulmonary arterial wedge V waves in assessing the presence and severity of mitral regurgitation. Am J Cardiol 1994;73:568–570.

76. Grossman W: Profiles in valvular heart disease. *In* Baim DS, Grossman W, eds. Cardiac Catheterization, Angiography and Intervention. Baltimore: Williams & Wilkins, 1996:735–756.

77. Tamari I, Borer JS, Goldberg HL, Moses JW, Fisher J, Wallis JB: Hemodynamic changes during retrograde left-heart catheterization in patients with aortic stenosis. Cardiology 1991;78:171–178.

78. Geigy Scientific Tables, vol 5: Heart and Circulation. Basel: Ciba-Geigy, 1990.

79. Braunwald E, Marcus M, Skorton DJ, Schelbert HR, Wolf GL, Brundage BH: Marcus Cardiac Imaging: A Companion to Braunwald's Heart Disease. Philadelphia: WB Saunders, 1996.

80. Topol EJ: Textbook of Interventional Cardiology. Philadelphia: WB Saunders, 1993.

81. Westaby S, Karp RB, Blackstone EH, Bishop SP: Adult human valve dimensions and their surgical significance. Am J Cardiol 1984;53:552–556.

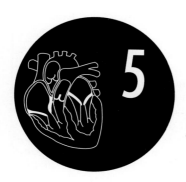

5 Other Diagnostic Approaches

Left Ventricular Volumes, Mass, and Systolic Function
  Magnetic Resonance Imaging
  Computed Tomography
  Radionuclide Ventriculography
Evaluation of Valve Dysfunction
  Valve Anatomy and Motion
  Valvular Regurgitation
    Spatial Distribution of Flow Disturbance
    Difference Between Left and Right Ventricular Stroke Volumes

Volume Flow Rates Using Velocity-Encoded Magnetic Resonance Imaging
Proximal Convergence Zone on Velocity-Encoded Images
  Valvular Stenosis
  Prosthetic Valves
Other Abnormalities
  Aortic Root Pathology
  Diastolic Left Ventricular Function
  Right Ventricular Volumes and Function
  Myocardial Metabolism

The standard clinical approach to the patient with valvular heart disease is a careful history and physical examination followed by transthoracic echocardiography. In some cases, transesophageal echocardiography, cardiac catheterization, or both may be needed. However, patients with valvular disease can be evaluated using other cardiac imaging modalities, such as radionuclide studies, computed tomography (CT), and magnetic resonance imaging (MRI). Although these procedures may provide additional useful clinical information in only selected cases, they are powerful research tools that can increase our understanding of the natural history of valvular disease. Further technical advances in these cardiac imaging procedures may lead to increased clinical use in the future.

Several areas of diagnostic concern about the patient with valvular disease can be addressed with these imaging techniques. The study may focus directly on valve anatomy and provide quantitative measures of the severity of valve dysfunction, similar to the types of data obtained by echocardiography and at cardiac catheterization. Alternatively, the study may provide quantitative data on the left ventricular (LV) response to volume or pressure overload, corresponding to the volume and ejection fraction calculations made from two-dimensional echocardiography or ventricular angiography.

Radionuclide techniques predominantly have been used for evaluation of ventricular function rather than direct assessment of valve anatomy and function. For example, radionuclide ventriculography has been used to evaluate LV and right ventricular (RV) function at rest and after exercise in patients with mitral or aortic valve regurgitation.[1–5]

MRI has great potential for evaluation of valvular disease in terms of valve anatomy and function and in terms of the LV response to chronic pressure or volume overload.[6] Conventional spin-echo images provide detailed three-dimensional (3D) views of cardiac anatomy, cine MRI allows recognition of areas of abnormal blood flow, and velocity-encoded techniques allow precise measurement of intracardiac velocities.[7–14] Together, these three MRI techniques have the potential to provide data analogous to that provided by two-dimensional echocardiography, color Doppler flow imaging, and pulsed and continuous wave Doppler velocity recordings.

CT techniques have primarily been used for evaluation of associated aortic root disease, as in patients with Marfan's syndrome. However, there has been some interest in the role of CT for direct imaging of valvular disease, particularly for quantitation of the degree of calcification using electron beam tomography.[15, 16]

Although of historical interest, phonocardiography is no longer used for evaluation of patients with valvular heart disease. Nonetheless, phonocardiography tracings can be a valuable teaching tool, especially when integrated with other diagnostic modalities.

LEFT VENTRICULAR VOLUMES, MASS, AND SYSTOLIC FUNCTION

Magnetic Resonance Imaging

The timing of surgical intervention for chronic valvular regurgitation largely is based on the LV response to chronic volume overload; the goal is identification of the onset of myocardial contractile dysfunction. Although there is no ideal clinical measure of contractility, relevant surrogate measures include LV volumes, mass, ejection fraction, and wall stress. MRI is especially well suited for evaluation of ventricular volumes and mass. Endocardial borders are clear due to the natural contrast between the blood and myocardium, epicardial borders are fully included in the image due to the wide field of view, and the data set is inherently three-dimensional (3D). For cardiac applications, temporal gating based on the electrocardiogram allows image acquisition at a specific point in the cardiac cycle (with standard spin-echo images) or as a continuous series of images (with cine MRI techniques).

Because images can be obtained in any 3D orientation and because the relationship of each image plane to the 3D data set is known, it is relatively straightforward to calculate LV volumes from endocardial borders traced at end-diastole or end-systole. Endocardial borders can be traced in multiple parallel short-axis images planes, with summation of the planar volumes to obtain the 3D volume. Alternatively, borders can be traced in two orthogonal long-axis planes, with calculation of volumes using formulas analogous to those used for echocardiographic images (Fig. 5–1). LV mass is determined by tracing endocardial and epicardial borders, calculating the volume between these two border sets, and multiplying by the mass density of myocardium.

LV volumes calculated by MRI are accurate compared with latex casts of the ventricle and compared with other imaging techniques.[17–30] Similar accuracy has been shown for LV mass calculations. MRI data also are highly repro-

ducible, with an intertest variability of less than 5%.[26, 31–36] Many investigators consider MRI as the reference standard for measurement of LV volumes, ejection fraction, and mass.

LV volumes, ejection fraction, and mass also can be calculated from cine MRI images, which provide better temporal resolution and faster acquisition times than conventional spin-echo images.[35, 37 38] Even shorter acquisition times are possible with ultrafast computed MRI and with breath-hold cine MRI.[39, 40] Because MRI images are acquired as a 3D data set, the images are particularly well suited for evaluation of ventricular shape. For example, MRI was used to study the sequential changes in LV and RV geometry in an animal model of chronic mitral regurgitation.[41]

LV wall stress can be calculated on the basis of MRI measurements of wall thickness and chamber dimensions in conjunction with cuff blood pressures and a carotid pulse tracing recorded immediately after MR image acquisition. MRI studies of patients with chronic regurgitation have shown that severe regurgitation is associated with increased wall stress.[38] MRI data also allow evaluation of the relationship between LV wall stress and ventricular mass. One disadvantage of wall stress measurements using MRI, compared with echocardiography, is that the blood pressure measurement and carotid pulse tracings cannot be recorded simultaneously with the wall thickness and chamber dimensions data. Both approaches are limited by the need to estimate end-systolic pressure from the carotid pulse tracing, a limitation that often is circumvented by calculation of peak-systolic, rather than end-systolic, wall stress.

The documented accuracy and reproducibility of MRI measurements of LV volumes, ejection fraction, and mass suggest that this modality may be particularly valuable for serial evaluations of patients with valvular heart disease and for assessment of therapeutic interventions. However, despite the potential advantages of this approach, it rarely is used for clinical patient management. Factors limiting the more widespread use of MRI in cases of valve disease include cost, nonportability, inconvenience, and imaging time. MRI cannot be performed for some patients with valvular disease, such as for those with a permanent pacer or implanted defibrillator or for medically unstable patients.

Echocardiography provides detailed images of valve anatomy and quantitation of the severity of valve stenosis and regurgitation in addi-

Biplane Long Axis

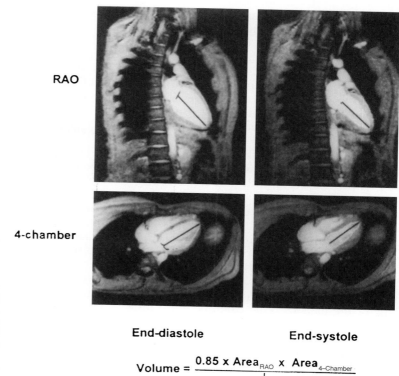

RAO

4-chamber

End-diastole   End-systole

$$Volume = \frac{0.85 \times Area_{RAO} \times Area_{4-Chamber}}{L_{min}}$$

Figure 5·1 Calculation of ventricular volumes with biplane cine MRI and the area-length method. RAO, right anterior oblique; L_{min}, minimum length. (From Blackwell GG, Pohost GM: The usefulness of cardiovascular magnetic resonance imaging. Curr Probl Cardiol 1994; 19:117–176.)

tion to reliable measures of LV size and systolic function. This advantage, in conjunction with a lower cost and greater portability, suggests that echocardiography will remain the procedure of choice for management of patients with valvular disease. However, MRI may have an important role in detailed studies of 3D cardiac anatomy and as a surrogate end point in clinical trials.

Computed Tomography

CT images gated to the cardiac cycle also can be used to calculate LV volumes, ejection fraction, and mass,[15] but they are rarely used clinically because of the need for radiographic contrast to provide delineation between the blood pool and myocardium. Cine CT offers the advantages of rapid scanning and accurate measurement of ventricular volumes and ejection fraction.[42] Cine CT also is a useful reference standard for evaluation of other methods for calculating LV volumes, such as echocardiography, in patients with valvular heart disease.[43]

Radionuclide Ventriculography

Radionuclide ventriculography provides reliable measurement of LV ejection fraction. In patients with chronic valvular disease, radionuclide ventriculography has been used for calculation of ejection fraction at rest and with exercise. Although some studies suggested that the change in ejection fraction from rest to exercise might predict the onset of contractile dysfunction in patients with chronic aortic regurgitation,[1-4] this approach is limited by the effect of loading conditions on ejection fraction. The inability to visualize valves or evaluate regurgitant severity directly with radionuclide techniques are significant disadvantages of this approach.[1, 44] Even so, there is continued interest in the use of radionuclide techniques to evaluate RV and LV systolic function after exercise in patients with mitral regurgitation.[5]

EVALUATION OF VALVE DYSFUNCTION
Valve Anatomy and Motion

Echocardiography provides real-time images of cardiac valves that are unrivaled by any other imaging modality (Table 5–1). Although cardiac-gated MRI allows visualization of aortic and mitral valve leaflets in some cases, it does not enable detailed evaluation of valve anatomy and motion.[15, 45] For example, in patients with mitral stenosis, the thickened leaflets and reduced diastolic opening of the valve can be recognized, and the maximal extent of leaflet opening correlates with stenosis severity.[46, 47] On cine CT imaging, identification of the calcified leaflets of aortic stenosis has been reported with the ability to planimeter valve area in some cases.[48] Thickened tricuspid valve leaflets in patients with carcinoid heart disease can be recognized on MRI and CT imaging.[49] Aortic valve vegetations[50] and complications of endocarditis may be recognized on MRI in some cases.[51, 52] Despite these examples, MRI and CT are rarely used clinically for evaluation of valve anatomy because of the ready availability of real-time echocardiographic imaging.

MRI has significant advantages as a research tool because of the inherent three dimensionality of the data set. One example illustrating its research potential is a study using MRI to demonstrate the normal 3D flexibility and motion of the mitral annulus during systole.[53]

Rapid CT imaging and electron beam tomography offer another potentially useful research tool because of the ability of these techniques to quantitate the extent of cardiac calcification. On CT scans, aortic valve calcification is seen incidentally in 30% of subjects, and the degree of calcification correlates with the severity of stenosis by echocardiography.[54] Electron beam CT of 49 chronic hemodialysis patients showed mitral valve calcification in 59% and aortic valve calcification in 55%, with evidence of progression over a 1-year period.[16] Noninvasive quantitation of the degree of valve calcification may provide an alternate approach to following disease progression and for assessing the response to therapeutic interventions to prevent or reverse the disease process in patients with calcific aortic stenosis.

Valvular Regurgitation

There are four basic approaches to quantitation of regurgitant severity using MRI, CT, and radionuclide techniques. First, the spatial area of the regurgitant flow disturbance can be evaluated, analogous to color Doppler flow imaging. Second, regurgitant volume can be calculated as the difference between LV and RV stroke volumes, based on endocardial border tracings for determination of ventricular volumes. Third, volume flow rate at two intracardiac sites can be used to calculate regurgitant volume and fraction. Fourth, the proximal isovelocity signal can be imaged for calculation of regurgitant flow rates.[45, 55]

Spatial Distribution of Flow Disturbance

Cine gradient-echo MRI can identify the severity of regurgitation. Areas of turbulent flow create a signal void in the high-intensity blood pool (Figs. 5–2 and 5–3), allowing identification of the presence of aortic or mitral regurgitation.[56, 57] The presence of a signal void as a marker of regurgitation is very accurate, with

TABLE 5·1 COMPARISON OF TYPES OF INFORMATION OBTAINED WITH OTHER DIAGNOSTIC APPROACHES IN PATIENTS WITH VALVULAR HEART DISEASE						
	Echocardiography	Cardiac Catheterization	MRI	CT	Radionuclide	MR-Spectroscopy
Valve anatomy and motion	+ + + +	+ +	+ +	+	−	−
Stenosis severity	+ + + +	+ + + +	+ +	+	−	−
Regurgitant severity	+ + + +	+ + + +	+ +	+	+	−
Pulmonary pressures	+ + +	+ + + +	−	−	−	−
Left ventricular size and systolic function	+ + +	+ + +	+ + + +	+ + + +	+ + +	−
Right ventricular size and function	+ + +	+ +	+ + + +	+ + +	+ + +	−
Aortic pathology	+ + + + (TEE)	+	+ + + +	+ + + +	−	−
Diastolic function	+ +	+ +	+ +	−	−	−
Myocardial metabolism	−	−	−	−	−	+ + + +

Utility on a scale of none (−) to extremely helpful (+ + + +).
TEE, transesophageal echocardiography.

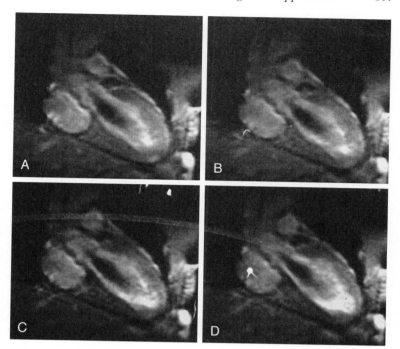

Figure 5·2 Coronal cine MRI images of a patient with severe aortic regurgitation at four time points in the cardiac cycle: end-systole *(A)*, early diastole *(B)*, mid-diastole *(C)*, late diastole *(D)*. The area of signal loss represents the regurgitant jet extending from the aortic valve into the left ventricle. (From Globits S, Higgins CB: Assessment of valvular heart disease by magnetic resonance imaging. Am Heart J 1995;129:371.)

a sensitivity of more than 93% and a specificity of more than 89% compared with Doppler flow imaging or angiography. As with color Doppler flow imaging, the 3D spatial distribution of the signal void is related to regurgitant severity, allowing separation of mild, moderate, and severe degrees of regurgitation.[58–68] Cine MRI has been used to convincingly show that the Austin-Flint murmur in patients with

aortic regurgitation is related to the extent of contact of the regurgitant jet with the LV free wall and not with impairment of mitral valve opening.[69]

As with color flow imaging, the spatial distribution of flow may be complex in three dimensions, such that evaluation in at least two orthogonal planes is necessary. The relatively low frame rates of cine MRI may complicate

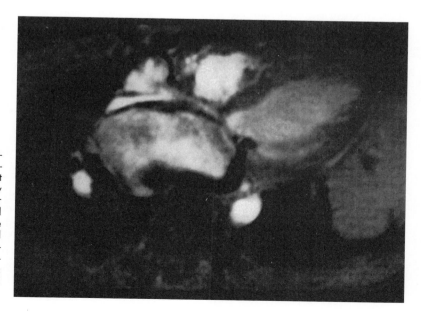

Figure 5·3 Eccentric jet of mitral regurgitation from a four-chamber cine MRI acquisition. The jet (signal void) is directed posteriorly and extends almost to the posterior atrial wall. Notice the signal void on the left ventricular side of the valve that results from the proximal convergence zone. (From Blackwell GG, Pohost GM: The usefulness of cardiovascular magnetic resonance. Curr Probl Cardiol 1994;19:117–176.)

evaluation of regurgitant severity.[56, 57] As with Doppler color flow imaging, the area of signal void on cine MRI may appear larger or smaller, depending on instrument settings, physiologic variability, and the severity of regurgitation. Standardized acquisition parameters, including echo time and window level and width, are needed for consistent results. Physiologic variability due to loading conditions must be taken into consideration, such as by recording heart rate and blood pressure at the time of the examination. Normal areas of signal void on cine MRI must not be mistaken for pathologic regurgitation.[70]

Although CT images rarely are used for evaluation of valvular regurgitation, cases of early opacification of the inferior vena cava and hepatic veins in patients with tricuspid regurgitation have been reported.[71] Although it is unlikely this approach will be useful for evaluation of patients with known valvular disease, this observation may be the first indication of valve disease in patients with an unsuspected diagnosis.

Difference Between Left and Right Ventricular Stroke Volumes

In patients with regurgitation of a single valve, regurgitant volume and fraction can be calculated from the difference between LV and RV stroke volumes. While any imaging approach potentially can be used for volume calculation, this method rarely is used with echocardiographic images because of the difficulty in accurately measuring RV stroke volume. In contrast, MRI data allow accurate calculation of RV and LV volumes. The use of conventional and cine MRI for calculation of regurgitant volume using this approach has been demonstrated for isolated mitral or aortic regurgitation.[72–74]

This approach also can be used with CT measurement of RV and LV volumes[75] or with radionuclide measures of ventricular volumes.[76–88] With ultrafast CT, regurgitant volume can be calculated as the difference between the LV stroke volume determined from cine images and the forward stroke volume determined using the indicator dilution method in the ascending aorta.[79]

In the patient with more than one affected valve, this approach provides only a measure of total regurgitant volume; the amount attributable to each valve cannot be determined. Although this approach rarely is needed for clinical decisions about patients, it has great

potential as a research tool for accurate determination of regurgitant severity in sequential studies or as a descriptor of disease severity at study entry.

Volume Flow Rates Using Velocity-Encoded Magnetic Resonance Imaging

Accurate noninvasive measurement of intracardiac velocities is possible using velocity-encoded MRI. Typically, a pair of images is generated; one shows the velocity data, and the other serves as an anatomic reference.[25] In these images, the velocity-encoded data represent average values,[45] rather than instantaneous beat-by-beat data, as are obtained with Doppler echocardiography (Fig. 5–4).

Using the principle that volume flow rate equals the flow cross-sectional area times velocity, these image pairs can be used to calculate instantaneous volume flow rates from the anatomic image (for cross-sectional area) and the velocity-encoded image (for spatial mean velocity). These data are integrated over the flow period to obtain stroke volume.

In patients with aortic regurgitation, regurgitant volume can be calculated as the difference between forward systolic flow and retrograde diastolic flow in the ascending aorta, measured by velocity-encoded MRI.[12, 80, 81] This approach has been used to monitor the response to afterload reduction in patients with chronic aortic regurgitation.[82] Analogous to the correlation between Doppler evidence of holodiastolic flow reversal in the descending aorta and severe aortic regurgitation, velocity-encoded MRI imaging of the descending aorta has been used to identify patients with severe aortic regurgitation. In a series of 20 controls and 24 patients with aortic regurgitation, the presence of marked retrograde motion in a transverse saturation band positioned 30 to 40 mm above the aortic valve indicated severe aortic regurgitation.[83]

In patients with mitral regurgitation, regurgitant volume is the difference between antegrade flow across the mitral annulus in diastole and LV ejection across the aortic valve in systole (Fig. 5–5).[84] Alternatively, the difference in flow between the aorta and pulmonary artery can be used to quantitate the severity of aortic or mitral regurgitation.[84] Each of these approaches has been validated when compared with Doppler flow mapping, angiography, or cine MRI calculations of regurgitant volume.[65, 81]

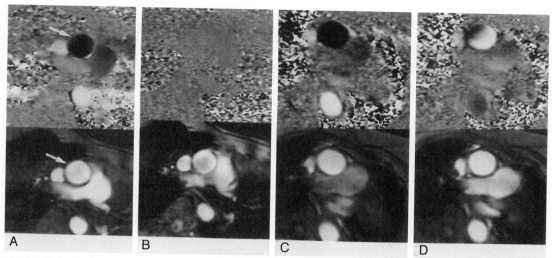

Figure 5·4 Peak systolic *(A and C)* and mid-diastolic *(B and D)* phase *(top)* and magnitude *(bottom)* MR images in a plane perpendicular to the ascending aorta *(arrow)* in a volunteer *(A and B)* and in a patient *(C and D)* with aortic regurgitation. In both persons, the ascending aorta shows a dark signal in systole, indicative of antegrade flow *(top in A and C)*. In diastole, the lack of a signal in the ascending aorta of the volunteer indicates nearly zero flow *(B)*. The white signal in the ascending aorta during diastole in the patient indicates retrograde flow *(D)*. (From Mostbeck GH, Caputo GR, Higgins CB: Am J Roentgenol 1992;159:453–461.)

Proximal Convergence Zone on Velocity-Encoded Images

The increase in velocity proximal to a regurgitant orifice can be visualized with cine MRI as an area of signal loss, similar to the proximal isovelocity surface area (PISA) seen on color Doppler flow images (see Fig. 5–3). It has been suggested that the size and persistence of the detected proximal convergence zone on cine MRI is a marker of regurgitant severity.[85–87] As with the Doppler PISA approach, the complex spatial and temporal geometry of the proximal acceleration region probably affects this measurement. A similar method that is independent of the geometry of the proximal flow field uses a "control volume" to measure volume flow rate retrograde through the regurgitant valve.[88] In vitro and preliminary in vivo validations of this approach are promising.

Valvular Stenosis

Signal loss on conventional gradient-echo or cine MRI images may allow identification of the site of obstruction, for example, subvalvular versus valvular stenosis.[12] On MRI, aortic stenosis is associated with a high-velocity jet distal to the valve, downstream turbulence, a proximal signal void related to flow acceleration, and a void at the valve plane due to

calcification (Fig. 5–6).[89] The length of the signal void in the ascending aorta allowed differentiation of sclerosis from stenosis in a small series of patients.[90] In addition, velocity-encoded MRI enables reliable measurement of the velocity across the stenotic region.[45] As with Doppler velocity data, maximal and mean transvalvular gradients can be calculated using the Bernoulli equation. The accuracy of MRI velocity data for patients with valvular stenosis has been demonstrated in small series of patients with mitral stenosis or with aortic stenosis when compared with Doppler or catheterization data (Fig. 5–7).[91–93]

Compared with Doppler echocardiography, velocity-encoded MRI has the advantages that acoustic access is not needed and alignment with jets of any direction is possible. However, the disadvantages of MRI, including cost, inconvenience, and time constraints, tend to outweigh these advantages, especially since diagnostic Doppler data can be obtained by transthoracic echocardiography in most cases. Thus, velocity-encoded MRI has not gained widespread acceptance. Other limitations of the MRI approach include image artifacts caused by flow-velocity components within the acquisition plane.[12]

MRI has been used for planimetry of aortic valve area from a short-axis anatomic image of the valve, similar to direct planimetry on transesophageal echocardiography.[94] In a

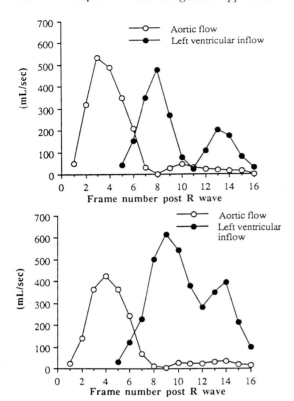

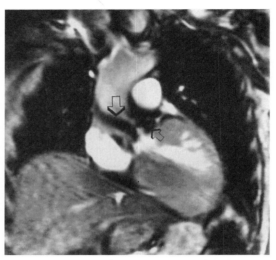

Figure 5·6 Coronal cine MRI image demonstrates a typical systolic signal void *(large arrow)* in a patient with valvular aortic stenosis. Low-signal aortic structures result from calcification *(small arrow)* and marked left ventricular hypertrophy. (From Globits S, Higgins CB: Assessment of valvular heart disease by magnetic resonance imaging. Am Heart J 1995;129:374.)

Figure 5·5 Typical left ventricular inflow and aortic flow velocity patterns derived from velocity encoded MRI images for a normal subject *(top)* and a patient with severe mitral regurgitation *(bottom)*. The normal velocity time integral for left ventricular inflow is the same as that for aortic flow over time. In mitral regurgitation, the integral of mitral inflow exceeds that of aortic flow. (From Fujita N, Chazouilleres AF, Hartiala JJ, et al: Quantification of mitral regurgitation by velocity-encoded cine nuclear magnetic resonance imaging. J Am Coll Cardiol 1994;23:951–958.)

tion of valve morphology was more helpful than the echocardiographic score for these 12 patients, the overwhelming advantages of echocardiography in providing assessment of the severity of stenosis and regurgitation dur-

small series of patients with aortic stenosis, aortic valve area measured from velocity-encoded images oriented perpendicular to the stenotic jet at the valve level correlated well with results from catheterization.[95]

Since diagnostic Doppler data are readily obtained for most patients with valvular stenosis from a transthoracic approach, velocity-encoded MRI data are likely to be clinically helpful only in rare cases. However, the ability to obtain a 3D velocity data set may have important research applications, for example, in evaluating the flow-velocity profiles proximal to and in a stenotic orifice.[96]

In a small series of patients, aortic valve area could be visualized on ultrafast CT.[48] Cine CT has been useful in evaluating mitral valve morphology in patients undergoing balloon mitral commissurotomy.[97] Although cine CT evalua-

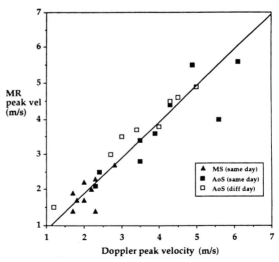

Figure 5·7 Peak jet velocity measurements determined by MRI are plotted against those determined by Doppler ultrasound for patients with aortic valve stenosis (AoS) or mitral valve stenosis (MS). (From Kilner PJ, Manzara CC, Mohiaddin RH, et al: Magnetic resonance jet velocity mapping in mitral and aortic valve stenosis. Circulation 1993;87:1239–1248.)

ing the valvuloplasty procedure suggest there is little role for cine CT in this setting.

Prosthetic Valves

MRI is considered safe for patients with prosthetic valves.[98, 99] The only exceptions are the Starr-Edwards mitral pre-6000 series valves (implanted between 1960 and 1964), which should not be scanned at field strengths greater than 0.35 Tesla.[100]

The use of cine MRI for detection of pathologic prosthetic regurgitation has been described with good correlation between cine MRI and transesophageal echocardiography in separating pathologic from physiologic regurgitation.[101, 102] Velocity-encoded MRI data have been used to measure prosthetic valve gradients and evaluate flow profiles.[103, 104]

OTHER ABNORMALITIES

MRI, CT, and radionuclide imaging may provide other useful clinical information about patients with valvular heart disease. These techniques can be used to evaluate the entire length of the aorta for aneurysm or dissection, to assess LV diastolic function, to measure RV size and systolic function, and to evaluate myocardial metabolism.

Aortic Root Anatomy

Like echocardiography, MRI and CT are noninvasive techniques. MR imaging of the aorta does not require injection of a contrast agent, and MRI and CT have the advantage of a wide field of view compared with transthoracic and transesophageal echocardiography. These properties, in conjunction with clear views of the entire aorta, make these approaches particularly valuable in assessing valve disease patients with associated aortic disease. For example, MRI has been used to evaluate aortic root graft anatomy after composite replacement of the aortic root,[105] and it is a standard method of follow-up for patients with Marfan's syndrome or previous aortic root surgery.[106, 107]

Diastolic Left Ventricular Function

Evaluation of diastolic function in patients with valvular disease remains problematic. MRI has been used to evaluate diastolic filling on the basis of the regional myocardial long-axis velocity in diastole,[108] the 3D pattern of diastolic filling evaluated with velocity-encoded MRI,[109, 110] and the transmitral and pulmonary vein filling patterns, analogous to Doppler measures of filling rates.[111]

In a small group of patients with aortic stenosis, velocity-encoded MRI evaluation of early and late diastolic filling velocities correlated well with Doppler measures, and a higher atrial contribution to ventricular filling (compared with normal controls) was demonstrated.[112] Although MRI evaluation of diastolic filling is unlikely to gain wide clinical use, this approach may provide useful data on the sequence of changes in diastolic function as the severity of valve disease increases and may allow evaluation of changes in diastolic function after therapeutic interventions.

Right Ventricular Volumes and Function

Many patients with valvular disease have RV enlargement and systolic dysfunction secondary to left-sided valve disease with consequent pulmonary hypertension. Echocardiographic evaluation of the right ventricle typically is limited to qualitative descriptions of RV size and systolic function, usually on a scale of mild, moderate, or severe.

RV volumes, ejection fraction, and mass can be reliably evaluated using MRI data.[12, 113–116] This approach offers the potential for more reliable evaluation of RV involvement in patients with valvular disease. However, since these data rarely are needed for clinical decision making, quantitative evaluation of the right ventricle cannot be considered routine.

Cine CT evaluation of cardiac volumes before and after mitral commissurotomy in 11 patients showed a decrease in left atrial volume and increase in RV and LV diastolic volumes 5 days after the procedure, with continued changes in cardiac volumes detected at the 1-year follow-up examination.[117] Another example of the use of CT techniques for patients with valvular disease is a study of 35 patients with mitral regurgitation in which regurgitant fraction calculated by electron beam tomography was negatively correlated with the RV ejection fraction.[118]

Radionuclide assessment of RV function can be helpful in patients with mitral regurgitation. For example, in one study of patients with severe mitral regurgitation, the RV ejection fraction response to exercise was more predictive of disease progression than LV parameters.[5] In a more detailed approach to evaluation of RV function, another group used

Fourier phase transforms of radionuclide ventriculograms for evaluation of the pattern of RV wall motion. There was marked heterogeneity in the pattern of RV contraction in patients with mitral valve prolapse compared with normal subjects in this study.[119]

Myocardial Metabolism

The potential use of MR spectroscopy or positron emission tomography for evaluation of myocardial metabolism in patients with LV volume or pressure overload caused by valvular disease has received less attention, although a few interesting studies have been published. For example, MR spectroscopy in an animal model of chronic mitral regurgitation showed that, compared with normal hearts, LV dilation was associated with low myocardial creatine phosphate to ATP ratio in each layer of the ventricular wall. These findings may explain the impaired contractile reserve with exercise observed in this model.[120]

Positron emission tomography has been used in studies of myocardial oxidative metabolism of the left and right ventricles in patients with aortic valve disease.[121, 122] Global myocardial C-11 labeled acetate clearance was higher in patients with aortic valve disease, and the degree of abnormality correlated with the severity of aortic stenosis. The authors suggest that these changes may reflect myocardial adaption or impaired contractility and further suggest that indices of myocardial oxygen demand may provide useful information on disease progression in patients with pressure overload. Others have also suggested that abnormalities in myocardial metabolism might serve as early markers of contractile dysfunction, allowing optimization of the timing of surgical intervention in patients with chronic pressure or volume overload due to valvular heart disease.[45]

References

1. Bonow RO, Lakatos E, Maron BJ, Epstein SE: Serial long-term assessment of the natural history of asymptomatic patients with chronic aortic regurgitation and normal left ventricular systolic function. Circulation 1991;84:1625–1635.
2. Massie BM, Kramer BL, Loge D, et al: Ejection fraction response to supine exercise in asymptomatic aortic regurgitation: relation to simultaneous hemodynamic measurements. J Am Coll Cardiol 1985;5:847–855.
3. Greenberg B, Massie B, Thomas D, et al: Association between the exercise ejection fraction response and systolic wall stress in patients with chronic aortic insufficiency. Circulation 1985;71:458–465.
4. Iskandrian AS, Heo J: Radionuclide angiographic evaluation of left ventricular performance at rest and during exercise in patients with aortic regurgitation. Am Heart J 1986;111:1143–1149.
5. Rosen SE, Borer JS, Hochreiter C, et al: Natural history of the asymptomatic/minimally symptomatic patient with severe mitral regurgitation secondary to mitral valve prolapse and normal right and left ventricular performance. Am J Cardiol 1994;74:374–380.
6. Blackwell GG, Pohost GM: The usefulness of cardiovascular magnetic resonance imaging. Curr Probl Cardiol 1994;19:117–175.
7. Rebergen SA, van-der-Wall EE, Doornbos J, de Roos A: Magnetic resonance measurement of velocity and flow: technique, validation, and cardiovascular applications. Am Heart J 1993;126:1439–1456.
8. MacMillan RM: Cardiac magnetic resonance imaging. Cardiovasc Clin 1993;23:125–35.
9. Rehr RB: Cardiovascular nuclear magnetic resonance imaging and spectroscopy. Curr Probl Cardiol 1991;16:125–215.
10. Kayser HW, Stoel BC, van der Wall EE, van der Geest RJ, de Roos A: MR velocity mapping of tricuspid flow: correction for through-plane motion. J Magn Reson Imaging 1997;7:669–673.
11. Haacke EM, Li D, Kaushikkar S: Cardiac MR imaging: principles and techniques. Top Magn Reson Imaging 1995;7:200–217.
12. Globits S, Higgins CB: Assessment of valvular heart disease by magnetic resonance imaging. Am Heart J 1995;129:369–381.
13. Duerinckx AJ, Higgins CB: Valvular heart disease. Radiol Clin North Am 1994;32:613–630.
14. Cranney GB, Lotan CS, Pohost GM: Nuclear magnetic resonance imaging for assessment and follow-up of patients with valve disease. Circulation 1991;84:I216–I227.
15. Bateman TM: X-ray computed tomography of the cardiovascular system. Curr Probl Cardiol 1991;16:765–829.
16. Braun J, Oldendorf M, Moshage W, Heidler R, Zeitler E, Luft FC: Electron beam computed tomography in the evaluation of cardiac calcification in chronic dialysis patients. Am J Kidney Dis 1996;27:394–401.
17. Rehr RB, Malloy CR, Filipchuk NG, Peshock RM: Left ventricular volumes measured by MR imaging. Ann Thorac Surg 1985;156:717–719.
18. Utz JA, Herfkens RJ, Heinsimer JA, et al: Cine MR determination of left ventricular ejection fraction. AJR Am J Roentgenol 1987;148:839–843.
19. Buser PT, Auffermann W, Holt WW, et al: Noninvasive evaluation of global left ventricular function with use of cine nuclear magnetic resonance. J Am Coll Cardiol 1989;13:1294–1300.
20. Buckwalter KA, Aisen AM, Dilworth LR, Mancini GB, Buda AJ: Gated cardiac MRI: ejection-fraction determination using the right anterior oblique view. Am J Roentgenol 1986;147:33–37.
21. Markiewicz W, Sechtem U, Kirby R, Derugin N, Caputo GC, Higgins CB: Measurement of ventricular volumes in the dog by nuclear magnetic resonance imaging. J Am Coll Cardiol 1987;10:170–177.
22. Dilworth LR, Aisen AM, Mancini GB, Lande I, Buda AJ: Determination of left ventricular volumes and ejection fraction by nuclear magnetic resonance imaging. Am Heart J 1987;113:24–32.
23. Longmore DB, Klipstein RH, Underwood SR, et al:

Dimensional accuracy of magnetic resonance in studies of the heart. Lancet 1985;1:1360–1362.

24. Underwood SR, Gill CR, Firmin DN, et al: Left ventricular volume measured rapidly by oblique magnetic resonance imaging. Br Heart J 1988;60:188–195.

25. Cranney GB, Lotan CS, Dean L, Baxley W, Bouchard A, Pohost GM: Left ventricular volume measurement using cardiac axis nuclear magnetic resonance imaging. Validation by calibrated ventricular angiography. Circulation 1990;82:154–163.

26. Ostrzega E, Maddahi J, Honma H, et al: Quantification of left ventricular myocardial mass in humans by nuclear magnetic resonance imaging. Am Heart J 1989;117:444–452.

27. Sechtem U, Pflugfelder PW, Gould RG, Cassidy MM, Higgins CB. Measurement of right and left ventricular volumes in healthy individuals with cine MR imaging. Ann Thorac Surg 1987;163:697–702.

28. Stratemeier EJ, Thompson R, Brady TJ, et al: Ejection fraction determination by MR imaging: comparison with left ventricular angiography. Ann Thorac Surg 1986;158:775–777.

29. van-Rossum AC, Visser FC, van-Eenige MJ, Valk J, Roos JP: Magnetic resonance imaging of the heart for determination of ejection fraction. Int J Cardiol 1988;18:53–63.

30. van-Rossum AC, Visser FC, Sprenger M, van-Eenige MJ, Valk J, Roos JP: Evaluation of magnetic resonance imaging for determination of left ventricular ejection fraction and comparison with angiography. Am J Cardiol 1988;62:628–633.

31. Maddahi J, Crues J, Berman DS, et al: Noninvasive quantification of left ventricular myocardial mass by gated proton nuclear magnetic resonance imaging. J Am Coll Cardiol 1987;10:682–692.

32. Florentine MS, Grosskreutz CL, Chang W, et al: Measurement of left ventricular mass in vivo using gated nuclear magnetic resonance imaging. J Am Coll Cardiol 1986;8:107–112.

33. Keller AM, Peshock RM, Malloy CR, et al: In vivo measurement of myocardial mass using nuclear magnetic resonance imaging. J Am Coll Cardiol 1986;8:113–117.

34. Caputo GR, Tscholakoff D, Sechtem U, Higgins CB. Measurement of canine left ventricular mass by using MR imaging. Am J Roentgenol 1987;148:33–38.

35. Shapiro EP, Rogers WJ, Beyar R, Soulen RL, et al: Determination of left ventricular mass by magnetic resonance imaging in hearts deformed by acute infarction. Circulation 1989;79:706–711.

36. Semelka RC, Tomei E, Wagner S, et al. Normal left ventricular dimensions and function: interstudy reproducibility of measurements with cine MR imaging. Ann Thorac Surg 1990;174:8.

37. Semelka RC, Tomei E, Wagner S, et al: Interstudy reproducibility of dimensional and functional measurements between cine magnetic resonance studies in the morphologically abnormal left ventricle. Am Heart J 1990;119:1367–1373.

38. Auffermann W, Wagner S, Holt WW, et al: Noninvasive determination of left ventricular output and wall stress in volume overload and in myocardial disease by cine magnetic resonance imaging. Am Heart J 1991;121:8.

39. Soldo SJ, Haywood LJ, Norris SL, Gober JR, Colletti PM, Terk MR: Method for assessing cardiac function using magnetic resonance imaging. Biomed Instrum Technol 1996;30:359–363.

40. Sakuma H, Fujita N, Foo TK, et al: Evaluation of left ventricular volume and mass with breath-hold cine MR imaging. Ann Thorac Surg 1993;188:377–380.

41. Young AA, Orr R, Smaill BH, Dell'Italia LJ: Three-dimensional changes in left and right ventricular geometry in chronic mitral regurgitation. Am J Physiol 1996;271:700.

42. Rumberger JA, Reiring AJ, Rees MR, et al: Quantitation of left ventricular mass and volume in normal patients using cine computed tomography. J Am Coll Cardiol 1986;7:173.

43. Rihal CS, Nishimura RA, Rumberger JA, Tajik AJ: Quantitative echocardiography: a comparison with ultrafast computed tomography in patients with chronic aortic regurgitation. J Heart Valve Dis 1994;3:417–424.

44. Starling MR, Kirsh MM, Montgomery DG, Gross MD: Mechanisms for left ventricular systolic dysfunction in aortic regurgitation: importance for predicting the functional response to aortic valve replacement. J Am Coll Cardiol 1991;17:887–897.

45. Schmidt M, Crnac J, Dederichs B, Theissen P, Schicha H, Sechtem U: Magnetic resonance imaging in valvular heart disease. Int J Card Imaging 1997;13:219–231.

46. Casolo GC, Zampa V, Rega L, et al: Evaluation of mitral stenosis by cine magnetic resonance imaging. Am Heart J 1992;123:1252–1260.

47. Rees MR, MacMillan RM, Lopez M, et al: Demonstration of mitral valve function by cine computed tomography using a new long axis view. Angiology 1986;37:79–85.

48. MacMillan RM, Rees MR, Lumia FJ, Maranhao V: Preliminary experience in the use of ultrafast computed tomography to diagnose aortic valve stenosis. Am Heart J 1988;115:665–671.

49. Mirowitz SA, Gutierrez FR: MR and CT diagnosis of carcinoid heart disease. Chest 1993;103:630–631.

50. Caduff JH, Hernandez RJ, Ludomirsky A: MR visualization of aortic valve vegetations. J Comput Assist Tomogr 1996;20:613–615.

51. Schwartz DR, Belkin RN, Pucillo AL, et al: Aneurysm of the mitral-aortic intervalvular fibrosa complicating infective endocarditis: preoperative characterization by two-dimensional and color flow Doppler echocardiography, magnetic resonance imaging, and cineangiography. Am Heart J 1990;119:196–199.

52. Winkler ML, Higgins CB: MRI of perivalvular infectious pseudoaneurysms. Am J Roentgenol 1986;147:253–256.

53. Komoda T, Hetzer R, Oellinger J, et al: Mitral annular flexibility. J Card Surg 1997;12:102–109.

54. Lippert JA, White CS, Mason AC, Plotnick GD: Calcification of aortic valve detected incidentally on CT scans: prevalence and clinical significance. Am J Roentgenol 1995;164:73–77.

55. Cranney GB, Lotan CS, Pohost GM: Evaluation of aortic regurgitation by nuclear magnetic resonance imaging. Curr Probl Cardiol 1990;15:87–114.

56. Evans AJ, Blinder RA, Herfkens RJ, et al: Effects of turbulence on signal intensity in gradient echo images. Invest Radiol 1988;23:512–518.

57. Evans AJ, Hedlund LW, Herfkens RJ, Utz JA, Fram EK, Blinder RA: Evaluation of steady and pulsatile flow with dynamic MRI using limited flip angles and gradient refocused echoes. Magn Reson Imaging 1987;5:475–482.

58. Utz JA, Herfkens RJ, Heinsimer JA, Shimakawa A, Glover G, Pelc N: Valvular regurgitation: dynamic MR imaging. Ann Thorac Surg 1988;168:91–94.

59. Wagner S, Auffermann W, Buser P, et al: Diagnostic accuracy and estimation of the severity of valvular regurgitation from the signal void on cine magnetic resonance images. Am Heart J 1989;118:760–767.

60. Aurigemma G, Reichek N, Schiebler M, Axel L: Evaluation of aortic regurgitation by cardiac cine magnetic resonance imaging: planar analysis and comparison to Doppler echocardiography. Cardiology 1991;78:340–347.

61. Nishimura F: Oblique cine MRI for the evaluation of aortic regurgitation: comparison with cineangiography. Clin Cardiol 1992;15:73–78.

62. Nishimura T, Yamada N, Itoh A, Miyatake K: Cine MR imaging in mitral regurgitation: comparison with color Doppler flow imaging. Am J Roentgenol 1989;153:721–724.

63. Pflugfelder PW, Sechtem UP, White RD, Cassidy MM, Schiller NB, Higgins CB: Noninvasive evaluation of mitral regurgitation by analysis of left atrial signal loss in cine magnetic resonance. Am Heart J 1989;117:1113–1119.

64. Aurigemma G, Reichek N, Schiebler M, Axel L: Evaluation of mitral regurgitation by cine magnetic resonance imaging. Am J Cardiol 1990;66:621–625.

65. Hundley WG, Li HF, Willard JE, et al: Magnetic resonance imaging assessment of the severity of mitral regurgitation. Comparison with invasive techniques. Circulation 1995;92:1151–1158.

66. Pflugfelder PW, Landzberg JS, Cassidy MM, et al: Comparison of cine MR imaging with Doppler echocardiography for the evaluation of aortic regurgitation. Am J Roentgenol 1989;152:729–735.

67. Ohnishi S, Fukui S, Kusuoka H, Kitabatake A, Inoue M, Kamada T: Assessment of valvular regurgitation using cine magnetic resonance imaging coupled with phase compensation technique: comparison with Doppler color flow mapping. Angiology 1992;43:913–924.

68. Underwood SR, Klipstein RH, Firmin DN, et al: Magnetic resonance assessment of aortic and mitral regurgitation. Br Heart J 1986;56:455–462.

69. Landzberg JS, Pflugfelder PW, Cassidy MM, Schiller NB, Higgins CB, Cheitlin MD: Etiology of the Austin Flint murmur. J Am Coll Cardiol 1992;20:408–413.

70. Mirowitz SA, Lee JK, Gutierrez FR, Brown JJ, Eilenberg SS: Normal signal-void patterns in cardiac cine MR images. Ann Thorac Surg 1990;176:49–55.

71. Collins MA, Pidgeon JW, Fitzgerald R: Computed tomography manifestations of tricuspid regurgitation. Br J Radiol 1995;68:1058–1060.

72. Glogar D, Globits S, Neuhold A, Mayr H: Assessment of mitral regurgitation by magnetic resonance imaging. Magn Reson Imaging 1989;7:611–617.

73. Globits S, Frank H, Mayr H, Neuhold A, Glogar D: Quantitative assessment of aortic regurgitation by magnetic resonance imaging. Eur Heart J 1992;13:78–83.

74. Sechtem U, Pflugfelder PW, Cassidy MM, et al: Mitral or aortic regurgitation: quantification of regurgitant volumes with cine MR imaging. Ann Thorac Surg 1988;167:425–430.

75. Reiter SJ, Rumberger JA, Stanford W, Marcus ML: Quantitative determination of aortic regurgitant volumes in dogs by ultrafast computed tomography. Circulation 1987;76:728–735.

76. Rigo P, Alderson PO, Robertson RM, Becker LC, Wagner HNJ: Measurement of aortic and mitral regurgitation by gated cardiac blood pool scans. Circulation 1979;60:306–312.

77. Sorensen SG, O'Rourke RA, Chaudhuri TK: Noninvasive quantitation of valvular regurgitation by gated equilibrium radionuclide angiography. Circulation 1980;62:1089–1098.

78. Lam W, Pavel D, Byrom E, Sheikh A, Best D, Rosen K: Radionuclide regurgitant index: value and limitations. Am J Cardiol 1981;47:292–298.

79. Kaminaga T, Naito H, Takamiya M, Nishimura T: Quantitative evaluation of mitral regurgitation with ultrafast CT. J Comput Assist Tomogr 1994;18:239–242.

80. Dulce MC, Mostbeck GH, O'Sullivan M, Cheitlin M, Caputo GR, Higgins CB: Severity of aortic regurgitation: interstudy reproducibility of measurements with velocity-encoded cine MR imaging. Ann Thorac Surg 1992;185:235–240.

81. Sondergaard L, Lindvig K, Hildebrandt P, et al: Quantification of aortic regurgitation by magnetic resonance velocity mapping. Am Heart J 1993;125:1081–1090.

82. Globits S, Blake L, Bourne M, et al: Assessment of hemodynamic effects of angiotensin converting enzyme inhibitor therapy in chronic aortic regurgitation by using velocity-encoded cine magnetic resonance imaging. Am Heart J 1996;131:289–293.

83. Ambrosi P, Faugere G, Desfossez L, et al: Assessment of aortic regurgitation severity by magnetic resonance imaging of the thoracic aorta. Eur Heart J 1995;16:406–409.

84. Fujita N, Chazouilleres AF, Hartiala JJ, et al: Quantification of mitral regurgitation by velocity-encoded cine nuclear magnetic resonance imaging. J Am Coll Cardiol 1994;23:951–958.

85. Yoshida K, Yoshikawa J, Hozumi T, et al: Assessment of aortic regurgitation by the acceleration flow signal void proximal to the leaking orifice in cine-magnetic resonance imaging. Circulation 1991;83:1951–1955.

86. Cranney GB, Benjelloun H, Perry GJ, et al: Rapid assessment of aortic regurgitation and left ventricular function using cine nuclear magnetic resonance imaging and the proximal convergence zone. Am J Cardiol 1993;71:1074–1081.

87. Simpson IA, Maciel BC, Moises V, et al: Cine magnetic resonance imaging and color Doppler flow mapping displays of flow velocity, spatial acceleration, and jet formation: a comparative in vitro study. Am Heart J 1993;126:1165–1174.

88. Walker PG, Oyre S, Pedersen EM, Houlind K, Guenet FS, Yoganathan AP: A new control volume method for calculating valvular regurgitation. Circulation 1995;92:579–586.

89. DeRoos A, Reichek N, Axel L, Kressel HY: Cine MR imaging in aortic stenosis. J Comput Assist Tomogr 1989;13:421–425.

90. Mitchell L, Jenkins JP, Watson Y, Rowlands DJ, Isherwood I: Diagnosis and assessment of mitral and aortic valve disease by cine-flow magnetic resonance imaging. Magn Reson Med 1989;12:181–197.

91. Heidenreich PA, Steffens J, Fujita N, et al: Evaluation of mitral stenosis with velocity-encoded cine-magnetic resonance imaging. Am J Cardiol 1995;75:365–369.

92. Eichenberger AC, Jenni R, von-Schulthess GK: Aortic valve pressure gradients in patients with aortic

valve stenosis: quantification with velocity-encoded cine MR imaging. Am J Roentgenol 1993;160:971–977.

93. Kilner PJ, Manzara CC, Mohiaddin RH, et al: Magnetic resonance jet velocity mapping in mitral and aortic valve stenosis. Circulation 1993;87:1239–1248.

94. Kupari M, Hekali P, Keto P, et al: Assessment of aortic valve area in aortic stenosis by magnetic resonance imaging. Am J Cardiol 1992;70:952–955.

95. Sondergaard L, Hildebrandt P, Lindvig K, et al: Valve area and cardiac output in aortic stenosis: quantification by magnetic resonance velocity mapping. Am Heart J 1993;126:1156–1164.

96. Kilner PJ, Firmin DN, Rees RS, et al: Valve and great vessel stenosis: assessment with MR jet velocity mapping. Ann Thorac Surg 1991;178:229–235.

97. White ML, Grover MM, Weiss RM, et al: Prediction of change in mitral valve area after mitral balloon commissurotomy using cine computed tomography. Invest Radiol 1994;29:827–833.

98. Soulen RL, Budinger TF, Higgins CB: Magnetic resonance imaging of prosthetic heart valves. Ann Thorac Surg 1985;154:705–707.

99. Randall PA, Kohman LJ, Scalzetti EM, Szeverenyi NM, Panicek DM: Magnetic resonance imaging of prosthetic cardiac valves in vitro and in vivo. Am J Cardiol 1988;62:973–976.

100. Shellock FG, Morisoli S, Kanal E: MR procedures and biomedical implants, materials, and devices: 1993 update. Ann Thorac Surg 1993;189:587–599.

101. Deutsch HJ, Bachmann R, Sechtem U, et al: Regurgitant flow in cardiac valve prostheses: diagnostic value of gradient echo nuclear magnetic resonance imaging in reference to transesophageal two-dimensional color Doppler echocardiography. J Am Coll Cardiol 1992;19:1500–1507.

102. Bachmann R, Deutsch HJ, Jungehulsing M, Sechtem U, Hilger HH, Schicha H: Magnetic resonance tomography in patients with a heart valve prosthesis [in German]. Rofo Fortschr Geb Rontgenstr Neuen Bildgeb Verfahr 1991;155:499–505.

103. DiCesare E, Enrici RM, Paparoni S, et al: Low-field magnetic resonance imaging in the evaluation of mechanical and biological heart valve function. Eur J Radiol 1995;20:224–228.

104. Walker PG, Pedersen EM, Oyre S, et al: Magnetic resonance velocity imaging: a new method for prosthetic heart valve study. J Heart Valve Dis 1995;4:296–307.

105. Lepore V, Lamm C, Bugge M, Larsson S: Magnetic resonance imaging in the follow-up of patients after aortic root reconstruction. Thorac Cardiovasc Surg 1996;44:188–192.

106. Smith JA, Fann JI, Miller DC, et al: Surgical management of aortic dissection in patients with the Marfan syndrome. Circulation 1994;90:235–42.

107. Finkbohner R, Johnston D, Crawford ES, Coselli J, Milewicz DM: Marfan syndrome. Long-term survival and complications after aortic aneurysm repair. Circulation 1995;91:728–733.

108. Karwatowski SP, Brecker SJ, Yang GZ, Firmin DN, St. John SM, Underwood SR: A comparison of left ventricular myocardial velocity in diastole measured by magnetic resonance and left ventricular filling measured by Doppler echocardiography. Eur Heart J 1996;17:795–802.

109. Walker PG, Cranney GB, Grimes RY, et al: Three-dimensional reconstruction of the flow in a human left heart by using magnetic resonance phase velocity encoding. Ann Biomed Eng 1996;24:139–147.

110. Kim WY, Walker PG, Pedersen EM, et al: Left ventricular blood flow patterns in normal subjects: a quantitative analysis by three-dimensional magnetic resonance velocity mapping. J Am Coll Cardiol 1995;26:224–238.

111. Hartiala JJ, Mostbeck GH, Foster E, et al: Velocity-encoded cine MRI in the evaluation of left ventricular diastolic function: measurement of mitral valve and pulmonary vein flow velocities and flow volume across the mitral valve. Am Heart J 1993;125:1054–1066.

112. Hartiala JJ, Foster E, Fujita N, et al: Evaluation of left atrial contribution to left ventricular filling in aortic stenosis by velocity-encoded cine MRI. Am Heart J 1994;127:593–600.

113. Doherty NE, Fujita N, Caputo GR, Higgins CB: Measurement of right ventricular mass in normal and dilated cardiomyopathic ventricles using cine magnetic resonance imaging. Am J Cardiol 1992;69:1223–1228.

114. Mackey ES, Sandler MP, Campbell RM, et al: Right ventricular myocardial mass quantification with magnetic resonance imaging. Am J Cardiol 1990;65:529–532.

115. Mogelvang J, Stubgaard M, Thomsen C, Henriksen O: Evaluation of right ventricular volumes measured by magnetic resonance imaging. Eur Heart J 1988;9:529–533.

116. McDonald KM, Parrish T, Wennberg P, et al: Rapid, accurate and simultaneous noninvasive assessment of right and left ventricular mass with nuclear magnetic resonance imaging using the snapshot gradient method. J Am Coll Cardiol 1992;19:1601–1607.

117. Grover MM, Weiss RM, Vandenberg BF, et al: Assessment of cardiac volumes and left ventricular mass by cine computed tomography before and after mitral balloon commissurotomy. Am Heart J 1994;128:533–539.

118. Shields JP, Watson P, Mielke CH Jr: The right ventricle in mitral regurgitation: evaluation by electron beam tomography. J Heart Valve Dis 1995;4:490–494.

119. Delhomme C, Casset-Senon D, Babuty D, et al: A study of 36 cases of mitral valve prolapse by isotopic ventricular tomography. Arch Mal Coer Vaiss 1996;89:1127–1135.

120. Zhang J, Toher C, Erhard M, et al: Relationships between myocardial bioenergetic and left ventricular function in hearts with volume-overload hypertrophy. Circulation 1997;96:334–343.

121. Hicks RJ, Savas V, Currie PJ, et al: Assessment of myocardial oxidative metabolism in aortic valve disease using positron emission tomography with C-11 acetate. Am Heart J 1992;123:653–664.

122. Hicks RJ, Kalff V, Savas V, Starling MR, Schwaiger M: Assessment of right ventricular oxidative metabolism by positron emission tomography with C-11 acetate in aortic valve disease. Am J Cardiol 1991;67:753–757.

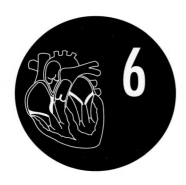

6 Principles of Medical Therapy for Valvular Heart Disease

Diagnosis of Valve Disease
Preventative Measures
   Diagnosis and Prevention of Rheumatic
     Fever
   Prevention of Bacterial Endocarditis
   Prevention of Embolic Events
     Anticoagulation Service
     Anticoagulation for Native Valve
      Disease
   General Health Maintenance
Slowing Disease Progression
   Prevention of Left Ventricular
     Contractile Dysfunction
   Prevention of Left Atrial Enlargement
     and Atrial Fibrillation
   Prevention of Pulmonary Hypertension
   Prevention of Progressive Valve Disease

Patient Education
Medical Treatment of Symptomatic
   Disease
Timing and Choice of Surgical
   Intervention
Medical Management of the
   Postoperative Patient
   Anticoagulation for Prosthetic Valves
     Chronic Warfarin Therapy
     Management of Patients Undergoing
      Surgical Procedures
     Management During Pregnancy
   Noninvasive Monitoring After Valve
     Surgery

DIAGNOSIS OF VALVE DISEASE

Valvular heart disease may first be diagnosed in the setting of an acute medical event, such as heart failure, pulmonary edema, atrial fibrillation, or infective endocarditis. More often, the diagnosis of valvular heart disease is initially suspected before the onset of overt symptoms on the basis of the physical examination finding of a cardiac murmur, during screening of relatives in a family with a history of a genetic disorder, or because of abnormal findings on an electrocardiogram, chest radiograph, or echocardiogram requested for unrelated reasons. Worldwide, many patients are first diagnosed with valvular heart disease when a cardiac murmur is heard during an episode of acute rheumatic fever.

For a patient with a cardiac murmur, the first step is clinical assessment based on the history and physical examination findings.[1–3] If clinical evaluation indicates probable significant valvular disease, the next step is echocar-

diography to confirm the diagnosis and evaluate valve anatomy and function.[4, 5] Clinical guidelines for indications for echocardiography have been published,[6] and a condensed version of the recommendations for patients with suspected or known valve disease is shown in Table 6–1.

In a patient with cardiac or respiratory symptoms and a cardiac murmur heard on auscultation, it is prudent to obtain an echocardiogram to evaluate possible valvular disease (Fig. 6–1). When the patient has symptoms, it is difficult to reliably exclude significant valvular disease on physical examination as findings may be subtle.[7] For example, some patients with severe aortic stenosis have only a grade 2 or 3 murmur on examination, and the carotid upstroke may appear normal because of coexisting atherosclerosis.[8–10] Diagnosis may be even more difficult in other situations. For example, only 50% of patients with acute mitral regurgitation have an audible murmur.[11]

TABLE 6·1	**SUMMARY OF ACC/AHA GUIDELINES[6] FOR ECHOCARDIOGRAPHY IN PATIENTS WITH SUSPECTED OR KNOWN VALVULAR HEART DISEASE (CLASS I INDICATIONS)**

Suspected Valvular Disease

Cardiac murmur in a patient with cardiorespiratory symptoms
Murmur suggestive of structural heart disease, even if asymptomatic
Chest pain with evidence of valve disease
Screening studies in asymptomatic patients with
    Family history of genetically transmitted cardiovascular disease
    Phenotypic features of Marfan's syndrome or related connective tissue disorders

Native Valve Disease

Stenosis
    Initial diagnosis and assessment of hemodynamic severity
    Assessment of left and right ventricular size, function, and hemodynamics
    Assessment of changes in valve or ventricular function during pregnancy
Regurgitation
    All patients
        Initial diagnosis and assessment of hemodynamic severity
        Initial evaluation of left and right ventricular size, function, and hemodynamics
    Mild to moderate regurgitation
        Reevaluation with a change in symptoms
        Reevaluation in patients with ventricular dilation
    Severe regurgitation
        Periodic reevaluation, even in asymptomatic patients
        Assessment of the effects of medical therapy on regurgitant severity and ventricular size and
            function
        Reassessment of valve and ventricular function during pregnancy
Mitral valve prolapse
    Assessment of leaflet morphology, hemodynamic severity, and ventricular compensation
Infective endocarditis
    Diagnosis of valvular lesion, hemodynamic severity, and ventricular compensation*
    Detection of vegetations in congenital heart disease patients with suspected endocarditis
    Detection of complications, such as abscesses and fistulas*
    Reevaluation in patients with complex endocarditis (eg, virulent organism, severe regurgitation,
        aortic valve involvement, persistent fever or bacteremia)
    High clinical suspicion of culture negative endocarditis*
Interventions for valvular disease
    Timing of valvular intervention when based on ventricular compensation, function, or severity of
        primary valvular lesion or secondary hemodynamic changes
    Selection of alternate therapies for mitral valve disease (balloon valvuloplasty, surgical valve repair
        vs replacement)*
    Monitoring interventional techniques
    Postintervention baseline study
    (Intraoperative echocardiography not addressed in this document)

Prosthetic Valves

Baseline after intervention for valve function (early) and ventricular remodeling (late)
Changing clinical signs and symptoms or suspected prosthetic valve dysfunction*
Prosthetic valve endocarditis
    Detection of endocarditis and characterization of valve and ventricular function*
    Detection of endocarditis complications and reevaluation in complex endocarditis*
    Suspected endocarditis and negative blood cultures*
    Bacteremia without known source*

*Transesophageal echocardiography usually is required.

Among asymptomatic patients with murmurs detected during physical examination, those with benign flow murmurs should be differentiated from those with pathologic murmurs. Although there are no absolutely reliable criteria for making this distinction, a reasonable pretest estimate of the likelihood of disease can be derived from the history and physical examination findings. Flow murmurs, defined as audible systolic murmurs in the absence of structural heart disease, are most common in younger patients and those with high-output states. A flow murmur is a normal finding in pregnancy and is heard in more

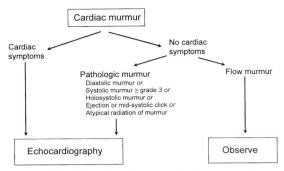

Figure 6·1 Flow chart illustrates the diagnostic pathway for evaluation of a cardiac murmur.

than 80% of pregnant women.[4, 5] Flow murmurs also are likely in patients who are anemic or febrile. Typically, a flow murmur is systolic, low intensity (grade 1 to 2), loudest at the base with little radiation, ends before the second heart sound, and is crescendo-decrescendo or "ejection" shaped with an early systolic peak. These murmurs are related to rapid ejection into the aorta or pulmonary artery in patients with normal valve function, high flow rates, and good transmission of sound to the chest wall.[2, 3] The yield of echocardiography is very low for asymptomatic patients with typical flow murmurs detected on examination, no cardiac history, and no cardiac symptoms elicited on careful questioning.

In contrast, echocardiographic examination usually is helpful for an asymptomatic patient with a diastolic murmur, a systolic murmur of grade 3 or higher, an ejection click or mid-systolic click, a holosystolic (rather than ejection) murmur, or an atypical pattern of radiation. To some extent, the loudness of the murmur correlates with disease severity.[12, 13] Echocardiography allows differentiation of valve disease from a flow murmur, identification of the specific valve involved, definition of the etiology of valve disease, and quantitation of the hemodynamic severity of the lesion along with left ventricular size and function. Based on these data, the expected prognosis, need for preventative measures, and timing of subsequent examinations (if any) can be determined.

In older adults, differentiating a benign from a pathologic murmur is more difficult than in younger patients, because many older patients have some degree of aortic valve sclerosis or mild mitral regurgitation, which can be appreciated on auscultation.[9, 14–16] Again, the basic principle is that a low-intensity systolic murmur in asymptomatic patients does not necessarily warrant echocardiographic evaluation. While progression of aortic sclerosis to significant obstruction may occur in elderly patients with an asymptomatic systolic murmur, clinical outcome remains excellent until symptom onset. Similarly, a soft mitral regurgitant murmur is most likely associated with mild to moderate regurgitation caused by mitral annular calcification and does not necessarily require further evaluation. Most elderly adults with significant mitral regurgitation have a louder murmur or cardiac symptoms warranting echocardiographic examination.

For patients with asymptomatic valvular heart disease, the basic principles of management are to (1) obtain an accurate diagnosis of the specific valvular lesion and quantitative disease severity using Doppler echocardiography; (2) prevent complications of the disease process, such as endocarditis,[17] atrial fibrillation, and embolic events; (3) periodically re-evaluate ventricular size and function to identify early ventricular dysfunction and optimize the timing of surgical intervention; and (4) provide patient education regarding the disease process, expected outcomes, and potential medical or surgical therapies.

PREVENTATIVE MEASURES
Diagnosis and Prevention of Rheumatic Fever

Rheumatic fever is a multiorgan inflammatory disease that occurs 10 days to 3 weeks after group A streptococcal pharyngitis. The clinical diagnosis is based on the conjunction of an antecedent streptococcal throat infection and classic manifestations of the disease, including carditis, polyarthritis, chorea, erythema marginatum, and subcutaneous nodules.[17a] Clinical guidelines for the diagnosis of rheumatic fever allow increased specificity, because many of the manifestations of rheumatic fever are seen in other conditions (Table 6–2). Although these guidelines are helpful in the initial diagnosis of rheumatic fever, exceptions do occur, and consideration of the diagnosis remains of central importance in the recognition of this disease.

The carditis associated with rheumatic fever is a pancarditis; the process may involve the pericardium, myocardium, and valvular tissue. Rheumatic disease preferentially affects the mitral valve, with mitral regurgitation being characteristic of the acute episode, while mitral stenosis is characteristic of the long-term

TABLE 6·2 UPDATED JONES CRITERIA FOR THE DIAGNOSIS OF INITIAL ATTACKS OF RHEUMATIC FEVER

Major Criteria

Carditis (may involve endocardium, myocardium, and pericardium)
Polyarthritis (most frequent manifestation, usually migratory)
Chorea (documentation of recent group A streptococcal infection may be difficult)
Erythema marginatum (distinctive, evanescent rash on trunk and proximal extremities)
Subcutaneous nodules (firm, painless nodule on extensor surfaces of elbows, knees, and wrists)

Minor Criteria

Clinical findings (arthralgia, fever)
Laboratory findings (elevated erythrocyte sedimentation rate or C-reactive protein level)
Electrocardiography (prolonged PR interval)

Evidence of Antecedent Group A Streptococcal Infection

Positive throat culture or rapid streptococci antigen test
Elevated or rising streptococcal antibody titer

Rheumatic Fever

High probability of rheumatic fever: 2 major criteria or 1 major plus 2 minor criteria *plus* evidence
   of preceding group A streptococcal infection

Modified from Guidelines for the diagnosis of rheumatic fever. Jones criteria, 1992 update. Special Writing Group of the Committee on Rheumatic Fever, Endocarditis, and Kawasaki Disease of the Council on Cardiovascular Disease in the Young of the American Heart Association. JAMA 1992;268:2069–2073.

effect of the disease process.[18-20] It has been suggested that echocardiography may improve the early diagnosis of rheumatic fever by detection of valvular regurgitation.[21] However, because a slight degree of mitral regurgitation is common in normal individuals, overdiagnosis should be avoided.

Primary prevention of rheumatic fever is based on treatment of streptococcal pharyngi-

tis with appropriate antibiotics for a sufficient period.[22] Patients with a history of rheumatic fever are at high risk for recurrent disease leading to repeated episodes of valvulitis and increased damage to the valvular apparatus. Since recurrent streptococcal infections may be asymptomatic, secondary prevention is based on the use of continuous antibiotic therapy (Table 6–3). The risk of recurrent disease

TABLE 6·3 RECOMMENDATIONS FOR PREVENTION OF RHEUMATIC FEVER

Primary Prevention (Treatment of Group A Streptococcal Tonsillopharyngitis)

Benzathine penicillin G, 600,000 U (pts ≤27 kg) or 1.2 million U (pts >27 kg) IM once *or*
Penicillin V, 250 mg (children) or 500 mg (adolescents and adults) orally 2–3 times daily for 10 days
For patients allergic to penicillin: erythromycin estolate, 20–40 mg/kg/d (maximum 1 g/d), or
   erythromycin ethylsuccinate, 40 mg/kg/d (maximum 1 g/d) in 2–4 divided oral doses daily for
   10 days

Secondary Prevention of Recurrent Rheumatic Fever

Benzathine penicillin G, 1.2 million U IM every 4 weeks (every 3 weeks in high-risk situations)
or
Penicillin V, 250 mg twice daily PO
or
Sulfadiazine, 0.5 mg daily (pts ≤27 kg) or 1.0 g daily (pts >27 kg)
For patients allergic to penicillin and sulfadiazine: erythromycin, 250 mg twice daily PO

Duration of Secondary Prophylaxis

Rheumatic fever with persistent valve disease: ≥10 y since last episode and to age ≥40 y, sometimes
   lifelong
Rheumatic fever with carditis but no valve disease: 10 y or well into adulthood, whichever is longer
Rheumatic fever without carditis: 5 y or until age 21 y, whichever is longer

Modified from Dajani AS, Taubert K, Ferrieri P, Peter G, Shulman S: Treatment of acute streptococcal pharyngitis and prevention of rheumatic fever: a statement for health professionals. Committee on Rheumatic Fever, Endocarditis, Kawasaki Disease of the Council on Cardiovascular Disease in the Young, the American Heart Association. Pediatrics 1995;96:1758–1764.

is highest for those exposed to streptococcal infections (eg, contact with children, crowded situations) and in economically disadvantaged groups. The recommended duration of secondary prevention is longer for patients with evidence of carditis or persistent valvular disease than those without evidence of valvular damage.

Prevention of Bacterial Endocarditis

Patients with valvular heart disease are at increased risk for infective endocarditis because of endothelial disruption on the valve leaflets caused by high-velocity and turbulent blood flow patterns (see Chapter 18). About 50% of patients with endocarditis have underlying native valve disease, and endocarditis may precipitate the diagnosis of valve disease in a previously asymptomatic patient.

Prevention of bacterial endocarditis is based on prophylactic antibiotic therapy at times of anticipated bacteremia in patients with known structural heart disease associated with an increased risk of endocarditis. The American Heart Association has published guidelines for groups of patients at risk (Table 6–4), procedures likely to cause bacteremia (Table 6–5), and appropriate antibiotic regimens (Table 6–6).[17] Other methods to decrease the risk of

TABLE 6·5 DENTAL OR SURGICAL PROCEDURES FOR WHICH ENDOCARDITIS PROPHYLAXIS IS RECOMMENDED

Dental procedures known to induce gingival or mucosal bleeding, including professional cleaning, extractions, and periodontal procedures
Tonsillectomy or adenoidectomy
Surgical operations that involve intestinal or respiratory mucosa
Bronchoscopy with a rigid bronchoscope
Sclerotherapy for esophageal varices
Esophageal dilatation
Endoscopic retrograde cholangiography with biliary obstruction
Biliary tract surgery
Prostatic surgery
Cystoscopy
Urethral dilatation

From Dajani AS, et al: Circulation 1997;96:358–366.

endocarditis include maintenance of oral hygiene with regular dental cleaning, use of antiseptic mouthwashes, less traumatic approaches to dental procedures, and avoidance of indwelling intravascular catheters in patients at risk. Even patients with rheumatic mitral stenosis on antibiotics to prevent recurrent rheumatic fever should receive standard antibiotic prophylaxis for prevention of bacterial endocarditis, because the doses used for secondary

TABLE 6·4 CARDIAC CONDITIONS FOR WHICH ENDOCARDITIS PROPHYLAXIS IS RECOMMENDED

Endocarditis Prophylaxis Recommended

High-risk category
   Prosthetic cardiac valves, including bioprosthetic and homograft valves
   Previous bacterial endocarditis, even in the absence of heart disease
   Complex cyanotic congenital heart disease
   Surgically constructed systemic-pulmonary shunts or conduits
Moderate-risk category
   Most other congenital cardiac malformations
   Acquired valvular dysfunction
   Hypertrophic cardiomyopathy
   Mitral valve prolapse with valvular regurgitation and/or thickened leaflets

Endocarditis Prophylaxis Not Recommended

Isolated secundum atrial septal defect
Surgical repair of secundum atrial septal defect, ventricular septal defect, or patent ductus arteriosus (without residua beyond 6 months)
Previous coronary artery bypass graft surgery
Mitral valve prolapse without valvular regurgitation*
Physiologic, functional, or innocent heart murmurs
Previous Kawasaki disease without valvular dysfunction
Previous rheumatic fever without valvular dysfunction
Cardiac pacemakers and implanted defibrillators

*Individuals who have mitral valve prolapse associated with thickening and/or redundancy of the valve leaflets may be at increased risk for bacterial endocarditis, particularly men who are 45 years of age or older.
From Dajani AS, et al: Circulation 1997;96:368–366.

TABLE 6·6   PROPHYLACTIC REGIMENS

Situation	Agents*	Regimen*
Dental, Oral, Respiratory Tract, or Esophageal Procedures†		
Standard general prophylaxis	Amoxicillin	Adults: 2.0 g orally 1 h before procedure Children: 50 mg/kg PO 1 h before procedure
Unable to take oral medications	Ampicillin	Adults: 2.0 g IM or IV within 30 min before procedure Children: 50 mg/kg IM or IV within 30 min before procedure
Allergic to penicillin	Clindamycin *or* Cephalexin‡ or cefadroxil‡ *or* Azithromycin or clarithromycin	Adults: 600 mg; children: 20 mg/kg orally 1 h before procedure Adults: 2.0 g; children: 50 mg/kg orally 1 h before procedure Adults: 500 mg; children: 15 mg/kg orally 1 h before procedure
Allergic to penicillin and unable to take oral medications	Clindamycin *or* Cefazolin‡	Adults: 600 mg; children: 20 mg/kg IV within 30 min before procedure Adults: 1.0 g; children: 25 mg/kg IM or IV within 30 min before procedure
Genitourinary and Gastrointestinal (Excluding Esophageal) Procedures		
High-risk patients	Ampicillin plus gentamicin	Adults: ampicillin, 2.0 g IM or IV, plus gentamicin, 1.5 mg/kg (not to exceed 120 mg) within 30 min of starting procedure; 6 h later, ampicillin, 1 g IM/IV, or amoxicillin, 1 g orally Children: ampicillin, 50 mg/kg IM or IV (not to exceed 2.0 g), plus gentamicin, 1.5 mg/kg, within 30 min of starting the procedure; 6 h later, ampicillin, 25 mg/kg IM/IV, or amoxicillin, 25 mg/kg orally
High-risk patients allergic to ampicillin/amoxicillin	Vancomycin plus gentamicin§	Adults: vancomycin, 1.0 g IV, over 1–2 h plus gentamicin, 1.5 mg/kg IV/IM (not to exceed 120 mg); complete injection/infusion within 30 min of starting procedure Children: vancomycin, 20 mg/kg IV, over 1–2 h plus gentamicin, 1.5 mg/kg IV/IM; complete injection/infusion within 30 min of starting procedure
Moderate-risk patients	Amoxicillin or ampicillin	Adults: amoxicillin, 2.0 g orally 1 h before procedure, or ampicillin, 2.0 g IM/IV within 30 min of starting procedure Children: amoxicillin, 50 mg/kg orally 1 h before procedure, or ampicillin, 50 mg/kg IM/IV within 30 min of starting procedure
Moderate-risk patients allergic to ampicillin/ amoxicillin	Vancomycin	Adults: vancomycin, 1.0 g IV over 1–2 h; complete infusion within 30 min of starting procedure Children: vancomycin, 20 mg/kg IV over 1–2 h; complete infusion within 30 min of starting procedure

* Total children's dose should not exceed adult dose.

† American Heart Association recommendations for endocarditis prophylaxis; adapted from Dajani AS, et al: Circulation 1997;96:358–366.

‡ Cephalosporins should not be used for persons with immediate-type hypersensitivity reactions (eg, urticaria, angioedema, anaphylaxis) to penicillin.

§ No second dose of vancomycin or gentamicin is recommended.

prevention of rheumatic fever are inadequate for prevention of endocarditis.

Prevention of Embolic Events

Prevention of embolic events in patients with valvular heart disease, particularly those with mitral stenosis or atrial fibrillation, is a key component of optimal medical therapy. The consequences of a systemic embolic event can be devastating and may occur even in previously asymptomatic patients. Systemic embolism usually results from left atrial thrombus formation in patients with low blood flow in a dilated left atrial chamber, with or without concurrent atrial fibrillation.[23–30] Embolic events due to calcific debris from the aortic or mitral valves are much less common.[31, 32]

Anticoagulation Service

Therapy for prevention of embolic events in patients with valvular heart disease may include antiplatelet agents, such as aspirin or dipyridamole, or chronic warfarin anticoagulation (Table 6–7). Warfarin therapy requires meticulous monitoring and patient education. Several studies show that optimal long-term warfarin therapy is best provided by pharmacists in an established anticoagulation clinic.[33–35] The rate of complications with a pharmacist-managed anticoagulation service is 65% to 95% lower than with routine medical care.[33, 35] An anticoagulation service is cost effective, with estimates of cost savings ranging from $1200 to $4000 per patient-year because of decreased rates of complications, hospitalization, and emergency room visits.[33, 35]

TABLE 6·7   RECOMMENDATIONS FOR ANTICOAGULATION IN PATIENTS WITH VALVULAR HEART DISEASE

Valve Lesion	Recommendation
Any valve disease with atrial fibrillation	Warfarin, INR 2.0–3.0
Rheumatic mitral valve disease	
Chronic or intermittent atrial fibrillation	Warfarin, INR 2.0–3.0
Previous embolic event	Warfarin, INR 2.0–3.0
Left atrial enlargement >55 mm	Consider warfarin, INR 2.0–3.0
Recurrent systemic emboli despite adequate anticoagulation	Add aspirin 80–100 mg qd *or* dipyridamole 400 mg qd *or* ticlopidine 250 mg bid
Aortic valve disease	Long-term anticoagulation not indicated
Mitral valve prolapse	
No embolic events, unexplained TIAs, or atrial fibrillation	Long-term anticoagulation not indicated
Documented but unexplained TIAs	Long-term (160–325 mg qd) aspirin
Documented systemic embolism, atrial fibrillation, or recurrent TIAs despite aspirin therapy	Warfarin, INR 2.0–3.0
Mitral annular calcification	Long-term anticoagulation not indicated unless atrial fibrillation is present or systemic emboli have been documented
Infective endocarditis	
Native valve or tissue prosthesis	Anticoagulation therapy contraindicated
Mechanical valve	Continue warfarin anticoagulation
Nonbacterial thrombotic endocarditis	
With systemic emboli	Heparin anticoagulation
Debilitating disease with aseptic vegetations on echocardiography	Heparin anticoagulation
Prosthetic valves	
Mechanical valves	
Bileaflet valves	Long-term warfarin, INR 2.5–3.5
Tilting disk valves	Long-term warfarin, INR 3.0–4.0
Ball-cage valves	Long-term warfarin, INR 4.0–4.9
Mechanical valve with systemic emboli despite anticoagulation	Add aspirin 100 mg/d *or* Add dipyridamole 400 mg/d
Biologic valves	Warfarin for 3 mo postoperatively, INR 2.0–3.0
Biologic valves with atrial fibrillation or history of systemic embolization	Long-term warfarin, INR 2.0–3.0

INR, international normalized ratio; TIAs, transient ischemic attacks.
Data from references 100, 109–111, 113, and 114.

The typical anticoagulation clinic is staffed by pharmacists with special expertise in anticoagulation management who use written policies and procedures developed in collaboration with the responsible physicians. Prompt and effective communication must be maintained between the referring physicians and the anticoagulation pharmacists. Responsibilities must be clearly defined, and any needed approvals at the institutional, state, and federal level should be obtained before beginning operation.

Monitoring warfarin therapy with prothrombin times has largely been abandoned because of intertest variability related to each specific batch of reagent. Instead, the international normalized ratio (INR) standard is used for all patients because it provides a consistent measure of the degree of anticoagulation. This allows maintenance of therapy within a narrow range, avoiding the risks of deficient or excessive anticoagulation.

At the initiation of therapy, a target INR and acceptable range are defined by the referring physician for each patient based on published guidelines and clinical factors unique to that patient. The pharmacist interviews each patient with specific attention to current medications, diet, lifestyle, and any other factors that may affect long-term anticoagulation therapy. Patient education about anticoagulation, possible dietary and drug interactions, complications of therapy, and the need for careful monitoring of the INR is provided verbally and using a variety of media such as pamphlets, videotapes, and computer-based material.

The anticoagulation clinic staff then initiate therapy and monitor the INR at appropriate intervals using systemic processes and guidelines. The INR is measured weekly or more frequently early after initiation of therapy, with a typical interval of 4 to 6 weeks for patients on a stable therapeutic regimen. At each visit, the timing of the next INR measurement is determined on the basis of the current INR and any trends over the past several visits. Further patient education and counseling are provided as needed. The pharmacist monitors concurrent medical therapy for any potential drug interaction, and the patient or physician can contact the pharmacist before starting new prescription or nonprescription medications to avoid possible interactions by choosing an alternate agent or to alert the pharmacist about the need for more frequent INR determinations if an effect is likely.

Minor bleeding complications may be managed by the anticoagulation clinic in consultation with the physician, depending on the specific protocol at each institution. If major bleeding episodes or thromboembolic events occur, the patient is triaged promptly for acute medical care. The anticoagulation clinic also manages changes in therapy necessitated by surgical or invasive procedures, using procedures developed in conjunction with the referring physician.

Anticoagulation for Native Valve Disease

Valvular heart disease patients with atrial fibrillation should be treated with warfarin to maintain an INR of 2.0 to 3.0.[36] In cases of mitral stenosis, warfarin anticoagulation is strongly recommended for patients with chronic or paroxysmal atrial fibrillation or a previous embolic event (Figs. 6–2 and 6–3).[37-44] Some data support the use of warfarin anticoagulation in mitral stenosis patients in sinus rhythm with a left atrial dimension larger than 55 mm because of the high risk of atrial thrombus formation, even in the absence of atrial fibrillation,[45] but this clinical decision is influenced by the severity of stenosis and the presence of comorbid conditions. In mitral stenosis patients with recurrent embolic events despite adequate anticoagulation, an antiplatelet agent (ie, aspirin, dipyridamole, or ticlopidine) should be added to the medical regimen. Anticoagulation is not indicated for patients with aortic valve disease or asympto-

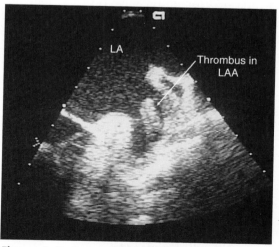

Figure 6·2 Transesophageal echocardiographic view shows a thrombus *(arrow)* in the left atrial appendage (LAA) of a patient with mitral stenosis and atrial fibrillation. LA, left atrium.

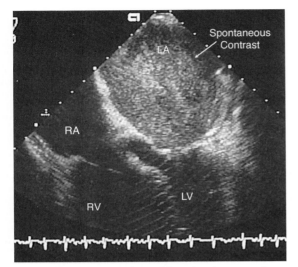

Figure 6·3 Transesophageal four-chamber view shows marked spontaneous contrast in a patient with mitral stenosis resulting from low-velocity blood flow. Spontaneous contrast (arrow) is associated with an increased risk of embolic events. LA, left atrium; RA, right atrium; LV, left ventricle; RV, right ventricle.

matic mitral valve prolapse because of the low risk of embolic events with these lesions. Although elderly patients with mitral annular calcification appear to be at higher risk for embolic events, there is no evidence that anticoagulation is beneficial in the absence of concurrent atrial fibrillation.[46–49] If mitral prolapse patients have unexplained transient ischemic attacks, treatment with aspirin is recommended. Long-term warfarin anticoagulation is indicated for mitral valve prolapse patients only after a documented systemic embolic event, for patients with recurrent, unexplained transient ischemic attacks despite antiplatelet therapy, and for those with atrial fibrillation.

In patients with infective endocarditis, anticoagulation should be avoided in general, given an increased risk of hemorrhage.[50–52] The major exception to the avoidance of anticoagulation in patients with endocarditis is the presence of a mechanical valve. In this situation, most studies suggest that chronic anticoagulation should be continued.[53–56] In addition, the use of heparin in nonbacterial thrombotic endocarditis appears to prevent embolic events.[57–59]

General Health Maintenance

Pneumococcal and annual influenza vaccinations are recommended for all adults older than 65 years of age and are especially important for patients with valvular disease, because the increased hemodynamic demands of an acute infection may lead to cardiac decompensation.[60] For younger patients with valve disease, routine immunization is indicated only if they have coexisting conditions associated with immunocompromise.

Patients with valvular disease should have an assessment of risk factors for coronary artery disease and aggressive risk factor modification as appropriate. Many patients with valvular disease eventually need surgical intervention, and the surgical mortality and morbidity rates are markedly increased when coronary disease complicates valvular heart disease. The negative impact of coexisting coronary disease is particularly striking for mitral regurgitation, with coronary disease conferring a fourfold increase in surgical mortality[61] and a 5-year survival rate one half that of patients without coronary disease.[62] For patients with aortic stenosis, concurrent coronary disease is associated with an approximate doubling of surgical mortality.[61, 63–66]

SLOWING DISEASE PROGRESSION

Ideally, the treatment of valvular heart disease should be directed toward the underlying disease affecting valve anatomy and function. However, other than prevention of rheumatic fever, no specific therapies are available to prevent or reverse the primary disease processes.

A secondary goal is prevention of the often irreversible consequences of the hemodynamic abnormality, including prevention of left ventricular dilation and systolic dysfunction, left atrial enlargement, atrial fibrillation, and pulmonary hypertension. This goal is primarily achieved through sequential noninvasive monitoring that allows surgical intervention before irreversible changes have occurred. Only recently have medical therapies been shown to slow disease progression, specifically in the case of afterload reduction for chronic aortic regurgitation.

Prevention of Left Ventricular Contractile Dysfunction

The basic response of the left ventricle to the chronic volume overload imposed by aortic or mitral regurgitation is an increase in chamber size (see Chapter 7). Initially, left ventricular systolic function is normal, but with long-standing disease, contractile dysfunction may supervene and may not improve after intervention to correct the regurgitant lesion. Although most patients develop symptoms that prompt consideration of valve surgery, in a subset of patients, left ventricular dysfunction occurs before symptom onset.[67] A major focus of the medical management of patients with chronic valvular regurgitation is periodic noninvasive evaluation to monitor left ventricular size and systolic function. The rationale for sequential monitoring is that surgical intervention can be performed just before or soon after the onset of contractile dysfunction.

A more elusive goal of medical therapy for patients with chronic regurgitation is to prevent or delay progressive left ventricular dilation and contractile dysfunction, thereby delaying the need for surgical intervention. In patients with aortic regurgitation, medical therapy with an afterload-reducing agent appears beneficial, leading to a reduction in ventricular dimensions and delaying the need for surgical intervention (see Chapter 12). For patients with mitral regurgitation, the data are less convincing, and afterload reduction cannot be routinely recommended for all patients with this lesion, (see Chapter 13).

In patients with valvular aortic stenosis, development of left ventricular contractile dysfunction is rare, and the timing of surgical intervention is based on symptom onset, rather than on changes in left ventricular geometry or function.[68] There are no known medical therapies to prevent or modify the development of left ventricular hypertrophy in adults with aortic stenosis, and it is not clear that preventing this adaptive response would improve outcome. Recently, there has been considerable interest in the changes in diastolic ventricular dysfunction that occur in aortic stenosis patients.[69–71] It has been hypothesized that surgical intervention before the development of irreversible changes in the myocardium might improve long-term clinical outcome.[72, 73] However, there is no medical therapy known to prevent diastolic dysfunction in patients with pressure overload hypertrophy.

Prevention of Left Atrial Enlargement and Atrial Fibrillation

Progressive left atrial enlargement and atrial fibrillation typically complicate the clinical course of mitral valve disease. Mitral regurgitation and mitral stenosis are associated with left atrial dilation due to the pressure or volume overload of the left atrium.[74–76] Atrial fibrillation occurs frequently, particularly in older patients and in those with severe and long-standing disease.[77–80] Atrial enlargement and fibrillation occasionally complicate aortic valve disease, typically late in the disease course, and may worsen hemodynamics substantially through loss of the atrial contribution to ventricular filling.[81]

No specific medical therapy can prevent these complications of the disease process, although it has been proposed that earlier surgical or percutaneous intervention might prevent atrial enlargement and eventual atrial fibrillation. Surgical intervention for mitral regurgitation soon after the onset of atrial fibrillation (within 3 months) is more likely to restore sinus rhythm than surgical intervention in patients with atrial fibrillation of longer duration, but this approach is not uniformly successful.[82] In patients with mitral stenosis, atrial fibrillation usually recurs or persists after intervention.[79, 83, 84]

Prevention of Pulmonary Hypertension

The chronic elevation in left atrial pressure associated with mitral valve disease results in a passive increase in pulmonary pressures that resolves when left atrial pressure decreases after surgical or percutaneous intervention. However, reactive changes in the pulmonary vasculature may become superimposed on this passive rise in pressure, with secondary histologic changes leading to irreversible pulmonary hypertension (see Chapter 10). Intervention before the onset of irreversible changes is desirable to avoid the long-term complications of right heart failure. In some patients, an excessive rise in pulmonary pressures with exercise may be the first clue that intervention is needed to prevent further irreversible changes in the pulmonary vasculature.[85, 86]

Prevention of Progressive Valve Disease

Worldwide, primary prevention of rheumatic heart disease would have a dramatic impact on the incidence of valvular heart disease. For patients with rheumatic heart disease, prevention of recurrent episodes of rheumatic fever is critical for preventing further valve damage and progressive disease.

Until recently, there has been little interest in the pathogenesis of nonrheumatic valve disease. In fact, some types of valve disease, such as calcific aortic stenosis, have been considered a nonspecific response to aging.[87, 88] However, even when valve lesions result from congenital structural abnormalities (eg, bicuspid aortic valve) or a genetic abnormality (eg, mitral valve prolapse), progressive valve dysfunction and symptom onset often are related to superimposed histopathologic changes. It now is recognized that the "degenerative" changes associated with calcific aortic stenosis, and superimposed on the leaflets of patients with a bicuspid aortic valve, represent an active disease process. This disease process has some similarities and some striking differences with atherosclerosis.[89–93] It is probable that specific disease processes involved in the progression of other types of valve disease will be identified. In the future, prevention based on risk factor modification[94, 95] or therapies targeted at specific steps in the disease process may be used in patients with valvular disease (see Table 1–4).

PATIENT EDUCATION

Patient education is the key to compliance with periodic noninvasive monitoring, prevention of complications, and the early recognition of symptoms in patients with valvular heart disease. Each patient should understand the long-term prognosis, potential complications, typical symptoms, rationale for sequential monitoring, and indications for surgical intervention. Appropriate education avoids needless concern and prompts early reporting of symptoms, allowing optimal timing of surgical intervention.

Patients also should be knowledgeable about the risk of infective endocarditis, situations in which endocarditis prophylaxis is needed, and the specific antibiotic regimen to be taken. Patients on long-term anticoagulation need education and a reliable source for consultation regarding warfarin dose, interactions with other medications, and prompt evaluation of any complications. All patients with valvular heart disease should be evaluated for risk factors for coronary artery disease and should receive education and appropriate therapy for coronary risk factor reduction.

Because the risk of pregnancy for women with valvular heart disease ranges from normal to very high, this risk should be estimated and discussed with the patient. In patients with very-high-risk valve lesions, surgical correction should be considered before a planned pregnancy. In women on long-term anticoagulation, the issue of warfarin versus heparin anticoagulation during pregnancy should be addressed. Contraception options should be reviewed for all women with valvular disease.

For patients with inherited forms of valve disease, such as Marfan's syndrome, the physician should make every effort to ensure that genetic counseling is available and other family members are screened for the disease.

MEDICAL TREATMENT OF SYMPTOMATIC DISEASE

Although the goal in management of patients with valvular disease is to avoid symptoms and the need for medical therapy by optimizing the timing of surgical intervention, some patients develop symptoms that do not yet warrant surgical intervention, persist after surgery, or occur only in response to a superimposed hemodynamic stress (eg, pregnancy). In these situations, medial therapy is based primarily on adjustment of loading conditions and control of heart rate and rhythm.

Patients with pulmonary congestion are treated with diuretics to decrease left atrial and pulmonary venous pressures, whether elevated left atrial pressures are caused by left ventricular dysfunction, mitral regurgitation, or mitral stenosis. However, for a patient with mitral stenosis, care is needed to ensure that left atrial pressures allow adequate left ventricular diastolic filling across the narrowed valve. In patients with aortic stenosis, diuretics should be used cautiously, as pulmonary congestion often is caused by diastolic dysfunction rather than volume overload. The further decrease in ventricular diastolic volume induced by diuretics may worsen symptoms as mid-cavity obstruction develops in the small, hypertrophied, hyperdynamic left ventricle.

Afterload reduction is most beneficial for treatment of heart failure symptoms in patients with aortic or mitral regurgitation. For patients with acute regurgitation, a continuous intravenous infusion of nitroprusside may be used. In the case of acute mitral regurgitation, intraaortic balloon counterpulsation provides effective afterload reduction while maintaining coronary diastolic perfusion pressures. In contrast, intraaortic balloon counterpulsation has the potential to worsen aortic regurgitant severity, since the increase in aortic diastolic pressure also increases the aortic to left ventricular diastolic pressure gradient. For patients with chronic aortic regurgitation, oral afterload reduction therapy with an angiotensin-converting enzyme inhibitor or nifedipine is beneficial.[96–99] Chronic afterload reduction therapy also may be beneficial in some patients with mitral regurgitation, particularly when associated with left ventricular dilation or systolic dysfunction.[99–101] In patients with mitral stenosis, afterload reduction is not helpful, because the ventricle typically is small with normal systolic function.

Afterload reduction should be used with caution or not at all in patients with valvular aortic stenosis. Although in theory vasodilators will reduce total left ventricular afterload, this assumption only holds true if the valvular obstruction is mild or moderate and there is coexisting left ventricular systolic dysfunction.[102] In this situation, the decrease in systemic vascular resistance leads to improved left ventricular contractility and an increase in left ventricular output due to increased opening of the valve leaflets. However, when valvular obstruction is severe, peripheral vasodilation may be accompanied by a precipitous fall in blood pressure, because only a fixed stroke volume can be pumped though the rigid orifice.[103, 104]

In patients with valvular heart disease and atrial fibrillation, restoration and maintenance of sinus rhythm is a high priority both to prevent atrial thrombus formation and to preserve the atrial contribution to left ventricular diastolic filling. Approaches to restoring and maintaining sinus rhythm are no different from those for patients without valve disease, other than the increased awareness of embolic risk and need for appropriate anticoagulation. When sinus rhythm cannot be maintained, ventricular rate is controlled using standard approaches. Rate control is especially important in mitral stenosis patients, because a shortened diastolic filling time may result in a symptomatic decrease in forward cardiac output.[105, 106]

Even when sinus rhythm is present, heart rate control may be needed in patients with valvular heart disease. For example, the increased heart rate and shortened diastolic filling time associated with pregnancy in a patient with mitral stenosis leads to inadequate ventricular filling and a reduced cardiac output. Slowing the heart rate with a β blocker improves diastolic filling and restores a normal cardiac output.[107, 108] Another example is the elderly patient with aortic stenosis. These elderly patients may develop bradycardia due to calcification of the conduction system with heart block or sick sinus syndrome, which further reduces the total cardiac output across the stenotic valve, leading to cardiac symptoms. Symptoms due to bradycardia resolve after placement of a pacer, possibly allowing deferral of aortic valve surgery.

TIMING AND CHOICE OF SURGICAL INTERVENTION

The optimal timing and choice of surgical intervention for each type of valvular heart disease are discussed in subsequent chapters. The feature common to all of these approaches is periodic noninvasive monitoring of the valvular lesion, the left ventricular response to pressure and/or volume overload, and secondary abnormalities caused by the valvular lesion. The frequency of periodic evaluations is tailored to each case, depending on the severity of the lesion at the initial evaluation, the natural history of the disease, indications for surgical intervention, and other clinical factors in each patient. Clearly, there is no simple set of rules that defines the optimal or most cost-effective frequency of evaluations. However, based on our current understanding of the natural history of valve disease, a framework for periodic evaluation can be devised (Table 6–8).

First, an initial complete diagnostic echocardiographic study is performed to define disease severity, left ventricular size and systolic function, pulmonary pressures, and any associated abnormalities. Next, a basic frequency of repeat examinations is suggested for each valve lesion, depending on the severity of valve disease and, for valve regurgitation, the left ventricular response to chronic volume overload.

However, the specific timing of repeat studies may need to be modified because of interim changes in symptoms or physical examination findings, new-onset atrial fibrillation, evidence for progressive left ventricular dilation or early contractile dysfunction, or evidence of increasing pulmonary pressures. For example, an apparent increase in ventricular dimensions in a patient with chronic regurgitation prompts a repeat evaluation at a shorter time interval to differentiate a pathologic change from normal physiologic or measurement variation. Similarly, a change in symptom status in a patient with myxomatous mitral valve disease warrants reevaluation because a sudden change in regurgitant severity caused by chordal rupture may have occurred. More frequent examinations also are warranted when quantitative parameters are approaching

TABLE 6·8   PERIODIC ECHOCARDIOGRAPHY FOR PATIENTS WITH VALVULAR HEART DISEASE

Step 1: Initial Diagnostic Study

Comprehensive baseline echocardiographic and Doppler examination
Transesophageal imaging should be considered if transthoracic images are nondiagnostic.

Step 2: Basic Frequency of Examination

The basic frequency of echocardiographic examination provides a starting point for each patient that is modified as appropriate in Steps 3 and 4.

Valve Lesion	*Severity*	*Basic Frequency*
Aortic stenosis	Mild (V_{max} <3.0 m/s)	Every 2–3 y
	Moderate (V_{max} 3–4 m/s)	Annually
	Severe (V_{max} > 4.0 m/s)	Annually
Aortic regurgitation	Mild	Every 2–3 y
	Moderate, normal LV size	Every 1–2 y
	Moderate, LV dilation	Annually
	Severe	Every 6–12 mo
Mitral stenosis	Mild (MVA >2.0 cm²)	Every 2–3 y
	Moderate (MVA 1–2 cm²)	Annually
	Severe (MVA <1.0 cm²)	Every 6–12 mo
Mitral regurgitation	Mild	Every 2–3 y
	Moderate, normal LV size	Every 1–2 y
	Moderate, LV dilation	Annually
	Severe	Every 6–12 mo

Step 3: Modifiers of Examination Frequency

Increase frequency
   Interim change in symptoms or physical examination findings
   New-onset atrial fibrillation
   Evidence for progressive LV dilation and/or early contractile dysfunction
   Evidence for increasing pulmonary pressures
Decrease frequency
   Stable findings over 2–3 examination intervals

Step 4: Special Situations

Preoperative for noncardiac surgery
Pregnancy
Monitoring interventional procedures
Assessment of complications and hemodynamic results after an intervention
Intraoperative transesophageal monitoring

LV, left ventricular; MVA, mitral valve area.

the values defined as optimal for timing of surgical intervention.

In other clinical situations, reexamination may be indicated to evaluate hemodynamics under changing physiologic conditions (eg, during pregnancy), to guide a surgical or interventional procedure, or to assess results and complications after an intervention. In patients with comorbid diseases, such as those undergoing noncardiac surgery, a repeat echocardiographic examination may be needed to assist in medical or surgical management.

MEDICAL MANAGEMENT OF THE POSTOPERATIVE PATIENT

Medical management after valve repair or replacement is similar to management of the patient who has not undergone surgical intervention. Because none of the valve substitutes results in normal valve anatomy or function, the patient continues to have significant, albeit less severe, valvular disease after the surgical procedure. The basic goals of medical therapy continue to be prevention of complications of the disease process and periodic monitoring of valve function. Prevention of bacterial endocarditis is especially important given the poor prognosis associated with prosthetic valve endocarditis.

Anticoagulation for Prosthetic Valves
Chronic Warfarin Therapy
MECHANICAL VALVE

Patients with a mechanical valve replacement require chronic anticoagulation for pre-

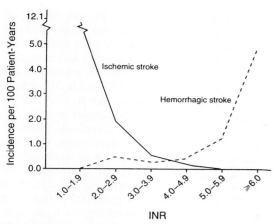

Figure 6·4 Incidence of ischemic and hemorrhagic stroke according to the international normalized ratio (INR) category. (From Cannegieter SC, Rosendaal FR, Wintzen AR, van der Meer FJ, Vandenbroucke JP, Briet E: Optimal oral anticoagulant therapy in patients with mechanical heart values. N Engl J Med 1995;333:11–17.)

vention of embolic events or valve dysfunction (Figs. 6–4 and 6–5). Although the target INR for each patient may be adjusted depending on other clinical factors, the current consensus recommendation for patients with a bileaflet mechanical valve is an INR of 2.5 to 3.5.[109, 110] Using this INR target, close monitoring, preferably by an anticoagulation clinic, is important to ensure the INR does not fall below 2.5. Given the higher embolic risk with other mechanical valve types, an INR or 3.0 to

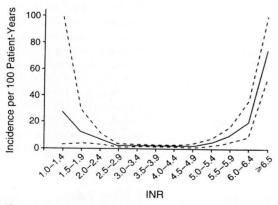

Figure 6·5 International normalized ratio (INR)–specific incidence of all adverse events: all episodes of thromboembolism, all major bleeding episodes, and unclassified stroke. The *dotted lines* indicate the 95% confidence interval. (From Cannegieter SC, Rosendaal FR, Wintzen AR, van der Meer FJ; Vandenbroucke JP, Briet E: Optimal oral anticoagulant therapy in patients with mechanical heart valves. N Engl J Med 1995;333:11–17.)

4.0 for tilting-disk valves and an INR of 4.0 to 4.9 for ball-cage valves are recommended.[109–111]

The goal INR may be increased for patients with mechanical valves if there is a higher risk for thromboembolic events, such as the presence of more than one prosthetic valve or concurrent atrial fibrillation. For example, the goal INR may be set at 3.0 to 4.5 for a patient with aortic and mitral valve prostheses. Increasing the INR beyond 4.9 should be avoided, because the risk of hemorrhagic complications increases with no additional benefit in prevention of embolic events.[109–112] If a thromboembolic event occurs despite adequate anticoagulation in a patient with a mechanical valve, an antiplatelet agent should be added to the anticoagulation regimen. Aspirin (100 mg/d) or dipyridamole (400 mg/d) is effective.[109, 113]

Some patients with mechanical valves are at lower risk for embolic complications, especially patients younger than 75 years of age with a single bileaflet valve replacement who are in sinus rhythm and have little left atrial enlargement. In this subgroup of patients, a randomized trial of standard-dose (INR 3.0 to 4.0) compared with lower-dose (INR 2.0 to 3.0) warfarin therapy showed no difference in thromboembolic events, but an increased incidence of hemorrhagic events in the standard-dose group.[114] These data suggest that lower-dose anticoagulation may be acceptable in carefully selected patients, although, in fact, the mean INR of the low-dose group was 2.74 ± 0.35, which falls within the current recommendations of an INR of 2.5 to 3.5 for bileaflet mechanical valves.

BIOPROSTHETIC VALVES

In patients with a bioprosthetic valve, warfarin anticoagulation to maintain an INR of 2.0 to 3.0 for the first 3 months after implantation is recommended. After 3 months, the patient may be maintained on aspirin (325 mg daily), although the evidence for this recommendation is weak. Of course, patients with bioprosthetic valves and other indications for chronic anticoagulation, such as a previous embolic event, atrial fibrillation, or left ventricular systolic dysfunction, should be continued on appropriate anticoagulant therapy.

Management of Patients Undergoing Surgical Procedures

One of several approaches may be used for the management of anticoagulation in a patient with a mechanical valve undergoing a surgical procedure. For procedures with minor bleeding that can be easily controlled, such as dental extractions, anticoagulation usually is continued at therapeutic levels. If interruption of anticoagulation is needed for the procedure, warfarin is stopped 3 to 4 days before the procedure to allow return of coagulation parameters to normal. If the INR remains elevated, a small dose of vitamin K (0.5 to 1.0 mg subcutaneously) provides reversal of the warfarin effects within 24 hours. Larger doses of vitamin K should be avoided to prevent resistance to anticoagulation postoperatively. Warfarin therapy is resumed after surgery.[110, 115]

Because this approach results in a period of about 1 day before and 1 to 2 days after surgery in which anticoagulation is subtherapeutic, some clinicians recommend the use of intravenous heparin therapy preoperatively after the INR has normalized, with discontinuation of heparin only a few hours before surgery for high-risk patients. Postoperatively, heparin is restarted as soon possible, based on the risk of surgical bleeding. Although the use of intravenous heparin markedly increases the cost of the surgical procedure, this approach should be considered in patients with prosthetic mechanical valves who are at high risk for thromboembolism, including patients with mitral valve prostheses, atrial fibrillation, ball-cage valves, left ventricular systolic dysfunction, or a history of prior embolization.[110, 115] For other prosthetic valve patients, the decision regarding perioperative heparin therapy must be individualized based on other clinical factors.

Management During Pregnancy

Although the importance of maintaining adequate anticoagulation during pregnancy in women with prosthetic valves is clear,[116, 117] the specific approach to management of anticoagulation remains controversial.[110] The risks of warfarin therapy during pregnancy include first-trimester teratogenicity, particularly between the 6th and 12th weeks of gestation.[118–120] There also may be an increased risk of central nervous system abnormalities with exposure to warfarin at any time during pregnancy.[118] In addition, there is a substantial risk of bleeding in the anticoagulated fetus, especially at the time of delivery.

In contrast, heparin does not cross the placenta and has not been associated with teratogenic effects or fetal bleeding.[121, 122] The disadvantages of heparin therapy include the need for twice-daily subcutaneous injections and the development of osteoporosis, with a small risk (<2%) of symptomatic fractures but a higher risk of a detectable decrease in bone density (in one third of women).[123–126] With either warfarin or heparin anticoagulation, the risk of bleeding complications is similar to that in nonpregnant patients with prosthetic valves.[121]

Based on these considerations, two approaches to the management of anticoagulation in pregnancy have been proposed. One approach is to use subcutaneous heparin from the 6th to 12th week of pregnancy and near the time of delivery, switching back to standard warfarin therapy for the remainder of pregnancy. The other approach is to start subcutaneous heparin therapy at soon as pregnancy is recognized and maintain therapeutic anticoagulation with heparin throughout pregnancy. Given the persistence of an anticoagulation effect for more than 24 hours after the last dose of heparin, therapy is discontinued 24 hours prior to elective induction of labor.[127, 128] Although there have been no randomized trials of the effectiveness of either of these approaches, the preference at our medical center is to use heparin throughout pregnancy given the potential risks of teratogenicity and fetal bleeding with warfarin. At other institutions, the alternate approach is used due to concern about heparin-induced osteoporosis and the difficulty of monitoring heparin therapy.[117]

With either approach, close control and monitoring of anticoagulation is essential to maintain a therapeutic level and to avoid bleeding or thrombotic complications. In the absence of a meticulous approach to anticoagulation, the rate of complications is high.[129] With subcutaneous heparin, the dose is adjusted to achieve an activated partial thromboplastin time of two times control, 6 hours after each dose.[127, 130] With warfarin, the INR is maintained between 2.5 and 3.5. Aspirin can be added to the regimen for patients with atrial fibrillation or previous thromboembolic events.[45, 131]

Noninvasive Monitoring After Valve Surgery

A baseline echocardiographic study is obtained after valve surgery to determine the degree of functional stenosis and valve regurgitation and to assess left ventricular chamber size, mass, and systolic function after the surgical procedure. Given the wide range of normal values for valvular hemodynamics, depending on valve type, position, size, and cardiac output, the Doppler velocities obtained at the postoperative study are used as the patient's normal values. Typically, this baseline examination is performed 3 to 4 months postoperatively for the asymptomatic patient to avoid the increased cardiac output state of the early postoperative period and to minimize patient discomfort. The examination should be performed earlier in the clinical course if prosthetic valve dysfunction is suspected.

Repeat echocardiographic studies are performed every 1 to 3 years initially. The frequency of examination is increased for biologic valves implanted for more than 10 years given their limited durability. Repeat evaluation also may be prompted by a change in clinical symptoms or physical examination findings. In addition, repeat evaluations may be needed to assess postoperative regression of left ventricular hypertrophy, changes in left ventricular chamber size and systolic function, or changes in pulmonary pressures.

References

1. Giuliani ER, Brandenburg RO, Fuster V: Evaluation of cardiac murmurs. Cardiovasc Clin 1980;10:1–18.
2. Perloff JK: Physical Examination of the Heart and Circulation. Philadelphia: WB Saunders, 1982.
3. Abrams J: Synopsis of Cardiac Physical Diagnosis. Philadelphia: Lea & Febiger, 1989.
4. Mishra M, Chambers JB, Jackson G: Murmurs in pregnancy: an audit of echocardiography. BMJ 1992;304:1413–1414.
5. Northcote RJ, Knight PV, Ballantyne D: Systolic murmurs in pregnancy: value of echocardiographic assessment. Clin Cardiol 1985;8:327–328.
6. Cheitlin MD, Alpert JS, Armstrong WF, et al: ACC/AHA guidelines for the clinical application of echocardiography: a report of the American College of Cardiology/American Heart Association Task Force on Practice Guidelines (Committee on Clinical Application of Echocardiography). Circulation 1997;95:1686–1744.
7. Jaffe WM, Roche AHG, Coverdale HA, McAlister HF, Ormiston JA, Greene ER: Clinical evaluation versus Doppler echocardiography in the quantitative assessment of valvular heart disease. Circulation 1988;78:267–275.
8. Lombard JT, Selzer A: Valvular aortic stenosis: a clinical and hemodynamic profile of patients. Ann Intern Med 1987;106:292–298.
9. Aronow WS, Kronzon I: Correlation of prevalence and severity of valvular aortic stenosis determined by continuous-wave Doppler echocardiography with physical signs of aortic stenosis in patients aged 62 to 100 years with aortic systolic ejection murmurs. Am J Cardiol 1987;60:399–401.
10. Forssell G, Jonasson R, Orinius E: Identifying severe aortic valvular stenosis by bedside examination. Acta Med Scand 1985;218:397–400.
11. Sutton GC, Craige E: Clinical signs of severe acute mitral regurgitation. Am J Cardiol 1967;20:141–144.
12. Desjardins VA, Enriquez Sarano M, Tajik AJ, Bailey KR, Seward JB: Intensity of murmurs correlates with severity of valvular regurgitation. Am J Med 1996;100:149–156.
13. Otto CM, Munt BI, Legget ME, Kraft CD, Miyake-Hull CY, Fujioka M: Correlation between physical examination findings and Doppler echocardiography in adults with aortic stenosis. Circulation 1997;96 (abstract).
14. Sainsbury R, White T, Wray R: Echocardiography in elderly patients with systolic murmurs. Age Ageing 1981;10:225–230.
15. Vigna C, Impagliatelli M, Russo A, et al: Systolic ejection murmurs in the elderly: aortic valve and carotid arteries echo-Doppler findings. Angiology 1991;42:455–461.
16. Wong M, Tei C, Shah PM: Degenerative calcific valvular disease and systolic murmurs in the elderly. J Am Geriatr Soc 1983;31:156–163.
17. Dajani AS, Taubert KA, Wilson W, et al: Prevention of bacterial endocarditis: recommendations by the American Heart Association. JAMA 1997;277:1794–1801.
17a. Guidelines for the diagnosis of rheumatic fever. Jones criteria, 1992 update. Special Writing Group of the Committee on Rheumatic Fever, Endocarditis, and Kawasaki Disease of the Council on Cardiovascular Disease in the Young of the American Heart Association. JAMA 1992;268:2069–2073.
18. Marcus RH, Sareli P, Pocock WA, Barlow JB: The spectrum of severe rheumatic mitral valve disease in a developing country: correlations among clinical presentation, surgical pathologic findings, and hemodynamic sequelae. Ann Intern Med 1994;120:177–183.
19. Bowe JC, Bland F, Sprague HB, White PD: Course of mitral stenosis without surgery: 10 and 20 year perspectives. Ann Intern Med 1960;52:741.
20. Chopra P, Tandon HD, Raizada V, Gopinath N, Butler C, Williams RC Jr: Comparative studies of mitral valves in rheumatic heart disease. Arch Intern Med 1983;143:661–666.
21. Abernethy M, Bass N, Sharpe N, et al: Doppler echocardiography and the early diagnosis of carditis in acute rheumatic fever. Aust N Z J Med 1994;24:530–535.
22. Dajani A, Taubert K, Ferrieri P, Peter G, Shulman S: Treatment of acute streptococcal pharyngitis and prevention of rheumatic fever: a statement for health professionals. Committee on Rheumatic Fever, Endocarditis, and Kawasaki Disease of the Council on Cardiovascular Disease in the Young, the American Heart Association. Pediatrics 1995;96:1758–1764.
23. Waller BF: Etiology of mitral stenosis and pure mitral regurgitation. *In* Waller BF, ed. Pathology of the Heart and Great Vessels. New York: Churchill Livingstone, 1988:101–148.
24. Aberg H: Atrial fibrillation. I. A study of atrial thrombosis and systemic embolism in a necropsy material. Acta Med Scand 1969;185:373–379.
25. Hwang JJ, Li YH, Lin JM, et al: Left atrial appendage function determined by transesophageal echocardiography in patients with rheumatic mitral valve disease. Cardiology 1994;85:121–128.
26. Coulshed N, Epstein EJ, McKendrick CS, Galloway RW, Walker E: Systemic embolism in mitral valve disease. Br Heart J 1970;32:26–34.

27. Hinton RC, Kistler JP, Fallon JT, Friedlich AL, Fisher CM: Influence of etiology of atrial fibrillation on incidence of systemic embolism. Am J Cardiol 1977;40:509–513.

28. Wolf PA, Dawber TR, Thomas HE Jr, Kannel WB: Epidemiologic assessment of chronic atrial fibrillation and risk of stroke: the Framingham Study. Neurology 1978;28:973–977.

29. Horstkotte D, Niehues R, Strauer BE: Pathomorphological aspects, aetiology and natural history of acquired mitral valve stenosis. Eur Heart J 1991;12 (suppl B):55–60.

30. Chiang CW, Lo SK, Kuo CT, Cheng NJ, Hsu TS: Noninvasive predictors of systemic embolism in mitral stenosis: an echocardiographic and clinical study of 500 patients. Chest 1994;106:396–399.

31. Brockmeier LB, Adolph RJ, Gustin BW, Holmes JC, Sacks JG: Calcium emboli to the retinal artery in calcific aortic stenosis. Am Heart J 1981;101:32–37.

32. Pleet AB, Massey EW, Vengrow ME: TIA, stroke, and the bicuspid aortic valve. Neurology 1981;31:1540–1542.

33. Wilt VM, Gums JG, Ahmed OI, Moore LM: Outcome analysis of a pharmacist-managed anticoagulation service. Pharmacotherapy 1995;15:732–739.

34. Lee YP, Schommer JC: Effect of a pharmacist-managed anticoagulation clinic on warfarin-related hospital readmissions. Am J Health Syst Pharm 1996;53:1580–1583.

35. Bussey HI, Chiquette E, Amato MG: Anticoagulation clinic care versus routine medical care: a review and interim report. J Thrombosis Thrombolysis 1996;2:315–319.

36. Hylek EM, Skates SJ, Sheehan MA, Singer DE: An analysis of the lowest effective intensity of prophylactic anticoagulation for patients with nonrheumatic atrial fibrillation. N Engl J Med 1996;335:540–546.

37. Szekely P: Systemic embolism and anticoagulant prophylaxis in rheumatic heart disease. BMJ 1964;1:209–212.

38. Hay WE, Levine SA: Age and atrial fibrillation as independent factors in auricular mural thrombus formation. Am Heart J 1942;24:1–4.

39. Fleming HA: Anticoagulants in rheumatic heart disease. Lancet 1971;2:486.

40. Petersen P, Boysen G, Godtfredsen J, Andersen ED, Andersen B: Placebo-controlled, randomised trial of warfarin and aspirin for prevention of thromboembolic complications in chronic atrial fibrillation: the Copenhagen AFASAK study. Lancet 1989;1:175–179.

41. Preliminary report of the Stroke Prevention in Atrial Fibrillation Study. N Engl J Med 1990;322:863–868.

42. Warfarin versus aspirin for prevention of thromboembolism in atrial fibrillation: Stroke Prevention in Atrial Fibrillation II Study. Lancet 1994;343:687–691.

43. The effect of low-dose warfarin on the risk of stroke in patients with nonrheumatic atrial fibrillation: the Boston Area Anticoagulation Trial for Atrial Fibrillation Investigators. N Engl J Med 1990;323:1505–1511.

44. Ezekowitz MD, Bridgers SL, James KE, et al: Warfarin in the prevention of stroke associated with nonrheumatic atrial fibrillation. Veterans Affairs Stroke Prevention in Nonrheumatic Atrial Fibrillation Investigators [published erratum appears in N Engl J Med 1993;328:148]. N Engl J Med 1992;327:1406–1412.

45. Turpie AG, Gent M, Laupacis A, et al: A comparison of aspirin with placebo in patients treated with warfarin after heart-valve replacement. N Engl J Med 1993;329:524–529.

46. de Bono DP, Warlow CP: Mitral-annulus calcification and cerebral or retinal ischaemia. Lancet 1979;2:383–385.

47. Fulkerson PK, Beaver BM, Auseon JC, Graber HL: Calcification of the mitral annulus: etiology, clinical associations, complications and therapy. Am J Med 1979;66:967–977.

48. Benjamin EJ, Plehn JF, D'Agostino RB, et al: Mitral annular calcification and the risk of stroke in an elderly cohort. N Engl J Med 1992;327:374–379.

49. Hart RG, Easton JD: Mitral valve prolapse and cerebral infarction. Stroke 1982;13:429–430.

50. McLean J, Meyer BBM, Griffith JM: Heparin in subacute bacterial endocarditis: report of a case and critical review of literature. JAMA 1941;117:1870–1879.

51. Katz LN, Elek SR: Combined heparin and chemotherapy in subacute bacterial endocarditis. JAMA 1944;124:149–152.

52. Kanis JA: Anticoagulants in infective endocarditis [letter]. Br Med J 1973;4:233.

53. Pruitt AA, Rubin RH, Karchmer AW, Duncan GW: Neurologic complications of bacterial endocarditis. Medicine (Baltimore) 1978;57:329–343.

54. Carpenter JL, McAllister CK: Anticoagulation in prosthetic valve endocarditis. South Med J 1983;76:1372–1375.

55. Block PC, DeSanctis RW, Weinberg AN, Austen WG: Prosthetic valve endocarditis. J Thorac Cardiovasc Surg 1970;60:540–548.

56. Lieberman A, Hass WK, Pinto R, et al: Intracranial hemorrhage and infarction in anticoagulated patients with prosthetic heart valves. Stroke 1978;9:18–24.

57. Lopez JA, Ross RS, Fishbein MC, Siegel RJ: Nonbacterial thrombotic endocarditis: a review. Am Heart J 1987;113:773–784.

58. Sack GH Jr, Levin J, Bell WR: Trousseau's syndrome and other manifestations of chronic disseminated coagulopathy in patients with neoplasms: clinical, pathophysiologic, and therapeutic features. Medicine (Baltimore) 1977;56:1–37.

59. Rogers LR, Cho ES, Kempin S, Posner JB: Cerebral infarction from non-bacterial thrombotic endocarditis: clinical and pathological study including the effects of anticoagulation. Am J Med 1987;83:746–756.

60. ACP Task Force on Adult Immunization, Infectious Disease Society of America, eds: Guide for Adult Immunization. Philadelphia: American College of Physicians, 1994.

61. Fremes SE, Goldman BS, Ivanov J, Weisel RD, David TE, Salerno T: Valvular surgery in the elderly. Circulation 1989;80:I:77–90.

62. Hendren WG, Nemec JJ, Lytle BW, et al: Mitral valve repair for ischemic mitral insufficiency. Ann Thorac Surg 1991;52:1246–1251.

63. Craver JM, Weintraub WS, Jones EL, Guyton RA, Hatcher CR Jr: Predictors of mortality, complications, and length of stay in aortic valve replacement for aortic stenosis. Circulation 1988;78:I85–90.

64. Freeman WK, Schaff HV, O'Brien PC, Orszulak TA, Naessens JM, Tajik AJ: Cardiac surgery in the octogenarian: perioperative outcome and clinical follow-up. J Am Coll Cardiol 1991;18:29–35.

65. Culliford AT, Galloway AC, Colvin SB, et al: Aortic valve replacement for aortic stenosis in persons aged 80 years and over. Am J Cardiol 1991;67:1256–1260.

66. Elayda MA, Hall RJ, Reul RM, et al: Aortic valve replacement in patients 80 years and older: operative risks and long-term results. Circulation 1993;88:II-11–16.

67. Donovan CL, Starling MR: Role of echocardiography in the timing of surgical intervention for chronic mitral and aortic regurgitation. *In* Otto CM, ed.: The Practice of Clinical Echocardiography. Philadelphia: WB Saunders, 1997:327–354.

68. Otto CM, Burwash IG, Legget ME, et al: A prospective study of asymptomatic valvular aortic stenosis: clinical, echocardiographic, and exercise predictors of outcome. Circulation 1997;95:2262–2270.

69. Douglas PS, Berko B, Lesh M, Reichele N: Alterations in diastolic function in response to progressive left ventricular hypertrophy. J Am Coll Cardiol 1989;13:461–467.

70. Villari B, Campbell SE, Hess OM, et al: Influence of collagen network on left ventricular systolic and diastolic function in aortic valve disease. J Am Coll Cardiol 1993;22:1477–1484.

71. Villari B, Campbell SE, Schneider J, Vassalli G, Chiariello M, Hess OM: Sex-dependent differences in left ventricular function and structure in chronic pressure overload. Eur Heart J 1995;16:1410–1419.

72. Lund O, Nielsen TT, Pilegaard HK, Magnussen K, Knudsen MA: The influence of coronary artery disease and bypass grafting on early and late survival after valve replacement for aortic stenosis. J Thorac Cardiovasc Surg 1990;100:327–337.

73. Carabello BA: Timing of valve replacement in aortic stenosis: moving closer to perfection [editorial]. Circulation 1997;95:2241–2243.

74. Pape LA, Price JM, Alpert JS, Ockene IS, Weiner BH: Relation of left atrial size to pulmonary capillary wedge pressure in severe mitral regurgitation. Cardiology 1991;78:297–303.

75. Burwash IG, Blackmore GL, Koilpillai CJ: Usefulness of left atrial and left ventricular chamber sizes as predictors of the severity of mitral regurgitation. Am J Cardiol 1992;70:774–779.

76. Sanfilippo AJ, Abascal VM, Sheehan M, et al: Atrial enlargement as a consequence of atrial fibrillation: a prospective echocardiographic study. Circulation 1990;82:792–797.

77. Deverall PB, Olley PM, Smith DR, Watson DA, Whitaker W: Incidence of systemic embolism before and after mitral valvotomy. Thorax 1968;23:530–536.

78. Arora R, Kalra GS, Murty GS, et al: Percutaneous transatrial mitral commissurotomy: immediate and intermediate results. J Am Coll Cardiol 1994;23:1327–1332.

79. Multicenter experience with balloon mitral commissurotomy: NHLBI Balloon Valvuloplasty Registry Report on immediate and 30-day follow-up results. The National Heart, Lung, and Blood Institute Balloon Valvuloplasty Registry Participants. Circulation 1992;85:448–461.

80. Tuzcu EM, Block PC, Griffin BP, Newell JB, Palacios IF: Immediate and long-term outcome of percutaneous mitral valvotomy in patients 65 years and older. Circulation 1992;85:963–971.

81. Braunwald E, Frahm CJ: Studies on Starling's law of the heart. IV. Observations on the hemodynamic functions of the left atrium in man. Circulation 1961;24:633.

82. Chua YL, Schaff HV, Orszulak TA, Morris JJ: Outcome of mitral valve repair in patients with preoperative atrial fibrillation: should the maze procedure be combined with mitral valvuloplasty? J Thorac Cardiovasc Surg 1994;107:408–415.

83. Pan M, Medina A, Suarez de Lezo J, et al: Factors determining late success after mitral balloon valvulotomy. Am J Cardiol 1993;71:1181–1185.

84. Vahanian A, Michel PL, Cormier B, et al: Immediate and mid-term results of percutaneous mitral commissurotomy. Eur Heart J 1991;12(suppl B):84–89.

85. Tunick PA, Freedberg RS, Gargiulo A, Kronzon I: Exercise Doppler echocardiography as an aid to clinical decision making in mitral valve disease. J Am Soc Echocardiogr 1992;5:225–230.

86. Leavitt JI, Coats MH, Falk RH: Effects of exercise on transmittal gradient and pulmonary artery pressure in patients with mitral stenosis or a prosthetic mitral valve: a Doppler echocardiographic study. J Am Coll Cardiol 1991;17:1520–1526.

87. Pomerance A: Pathology of the heart with and without cardiac failure in the aged. Br Heart J 1965;17:697–710.

88. Pomerance A, Darby AJ, Hodkinson HM: Valvular calcification in the elderly: possible pathogenic factors. J Gerontol 1978;33:672–675.

89. Otto CM, Kuusisto J, Reichenbach DD, Gown AM, O'Brien KD: Characterization of the early lesion of "degenerative" valvular aortic stenosis: histologic and immunohistochemical studies. Circulation 1994;90:844–853.

90. Olsson M, Dalsgaard CJ, Haegerstrand A, Rosenqvist M, Ryden L, Nilsson J: Accumulation of T lymphocytes and expression of interleukin-2 receptors in nonrheumatic stenotic aortic valves. J Am Coll Cardiol 1994;23:1162–1170.

91. Gotoh T, Kuroda T, Yamasawa M, et al: Correlation between lipoprotein(a) and aortic valve sclerosis assessed by echocardiography (the JMS cardiac echo and cohort study). Am J Cardiol 1995;76:928–932.

92. O'Brien KD, Kuusisto J, Reichenbach DD, et al: Osteopontin is expressed in human aortic valvular lesions. Circulation 1995;92:2163–2168.

93. O'Brien KD, Reichenbach DD, Marcovina SM, Kuusisto J, Alpers CE, Otto CM: Apolipoproteins B, (a) and E accumulate in the morphologically early lesion of "degenerative" valvular aortic stenosis. Arterioscler Thromb 1996;16:523–532.

94. Mohler ER, Sheridan MJ, Nichols R, Harvey WP, Waller BF: Development and progression of aortic valve stenosis: atherosclerosis risk factors—a causal relationship? A clinical morphologic study. Clin Cardiol 1991;14:995–999.

95. Stewart BF, Siscovick D, Lind BK, et al: Clinical factors associated with calcific aortic valve disease. J Am Coll Cardiol 1997;29:630–634.

96. Scognamiglio R, Fasoli G, Ponchia A, Dalla Volta S: Long-term nifedipine unloading therapy in asymptomatic patients with chronic severe aortic regurgitation. J Am Coll Cardiol 1990;16:424–429.

97. Lin M, Chiang HT, Lin SL, Chang MS, Chiang BN, Kuo HW, Cheitlin MD: Vasodilator therapy in chronic asymptomatic aortic regurgitation: enalapril versus hydralazine therapy. J Am Coll Cardiol 1994;24:1046–1053.

98. Schon HR: Hemodynamic and morphologic

changes after long-term angiotensin converting en-zyme inhibition in patients with chronic valvular re-gurgitation. J Hypertens Suppl 1994;12:S95–104.

99. Wisenbaugh T, Sinovich V, Dullabh A, Sareli P: Six month pilot study of captopril for mildly sympto-matic, severe isolated mitral and isolated aortic re-gurgitation. J Heart Valve Dis 1994;3:197–204.

100. Levine HJ, Gaasch WH: Vasoactive drugs in chronic regurgitant lesions of the mitral and aortic valves. J Am Coll Cardiol 1996;28:1083–1091.

101. Keren G, Pardes A, Eschar Y, et al: One-year clinical and echocardiographic follow-up of patients with congestive cardiomyopathy treated with captopril compared to placebo. Isr J Med Sci 1994;30:90–98.

102. Martinez SC, Henne O, Arceo A, et al: Hemody-namic effects of oral captopril in patients with criti-cal aortic stenosis [in Spanish]. Arch Inst Cardiol Mex 1996;66:322–330.

103. Richards AM, Nicholls MG, Ikram H, Hamilton EJ, Richards RD: Syncope in aortic valvular stenosis. Lancet 1984;2:1113–1116.

104. Johnson AM: Aortic stenosis, sudden death, and the left ventricular baroceptors. Br Heart J 1971;33:1–5.

105. Patel JJ, Dyer RB, Mitha AS: Beta adrenergic block-ade does not improve effort tolerance in patients with mitral stenosis in sinus rhythm. Eur Heart J 1995;16:1264–1268.

106. Ashcom TL, Johns JP, Bailey SR, Rubal BJ: Effects of chronic beta-blockade on rest and exercise hemo-dynamics in mitral stenosis. Cathet Cardiovasc Di-agn 1995;35:110–115.

107. Stoll BC, Ashcom TL, Johns JP, Johnson JE, Rubal BJ: Effects of atenolol on rest and exercise hemody-namics in patients with mitral stenosis. Am J Cardiol 1995;75:482–484.

108. al Kasab SM, Sabag T, al Zaibag M, et al: Beta-adren-ergic receptor blockade in the management of preg-nant women with mitral stenosis. Am J Obstet Gyne-col 1990;163:137–140.

109. Stein PD, Alpert JS, Copeland J, Dalen JE, Goldman S, Turpie AG: Antithrombotic therapy in patients with mechanical and biological prosthetic heart valves [published erratum appears in Chest 1996;109:592]. Chest 1995;108:371S–379S.

110. Vongpatanasin W, Hillis LD, Lange RA: Prosthetic heart valves. N Engl J Med 1996;335:407–416.

111. Cannegieter SC, Rosendaal FR, Wintzen AR, van der Meer FJ, Vandenbroucke JP, Briet E: Optimal oral anticoagulant therapy in patients with mechani-cal heart valves. N Engl J Med 1995;333:11–17.

112. Azar AJ, Cannegieter SC, Deckers JW, et al: Optimal intensity of oral anticoagulant therapy after myocar-dial infarction. J Am Coll Cardiol 1996;27:1349–1355.

113. Altman R, Rouvier J, Gurfinkel E, Scazziota A, Tur-pie AG: Comparison of high-dose with low-dose aspi-rin in patients with mechanical heart valve replace-ment treated with oral anticoagulant. Circulation 1996;94:2113–2116.

114. Acar J, Iung B, Boissel JP, et al: AREVA: multicenter randomized comparison of low-dose versus stan-dard-dose anticoagulation in patients with mechani-cal prosthetic heart valves. Circulation 1996;94:2107–2112.

115. Kearon C, Hirsh J: Management of anticoagulation before and after elective surgery. N Engl J Med 1997;336:1506–1511.

116. Sareli P, England MJ, Berk MR, et al: Maternal and fetal sequelae of anticoagulation during pregnancy in patients with mechanical heart valve prostheses. Am J Cardiol 1989;63:1462–1465.

117. Hanania G, Thomas D, Michel PL, et al: Pregnancy and prosthetic heart valves: a French cooperative retrospective study of 155 cases. Eur Heart J 1994;15:1651–1658.

118. Hall JG, Pauli RM, Wilson KM: Maternal and fetal sequelae of anticoagulation during pregnancy. Am J Med 1980;68:122–140.

119. Becker MH, Genieser NB, Finegold M, Miranda D, Spackman T: Chondrodysplasis punctata: is mater-nal warfarin therapy a factor? Am J Dis Child 1975;129:356–359.

120. Iturbe Alessio I, Fonseca MC, Mutchinik O, Santos MA, Zajarias A, Salazar E: Risks of anticoagulant therapy in pregnant women with artificial heart valves. N Engl J Med 1986;315:1390–1393.

121. Ginsberg JS, Hirsh J, Turner DC, Levine MN, Bur-rows R: Risks to the fetus of anticoagulant therapy during pregnancy. Thromb Haemost 1989;61:197–203.

122. Ginsberg JS, Kowalchuk G, Hirsh J, Brill Edwards P, Burrows R: Heparin therapy during pregnancy: risks to the fetus and mother. Arch Intern Med 1989;149:2233–2236.

123. Ginsberg JS, Kowalchuk G, Hirsh J, et al: Heparin effect on bone density. Thromb Haemost 1990;64:286–289.

124. Dahlman T, Lindvall N, Hellgren M: Osteopenia in pregnancy during long-term heparin treatment: a radiological study post partum. Br J Obstet Gynae-col 1990;97:221–228.

125. Barbour LA, Kick SD, Steiner JF, et al: A prospec-tive study of heparin-induced osteoporosis in preg-nancy using bone densitometry. Am J Obstet Gyne-col 1994;170:862–869.

126. Dahlman TC: Osteoporotic fractures and the recur-rence of thromboembolism during pregnancy and the puerperium in 184 women undergoing throm-boprophylaxis with heparin. Am J Obstet Gynecol 1993;168:1265–1270.

127. Ginsberg JS, Hirsh J: Use of antithrombotic agents during pregnancy. Chest 1995;108:305S–311S.

128. Anderson DR, Ginsberg JS, Burrows R, Brill Ed-wards P: Subcutaneous heparin therapy during preg-nancy: a need for concern at the time of delivery. Thromb Haemost 1991;65:248–250.

129. Sbarouni E, Oakley CM: Outcome of pregnancy in women with valve prostheses. Br Heart J 1994;71:196–201.

130. Brill Edwards P, Ginsberg JS, Johnston M, Hirsh J: Establishing a therapeutic range for heparin ther-apy. Ann Intern Med 1993;119:104–109.

131. CLASP (Collaborative Low-dose Aspirin Study in Pregnancy) Collaborative Group. CLASP: a randomi-sed trial of low-dose aspirin for the prevention and treatment of pre-eclampsia among 9364 pregnant women. Lancet 1994;343:619–629.

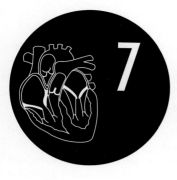

7

Left Ventricular Response to Chronic Pressure and Volume Overload

In patients with valvular heart disease, the left ventricular (LV) response to chronic volume or pressure overload, rather than the severity of the valve lesion alone, often is the primary determinant of clinical outcome. In this sense, the left ventricle is the "end organ" damaged by underlying valvular disease.

For patients with chronic aortic or mitral regurgitation, outcome after surgical intervention is best predicted by measures of LV systolic function, rather than by measures of regurgitant severity. Patients with evidence of impaired LV contractility at baseline evaluation have persistent or worsening ventricular dysfunction after correction of the valvular lesion.[1–7] Prediction of the onset of LV contractile dysfunction is key in the optimal timing of surgical intervention in patients with chronic regurgitation.

For patients with pressure overload due to aortic stenosis, outcome is most closely related to symptom status and the severity of valvular obstruction. Typically, LV hypertrophy regresses and systolic function improves after surgical intervention, even if systolic performance is impaired preoperatively. However, abnormalities in LV geometry and diastolic function are a significant cause of symptoms in patients with aortic stenosis. Diastolic dysfunc-

tion persists postoperatively and may be related to the continued suboptimal functional status and exercise capacity of these patients.[8–10] Moreover, a pattern of excessive LV hypertrophy is associated with a higher surgical risk.[11, 12]

In patients with isolated mitral stenosis, the left ventricle is relatively unaffected by the valvular lesion, other than low filling volumes and pressures due to impaired diastolic filling. However, mitral stenosis often is accompanied by aortic or mitral regurgitation, leading to LV volume overload.

This chapter reviews the overall LV response to chronic pressure and/or volume overload in patients with valvular heart disease. Further details of the ventricular response in patients with specific valve lesions are found in subsequent chapters.

MOLECULAR AND CELLULAR EVENTS IN RESPONSE TO CHRONIC OVERLOAD STATES

It is somewhat intuitive that volume overload stretches the myocardium, resulting in ventricular dilatation, whereas pressure overload increases wall stress, leading to increased myocardial thickness. However, the cellular and molecular mechanisms underlying the normal physiologic responses to chronic pressure or volume overload are not well understood. The processes leading to the transition from an appropriate hypertrophic response to contractile dysfunction have not been fully elucidated.[13] Most data on these issues have been derived from in vitro models or from in vivo models that approximate the clinical problems of systemic hypertension or dilated cardiomyopathy. Relatively few studies have been conducted on the effects of LV volume overload due to valvular regurgitation or pressure overload due to subcoronary aortic valve obstruction.

Overall, the response to pressure and volume overload can be divided into three phases (Fig. 7–1). Acutely, overload stimulates physiologic compensatory mechanisms and initiates the response at the cellular and molecular levels. With chronic disease, this phase presumably occurs in imperceptible steps, with each incremental increase in load resulting in appropriate compensatory mechanisms such that there is no clinical evidence for impaired

ventricular function. Concentric hypertrophy (with pressure overload) or eccentric hypertrophy (with volume overload) occurs, with preservation of ventricular contractility and ejection performance. The end-stage of the sequence of events initiated by pressure or volume overload is the transition to impaired LV contractility and cardiac failure.

The initial response to LV pressure or volume overload at the cellular and molecular level is complex. First, there must be a signal transduction pathway for "sensing" the mechanical overload state.[14–16] Although the specific molecules involved have not been identified, it is likely that the signal transduction pathways differ according to the type of ventricular load. For example, in an animal model of valvular disease, a 30% increase in the rate of myosin heavy-chain synthesis was seen after 6 hours of acute pressure overload but not after volume overload of similar hemodynamic severity and duration.[17]

Second, significant changes occur in gene expression and protein synthesis within cardiac myocytes in response to pressure or vol-

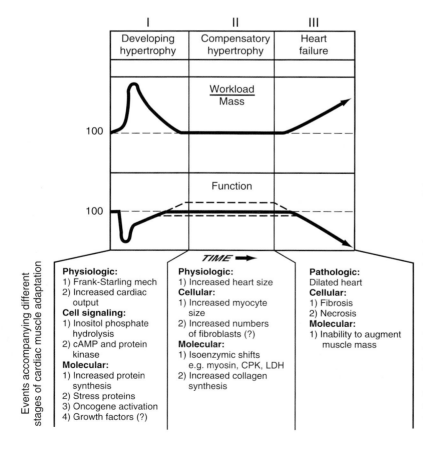

Figure 7·1 Phases of cardiac overload. In the diagram, 100 on the vertical axes and the dotted line indicate normal values of the respective parameters of the workload and function (ie, values obtained before the imposition of the overload). The solid line indicates the generalized response of the heart to the overload. The dashed line indicates that conflicting data have been obtained in various models or by various investigators. For example, in phase II, heart function was reported in various studies to be normal, increased, and depressed. (From Bugiasky LB, Gupta M, Gupta MP, Zak R: Cellular and molecular mechanisms of cardiac hypertrophy. *In The Heart and Cardiovascular System,* ed 2. New York: Raven Press, 1992: 1629.)

ume overload. In pressure overload induced by aortic banding in weanling rats, changes include reexpression of fetal gene products, including β-myosin heavy chain and skeletal α-actin.[18–23] Because mature cardiac myocytes do not undergo cell division, hypertrophy occurs by an increase in the volume of the existing myocytes. Volume overload and pressure overload lead to an increase in myocyte volume through increased synthesis of sarcomeres. With volume overload hypertrophy, sarcomeres are added in series, resulting in increased myocyte length and a dilated chamber, a pattern called eccentric hypertrophy. With pressure overload hypertrophy, sarcomeres are added in parallel, leading to increased myocyte diameter and a thick-walled chamber, a pattern defined as concentric hypertrophy.

Third, ventricular hypertrophy involves the extracellular matrix as well as the contractile elements of the myocardium. The interstitial fibers of the myocardium appear to be important in distributing and modulating the force generated by the myocytes, and they limit the maximal passive length of the myocytes.[24] Cardiac connective tissue is highly active metabolically,[24, 25] and mechanical stretch promotes cardiac fibroblast proliferation and enhances collagen production, possibly through integrin activation.[24, 26] In an in vitro model, mechanical stretch of cardiac fibroblasts led to an increased ratio of collagen type III to type I, with evidence for an increase in type III collagen mRNA after as little as 12 hours of mechanical stretch.[24] In vitro studies show that angiotensin II and aldosterone can stimulate transduction and migration of fibroblasts, stimulate collagen synthesis, and inhibit collagen breakdown by inhibition of matrix metalloproteinase I activity.[25–27]

Upregulation of cardiac neurohormonal systems occurs with cardiac hypertrophy, including increased levels of atrial natriuretic peptide and increased production of angiotensin-converting enzyme mRNA.[14] The clinical importance of this upregulation is underlined by the effects of long-term angiotensin 1 receptor blockade in improving LV end-diastolic pressure and normalizing angiotensin-converting enzyme mRNA levels.[19]

The transition from physiologic hypertrophy to contractile dysfunction remains an area of ongoing research. In patients with valvular disease, this transition occurs only with chronic, severe valve dysfunction, typically in the setting of substantial LV dilatation. At the cellular and molecular levels, the mechanism of impaired contractility is unknown. Lorell proposes that the "transition to failure relates to interactive changes in expression of multiple genes regulating composition of the motor unit, cytoskeleton and extracellular matrix, ion homeostasis, and myocyte cell loss due to both apoptosis and necrosis."[28]

MEASURES OF VENTRICULAR SYSTOLIC FUNCTION

In patients with valvular heart disease, hemodynamic decompensation is associated with the onset of LV systolic dysfunction. In some cases, systolic function improves after relief of the valvular lesion, but in other cases, LV function remains depressed or even worsens after surgical intervention. A goal in the management of patients with valvular heart disease is to identify the onset of hemodynamic decompensation and intervene before the development of irreversible changes.

Evaluation of ventricular function in the clinical setting is complicated by its dependence on loading conditions. Ventricular ejection performance (ie, ability of the ventricle to pump blood) should be differentiated from ventricular contractility (ie, intrinsic capacity of the myocardium to contract independent of loading conditions). Ejection performance varies with heart rate, preload, afterload, and ventricular geometry, even without changes in myocardial contractility. Thus, assessment of ventricular function is a particular problem in patients with valvular heart disease because loading conditions are uniformly abnormal. Unfortunately, no ideal independent clinical measure of contractility exists (Table 7–1).[29] Instead, surrogate measures, based on experimental models and observational clinical studies, have been used in the management of patients with valvular disease.

Ejection-Phase Indices

While stroke volume is a direct measure of the pumping action of the heart, it has little value as a measure of ventricular function in patients with valvular heart disease. First, the forward stroke volume delivered to the body must be differentiated from the total stroke volume pumped by the left ventricle, because total stroke volume includes regurgitant volume. Second, compensatory mechanisms ensure that stroke volume at rest is maintained in the normal range until very late in the disease course. Third, stroke volume depends

TABLE 7·1 PHYSIOLOGIC FRAMEWORK FOR ASSESSING PREOPERATIVE PREDICTORS OF SURGICAL OUTCOME FOR PATIENTS WITH CHRONIC AORTIC REGURGITATION				
Variable	Preload	Afterload	Heart Rate	Contractility
Severity of aortic regurgitation				
Regurgitant volume	+	+	+	0
Regurgitant fraction	+	+	+	0
End-diastolic indices				
Volume (dimension)	+	+	+	+/0
Pressure	+	+	+	+/0
Ejection-phase indices				
Rest data	+	+	+	+
Exercise response	+	+	+	+
End-systolic indices				
Volume (dimension)	0	+	+/0	+
Pressure-volume slope	0	0	+/0	+
Wall stress/volume ratio	0	+	0	+
Wall stress–ejection fraction relationship	+	0	+	+
Wall stress–Vcf_c relationship	0	0	0	+

Vcf_c, rate-corrected velocity of fiber shortening; +, dependent; 0, independent.

Adapted from Borow KM: Surgical outcome in chronic aortic regurgitation: a physiologic framework for assessing preoperative predictors. J Am Coll Cardiol 1987;10:1165–1170; reprinted with permission from the American College of Cardiology.

on ventricular size, heart rate, preload, and afterload, providing little information about the contractile state of the myocardium. Evaluation of stroke volume after exercise or the change in stroke volume from rest to exercise provides insight into the mechanisms of exertional symptoms, but these are not reliable measures for detection of the onset of contractile dysfunction.

Ejection fraction, the ratio of stroke volume to end-diastolic volume, also depends on preload, afterload, and heart rate. For example, an increase in end-diastolic fiber stretch (preload) increases ventricular contractility, resulting in a higher ejection fraction. This phenomenon is known as the Frank-Starling mechanism (Fig. 7–2). Ejection fraction also is affected by afterload, with increased afterload resulting in a reduced velocity of fiber shortening (Fig. 7–3). Afterload, the force developed by the myocardium by contraction, often is approximated by systemic blood pressure or vascular resistance, although end-systolic wall stress may be a more appropriate measure. Use of end-systolic wall stress as a descriptor of afterload is especially important for patients

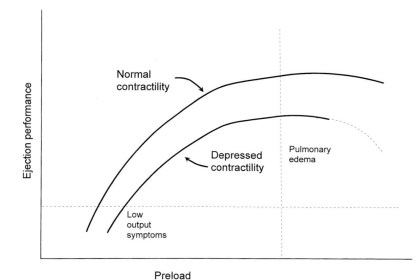

Figure 7·2 Relationship between preload (often approximated by left ventricular end-diastolic volume or pressure) and ejection performance (often approximated by stroke volume or ejection fraction) for a ventricle with normal and depressed contractility. At high levels of preload, the elevated left ventricular end-diastolic pressure leads to pulmonary congestion. At low preload levels, low cardiac output symptoms are seen. Low output symptoms occur at a higher preload level when contractility is impaired. It remains controversial whether ventricular function deteriorates at high preload levels *(curved dashed line)*.

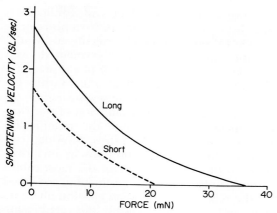

Figure 7·3 The inverse relation between isotonic afterload and shortening velocity is illustrated. Beats that begin at a long muscle length manifest a more rapid shortening velocity for any given afterload than beats that begin at a short length. (From Huntsman LL, Feigl EO: Cardiac mechanics. *In* Patton Hille B, Scher AM, Steiner R, eds. Textbook of Physiology, vol 2, ed 21. Philadelphia: WB Saunders, 1989:827.)

with valvular heart disease when LV systolic pressures are not approximated by systemic pressures, as in persons with valvular aortic stenosis.

Measurement of exercise ejection fraction and, more specifically, the change in ejection fraction from rest to exercise also has been proposed as a useful gauge of ventricular function in patients with chronic aortic or mitral regurgitation. Even though this measure is more robust than the resting ejection fraction, the effects of loading conditions still limit its utility. Overall, ejection-phase indices reflect the ejection performance of the ventricle but not the state of myocardial contractility.

Despite its load dependence, ejection fraction can be measured easily, reliably, and repeatedly using noninvasive techniques. Thus, ejection fraction continues to be one of the most useful clinical measures of systolic function in patients with valvular disease, especially when loading conditions and parameters of LV size are considered in the decision-making process.

End-Diastolic Indices

End-diastolic measures of ventricular dimension and volume depend on preload but are relatively independent of afterload. As an indicator of the degree of LV dilation, these measures are useful adjuncts in the evaluation of patients with chronic valvular regurgita-

tion.[2, 30] Sequential studies showing progressive increases in end-diastolic dimensions or volumes are particularly helpful clinically.

End-diastolic wall stress, derived from measurements of wall thickness, chamber dimension, and diastolic ventricular pressure, also has been useful in the experimental setting. Clinical applications are limited by the lack of a noninvasive method for determining LV diastolic pressures.

End-Systolic Indices

End-systolic measures of LV dimensions or volumes are relatively independent of heart rate and preload.[1, 3, 5, 30–36] Although end-systolic measures are affected to some extent by afterload, these parameters have been shown to be useful in optimizing the timing of surgical intervention in patients with chronic mitral or aortic regurgitation.

The end-systolic pressure-volume relationship (ESPVR), also called elastance (E_{max}), is the slope of the line connecting the end-systolic points on several pressure-volume loops as afterload is varied during a short period (Fig. 7–4).[37] The ESPVR is relatively independent of loading conditions and provides a rigorous experimental measure of ventricular contractility.[35, 36, 38–40] However, calculation of

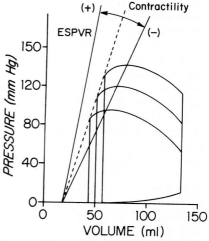

Figure 7·4 Short term variation of afterload (aortic pressure) can be used to generate a set of pressure-volume loops. The end-systolic points lie along a line that is called the end-systolic pressure-volume relation (ESPVR). The slope of this relation is an indicator of the contractile state of the ventricle. (From Huntsman LL, Feigl EO: Cardiac mechanics. *In* Patton Hille B, Scher AM, Steiner R, eds. Textbook of Physiology, vol 2, ed 21. Philadelphia: WB Saunders, 1989:831.)

elastance requires measurement of end-systolic volume and pressure at several levels of afterload. Measurement of instantaneous pressures and volumes throughout the cardiac cycle is difficult in the clinical setting. In addition, altering afterload in patients with significant valve dysfunction may be risky. Even though measurement of elastance has increased our understanding of the pathophysiology of valve disease in experimental models and in limited patient studies, this measure rarely is used for clinical patient management.

End-systolic wall stress incorporates the effects of ventricular wall thickness, chamber size, and ventricular pressure into a single measurement. Wall stress is the force per unit area of the myocardium. For a spherical chamber, wall stress (σ) is calculated as:

$$\sigma = PR/2Th$$

In the equation, P is the LV pressure, R is the radius of the LV, and Th is wall thickness. Thus, wall stress increases as the ratio of wall thickness to chamber dimension decreases or as LV pressure increases.

In view of the three-dimensional geometry of the ventricle, clinically relevant wall stress calculations are more complex than suggested by the simple formula for a sphere. Further, wall stress can be subdivided into the stresses acting in different directions within the myocardium. Circumferential wall stress reflects the stresses affecting the myocardial fibers in the ventricular short-axis dimension, whereas meridional wall stress reflects the forces acting in the long-axis dimension. Although both calculations are complex, the basic measurements required for these calculations are wall thickness, chamber dimensions, and ventricular pressure. Therefore, wall stress can be calculated using echocardiographic, angiographic, or magnetic resonance images of the left ventricle in conjunction with pressure data.[41, 42] Formulas for calculation of circumferential and meridional wall stress using echocardiographic data are given in Chapter 3, and formulas used with angiographic data are given by Mirsky.[41]

If ventricular pressures are not measured directly by catheter, the end-systolic ventricular pressure typically is noninvasively estimated in one of three ways: (1) end-systolic pressure is calculated from cuff systolic pressure in conjunction with calibrated carotid pulse tracings; (2) the mean systolic pressure is used instead of end-systolic pressure; or (3) peak systolic pressure is used instead of end-systolic pressure. Even in patients with aortic stenosis, peak systolic LV pressure can be calculated by adding the transaortic pressure gradient derived from Doppler data to the cuff blood pressure, and there is a close linear relationship between peak and end-systolic pressures.[43]

Another approach to evaluation of ventricular function is to examine the relationship between two of these measures, allowing "correction" for loading conditions by including them in the analysis. Perhaps the most robust measures of ventricular contractility are based on the relationship between ejection-phase indices and afterload. Typically, this relationship is shown as a graph, with the ejection-phase index on the vertical axis and afterload on the horizontal axis. Usually, mid-wall velocity of circumferential fiber shortening or ejection fraction is used as the measure of ejection performance[34, 44] and end or mean systolic wall stress is used for afterload.[44–46] Points on the graph are then compared with the normal range for this relationship (Fig. 7–5). Data points that fall below the normal range indicate impaired contractility, with an ejection performance less than expected for a given degree of afterload.

However, the calculation of these data is quite complex. Errors in any of the basic measurements result in error in the calculated value. In addition, the limits of reproducibility

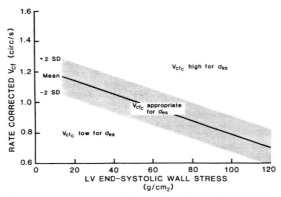

Figure 7·5 Diagram of the end-systolic wall stress (σ_{es})/rate-corrected velocity of fiber shortening (V_{cf}) relation. Depressed contractile state (V_{cfc} low for the level of σ_{es}) may be differentiated from situations in which contractility is normal but afterload is increased (V_{cfc} appropriate for the level of σ_{es}). Velocity of fiber shortening, which is high for the level of end-systolic wall stress, is characteristic of increased inotropic state. (From Colan SD, Borow KM, Neumann A: Left ventricular end-systolic wall stress-velocity of fiber shortening relation: a load-independent index of myocardial contractility. J Am Coll Cardiol 1984;4:715–724.)

for clinical use of these measures have not been defined. Despite the insight into the pathophysiology of disease provided by this approach, measurement of the relationship between fiber shortening and end-systolic wall stress in the clinical setting rarely is helpful.

Perhaps the simplest end-systolic measure is LV volume or dimension. Although this relatively unsophisticated measure may be affected by afterload, dimension and volume at end-systole both are independent of preload. Simple dimensions have the advantage that they can be measured on two-dimensional echocardiography with a low intertest variability and a high degree of accuracy, when recorded correctly. Compared with a simple linear dimension, end-systolic volume more accurately reflects the three-dimensional size of the ventricle, with the slight disadvantage that it is more difficult to measure and requires meticulous attention to technical details in an experienced laboratory. Both end-systolic dimensions and volumes have become standard approaches to evaluation of ventricular function in patients with valvular disease.

SERIAL CHANGES IN VENTRICULAR VOLUMES AND MASS

At the macroscopic level, the ventricular response to pressure and volume overload is heterogeneous. In comparing patients with pressure versus volume overload, distinct differences in the severity and timing of LV dilatation and hypertrophy and the onset of contractile dysfunction are seen.[39] In addition, the ventricular response within groups of patients with the same valvular lesion is modulated by factors such as age and gender. However, even when other known factors are taken into account, considerable individual variability in the ventricular response is seen.[47]

Pressure Overload

Acute aortic stenosis is not tolerated hemodynamically. The abrupt increase in LV systolic pressures in the absence of compensatory hypertrophy leads to a marked increase in end-systolic wall stress. Ejection performance is depressed, and the resultant inability of the ventricle to pump blood across the obstruction leads to an acute decline in cardiac output and systemic hypotension. The compensatory increase in filling volumes into a noncompliant ventricle leads to elevated ventricular diastolic pressures and pulmonary edema. Fortu-

nately, acute stenosis is rare in the clinical setting; the only example is acute thrombosis of a prosthetic valve.

In patients with native valvular aortic stenosis, the basic response to chronic LV pressure overload is concentric hypertrophy, specifically an increase in the thickness of the myocardium with little change in the dimensions or volume of the ventricular chamber. Concentric hypertrophy in adults with aortic stenosis primarily is caused by an increase in muscle fiber diameter, with a smaller increase in interstitial fibrosis. In patients with native valvular aortic stenosis, LV hypertrophy develops gradually over many years, corresponding to the gradual increase in the degree of valvular obstruction. However, in animal models of "chronic" valvular or supravalvular aortic stenosis, LV hypertrophy occurs rapidly, with an increase in LV mass of 30% to 45% after only 6 to 8 weeks.[44, 48] In animal models and in patients with aortic stenosis, the increase in LV mass directly correlates with the transaortic pressure gradient, although considerable individual variability is seen.[49]

With compensated aortic stenosis, wall stress remains normal despite increased LV pressure from the increased ratio of wall thickness to chamber dimension. When compensatory hypertrophy is adequate, LV afterload is normal, despite the presence of aortic stenosis.[39, 50] As stenosis severity gradually increases, compensatory LV hypertrophy maintains wall stress in the normal range, allowing preserved ventricular ejection performance for a long period of time, typically many years, in adults with slowly progressive disease.

Another way to examine the LV response to valvular heart disease is in terms of the LV pressure-volume curve. Compensated aortic stenosis is characterized by normal ventricular volumes, higher systolic pressures, and a normal ejection fraction. The end-systolic pressure-volume relationship is shifted to the left but remains parallel to the normal relationship (eg, with the same slope), reflecting normal ventricular contractility. There also may be a slight upward shift in the passive diastolic pressure-volume relationship because of the decreased compliance of the hypertrophied myocardium (Fig. 7–6). Decreased compliance in conjunction with a fixed maximal myocyte length leads to a phenomenon known as *limited preload reserve*. This term implies that only a limited increase in ventricular filling volumes is possible before the maximal myocyte length is reached. Thus, with exercise, stroke volume

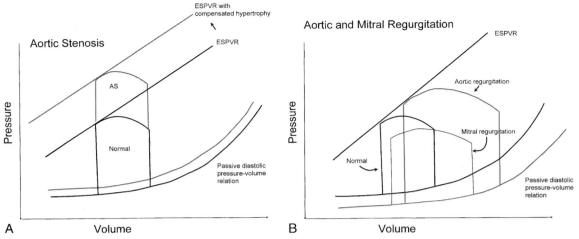

Figure 7·6 Schematic diagram of pressure-volume loops in left ventricular pressure and volume overload compared with normal values. *A*, With pressure overload from aortic stenosis (AS), despite higher systolic pressure, the ejection fraction is normal, and the slope of the end-systolic pressure volume relation (ESPVR) is unchanged, indicating normal contractility. Because of increased myocardial stiffness, the passive diastolic pressure-volume relation is shifted upward and to the left. *B*, With chronic volume overload, the passive diastolic pressure volume relationship is shifted downward and to the right. Ventricular volumes are increased, and the ejection fraction remains normal or is increased. The slope of the ESPVR remains normal until a decline in contractility occurs. Aortic regurgitation differs from mitral regurgitation in that ventricular volumes are larger and systolic pressures are higher, resulting in combined pressure and volume overload.

rises minimally or not at all, whereas LV diastolic pressures rise dramatically, leading to symptoms of exertional intolerance and pulmonary congestion.

As the disease progresses, even in patients with aortic stenosis and normal LV contractility, ejection fraction may be reduced because of the increased afterload from the valvular obstruction. After relief of aortic stenosis, ejection fraction returns to normal. Even in aortic stenosis patients with a normal ejection fraction, there is a small increase in ejection fraction after valve replacement.[51-54]

When the patient with aortic stenosis has a depressed ejection fraction, it often is problematic to separate LV dysfunction due to increased afterload from intrinsic myocardial disease. Although impaired ejection performance due to the elevated afterload of aortic stenosis should improve after valve replacement, the degree of improvement may be suboptimal if the patient has impaired contractility (see Chapter 9).[55, 56] Many patients with aortic stenosis have coexisting coronary disease, which may account for irreversible myocardial damage.[57] Measures such as the ratio of mid-wall fiber shortening to end-systolic wall stress help separate those with reversible from those with irreversible systolic dysfunction (Fig. 7–7).[58]

Considerable individual variability exists both in the extent of LV hypertrophy and in the onset of decompensation resulting in impaired ejection performance.[44, 48, 59] Some of these differences are gender related; studies of adults with aortic stenosis show that women typically have small ventricles with thick walls and preserved systolic function, but men have dilated ventricles with normal wall thickness and impaired ejection performance.[43, 60-63] Women have LV hypertrophy more often than men, and in addition, in women, the ratio of wall thickness to chamber dimension is increased, maintaining normal wall stress, while in men, the ratio of wall thickness to chamber dimension fails to rise adequately for the increase in LV pressure.[61]

A heterogeneous response to pressure overload, independent of gender differences, has been seen in a canine model of ascending aortic constriction. Dogs with a high ratio of LV mass to body weight at baseline developed compensatory ventricular hypertrophy and maintained normal contractile function as the severity of obstruction increased. In contrast, those with lower baseline ratio of ventricular mass to body weight had a smaller increase in LV mass and developed depressed contractility late in the study (Fig. 7–8).[44] The investigators suggest that the association of contractile dysfunction with higher wall stress and lower systolic ejection rates at baseline indicates the

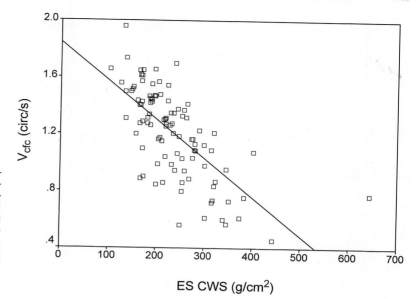

Figure 7·7 Graph of the velocity of circumferential fiber shortening (V_{cfc}) versus end-systolic meridional wall stress (ES CWS) in 123 patients with asymptomatic aortic stenosis shows the linear relationship between these two variables in patients with compensated pressure overload. (Figure courtesy of Malcolm E. Legget, MD, Auckland, NZ.)

possibility of variability in the set points for regulation of myocardial growth.[44] A decreasing ratio of LV mass to body weight also has been noted to precede the onset of systolic dysfunction in the weanling rat aortic banding model.[21, 64]

After valve replacement for aortic stenosis, LV wall thickness and mass decrease.[65] Although there is a 30% decrease in LV mass by 10 months, LV mass continues to decline over several years, with significant changes documented as late as 8 years after surgical intervention.[10] Elegant studies by Krayenbuehl and colleagues[10] have shown that the early decrease in ventricular mass is related to a decrease in the muscle fiber diameter and that the late decrease in ventricular mass reflects slower regression of interstitial fibrotic changes in the myocardium (Fig. 7–9).

Volume Overload

Mitral regurgitation results in LV volume overload due to the increase in total LV stroke volume as blood is ejected forward into the aorta and retrograde across the mitral valve. With acute mitral regurgitation, the left ventricle empties more completely (eg, LV ejection fraction increases) such that forward cardiac output is maintained (Table 7–2).[66]

With compensated chronic regurgitation, LV diastolic volume increases, and the ejection fraction is normal such that end-systolic volume is within the normal range or only mildly increased. Afterload often is considered to be decreased in patients with mitral regurgitation because of ejection into the low-impedance left atrium. In this setting, a lower afterload maintains ejection performance, masking contractile dysfunction.[67] However, wall stress, a better measure of afterload, remains in the normal range in patients with chronic mitral regurgitation, as the effect of decreased ejection force is counterbalanced by increased ventricular chamber size without an increase in wall thickness.[68–70] Thus, with chronic mitral regurgitation, ejection fraction typically is in

TABLE 7·2   MECHANICS OF VALVULAR REGURGITATION

Variable	AR Preop	Post AVR	MR Preop	Post MVR	Post MV Repair
Peak systolic pressure	↑ ↑	Nl	↓	Nl	Nl
LV ratio of radius to thickness	Nl	Nl	↑ ↑	↑ ↑	Nl
Systolic wall stress	↑ ↑	Nl	Nl	↑ ↑	Nl
Diastolic wall stress	↑ ↑	Nl	↑ ↑ ↑	↑ ↑	Nl
Ejection fraction	Nl or ↓	Nl	Nl or ↑	↓	Nl

LV, left ventricular; AR, aortic regurgitation; AVR, aortic valve replacement; MR, mitral regurgitation; MVR, mitral valve replacement; MV, mitral valve; Preop, preoperative; Nl, normal; arrows indicate relative degree of increase or decrease in each variable.

From Carabello BA: The changing unnatural history of valvular regurgitation. Ann Thorac Surg 1992;53:191–199.

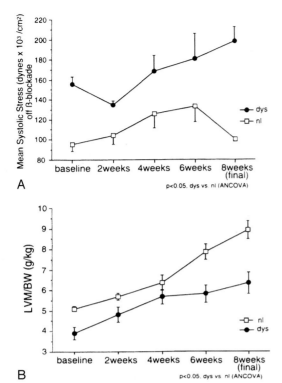

Figure 7·8 In an animal model of aortic stenosis, sequential measurements of left ventricular mass *(A)* and mean systolic wall stress *(B)* were obtained during β blockade. The group that maintained normal function (nl) has lower wall stress than the group that developed dysfunction (dys). Although the ratio of left ventricular mass (LVM) to body weight (BW), an index of hypertrophy, increased in both groups, the time course of development of hypertrophy was different for the two groups. (From Koide M, Nagatsu M, Zile M, et al: Premorbid determinants of left ventricular dysfunction in a novel model of gradually induced pressure overload in the adult canine. Circulation 1997;95:1601–1610; by permission of The American Heart Association, Inc.)

the normal range. While there is some increase in LV mass with chronic mitral regurgitation, the degree of increase is less than that with aortic stenosis or regurgitation.

With chronic mitral regurgitation, contractile dysfunction may occur relatively early in the disease course, often even before the onset of symptoms. Ventricular decompensation in chronic mitral regurgitation is characterized by an increase in end-diastolic and end-systolic dimensions. Ejection fraction declines but may still be within the normal range, making recognition of the onset of contractile dysfunction more difficult.[1, 29, 39, 71, 72] Eventually, wall stress increases, leading to further ventricular dilation and worsening ventricular systolic function.

Mitral valve replacement usually results in worsening of LV ejection performance, with an average decline of 5 to 10 ejection fraction units.[6, 73–75] To some extent, this decline in ventricular ejection performance can be prevented by preservation of mitral annular and papillary muscle continuity, as discussed in Chapter 15.[38, 46, 76–80]

However, with decreased contractility preoperatively, persistent LV dilatation, increased wall stress, and reduced ejection fraction can be expected postoperatively, even after mitral valve repair.[38, 81, 82] As discussed in Chapter 13, clinical, echocardiographic, and hemodynamic predictors of contractile dysfunction have been developed that allow early recognition of decompensation and optimal timing of surgical intervention.

Combined Pressure and Volume Overload

Aortic regurgitation results in volume and pressure overload of the left ventricle.[29, 83, 84] Volume overload is obvious because of the increase in total LV stroke volume from the addition of the regurgitant volume to the forward stroke volume. However, pressure overload also exists, because this increased stroke volume is ejected into the high-impedance aorta. Thus, there is both increased diastolic wall stress and increased systolic wall stress, resulting in features of volume overload (dilatation) and pressure overload (hypertrophy).[39, 46, 68]

With acute aortic regurgitation, the abrupt increase in ventricular diastolic filling leads to a dramatic increase in LV end-diastolic pressure and pulmonary edema. However, ventricular volumes and mass are not increased, since the time course is too rapid for compensatory changes to occur. Acute regurgitation may be accompanied by impaired ventricular ejection performance, despite normal contractility, due to the abrupt increase in afterload, a combination called *afterload mismatch.*[84]

With chronic aortic regurgitation, LV volumes increase substantially at end-diastole and at end-systole. The LV passive diastolic pressure-volume curve shifts upward and to the right, allowing accommodation of the increased ventricular volume with normal filling pressures. LV wall thickness often is increased, depending on LV systolic pressure, to maintain a normal systolic wall stress. Overall, LV mass is markedly increased, particularly compared with isolated pressure or volume overload (Fig. 7–10).

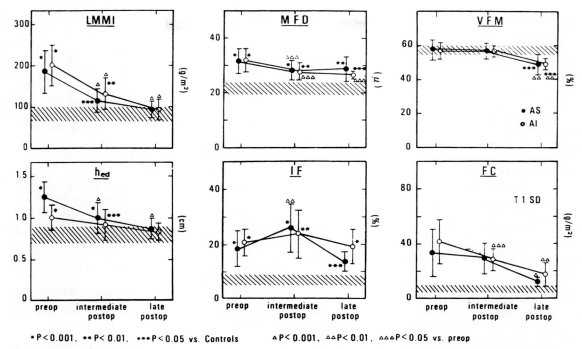

•P<0.001. ••P<0.01. •••P<0.05 vs. Controls   ▵P<0.001. ▵▵P<0.01. ▵▵▵P<0.05 vs. preop

Figure 7·9 Left ventricular macroscopic and microscopic morphometric findings in patients with aortic stenosis *(closed circles)* and aortic insufficiency *(open circles)* preoperatively and intermediate (18 months) and late (5 years) postoperatively. Control values are indicated by the shaded areas (mean ± SD). LMMI, left ventricular muscle mass index; MFD, muscle fiber diameter; VFM, volume fraction of myofibrils; h_{ed}, left ventricular end-diastolic wall thickness; IF, percent interstitial fibrosis; FC, left ventricular fibrous content. (From Krayenbuehl HP, Hess OM, Monrad ES, Schneider J, Mall G, Turina M: Left ventricular myocardial structure in aortic valve disease before, intermediate, and late after aortic valve replacement. Circulation 1989;79:748; by permission of The American Heart Association, Inc.)

As with other chronic overload states, normal ventricular ejection performance is maintained for many years in patients with aortic regurgitation. Eventually, prolonged, severe volume overload leads to contractile dysfunction, often without overt clinical symptoms.[40, 85] The transition to irreversible contractile dysfunction invariably occurs in the setting of substantial LV dilatation, albeit the criteria for severe dilation may vary for men and women.[2, 86–88] With decompensated aortic regurgitation, the ratio of chamber dimension to wall thickness increases, and end-systolic wall stress is elevated. LV ejection performance deteriorates, and contractile dysfunction develops with further ventricular dilation and worsening systolic function.[84, 89] Note that with both aortic and mitral regurgitation, a component of acute, superimposed on chronic, regurgitation may precipitate sudden hemodynamic de-

Figure 7·10 Left ventricular mass index is demonstrated for normal subjects, patients with mitral regurgitation (MR), patients with aortic stenosis (AS), and patients with aortic regurgitation (AR). Patients with mitral regurgitation have less extensive hypertrophy than those with aortic regurgitation. (Data from Dodge HT, Kennedy JW, Petersen JL: Prog Cardiovasc Dis 1973;16:1–23.)

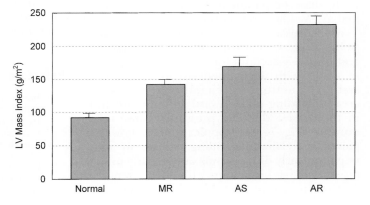

compensation in a patient with previously slowly progressive disease.

The LV response in patients with chronic aortic regurgitation can be altered by the use of afterload reduction therapy. Studies of acute and long-term disease suggest that afterload reduction decreases the rate of increase of LV dimensions and prevents an increase in LV mass.[90–92] Furthermore, afterload reduction therapy has been shown to prevent the onset of impaired ejection performance and delay the need for surgical intervention in a randomized controlled clinical trial.[93]

After surgical intervention for relief of aortic regurgitation, ventricular volumes and mass return toward normal. Much of the decrease occurs in the first 1 to 2 years, but LV mass continues to decrease up to 8 years postoperatively.[94–98]

Unlike the outcome for mitral regurgitation, LV function improves after valve replacement for aortic regurgitation, even if impaired contractility was present at baseline. As in patients with aortic stenosis, valve replacement favorably affects LV systolic performance due to a decrease in afterload.[4, 86, 94, 99–102] If contractility itself has deteriorated, LV systolic function still improves, albeit to a lesser degree.[2, 103]

CHANGES IN DIASTOLIC FUNCTION

Diastolic function of the left ventricle also is affected by the pressure and volume overload states due to valvular heart disease. With LV dilatation there is a rightward shift along the passive pressure-volume curve. In addition, with chronic volume overload caused by aortic or mitral regurgitation, diastolic compliance increases, producing a rightward and downward shift of the diastolic pressure-volume relationship. Thus, with compensated volume overload, larger LV volumes are accommodated at normal filling pressures. Postoperatively, diastolic parameters return toward normal as LV dilatation regresses.

With pressure overload hypertrophy, diastolic changes occur early in the disease course and probably account for exertional symptoms in adults with aortic stenosis and preserved systolic function. LV chamber stiffness increases, leading to a leftward and upward shift in the passive diastolic pressure-volume relationship (Fig. 7–11). Doppler studies show impaired early diastolic filling, consistent with impaired early diastolic relaxation, early in the disease course in patients with aortic stenosis. As the disease progresses, LV end-diastolic

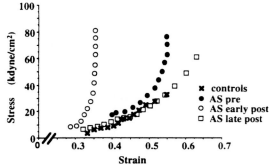

Figure 7·11   Representative plot of the diastolic stress-strain relation for a control subject and for a patient with severe aortic stenosis (AS) before surgery (pre) and early and late after valve replacement (post). Early after surgery (early postop), the curve is shifted to the left compared with the preoperative evaluation, and the constant of myocardial stiffness is increased. Late after valve replacement (late post), the curve is shifted to the right, and the constant of myocardial stiffness is normalized. (From Villari B, Vassalli G, Monrad ES, et al: Normalization of diastolic dysfunction in aortic stenosis late after valve replacement. Circulation 1995;91:2353–2358; by permission of The American Heart Association, Inc.)

pressure rises, and compliance decreases, resulting in a Doppler LV inflow curve characterized by rapid early diastolic filling, a steep deceleration slope, and a small atrial contribution to filling.[104, 105] Because the patient with aortic stenosis is operating with a higher resting diastolic pressure, the inability to increase cardiac output with exercise may partly result from limited preload reserve.[106]

The diastolic abnormalities in aortic stenosis are associated with an increase in the total collagen content of the myocardium and in the orthogonal collagen fiber network.[9, 107] After relief of aortic stenosis, systolic function improves promptly, but diastolic dysfunction continues because of persistent interstitial fibrosis.[10] The extent of myocardial fibrosis is affected by age, gender, and aortic valve obstruction.[63, 108] Normalization of the extent of myocardial fibrosis and diastolic stiffness occurs only 6 to 7 years after surgical intervention.[63, 109, 110]

References

1. Borow KM, Green LH, Mann T, et al: End-systolic volume as a predictor of postoperative left ventricular performance in volume overload from valvular regurgitation. Am J Med 1980;68:655–663.
2. Gaasch WH, Carroll JD, Levine HJ, Criscitiello MG: Chronic aortic regurgitation: prognostic value of left ventricular end-systolic dimension and end-diastolic radius/thickness ratio. J Am Coll Cardiol 1983;1:775–782.

3. Zile MR, Gaasch WH, Carroll JD, Levine HJ: Chronic mitral regurgitation: predictive value of preoperative echocardiographic indexes of left ventricular function and wall stress. J Am Coll Cardiol 1984;3:1235–1242.

4. Bonow RO, Rosing DR, Kent KM, Epstein SE: Timing of operation for chronic aortic regurgitation. Am J Cardiol 1982;50:325–336.

5. Carabello BA, Usher BW, Hendrix GH, Assey ME, Crawford FA, Leman RB: Predictors of outcome for aortic valve replacement in patients with aortic regurgitation and left ventricular dysfunction: a change in the measuring stick. J Am Coll Cardiol 1987;10:991–997.

6. Crawford MH, Souchek J, Oprian CA, et al: Determinants of survival and left ventricular performance after mitral valve replacement. Department of Veterans Affairs Cooperative Study on Valvular Heart Disease. Circulation 1990;81:1173–1181.

7. Greves J, Rahimtoola SH, McAnulty JH, et al: Preoperative criteria predictive of late survival following valve replacement for severe aortic regurgitation. Am Heart J 1981;101:300–308.

8. Villari B, Hess OM, Kaufmann P, Krogmann ON, Grimm J, Krayenbuehl HP: Effect of aortic valve stenosis (pressure overload) and regurgitation (volume overload) on left ventricular systolic and diastolic function. Am J Cardiol 1992;69:927–934.

9. Villari B, Campbell SE, Hess OM, et al: Influence of collagen network on left ventricular systolic and diastolic function in aortic valve disease. J Am Coll Cardiol 1993;22:1477–1484.

10. Krayenbuehl HP, Hess OM, Monrad ES, Schneider J, Mall G, Turina M: Left ventricular myocardial structure in aortic valve disease before, intermediate, and late after aortic valve replacement. Circulation 1989;79:744–755.

11. Orsinelli DA, Aurigemma GP, Battista S, Krendel S, Gaasch WH: Left ventricular hypertrophy and mortality after aortic valve replacement for aortic stenosis: a high risk subgroup identified by preoperative relative wall thickness. J Am Coll Cardiol 1993;22:1679–1683.

12. Aurigemma G, Battista S, Orsinelli D, Sweeney A, Pape L, Cuenoud H: Abnormal left ventricular intracavitary flow acceleration in patients undergoing aortic valve replacement for aortic stenosis: a marker for high postoperative morbidity and mortality. Circulation 1992;86:926–936.

13. Bugaisky LB, Gupta M, Gupta MP, Zak R: Cellular and molecular mechanisms of cardiac hypertrophy. *In* Fozzard HA, Haber E, Jennings RB, Katz AM, Morgan HE, eds. The Heart and Cardiovascular System: Scientific Foundations, ed 2. New York: Raven Press, 1992:1621–1640.

14. Izumo S, Nadal GB, Mahdavi V: Proto-oncogene induction and reprogramming of cardiac gene expression produced by pressure overload. Proc Natl Acad Sci USA 1988;85:339–343.

15. Schneider MD, Parker TG: Cardiac myocytes as targets for the action of peptide growth factors. Circulation 1990;81:1443–1456.

16. Simpson PC: Proto-oncogenes and cardiac hypertrophy. Annu Rev Physiol 1989;51:189–202.

17. Imamura T, McDermott PJ, Kent RL, Nagatsu M, Cooper G, Carabello BA: Acute changes in myosin heavy chain synthesis rate in pressure versus volume overload. Circ Res 1994;75:418–425.

18. Weinberg EO, Schoen FJ, George D, et al: Angiotensin-converting enzyme inhibition prolongs survival and modifies the transition to heart failure in rats with pressure overload hypertrophy due to ascending aortic stenosis. Circulation 1994;90:1410–1422.

19. Weinberg EO, Lee MA, Weigner M, et al: Angiotensin AT1 receptor inhibition. Effects on hypertrophic remodeling and ACE expression in rats with pressure-overload hypertrophy due to ascending aortic stenosis. Circulation 1997;95:1592–1600.

20. Feldman AM, Weinberg EO, Ray PE, Lorell BH: Selective changes in cardiac gene expression during compensated hypertrophy and the transition to cardiac decompensation in rats with chronic aortic banding. Circ Res 1993;73:184–192.

21. Schunkert H, Weinberg EO, Bruckschlegel G, Rieger AJ, Lorell BH: Alteration of growth responses in established cardiac pressure overload hypertrophy in rats with aortic banding. J Clin Invest 1995;96:2768–2774.

22. Ito N, Bartunek J, Spitzer KW, Lorell BH: Effects of the nitric oxide donor sodium nitroprusside on intracellular pH and contraction in hypertrophied myocytes. Circulation 1997;95:2303–2311.

23. Schunkert H, Jahn L, Izumo S, Apstein CS, Lorell BH: Localization and regulation of c-fos and c-jun proto-oncogene induction by systolic wall stress in normal and hypertrophied rat hearts. Proc Natl Acad Sci USA 1991;88:11480–11484.

24. Carver W, Nagpal ML, Nachtigal M, Borg TK, Terracio L: Collagen expression in mechanically stimulated cardiac fibroblasts. Circ Res 1991;69:116–122.

25. Sigusch HH, Campbell SE, Weber KT: Angiotensin II-induced myocardial fibrosis in rats: role of nitric oxide, prostaglandins and bradykinin. Cardiovasc Res 1996;31:546–554.

26. Booz GW, Baker KM: Molecular signaling mechanisms controlling growth and function of cardiac fibroblasts. Cardiovasc Res 1995;30:537–543.

27. Takemoto M, Egashira K, Usui M, et al: Important role of tissue angiotensin-converting enzyme activity in the pathogenesis of coronary vascular and myocardial structural changes induced by long-term blockade of nitric oxide synthesis in rats. J Clin Invest 1997;99:278–287.

28. Lorell BH: Transition from hypertrophy to failure. Circulation 1997;96:3824–3827.

29. Borow KM: Surgical outcome in chronic aortic regurgitation: a physiologic framework for assessing preoperative predictors. J Am Coll Cardiol 1987;10:1165–1170.

30. Kumpuris AG, Quinones MA, Waggoner AD, Kanon DJ, Nelson JG, Miller RR: Importance of preoperative hypertrophy, wall stress and end-systolic dimension as echocardiographic predictors of normalization of left ventricular dilatation after valve replacement in chronic aortic insufficiency. Am J Cardiol 1982;49:1091–1100.

31. Carabello BA, Williams H, Gash AK, et al: Hemodynamic predictors of outcome in patients undergoing valve replacement. Circulation 1986;74:1309–1316.

32. Carabello BA, Nolan SP, McGuire LB: Assessment of preoperative left ventricular function in patients with mitral regurgitation: value of the end-systolic wall stress–end-systolic volume ratio. Circulation 1981;64:1212–1217.

33. Carabello BA: Do all patients with aortic stenosis and left ventricular dysfunction benefit from aortic

valve replacement? Cathet Cardiovasc Diagn 1989;131–132.

34. Taniguchi K, Nakano S, Kawashima Y, et al: Left ventricular ejection performance, wall stress, and contractile state in aortic regurgitation before and after aortic valve replacement. Circulation 1990;82:798–807.

35. Iskandrian AS, Hakki AH, Kane MS: Left ventricular pressure/volume relationship in aortic regurgitation. Am Heart J 1985;110:1026–1032.

36. Schuler G, von OK, Schwarz F, et al: Noninvasive assessment of myocardial contractility in asymptomatic patients with severe aortic regurgitation and normal left ventricular ejection fraction at rest. Am J Cardiol 1982;50:45–52.

37. Suga HK, Sagawa K, Koustwick DP: Controls of ventricular contractility assessed by pressure-volume ratio, E_{max}. Cardiovasc Res 1976;10:582–592.

38. Starling MR, Kirsh MM, Montgomery DG, Gross MD: Impaired left ventricular contractile function in patients with long-term mitral regurgitation and normal ejection fraction. J Am Coll Cardiol 1993;22:239–250.

39. Grossman W, Jones D, McLaurin LP: Wall stress and patterns of hypertrophy in the human left ventricle. J Clin Invest 1975;56:56–64.

40. Starling MR, Kirsh MM, Montgomery DG, Gross MD: Mechanisms for left ventricular systolic dysfunction in aortic regurgitation: importance for predicting the functional response to aortic valve replacement. J Am Coll Cardiol 1991;17:887–897.

41. Mirsky I: Left ventricular stresses in the intact human heart. Biophys J 1969;9:189–208.

42. Aurigemma GP, Douglas PS, Gaasch WH: Quantitative evaluation of left ventricular structure, wall stress, and systolic function. In Otto CM, ed. The Practice of Clinical Echocardiography. Philadelphia: WB Saunders, 1997:1–24.

43. Legget ME, Kuusisto J, Healy NL, Fujioka M, Schwaegler RG, Otto CM: Gender differences in left ventricular function at rest and with exercise in asymptomatic aortic stenosis. Am Heart J 1996;131:94–100.

44. Koide M, Nagatsu M, Zile MR, et al: Premorbid determinants of left ventricular dysfunction in a novel model of gradually induced pressure overload in the adult canine. Circulation 1997;95:1601–1610.

45. Colan SD, Borow KM, Neumann A: Left ventricular end-systolic wall stress-velocity of fiber shortening relation: a load-independent index of myocardial contractility. J Am Coll Cardiol 1984;4:715–724.

46. Carabello BA: The changing unnatural history of valvular regurgitation. Ann Thorac Surg 1992;53:191–199.

47. Ross JJ: On variations in the cardiac hypertrophic response to pressure overload. Circulation 1997;95: 1349–1351.

48. Burwash IG, Forbes AD, Sadahiro M, et al: Echocardiographic volume flow and stenosis severity measures with changing flow rate in aortic stenosis. Am J Physiol 1993;265:1734–43.

49. Rockman HA, Wachhorst SP, Mao L, Ross JJ: ANG II receptor blockade prevents ventricular hypertrophy and ANF gene expression with pressure overload in mice. Am J Physiol 1994;266:75.

50. Gaasch WH: Left ventricular radius to wall thickness ratio. Am J Cardiol 1979;43:1189–1194.

51. Munt BI, Legget ME, Healy NL, Fujioka M, Schwaegler R, Otto CM: Effects of aortic valve re-

placement on exercise duration and functional status in adults with valvular aortic stenosis. Can J Cardiol 1997;13:346–350.

52. Smith N, McAnulty JH, Rahimtoola SH: Severe aortic stenosis with impaired left ventricular function and clinical heart failure: results of valve replacement. Circulation 1978;58:255–264.

53. Krayenbuehl HP, Turina M, Hess OM, Rothlin M, Senning A: Pre- and postoperative left ventricular contractile function in patients with aortic valve disease. Br Heart J 1979;41:204–213.

54. Harpole DH, Jones RH: Serial assessment of ventricular performance after valve replacement for aortic stenosis. J Thorac Cardiovasc Surg 1990;99:645–650.

55. Hwang MH, Hammermeister KE, Oprian C, et al: Preoperative identification of patients likely to have left ventricular dysfunction after aortic valve replacement. Participants in the Veterans Administration Cooperative Study on Valvular Heart Disease. Circulation 1989;80:165–176.

56. Connolly HM, Oh JK, Orszulak TA, et al: Aortic valve replacement for aortic stenosis with severe left ventricular dysfunction: prognostic indicators. Circulation 1997;95:2395–2400.

57. Georgeson S, Meyer KB, Pauker SG: Decision analysis in clinical cardiology: when is coronary angiography required in aortic stenosis. J Am Coll Cardiol 1990;15:751–762.

58. Carabello BA, Green LH, Grossman W, Cohn LH, Koster JK, Collins JJJ: Hemodynamic determinants of prognosis of aortic valve replacement in critical aortic stenosis and advanced congestive heart failure. Circulation 1980;62:42–48.

59. Otto CM, Burwash IG, Legget ME, et al: A prospective study of asymptomatic valvular aortic stenosis: clinical, echocardiographic, and exercise predictors of outcome. Circulation 1997;95:2262–2270.

60. Carroll JD, Carroll EP, Feldman T, et al: Sex-associated differences in left ventricular function in aortic stenosis of the elderly. Circulation 1992;86:1099–1107.

61. Douglas PS, Otto CM, Mickel MC, Labovitz A, Reid CL, Davis KB: Gender differences in left ventricular geometry and function in patients undergoing balloon dilation of the aortic valve for isolated aortic stenosis. Br Heart J 1995;73:548–554.

62. Aurigemma GP, Silver KH, McLaughlin M, Mauser J, Gaasch WH: Impact of chamber geometry and gender on left ventricular systolic function in patients >60 years of age with aortic stenosis. Am J Cardiol 1994;74:794–798.

63. Villari B, Campbell SE, Schneider J, Vassalli G, Chiariello M, Hess OM: Sex-dependent differences in left ventricular function and structure in chronic pressure overload. Eur Heart J 1995;16:1410–1419.

64. Litwin SE, Katz SE, Weinberg EO, Lorell BH, Aurigemma GP, Douglas PS: Serial echocardiographic-Doppler assessment of left ventricular geometry and function in rats with pressure-overload hypertrophy: chronic angiotensin-converting enzyme inhibition attenuates the transition to heart failure. Circulation 1995;91:2642–2654.

65. Morris JJ, Schaff HV, Mullany CJ, Morris PB, Frye RL, Orszulak TA: Gender differences in left ventricular functional response to aortic valve replacement. Circulation 1994;90:183–189.

66. Ross J Jr: Left ventricular function and the timing of surgical treatment in valvular heart disease. Ann Intern Med 1981;94:498–504.

67. Ross J Jr: Applications and limitations of end-systolic measures of ventricular performance. Fed Proc 1984;43:2418–2422.

68. Wisenbaugh T, Spann JF, Carabello BA: Differences in myocardial performance and load between patients with similar amounts of chronic aortic versus chronic mitral regurgitation. J Am Coll Cardiol 1984;3:916–923.

69. Braunwald E: Mitral regurgitation: physiologic, clinical and surgical considerations. N Engl J Med 1969;281:425–433.

70. Urschel CW, Covell JW, Sonnenblick EH, Ross J Jr, Braunwald E: Myocardial mechanics in aortic and mitral valvular regurgitation: the concept of instantaneous impedance as a determinant of the performance of the intact heart. J Clin Invest 1968;47:867–883.

71. Marsh JD, Green LH, Wynne J, Cohn PF, Grossman W: Left ventricular end-systolic pressure-dimension and stress-length relations in normal human subjects. Am J Cardiol 1979;44:1311–1317.

72. Mirsky I, Corin WJ, Murakami T, Grimm J, Hess OM, Krayenbuehl HP: Correction for preload in assessment of myocardial contractility in aortic and mitral valve disease: application of the concept of systolic myocardial stiffness. Circulation 1988;78:68–80.

73. Leung DY, Griffin BP, Stewart WJ, Cosgrove DM III, Thomas JD, Marwick TH: Left ventricular function after valve repair for chronic mitral regurgitation: predictive value of preoperative assessment of contractile reserve by exercise echocardiography. J Am Coll Cardiol 1996;28:1198–1205.

74. Kennedy JW, Doces JG, Stewart DK: Left ventricular function before and following surgical treatment of mitral valve disease. Am Heart J 1979;97:592–598.

75. Pitarys CJ II, Forman MB, Panayiotou H, Hansen DE: Long-term effects of excision of the mitral apparatus on global and regional ventricular function in humans. J Am Coll Cardiol 1990;15:557–563.

76. Rozich JD, Carabello BA, Usher BW, Kratz JM, Bell AE, Zile MR: Mitral valve replacement with and without chordal preservation in patients with chronic mitral regurgitation: mechanisms for differences in postoperative ejection performance. Circulation 1992;86:1718–1726.

77. David TE, Burns RJ, Bacchus CM, Druck MN: Mitral valve replacement for mitral regurgitation with and without preservation of chordae tendineae. J Thorac Cardiovasc Surg 1984;88:1718–1725.

78. David TE, Uden DE, Strauss HD: The importance of the mitral apparatus in left ventricular function after correction of mitral regurgitation. Circulation 1983;68:76–82.

79. Goldman ME, Mora F, Guarino T, Fuster V, Mindich BP: Mitral valvuloplasty is superior to valve replacement for preservation of left ventricular function: an intraoperative two-dimensional echocardiographic study. J Am Coll Cardiol 1987;10:568–575.

80. Wisenbaugh T: Does normal pump function belie muscle dysfunction in patients with chronic severe mitral regurgitation? Circulation 1988;77:515–525.

81. Gaasch WH, Zile MR: Left ventricular function after surgical correction of chronic mitral regurgitation. Eur Heart J 1991;12(suppl):48–51.

82. Starling MR: Effects of valve surgery on left ventricular contractile function in patients with long-term mitral regurgitation. Circulation 1995;92:811–818.

83. Carabello BA: Aortic regurgitation: a lesion with similarities to both aortic stenosis and mitral regurgitation. Circulation 1990;82:1051–1053.

84. Ross J Jr: Afterload mismatch in aortic and mitral valve disease: implications for surgical therapy. J Am Coll Cardiol 1985;5:811–826.

85. Bonow RO, Lakatos E, Maron BJ, Epstein SE: Serial long-term assessment of the natural history of asymptomatic patients with chronic aortic regurgitation and normal left ventricular systolic function. Circulation 1991;84:1625–1635.

86. Bonow RO, Dodd JT, Maron BJ, et al: Long-term serial changes in left ventricular function and reversal of ventricular dilatation after valve replacement for chronic aortic regurgitation. Circulation 1988;78:108–120.

87. Klodas E, Enriquez Sarano M, Tajik AJ, Mullany CJ, Bailey KR, Seward JB: Aortic regurgitation complicated by extreme left ventricular dilation: long-term outcome after surgical correction. J Am Coll Cardiol 1996;27:670–677.

88. Carabello BA: Aortic regurgitation in women: does the measuring stick need a change? Circulation 1996;94:2355–2357.

89. Ricci DR: Afterload mismatch and preload reserve in chronic aortic regurgitation. Circulation 1982;66:826–834.

90. Lin M, Chiang HT, Lin SL, et al: Vasodilator therapy in chronic asymptomatic aortic regurgitation: enalapril versus hydralazine therapy. J Am Coll Cardiol 1994;24:1046–1053.

91. Schon HR: Hemodynamic and morphologic changes after long-term angiotensin converting enzyme inhibition in patients with chronic valvular regurgitation. J Hypertens 1994;12(suppl):95–104.

92. Wisenbaugh T, Sinovich V, Dullabh A, Sareli P: Six month pilot study of captopril for mildly symptomatic, severe isolated mitral and isolated aortic regurgitation. J Heart Valve Dis 1994;3:197–204.

93. Scognamiglio R, Rahimtoola SH, Fasoli G, Nistri S, Dalla Volta S: Nifedipine in asymptomatic patients with severe aortic regurgitation and normal left ventricular function. N Engl J Med 1994;331:689–694.

94. Boucher CA, Bingham JB, Osbakken MD, et al: Early changes in left ventricular size and function after correction of left ventricular volume overload. Am J Cardiol 1981;47:991–1004.

95. Monrad ES, Hess OM, Murakami T, Nonogi H, Corin WJ, Krayenbuehl HP: Time course of regression of left ventricular hypertrophy after aortic valve replacement. Circulation 1988;77:1345–1355.

96. Carroll JD, Gaasch WH, Zile MR, Levine HJ: Serial changes in left ventricular function after correction of chronic aortic regurgitation: dependence on early changes in preload and subsequent regression of hypertrophy. Am J Cardiol 1983;51:476–482.

97. Gaasch WH, Andrias CW, Levine HJ: Chronic aortic regurgitation: the effect of aortic valve replacement on left ventricular volume, mass and function. Circulation 1978;58:825–836.

98. Schuler G, Peterson KL, Johnson AD, et al: Serial noninvasive assessment of left ventricular hypertrophy and function after surgical correction of aortic regurgitation. Am J Cardiol 1979;44:585–594.

99. Bonow RO, Picone AL, McIntosh CL, et al: Survival and functional results after valve replacement for aortic regurgitation from 1976 to 1983: impact of preoperative left ventricular function. Circulation 1985;72:1244–1256.

100. Bonow RO, Rosing DR, Maron BJ, et al: Reversal of left ventricular dysfunction after aortic valve replacement for chronic aortic regurgitation: influence of duration of preoperative left ventricular dysfunction. Circulation 1984;70:570–579.

101. Borer JS, Herrold EM, Hochreiter C, et al: Natural history of left ventricular performance at rest and during exercise after aortic valve replacement for aortic regurgitation. Circulation 1991;84:133–9.

102. Roman MJ, Klein L, Devereux RB, et al: Reversal of left ventricular dilatation, hypertrophy, and dysfunction by valve replacement in aortic regurgitation. Am Heart J 1989;118:553–563.

103. Henry WL, Bonow RO, Borer JS, et al: Observations on the optimum time for operative intervention for aortic regurgitation. I. Evaluation of the results of aortic valve replacement in symptomatic patients. Circulation 1980;61:471–483.

104. Otto CM, Pearlman AS, Amsler LC: Doppler echocardiographic evaluation of left ventricular diastolic filling in isolated valvular aortic stenosis. Am J Cardiol 1989;63:313–316.

105. Vanoverschelde JL, Essamri B, Michel X, et al: Hemodynamic and volume correlates of left ventricular diastolic relaxation and filling in patients with aortic stenosis. J Am Coll Cardiol 1992;20:813–821.

106. Clyne CA, Arrighi JA, Maron BJ, Dilsizian V, Bonow RO, Cannon RO III: Systemic and left ventricular responses to exercise stress in asymptomatic patients with valvular aortic stenosis. Am J Cardiol 1991;68:1469–1476.

107. Douglas PS, Berko B, Lesh M, Reichek N: Alterations in diastolic function in response to progressive left ventricular hypertrophy. J Am Coll Cardiol 1989;13:461–467.

108. Villari B, Vassalli G, Schneider J, Chiariello M, Hess OM: Age dependency of left ventricular diastolic function in pressure overload hypertrophy. J Am Coll Cardiol 1997;29:181–186.

109. Lorell BH, Grossman W: Cardiac hypertrophy: the consequences for diastole. J Am Coll Cardiol 1987;9:1189–1193.

110. Villari B, Vassalli G, Betocchi S, Briguori C, Chiariello M, Hess OM: Normalization of left ventricular nonuniformity late after valve replacement for aortic stenosis. Am J Cardiol 1996;78:66–71.

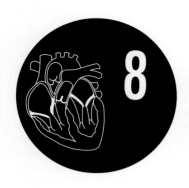

8

Valvular Heart Disease: The Surgical Approach

R. Pat Cochran and Edward D. Verrier

Valvular heart disease has been a primary catalyst for innovation since the inception of cardiac surgery. As surgical techniques and technology have evolved, so too has the approach to valvular heart disease. In the past decade, because of advances in myocardial protection, cardiac anesthesia, critical care management, and virtually all other aspects of cardiac surgery, higher-risk patients have been treated successfully. These advances have opened the door to other innovations, and patients with valvular heart disease increasingly are offered more complex operations that may yield a better quality of life and extended longevity. An example of this type of change in surgical philosophy and approach has been the marked worldwide increase in mitral valve repair compared with replacement

since the early 1980s. Other examples are aortic valve–sparing operations for aortic aneurysmal disease, pulmonary valve autotransplant for aortic valve lesions (ie, Ross procedure), and expanding indications for the use of cadaveric valve tissue for aortic, mitral, and tricuspid valve disease. The challenge for the cardiologist and the cardiac surgeon is to understand the advantages of these newer techniques, to realize where theoretical advantage and practicality converge, and to match the intervention with the patient.

This chapter presents the conventional and cutting-edge approaches to each valvular lesion. Although we also discuss our bias about the general algorithms we use, we emphasize that they are merely guidelines and that treatment of all cardiac surgical lesions and valvular

151

disease requires individualization to match the patient's needs with methods that ensure survival and improved quality of life.

BASIC SURGICAL APPROACH

All valve surgery is "open heart" surgery. All four cardiac valves are contained within the heart, and obtaining access to the valve or valves for repair or replacement requires opening the right- or left-sided circulation to atmospheric pressure. Isolated right-sided procedures can be done without aortic occlusion and cardioplegia, but left-sided procedures routinely require occlusion and cardioplegia. Virtually all valve procedures require some form of cardiopulmonary bypass. Innumerable variations in cannulation, incision, and procedure have been advocated to minimize the risk that opening the heart imposes, but no technical changes have significantly altered the risks of thromboembolic complications when the heart is opened and valves are manipulated. With the popularity of "port access" surgery, many claims have been made about improved comfort, faster recovery, and greater patient satisfaction, but these changes have not improved thromboembolic risks. Because of the necessity of opening the heart or aorta, all valve operations have inherently greater risks than coronary bypass operations.

One significant change has occurred. In the past, the choices for cannulation, incisional approach, degree of hypothermia, and flow rates for cardiopulmonary bypass were influenced largely by surgical training or prior negative experiences. More often than not, these choices are driven today by hopes for reduction in the cost of care or by desires for increasing market share.

RISK FACTORS

The process of deciding which valve operation is best for a patient must begin with assessment of surgical risk. Several risk factors have been repeatedly shown to affect surgical outcome, and the weight assigned to each factor requires significant clinical judgment. Individualization is crucial for successful valve surgery.

The single most important risk factor in all cardiac surgery reports has been ventricular function. In multiple previous studies, reduced ejection fraction has been shown to increase surgical risk and mortality.[1-3] However, like most variables in cardiac surgery, the impor-

tance of ejection fraction has changed as techniques have improved. The common wisdom in the 1980s was that surgery for patients with mitral regurgitation with an ejection fraction of less than 30%, particularly in those with ischemic disease, was ill advised. With improved perioperative management, mitral regurgitation is being successfully treated surgically, even in the very low ejection fraction range.[4] This success is a tribute to improved technique and improved patient selection (ie, judgment) and by no means diminishes the impact of reduced ejection fraction as a predictor of higher operative risks.

From the surgical perspective, operative time seems logically to be a risk factor. The crossclamp time, the time on cardiopulmonary bypass, and the operative time have proved in large clinical trials to be risk factors.[1] Increased complexity also has had statistical weight as a risk factor. Increased complexity in most series has correlated with combined procedures such as a valve and coronary bypass, multiple valves, or a valve with aneurysmal disease.

Age remains a risk factor, although a cutoff has not been established. The octogenarian barrier was broken in the 1980s, establishing that aortic valve replacement could be accomplished with acceptable mortality.[5-7] Subsequently, the nonagenarian barrier was broached with surgery for the same lesion.[8] Despite acceptable mortality rates for a patient population that has limited short-term survival without surgery because of aortic stenosis, age continues to be a surgical risk factor, with complication rates increasing starting as early as age 65. Risk of stroke and renal insufficiency increases after 70 years of age.[9] In the changing health care environment and as quality of life is deemed more important than raw survival issues, determining what the true risk-benefit ratio is as patients age remains a challenge for the cardiologist and cardiac surgeon.

Comorbid disease is the most difficult area of risk to assess. Diabetes, hypertension, renal insufficiency, peripheral vascular disease, cerebrovascular disease, pulmonary dysfunction, and a host of other diseases can adversely affect surgical outcome.[2, 10, 11] In addition, the presence of pulmonary hypertension increases the risk of valvular surgery. We have adopted from the literature our own risk stratification system that weights each of the known risk factors, and we have established a risk stratification scheme for all our cardiac surgical patients (Fig. 8–1). The relative risk assignment is divided into categories A through E. Patients

Cardiac Surgery Risk Stratification Worksheet

PATIENT...

ATTENDING

REFERRING...

OPERATIVE INDICATIONS...

SURGERY DATE....................

ISOLATED OPERATION
    CABG
    VALVE
    THORACIC

COMPLEX OPERATION
    VALVE + CABG
    REDO (valve or CABG)
    VENT. ANEURYSM
    MULTIPLE VALVE
    AICD OR PCD
    COMPLEX THORACIC

MAJOR RISK FACTORS
    AGE >75
    REST ANGINA
    CHF BY HISTORY
    RECENT MI (<14 DAYS)
    EMERGENCY OPERATION   TOTAL #..................
    LVEDP > 20 TORR
    PA MEAN > 25 TORR
    PREOP IABP
    CREATININE >3.0

MINOR RISK FACTORS
    AGE 70 - 75
    FEMALE
    URGENT PRIORITY
    CREATININE 2.0 - 2.9   TOTAL #...................
    PT >15 SEC
    DIABETES
    CAROTID DISEASE

RISK CATEGORIES (circle the letter most closely approximating the profile of the patient)

  A. ISOLATED OPERATION (IOP) + NO RISK FACTORS

  B. IOP + 1 MAJOR AND <2 MINOR

  C. IOP + 2 MAJOR AND <2 MINOR, or
       COMPLEX OPERATION (COP) AND NO RISK FACTORS

  D. IOP + 2 MAJOR AND 2 OR MORE MINOR
       IOP + 3 MAJOR AND <2 MINOR
       COP +1 MAJOR AND <2 MINOR

  E. IOP +3 MAJOR AND 2 OR MORE MINOR
       IOP + 4 MAJOR AND ANY MINOR
       COP +2 MAJOR AND ANY MINOR

Figure 8·1 Risk stratification worksheet for cardiac patients at the University of Washington Medical Center.

in risk stratification A have a mortality risk of 3% or less. Patients in risk stratification E have a mortality risk in excess of 20%.

Each of the risk factors can affect the decision to operate on an individual patient and influence what type of operation to do. The decision about which is the best and safest procedure, short and long term, has become more difficult as medical therapy and management have improved survival for all risk groups. The increased emphasis on quality of life may help to guide these decisions as more data become available. In addition, quality of life issues may bias the patient's decision process significantly and ultimately dictate surgical choice. The consumer of cardiac surgical services in the United States is increasingly better informed and often arrives with set guidelines for therapy. For example, patients commonly request no long-term anticoagulation after valve surgery. Fifteen years ago, this was a difficult request to honor, particularly for young patients, without guaranteeing a relatively early reoperation. With the advent of mitral repair, aortic valve sparing, pulmonary valve autotransplant, homografts, and stentless porcine valves, it has become a far more realistic request for short- and long-term successful therapy. There is increasing scientific evidence that alternative procedures may have added benefit in improving long-term ventricular function and ventricular remodeling. The threat of early (≤10 years) reoperation that was once expected with stented biologic valves appears to be less likely with the newer alternatives; however, long-term outcome data will not be available for at least another 5 years.

Other factors may direct the algorithm for deciding the best operation for each patient. Endocarditis in the native valves and particularly endocarditis of prosthetic valves add the risk of recurrent infection, which must be considered and planned for during the operation. In this situation, the use of minimal foreign material and the need for radical debridement may change the surgical approach or plan.

As all aspects of medical therapy improve, surgeons and cardiologists are asked to see patients with diseases that used to preclude operation. Increasingly, patients with blood dyscrasias and clotting abnormalities are being referred for surgery, and these diseases may affect the operative and long-term management of these patients. Patient choice may also have an impact. For example, Jehovah's Witnesses may dictate which therapeutic options are available by restricting the use of blood products. Patient idiosyncrasy or lifestyle choice also may modify or dictate therapeutic options. Patients commonly come to surgery with professional or recreational lifestyles that preclude certain options, such as anticoagulation, and are unwilling to consider a lifestyle change.

Real and patient-generated risk factors influence the decision-making process for all cardiac surgery, which is most profoundly seen in valvular heart disease when anticoagulation is an integral part of the algorithm. Fortunately, with advances in cardiac surgical care, most of these risk factors can be accommodated while attaining excellent short- and long-term results. Making treatment decisions about valvular heart disease cannot be addressed in a purely generic fashion, because the options available vary with the valve or valves involved. The remainder of this chapter discusses the specifics of surgical techniques and the impact that the technical aspects have on decision making.

AORTIC VALVE DISEASE

Aortic valve disease varies in its clinical presentation and course. Whether the valve is stenotic, insufficient, or both influences when surgery should be considered, but because those aspects are addressed in other portions of this text, we do not dwell on them here. However, it is worth pointing out that the degree of ventricular hypertrophy or dilatation affects myocardial protection and may influence the length of operation that the surgeon is willing to consider. Ventricular dilatation, particularly a long-standing condition with a reduced ejection fraction, may significantly influence long-term survival and therefore may preclude longer, preferable operations in favor of more expeditious surgery targeting short-term survival as the primary goal.

Aortic valve replacement began the modern era of adult cardiac surgery. Largely because of the expected improvement of ventricular function postoperatively, aortic stenosis has been the lesion that has continuously pushed the frontier. Treating older patients, addressing more complex disease, and undertaking longer operations have all been initiated for cases of aortic valve disease, particularly stenosis. Success has depended on the ability to offer expedient, reproducible surgical results for aortic valve lesions. These results have been attained with a standardized, conventional decision algorithm that remains a realistic approach for many patients despite the many innovative options that have become available.

Conventional Therapy

The gold standard in terms of surgical survival permits the use of only two valve types. Whether the valve chosen is a mechanical or a stented biologic valve is determined by age and lifestyle choices, but either valve type offers reproducible, expedient valve replacement that in experienced hands can be accomplished with remarkably low operative mortality. Both options allow a variety of suture techniques for surgeon preference and flexibility. The only limiting factor on the use of either valve is that stented bioprosthetic valves 23 mm in diameter or smaller leave a residual gradient. The need for additional aortic root enlargements in this setting, with concomitant increased operative time, opens the door for consideration of more complex valve replacement options with equivalent risks. The counterposition for conservative therapy for high-risk patients is the use of mechanical valves in all smaller aortic annuli, but this approach also has limitations at the smaller sizes.

The insertion or suturing techniques used are as varied as the surgeons. The techniques used for mechanical and stented biologic valves are remarkably similar. Simple interrupted, running, figure-eight, and horizontal mattress sutures, with and without pledgets and with inflow or outflow placement, have all been used successfully, with no proven difference other than the surgeon's preference.

Alternatives to the Conventional Approach

The burden is put on the surgeon to achieve equivalent results if other alternatives to conventional therapy are considered. Because this requires extremely cautious patient selection for the more challenging surgical techniques, these options have not been embraced by all practitioners. These alternative procedures are often restricted to academic centers and to large-volume, valve-oriented practices. However, increasing patient and cardiologist awareness is creating a greater demand for the more innovative and "improved lifestyle" options. In many cases, patients and cardiologists are in pursuit of valve replacement options that avoid anticoagulation, are durable, and improve long-term ventricular function. Three available options make a reasonable attempt at meeting these goals. These options are presented in progression of most to least technically difficult.

Autotransplantation of the Pulmonary Valve: Ross Procedure

The Ross procedure, or autotransplantation of the patient's pulmonary valve into the aortic position,[12, 13] is the most "natural" alternative and appeals to surgeons, patients, and cardiologists. Because the excised pulmonary valve must be replaced by a pulmonary or aortic homograft, this is a double-valve procedure. The obligatory double-valve replacement does increase the surgical risks, as does any increase in operative or crossclamp time. This increased risk has restricted this operation to a relatively young and healthy patient population. Moreover, several technical aspects of this procedure may increase surgical risk, which has prompted many modifications. We discuss briefly the necessary maneuvers that may add surgical risks and their impact on surgical technique and patient selection.

The pulmonary valve must be excised from its anatomic position and reimplanted in the aortic position to accomplish this procedure (Fig. 8–2). A replacement valve, usually a pulmonary homograft but occasionally an aortic homograft, must be sewn into the pulmonary position. The proximity of the first septal perforator to the base of the pulmonary valve is a potential mortal hazard if injured during excision or reimplantation. The position of this artery can be well defined by preoperative catheterization, or if catheterization is unnecessarily high risk, as in neonates and patients with endocarditis, the artery's location can be ascertained by meticulous surgical dissection.[14, 15] The surgeon must avoid the perfora-

Excise Pulmonary Valve... Pulmonary Valve To Aorta... Homograft To Pulmonary Artery...

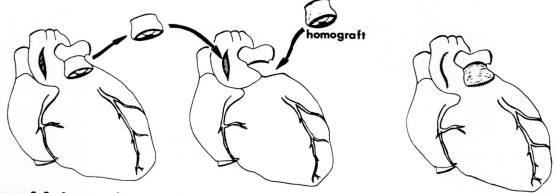

Figure 8·2   Sequence of Ross procedure. (From Ross D: Replacement of the aortic valve with a pulmonary autograft: the Switch operation. Ann Thorac Surg 1991;52:1346–1350.)

tor's injury or incorporation in the implantation sutures to prevent high septal infarction, an almost universally and quickly fatal event. It is this aspect of this otherwise appealing procedure that prevented its early popularization and still limits its wide-scale use.

Another technical aspect of the Ross procedure, which is not unique to this operation, is the need for removal and reimplantation of the right and left coronary artery ostia (Fig. 8–3). This is not an unusual maneuver for most cardiac surgeons and is common in a practice that involves a large volume of valves, aneurysms and dissections. However, removal of both coronary ostia without injury and reimplantation of both without distortion are crucial elements in this operation's success. The concerns about this aspect of the procedure are great enough that some surgeons advocate an inclusion technique. In the inclusion technique, the pulmonary valve is inserted into the intact aortic root without removal of the coronary ostia.[15, 16] Other surgeons sharing this concern, particularly about the posteriorly positioned left coronary, have developed a technique for leaving the left coronary ostium attached to the native distal aorta to achieve a "natural" alignment and to reduce the risk of postimplantation bleeding.[17]

The remainder of the technical considerations largely are matters of surgeon prefer-

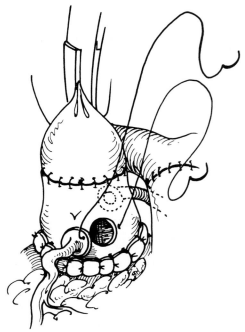

Figure 8·4 Completion of Ross procedure by attachment of a right coronary button. (From Ross D: Replacement of the aortic valve with a pulmonary autograft: the Switch operation. Ann Thorac Surg 1991;52:1346–1350.)

ence. Some surgeons interrupt the proximal suture row; others run that row. Some surgeons reinforce the proximal suture line with pericardium, and others use no reinforcement. The technical aspects of this double-valve procedure with increased operative time, proximity to the first septal perforator, and the need for coronary ostial implantation are what set this procedure apart from the other options and increase its risk (Fig. 8–4). We define an algorithm for its placement in the scheme of aortic valve replacement after the other alternatives have been discussed.

Aortic Homograft

A similar, but less complex option to the Ross procedure is the replacement of the aortic valve with an aortic homograft (ie, allograft).[18] This operation is an "old" operation, originating before prosthetic availability and evolving in terms of implantation technique and preparation of the homograft over the last four decades to a highly reproducible and durable procedure.[19] From a preparation and preservation standpoint, the valves used today are handled quite differently than the original valves. In the United States, there is only one

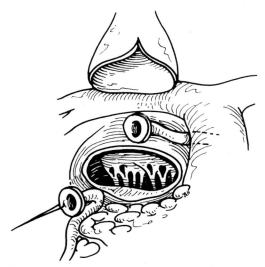

Figure 8·3 Demonstration of an excised aortic root, ready for pulmonary valve autotransplant. Note the coronary "buttons" for reimplantation. (From Ross D: Replacement of the aortic valve with a pulmonary autograft: the Switch operation. Ann Thorac Surg 1991;52:1346–1350.)

preparation available: cryopreserved. World-wide, some centers use "fresh" valves, and some centers use valves that are cryopreserved but thought to be nonvital. These differences should be considered when interpreting results from various centers.

In the United States, cryopreserved valves are available from several sources. The use of cryopreserved valves in the United States had a resurgence with the 1987 publication of the work of O'Brien and colleagues[20] in Brisbane, Australia. They assessed the results of using "fresh" (ie, antibiotic preserved) valves and cryopreserved valves and showed a profound superiority for cryopreservation at 10 years.[20] After this work appeared and cryopreserved valves became available in the United States, use of the valves rose steadily. Rapid spread of the use of cryopreserved valves, which theoretically are an ideal substitute and accomplish all the goals we have outlined, was prevented by the technical aspect of implantation and by tissue availability.

The original implantation techniques for aortic homografts were inclusion techniques. Numerous articles described various suturing

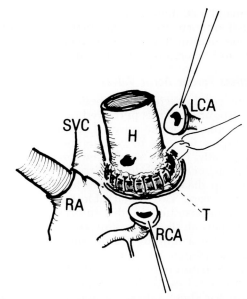

Figure 8·6   Attachment of coronary ostia to homograft in miniroot technique. SVC, superior vena cava; H, homograft; LCA, left coronary artery; T, Teflon felt; RCA, right coronary artery. (Permission [pending] from Okita Y, Franciosi G, Matsuki O, Robles A, Ross DN: Early and late results of aortic root replacement with antibiotic-sterilized aortic homograft. J Thorac Cardiovasc Surg 1988;95:696–704.)

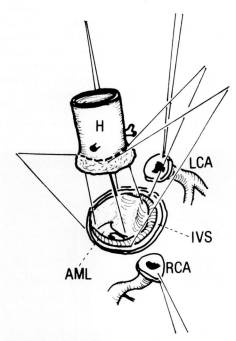

Figure 8·5   Miniroot homograft insertion technique. AML, anterior mitral leaflet; H, homograft; LCA, left coronary artery; RCA, right coronary artery; IVS, intraventricular septum. (From Okita Y, Franciosi G, Matsuki O, Robles A, Ross DN: Early and late results of aortic root replacement with antibiotic-sterilized aortic homograft. J Thorac Cardiovasc Surg 1988;95:696–704.)

methods (eg, running, interrupted), tailoring the homografts to fit the disparate annulus, and the relative and absolute contraindications of this approach.[21-25] As use of these valves became widespread, complications causing early failure, particularly if valvular insufficiency was involved, raised questions about technique, particularly whether tissue resorption required oversizing or whether commissural positioning was distorted, so that implantation techniques were modified.[26]

By the late 1980s, the "miniroot" replacement (ie, total excision of the valve and sinuses of Valsalva, followed by replacement of the "whole" valve apparatus with coronary implantation) evolved as the procedure of choice.[19] The miniroot procedure's popularity was probably enhanced by the increasing interest in the Ross procedure, because the implantation technique in the aortic position is the same for both procedures (Figs. 8–5 and 8–6). As surgeons became more comfortable with aortic root replacement, homograft miniroot replacement became more appealing. Despite the relative ease of homograft root replacement, particularly compared with the Ross procedure, not all patients, most notably the elderly, can tolerate the longer obligatory ischemia. Thus, there is still a need for a more expedient aortic valve replacement that avoids anticoagulation, gives good hemodynamic results, and has reasonable durability.

Stentless Porcine Aortic Valves

The cardiovascular prosthetics community has responded to this perceived need with several stentless porcine valves. The implantation techniques for this new generation of valve vary greatly, from a single row of sutures to inclusion techniques to miniroot techniques. Follow-up data on these valves are limited to about 8 years. Two remarkable features have been demonstrated in this intermediate follow-up period: slightly prolonged implantation time is not a limiting factor, and ventricular response (function) appears to be improved by the extremely low transvalvular gradient with these valves. With the relatively short follow-up for these valves, durability cannot be determined. However, there appears to be no early failure, and it is speculated that the stentless aspect will equal or extend durability of this valve over its stented predecessors. For the target population of persons older than 65 years of age, this may be adequate durability, particularly if ventricular function is maintained or improved. Conversely, improved ventricular function in this age group may improve long-term survival and allow patient survival to surpass valve survival.

Optimizing a Small Aortic Annulus

One of the great appeals of stentless valves, homografts, and autotransplantation of the pulmonary valve is that all these options optimize the orifice size after implantation. Mechanical and biologic stented valves reduce the orifice size or effective aortic area by the size of the stent (Fig. 8–7). Because stentless technology is still evolving and the stented valves are still the most commonly used valves, several techniques for insertion of a stented valve into a small annulus are worth mentioning.

The first consideration is what constitutes a small annulus. For two decades, the critical size has been 23 mm for bioprostheses and 19 mm for mechanical prostheses. These numbers, however, must be evaluated in terms of the patient's size and activity. If a stented valve is to be used in the aortic position in sizes at or below these critical levels, aortic root enlargement must be considered to avoid unacceptable postoperative hemodynamics. There are three classic ways to enlarge the aortic annulus and implant a stented valve.

If there is only a small size discrepancy between the desired valve and the size of the aortic annulus, root enlargement as described by Nicks can be performed (Fig. 8–8).[27] The aortotomy is extended into the aortic annulus in the region of the noncoronary sinus of Valsalva. This permits a triangular patch to be placed between the two sides of the aortotomy and the annulus, allowing 1 to 3 mm of annular increase, or an increase of one to two valve sizes. This straightforward technique allows significant flexibility in valve insertion.

If a greater increase in annular size is needed than can be accomplished by the Nicks

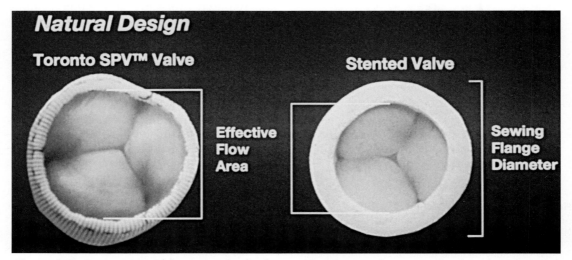

Figure 8·7 Demonstration of the increased orifice for a stentless porcine valve compared with an equivalent-sized stented valve. (Courtesy of St. Jude Medical Heart Valve Division, St. Paul, MN. Toronto SPV is a registered trademark of St. Jude Medical, Inc.)

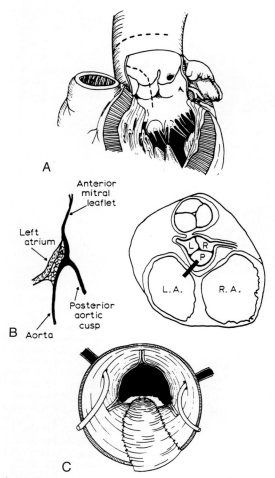

Anterior mitral leaflet

Left atrium

Posterior aortic cusp

A

B   Aorta

C

Figure 8·8   *A,* Incision for Nicks aortic enlargement. *B,* Structures involved in enlargement. *C,* Patch placement. (From Nicks R, Cartmill T, Bernstein L: Hypoplasia of the aortic root: the problem of aortic valve replacement. Thorax 1970;25:339–346. BMJ Publishing Group.)

procedure, a more extensive annular enlargement is necessary. Manouguian described curving the aortotomy more posteriorly than Nicks, enabling the incision to be carried completely across the annulus into the anterior leaflet of the mitral valve (Fig. 8–9).[28] The defect created is reconstructed with a diamond-shaped patch that allows an increase in the annular size by 3 to 5 mm, or an increase of two to three valve sizes. This maneuver is usually all that is necessary for increasing annular size in adults. It is a bit more complex and time consuming than the Nicks procedure, and it may present bleeding risks posteriorly below the left coronary artery. The increased time and risk of this procedure make using a stentless valve or a homograft a reason-

able alternative when the annulus requires this degree of enlargement.

The third and most radical root enlargement procedure, the Konno-Rastan procedure (Figs. 8–10 through 8–12), is not usually performed in adults.[29, 30] This procedure is usually reserved for severe congenital stenosis or unusual adult abnormalities that require a profound enlargement of the aortic annulus. With this procedure, whatever valve size the surgeon chooses can be used, because the size of the patch used to reconstruct the annulus establishes the new annular size. This procedure must be planned from the initiation of the operation because a different aortotomy is required. The previous two enlargement procedures modified a standard transverse or oblique aortotomy. With the Konno-Rastan procedure, a vertical aortotomy is required. This aortic incision is placed on the left side of the right coronary ostia and extends into the right ventricular outflow tract and into the ventricular septum. Reconstruction is classically a two-patch reconstruction with a large, diamond-shaped patch closing the aortoseptal defect; the patch's width defines the size of the new annulus for the valve. The second patch is triangular and closes the defect from the base of the aorta out onto the right ventricular outflow tract. These radical reconstructions have increasingly become replaced with the Ross procedure or a modification of the homograft reconstruction when possible, because these procedures have equivalent operative times and risks.

Aortic Valve Repair

No good long-term results for repair of aortic stenosis have been reported from several trial series.[31, 32] Conversely, there is growing interest in various repair techniques for aortic insufficiency,[33] particularly in combination with aortic aneurysmal disease. Because leaflet resuspension, re-creation of the sinotubular junction, and other successful aortic repair maneuvers are used more frequently in aneurysmal disease, we describe them in the next section on aortic valve disease associated with ascending aortic aneurysmal disease.

Algorithm for Aortic Valve Disease

The decision about which procedure is best for the patient who needs aortic valve replacement is multifactorial. The advantages of lifestyle choice, preserved or improved ventricu-

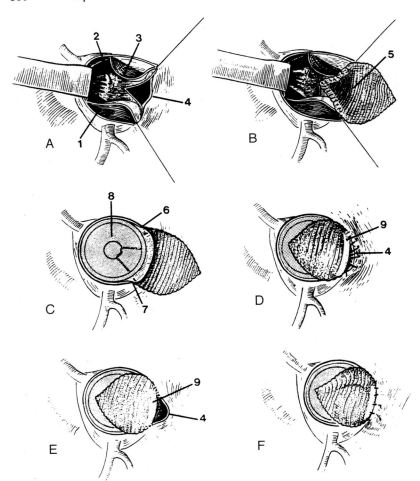

Figure 8·9 *A*, Incision into the anterior mitral leaflet for Manouguian enlargement. *B*, Patch reconstruction of the mitral leaflet. *C*, Valve implantation. *D, E, F,* Hemostatic closure of the cardiac defect to the patch. (From Manouguian S, Seybold-Epting W: Patch enlargement of the aortic valve ring by extending the aortic incision into the anterior mitral leaflet: new operative technique. J Thorac Cardiovasc Surg 1979;78:402–412.)

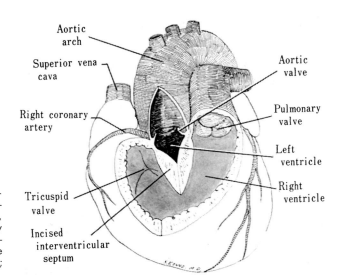

Figure 8·10 Incision from the aorta into the septum and right ventricular outflow tract for a Konno-Rastan aortic annular enlargement. (From Konno S, Imai Y, Iida Y, Nakajima M, Tatsuno K: A new method for prosthetic valve replacement in congenital aortic stenosis associated with hypoplasia of the aortic valve ring. J Thorac Cardiovasc Surg 1975; 70:909–917.)

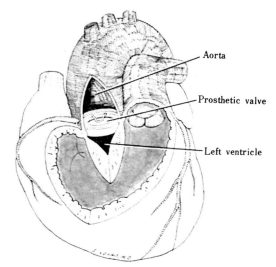

Figure 8·11 Valve insertion (Konno-Rastan) in an enlarged aortic annulus. (From Konno S, Imai Y, Iida Y, Nakajima M, Tatsuno K: A new method for prosthetic valve replacement in congenital aortic stenosis associated with hypoplasia of the aortic valve ring. J Thorac Cardiovasc Surg 1975;70:909–917.)

has favorable hemodynamics. All other factors affecting valve choices are lifestyle issues, albeit some are very compelling. For women of child-bearing age who desire pregnancy, for an athlete exposed to trauma, for persons in occupations commonly involving injury, and for patients from remote areas where follow-up is difficult, anticoagulation can be a significant problem.

In the algorithm of valve choice, age is the largest determining factor, followed closely by ventricular function and operative complexity. Figure 8–13 helps outline these interactions. Patient preference dictates much of the decision, but if the patient is open to all options, the following guidelines are used. The Ross procedure is the procedure of choice for patients younger than 50 years of age if the ventricular function can tolerate the longer procedure and the anatomy is favorable.

Between 50 and 65 years of age, patient choice plays the biggest role. The Ross procedure may be an option for active patients, but it is used selectively. For this age group, the aortic homograft or allograft as a miniroot replacement is an appealing option. However, many persons who want the most durable procedure and who are comfortable with anticoagulation choose the mechanical valve. Increasingly, the stentless porcine valve is being chosen by patients in this age range. If its long-term durability is good, it may become the valve of choice, because it keeps operative time reasonable, avoids anticoagulation, and attains reasonable longevity with preserved ventricular function.

lar function, and durability should be considered only if immediate and short-term survival can be relatively ensured. The first issue is whether there are relative or absolute contraindications to anticoagulation, such as active peptic ulcer disease or blood dyscrasias. If there is no reason to avoid anticoagulation, the next issue is whether to use a mechanical valve, as it is the most durable prosthesis and

Figure 8·12 Double-patch closure of defect. (From Konno S, Imai Y, Iida Y, Nakajima M, Tatsuno K: A new method for prosthetic valve replacement in congenital aortic stenosis associated with hypoplasia of the aortic valve ring. J Thorac Cardiovasc Surg 1975;70:909–917.)

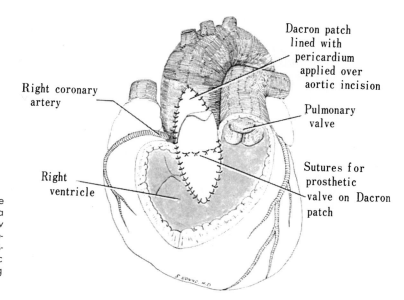

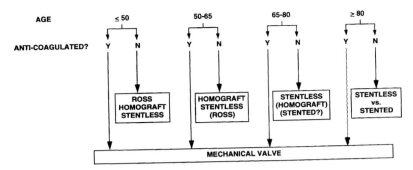

Figure 8·13 Algorithm for aortic valve disease.

For patients older than 65 years of age, the stentless porcine valve is gaining even more popularity, but the mechanical valve remains the primary valve of choice. At 80 years of age, the fear of spontaneous intracranial hemorrhage with anticoagulation and inadvertent falls while anticoagulated shifts interest from the mechanical valve to the porcine valves. If the patient can tolerate a slightly increased operative time, the stentless valve is favored, but the stented valve is still used if the ventricular function is questionable or if extensive coronary grafting is necessary. If a minimally invasive surgical approach is used, the emphasis is on simplicity. With this approach, stented bioprosthetic and mechanical valves tend to be preferred.

ASCENDING AORTIC ANEURYSMAL DISEASE INVOLVING THE AORTIC VALVE

Ascending aortic aneurysmal disease involving the aortic valve is covered separately because it raises a different set of decision criteria, represents a more complex patient population, and is the disease group for which aortic valve repair may have a role. The first level on this decision tree is whether there is primary or secondary damage to the aortic valve and whether the valve is salvageable. If so, the surgical options are more diverse. The options used depend on the surgeon's opinion about what the disease process is that must be corrected. If the valve is not salvageable, the surgical options are relatively small and straightforward.

Salvageable aortic valves are found primarily in aneurysmal disease and in dissection with or without aneurysmal disease. Aortic valve sparing was first described for aneurysmal disease. Type A or DeBakey type I and II dissections involve the ascending aorta and are considered surgical emergencies. Despite their high-risk nature and emergent presentation, techniques for sparing the aortic valve while repairing a dissection, even when there was significant prolapse of the aortic valve, were described as early as the 1970s (Fig. 8–14).[34] Resuspension of the commissural post within the repaired aortic dissection proved successful and durable.[35]

Ascending Aortic Aneurysm With Aortic Valve Insufficiency

Primary aneurysmal diseases of the ascending aorta do not necessarily affect the aortic valve. However, if the aneurysm persists long enough and grows large enough, aortic valve insufficiency often occurs as a secondary process. If aortic insufficiency from the aneurysm exists long enough, the valve ultimately becomes damaged, and the damage may put the valve beyond repair. With the desire to save native valves whenever possible, a more aggressive approach to this disease process has been undertaken in the past decade. Several techniques have been described for preserving the native aortic valve when repairing aortic aneurysms. The extent of the disease process—whether the involvement extends to the level of the annulus—remains the critical factor in determining which is the better technique.

All the aneurysmal disease processes involve the aortic wall tissue above the valve, including the sinuses of Valsalva. Supracoronary aneurysm replacement of the ascending aorta in aneurysmal disease is seldom done today because of the recurrence of sinus of Valsalva aneurysmal disease. We mention this technique for the sake of completeness and because some of these patients are still returning for reoperation.

The remainder of aortic valve–sparing procedures are technically categorized into three groups: inclusion techniques, resection with supra-annular reconstruction and resection with subannular reconstruction. The following

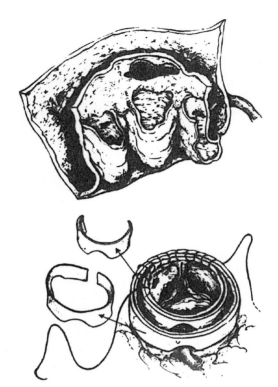

Figure 8·14 Key components of valve resuspension for aortic dissection, illustrating resuspension of commissural posts and buttressing with external and internal felt strips. (From Miller DC: Surgical management of acute aortic dissection: new data. Semin Thorac Cardiovasc Surg 1991;3:225–237.)

sections describe the current techniques, their merits, and their drawbacks.

Inclusion Technique

The inclusion technique acknowledges that the tissue of the sinuses of Valsalva are involved and relies on stabilization with a tailored external conduit (Fig. 8–15).[36] This technique spares the native valve, maintains the commissural orientation, and stabilizes the sinus of Valsalva tissue to prevent further sinus aneurysm formation. One disadvantage is that the annulus of the valve is not truly stabilized, and if the disease process involves the annulus (eg, Marfan's syndrome), the potential for further valve dilatation and failure exists. Because of tailoring of the conduit to accommodate the coronary ostia, the procedure is time consuming and must be individualized, which makes reproducibility difficult.

Supra-annular Reconstruction

The resection and supra-annular reconstruction techniques have been described by several surgeons and allow removal of all tissue down to a small rim in the sinus of Valsalva and along the commissural posts that are used for attaching the conduit for reconstruction (Figs. 8–16 and 8–17).[37, 38] These techniques enable tailoring of the replacement, which may spare one or two sinuses if they are thought to be uninvolved, or replacement of all three. These techniques may allow re-creation of the curvature of the sinuses of Valsalva if the conduit is tailored correctly. These techniques are similar to inclusion techniques in that they leave the annulus unstabilized, because the conduit is sewn above the annulus and exposes the valve to the risk of future dilatation.

Subannular Reconstruction

The resection and subannular reconstruction technique is the one favored by our group.[39, 40] This technique allows complete resection and stabilization of the diseased tissue

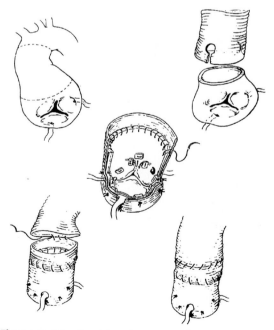

Figure 8·15 Conduit replacement with aortic root inclusion. The entire aortic root is included (resuspended) within a conduit with keyholes cut out for the coronary arteries. (From Ergin M, Griepp R: When, why and how should the native aortic valve be preserved in patients with annuloaortic ectasia or Marfan syndrome. Semin Thorac Cardiovasc Surg 1993;5:91–92.)

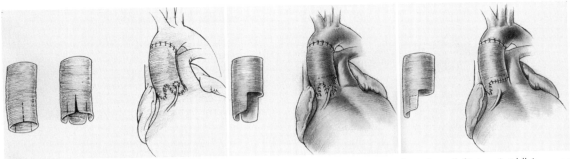

Figure 8·16   Conduit tailoring in a supravalvular position. The conduit is cut to replace three *(left)*, two *(middle)*, or one *(right)* individual sinuses. (From David TE, Feindel CM, Bos J: Repair of the aortic valve in patients with aortic insufficiency and aortic root aneurysm. J Thorac Cardiovasc Surg 1995;109:345–351.)

while sparing the valve. By suturing the conduit to the surgical annulus at the termination of the left ventricular outflow tract, this technique prevents further valvular dilatation (Fig. 8–18). Modification of the original technique also allows tailoring of the conduit to create pseudosinuses that should allow greater valve

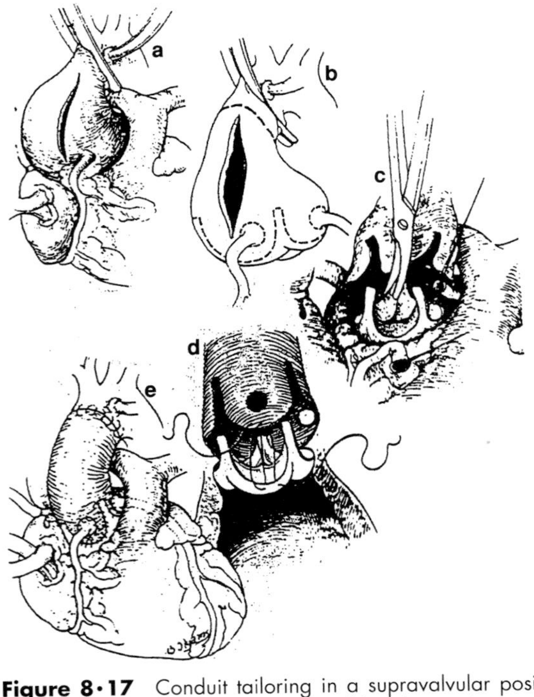

Figure 8·17   Conduit tailoring in a supravalvular position. After incision *(a)* and resection *(b)* of the aortic aneurysm, with preservation of the commissural posts *(c)*, the graft is prepared in a crown shape, tailored to individual sinuses of Valsalva anatomy *(d)*, and sutured to the aorta with reimplantation of coronary arteries *(e)*. (From Yacoub MN, Sundt TM, Rasmi N: Management of aortic valve incompetence in patients with Marfan syndrome. *In* Hetzer R, Gehle P, Ennker J, eds. Cardiovascular aspects of Marfan syndrome. New York: Springer-Verlag, 1995:75.)

durability (Fig. 8–19). We think this technique is preferable for aortic valve sparing because it allows the greatest degree of prophylaxis against future degeneration from aneurysm or valve failure.

For completeness, the Ross procedure and the aortic homograft also should be mentioned. These procedures are relatively contraindicated in treating aneurysmal disease because progression of annular dilatation or primary involvement of the autotransplant may lead to early failure. The exceptions are discussed later.

Valved-Conduit Replacement of the Aortic Valve and Root

The modified Bentall approach is an option for treating aneurysmal disease, even with an undamaged aortic valve.[41] The modified Bentall is a valved conduit replacement of the aortic root to the transverse arch and beyond. The procedure remains an excellent and reproducible procedure that may be chosen when other extensive surgery precludes the time-consuming reconstructive techniques of aortic valve sparing. For example, the Bentall approach should be considered when coronary grafting is necessary, when extensive aortic arch reconstruction is necessary, or when only an expedient procedure can be tolerated.

When ascending aneurysmal disease involves the aortic valve with valvular tissue damage as a primary or secondary process, the operative decision is more straightforward. Replacement of the valve and ascending aorta is a much simpler process than the reconstructive techniques needed for aortic valve sparing. Aortic aneurysm with valve involvement can be treated with the classic modified Bentall

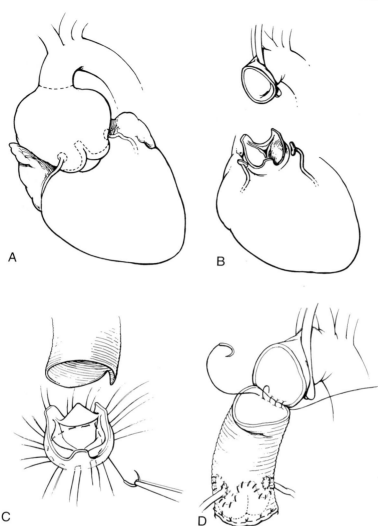

Figure 8·18 Valve resuspension in a tubular conduit. *A,* The dotted lines indicate lines of resection. *B,* The aortic valve and coronary buttons are left intact, and horizontal mattress sutures are placed subvalvularly. *C,* The valve is then resuspended within the graft. *D,* The distal end is anastomosed. (From David TE, Feindel CM: An aortic valve–sparing operation for patients with aortic incompetence and aneurysm of the ascending aorta. J Thorac Cardiovasc Surg 1992;103:617–612.)

procedure, two current alternatives, or another option that may soon be available, as described in the next section.

The original Bentall procedure represented a tremendous advance in treatment of a formidable surgical problem (Fig. 8–20).[41] Subsequent minor modifications in technique have created an expedient, reproducible procedure that has excellent durability and patient survival rates.[42] The modifications that have improved the original technique include excision of the aneurysm (ie, not wrapping the graft with aneurysmal tissue) and isolated implantation of the coronary ostia. These modifications allow more precise and hemostatic implantation and lead to fewer subsequent aneurysms and pseudoaneurysms.

Alternative Techniques for Aortic Aneurysmal Disease

Alternative techniques for replacement of a diseased aortic valve in conjunction with aneurysmal disease occasionally are necessary, particularly in the young patient or in any patient who cannot tolerate anticoagulation. In this setting, aortic homograft replacement with annular stabilization with felt or other prosthetic material is an excellent option. The availability of large homografts, which are frequently required, is the limiting factor for using this technique. If homograft replacement is not an option and anticoagulation is the limiting factor, a stented porcine valve in a conduit as a modification of the Bentall procedure or, in

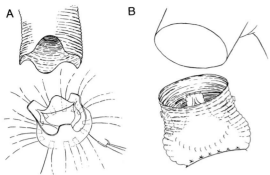

Figure 8·19   *A,* Creation of three symmetric scallops in the proximal conduit and circumferential subvalvular stitch placement. *B,* Completed conduit placement and valve re-suspension with the creation of pseudosinuses. (From Cochran RP, Kunzelman KS, Eddy AC, Hofer BO, Verrier ED: Modified conduit preparation creates a pseudosinus in an aortic valve–sparing procedure for aneurysm of the ascending aorta. J Thorac Cardiovasc Surg 1995;109: 1049–1057.)

rare circumstances, as a valve replacement with supracoronary aneurysm repair can be used. Because this procedure has a high failure rate, it is reserved for the elderly or the patient with limited longevity due to comorbid disease.

Stentless porcine valves are needed that can be combined with conduits to give a better alternative for aortic aneurysmal disease involving the aortic valve when anticoagulation is unacceptable. Such valves are only in the investigational phase.

Algorithm for Aneurysmal Disease With and Without Aortic Valve Disease

The algorithm that we use for treating the complex patient with aneurysmal disease hinges on three factors: a salvageable aortic valve, a patient who can tolerate long-term anticoagulation, and a patient who can tolerate a longer procedure (preferably without comorbid disease) (Fig. 8–21). The best candidates with a salvageable valve undergo an aortic valve–sparing procedure with creation of pseudosinuses. The patients with unsalvageable valves usually undergo a modified Bentall procedure. However, the surgeon must keep all options in mind and tailor the procedure to the patient's needs and desires.

MITRAL VALVE DISEASE

The past 15 years have seen a total change in the surgical management of mitral valve

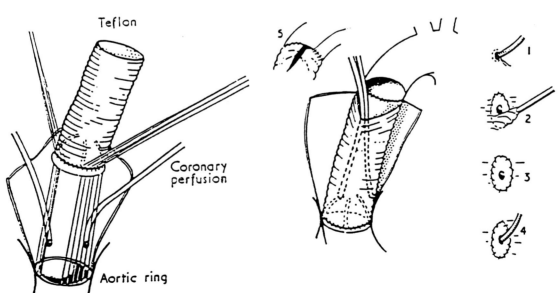

Figure 8·20   Original Bentall valved conduit technique. *Left,* The mechanical valve has been sutured to the aortic prosthesis; sutures have been placed in the aortic ring before fixing the combined prosthesis. *Right,* Combined prostheses in situ. The coronary arteries have been recannulated through the lumen of the aortic graft. Insets 1 to 4 show details of the holes fashioned in the side wall of the Teflon graft to reincorporate the coronary ostia within the lumen of the new ascending aorta. Inset 5 shows the vertical slit in the aortic graft which is closed only after the coronary cannulae are removed and air evacuated. (From Bentall H, De Bono A: A technique for complete replacement of the ascending aorta. Thorax 1968;23:338–339. BMJ Publishing Group.)

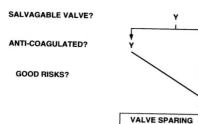
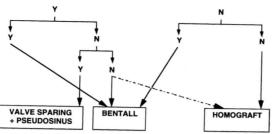

Figure 8·21 Algorithm for management of the aortic valve in aortic aneurysmal disease.

disease. Since Carpentier published his techniques[43–45] and long-term success with mitral valve repair,[46, 47] surgeons worldwide have changed their approach to this disease. Particularly in the last 10 years in the United States, the desire for mitral valve repair instead of replacement has spread to the cardiologist, internist, family practitioner, and patient. However, repair of the diseased mitral valve is not the best option for all patients, and choosing when repair is appropriate and durable instead of performing standard valve replacement is a challenge for the cardiac surgeon.

Mitral repair long predates mitral replacement, because in the early days of cardiac surgery, prostheses were not available. Rheumatic heart disease has been and remains a major factor in worldwide morbidity and mortality, and one of the first and still most widely practiced repair techniques is commissurotomy for stenosis. Increasingly, this is done by balloon techniques for isolated stenosis, but it is still an essential maneuver for repair, particularly in mixed stenosis and insufficiency lesions.

Early replacement efforts were quite imaginative, including "blindly" suturing an aortic homograft into the mitral position without the aid of cardiopulmonary bypass.[48] The first real breakthrough in surgical treatment of mitral valve disease came with the first generation of mechanical prostheses.[49, 50] However, because rheumatic heart disease, which affects younger patients, was a common etiology of valve dysfunction, the need for anticoagulation made these devices a less than ideal replacement for many patients, particularly women in the child-bearing years. The availability of bioprostheses represented the next great breakthrough in survival and improved lifestyle for patients with mitral valve disease.

Unfortunately, neither option proved optimal. Mechanical valves, although durable, require lifelong anticoagulation. Bioprostheses, although ideal for avoiding lifelong anticoagulation, are not durable, with failure requiring

reoperation and often occurring less than 10 years after surgery. Moreover, ventricular function after mitral valve replacement fails to improve or even declines.[51] The cause for this postoperative ventricular failure is disruption of papillary-annular continuity.[52–56] Surgical techniques to prevent ventricular dysfunction have been designed, so that interest in repair techniques was rekindled. Coincidentally, surgeons at a few centers, primarily Carpentier in Paris, had data to support successful, durable repair as an option.[46, 47] Thus, since the mid-1980s, the preferred procedure is mitral repair, with chord-sparing valve replacement as an excellent second alternative.

Mitral Valve Repair Techniques

The surgical approach to mitral repair for stenosis, insufficiency, or a combination uses the same series of maneuvers and attempts to accomplish the same final result. The first requirement for accomplishing a good result with a surgical repair is that the anterior leaflet must be mobile. Second, the posterior leaflet must be mobile but must be somewhat restricted in its position. Third, the mitral orifice must be reduced to a size and shape that the anterior leaflet can obliterate or cover. Fourth, coaptation must occur at a subannular level (eg, on the ventricular side of the annulus). If these goals are accomplished, a competent and durable repair can be completed. The techniques used to accomplish this goal were largely described in Carpentier's early papers. There have been some modifications and additions to these techniques in the last two decades.

Mobility

Several techniques can be used to accomplish each of the requirements for repair. Anterior and posterior leaflet mobility is accomplished by commissurotomy, chordal excision, fenestration, or a combination of these tech-

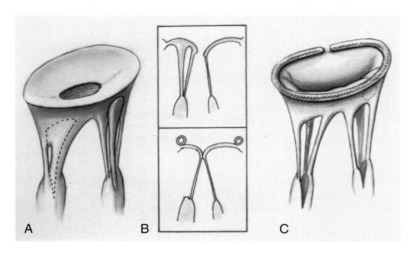

Figure 8·22 *A,* Dotted lines illustrate the incision for commissurotomy and fenestration. *B,* Increased mobility. *C,* Valve repair completed with an annuloplasty ring. (From Carpentier A: Mitral valve repair: the "French correction." J Thorac Cardiovasc Surg 1983;86:323–337.)

niques. Commissurotomy as an isolated procedure is done primarily percutaneously. However, it remains an essential part of operative repair when mobility of either or both leaflets is necessary (Fig. 8–22). The chordal apparatus commonly is bound or fused together, particularly in patients with rheumatic disease. To attain mobility, it is often necessary to excise chordae that are restricting motion. In the more severe types of leaflet restriction, all the chordae may be fused, and fenestration then may be necessary. Fenestration re-creates chordae by cutting openings in the fused chordal structure, allowing increased mobility.

Prolapse

Excessive mobility or prolapse can occur with either leaflet and may be dealt with by chordal shortening, chordal transfer, or chordal replacement. Chordal shortening requires meticulous subvalvular work, with creation of a "trench" in the papillary muscle into which the elongated chordae are placed. After the trench is created, the elongated chordae are folded into the trench and secured (Fig. 8–23). Chordal transfer is an easier maneuver,[57] in which the opposing chordal apparatus is moved from one leaflet to the

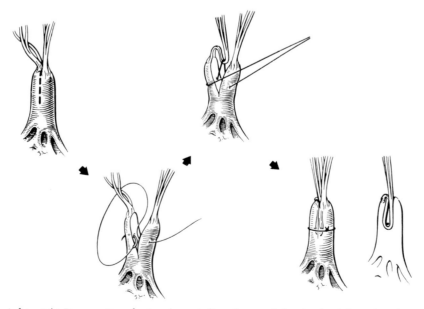

Figure 8·23 *Left to right,* Demarcation of a trench, encircling elongated chordae for delivery into the trench, positioning and securing chordae within the trench, and trench repair. (From Cosgrove DM: Surgery for degenerative mitral valve disease. Semin Thorac Cardiovasc Surg 1989;1:183–193.)

other, requiring far less estimation of length and tension (Fig. 8–24). Chordal replacement is gaining greater popularity[58, 59] and is probably the procedure of choice for complex prolapse. Polytetrafluoroethylene (PTFE) suture is durable and closest to native properties[60] and has been used extensively worldwide for chordal replacement.

Annular Reduction

Posterior leaflet restriction is accomplished by chordal shortening, chordal replacement, quadrangular resection and repair, or a combination of these techniques. Quadrangular resection is the most effective approach because it reduces the length and the redundancy of the leaflet. The originally described triangular resection of the anterior leaflet (to the annulus) has been abandoned because of failure.

The third requirement of annular reduction so that the anterior leaflet obliterates the orifice is accomplished by annuloplasty (Fig. 8–25). If the annulus is not enlarged and signifcant leaflet resection is not needed, annuloplasty may not be necessary. However, most repairs in the United States are accompanied by some form of annuloplasty. Techniques for annuloplasty vary widely, including circumferential ring placement, partial ring placement, autologous tissue augmentation, or suture plication.[61] The technique is probably not as important as the result. As long as the first two requirements are met and the annulus is reduced to the size and shape of the anterior leaflet, coaptation occurs subannularly, fulfilling the fourth requirement, so that competence should be ensured.

Mitral Valve Replacement

Not all mitral valves can be repaired. When repair is impossible, the standard procedure for most patients in the United States is mechanical valve replacement. A mechanical valve is superior to a bioprosthesis because of its excellent durability and because of the high frequency of atrial fibrillation that necessitates anticoagulation in this population in any case. Ventricular dysfunction is prevented by chordal and leaflet preservation during valve replacement. Techniques include posterior leaflet sparing and anterior and posterior leaflet sparing. The amount of subvalvular apparatus preserved is largely dictated by the degree of valvular destruction and the degree of concern for subvalvular obstruction of the mechanical valve. Use of these techniques has resolved most of the ventricular dysfunction seen previously.

Bioprostheses do have some indications in this setting. If the valve cannot be repaired and anticoagulation is contraindicated or declined, a bioprosthesis is a good short-term alternative. Chordal preservation is much easier with bioprostheses because there is no danger of retained chordae disrupting valve function.

Algorithm for Mitral Valve Disease

Many factors influence the decision-making process for mitral valve surgery. Ten-year dura-

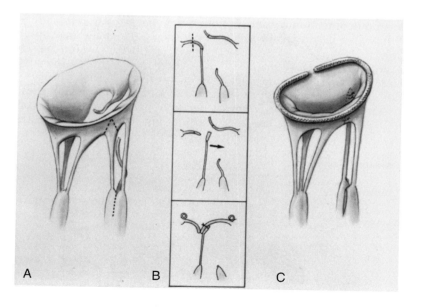

Figure 8·24 *A,* Ruptured chord, with dotted lines demarcating the chord for mobilization and transfer. *B,* Lateral view of the chordal transfer technique. *C,* Repair completed with an annuloplasty ring. (From Carpentier A: Mitral valve repair: the "French correction." J Thorac Cardiovasc Surg 1983;86:323–337.)

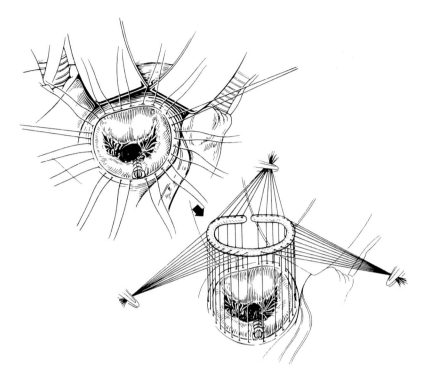

Figure 8·25 Demonstration of the annuloplasty ring technique. (From Cosgrove DM: Surgery for degenerative mitral valve disease. Semin Thorac Cardiovasc Surg 1989;1:183–193.)

bility with low complication rates are well documented for mitral repair.[47] However, for proven, long-term durability, the mechanical valves are clearly superior. We do not know how long repair techniques will last, because all repairs rely on diseased tissue. Despite a philosophic approach of evaluating every mitral valve with repair in mind, the judicious surgeon matches repair and replacement to the patient and to the best estimate of long-term outcome. Some examples using the algorithm may help explain this process (Fig. 8–26).

For a 50-year-old man with a slightly enlarged left atrium, one bout of atrial fibrillation that converted to sinus rhythm, and a flail posterior leaflet, repair is an easy decision. For a 70-year-old, petite female in chronic atrial

fibrillation who is tolerating warfarin without complications and has a stenotic heavily calcified valve, mechanical valve replacement is a relatively clear decision. The decision process becomes more difficult for an active 60-year-old man who does not want to take anticoagulation but who has rheumatic valvular disease, a markedly enlarged left atrium and several episodes of atrial fibrillation, with the last episode refractory to cardioversion. Although the valve may be reparable, the repair may not be durable. In addition, there may not be a true benefit from repair if he must ultimately be on warfarin because of atrial fibrillation. The process of sorting the options in these complex patients has become even more difficult with the success of the maze procedure for surgical correction of

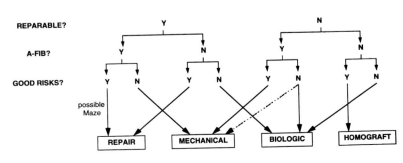

Figure 8·26 Algorithm for treating mitral valve disease.

atrial fibrillation. Although theoretically appealing, the magnitude of combining valve repair and this extensive surgical ablation must be weighed carefully in the selection process.[62]

Extension of Valve Repair Techniques

The growing use and popularity of mitral valve repair over the past decade has prompted extension of the techniques beyond the standard maneuvers described, particularly in unusual circumstances such as endocarditis for which prostheses are poor alternatives. These extended or radical maneuvers are proving relatively durable and are crossing into the realm of elective valve repair with greater frequency.

The most frequently used of these maneuvers are pericardial reconstructive techniques. Pericardium, fresh or treated briefly with glutaraldehyde, has been used to reconstruct leaflet perforations, for annular disruption, and for chordal replacement.[63–66] The commissural regions have long represented a reconstructive dilemma. Two techniques have been described to circumvent this problem. First, Hvass from France described using part of the tricuspid valve, resected intact with its papillary muscle attached, as a partial replacement implanted to fill mitral defects, particularly in the commissural region (Fig. 8–27).[67] Acar described total and partial homograft replacement of diseased mitral valves that cannot be repaired conventionally (Fig. 8–28).[68–72] These two maneuvers greatly increase the range of repair techniques available to the mitral valve surgeon. The tricuspid transfer technique is available to any surgeon. Mitral valve homografts are available only in a few centers in the United States.

In addition, the need for better mitral valve prostheses is being addressed by the development of several new devices. Some remain theoretical, but others are in clinical trials in various countries outside the United States. Bovine pericardial valves, "stentless" mitral valves, autologous pericardial valves, quadrileaflet design valves, and several others should be appearing in the near future if preliminary trials are successful.

TRICUSPID VALVE DISEASE

In contrast to congenital heart surgery, right-sided valvular disease in adults represents a relatively small portion of valve surgery. Except for use of the pulmonary valve for auto-

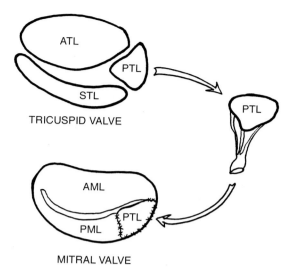

Figure 8·27 Technique for transfer of the posterior tricuspid leaflet (PTL) to reconstruct the mitral commissural region. AML, anterior tricuspid valve leaflet; ATL, anterior tricuspid leaflet; PML, posterior mitral valve leaflet; STL, superior tricuspid leaflet. (From Hvass U, Calliani J, Nataf I, Julliard JM, Vahanian A: Transfer of the posterior tricuspid leaflet and chordae for mitral valve repair. J Thorac Cardiovasc Surg 1995;110:859–861.)

transplantation in the Ross procedure and occasionally using a pulmonary homograft for aortic reconstruction, the pulmonary valve is rarely operated on in adults. The tricuspid valve similarly takes a minor role in adult cardiac surgery, and it is almost exclusively regurgitation that is dealt with when addressing the tricuspid valve. Because regurgitation is the primary lesion and the techniques of mitral valve repair transpose nicely to the tricuspid valve, repair is the procedure of choice for the tricuspid valve, an approach that has been strengthened by the overall poor performance of all prosthetics in the lower-pressure right heart.

Tricuspid valve regurgitation typically is encountered in two circumstances. The most common primary process that affects the tricuspid valve and requires surgical intervention is endocarditis. The most common secondary cause is mitral valve disease.

Tricuspid Regurgitation Caused by Endocarditis

Tricuspid regurgitation caused by endocarditis is most frequently the result of intravenous drug abuse. Because of the excellent outcome with medical therapy on most patients,

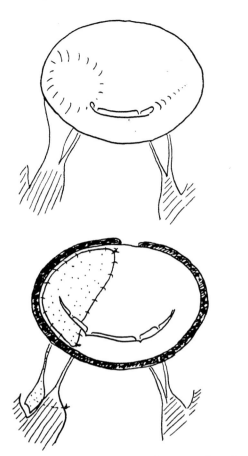

Figure 8·28   Parital homograft replacement of a mitral valve. (From Acar C, Gaer J, Chauvaud S, Carpentier A: Technique of homograft replacement of the mitral valve. J Heart Valve Dis 1995;4:31–34.)

and the risks of a prosthetic valve in this patient group, the medical approach to therapy is pursued much more diligently than for other valvular lesions.

If medical therapy fails, two surgical approaches are available. The first was popularized in Detroit and has met with variable success outside of that center. It advocates valve excision without replacement.[73] This technique relies on the relative tolerance and medical manageability of the residual problem of wide-open tricuspid regurgitation. The proponents further advocate that, even when not tolerated, this technique allows a staged approach with improved results by reduction in septic load, improved antibiotic responsiveness, and less likelihood of reinfection of a prosthesis placed days to weeks after excision. The conventional counter to this position offers relatively early radical excision of infected tissue and replacement with a bioprosthesis with aggressive medical therapy. This approach presumes individual reform that allows subsequent use of a mechanical prosthesis at reoperation or survival of the bioprosthesis to be in excess of that of the patient. Neither of these conventional approaches offers a good long-term solution.

Although not conventional, using radical, extended valve repair techniques in this population is an appealing option. Repair with extensive use of autologous pericardium for leaflet reconstruction, coupled with imaginative chordal replacement and various annuloplasty techniques, can offer complete resolution or marked reduction of regurgitation. The use of little or no foreign material coupled with radical debridement of all infected tissue offers a good short- and long-term solution in this difficult patient population.[74] Because these patients tolerate wide-open regurgitation fairly well, less than ideal valve competency should be tolerated quite well and offers much better long-term prognosis than reoperation or chronic anticoagulation.

Tricuspid Regurgitation With Mitral Valve Disease

Tricuspid regurgitation can occur in conjunction with mitral valve disease in two circumstances. First, the tricuspid valve may be involved in the same process as the mitral valve, for example, rheumatic heart disease. Second, the tricuspid valve may be purely involved secondarily; as pulmonary artery pressures rise due to mitral disease, right heart dilatation results in tricuspid annular dilatation and subsequent regurgitation.

Conventional therapy for both causes has included only two courses of action. One approach has been to ignore the tricuspid lesion and treat the mitral valve, assuming that the tricuspid regurgitation will improve or resolve by improving the mitral hemodynamics. The other course has been routine repair using numerous techniques. About 20 years ago, the repair option was considered excessively aggressive, even meddlesome, by many surgeons and cardiologists. However, with improved repair techniques and increased use of the biatrial incision (Giraudon incision), routine repair of the regurgitant tricuspid valve has become the procedure of choice.

The techniques for treating tricuspid regurgitation caused by mitral valve disease are varied. Replacement of the tricuspid valve in this setting is virtually never done, except in the rare case of rheumatic disease that has destroyed the valve beyond repair. Because wide-open regurgitation and complete excision is tolerated by some patients, repair can be pushed to the absolute limits of innovation and creativity in trying to improve manageability rather than absolute competency of the valve. Only the destroyed valve with no components for reconstruction is replaced, and even some of these may be left for medical management because of the poor track record for prostheses in this position.

Repair techniques are used liberally for tricuspid valves. Because the techniques share the same basis as those for mitral repair, they are very similar to those used and described previously, with a few modifications. Regurgitation is the primary lesion treated, and annuloplasty is the mainstay of repair. Prosthetic ring annuloplasty, particularly with the Carpentier semirigid, shaped annuloplasty ring, is popular for restoration of the shape. This design avoids suture placement near the conducting system.[45] Various flexible rings and partial rings also can be used, but the degree to which they reshape the annulus depends on the surgeon. All annuloplasty techniques reduce the orifice, and in an otherwise normal valve, this should restore or improve competence.

The classic annular reduction procedure, which remains an option, is the DeVega suture annuloplasty.[75] The suture annuloplasty, although appealing for treating endocarditis because it avoids insertion of foreign material, is somewhat time consuming and "uncontrolled" as far as sizing. It therefore has lost popularity with the availability of standard ring repairs. Another older technique that surgeons may still find clinically applicable is the annular reduction by posterior leaflet obliteration or "bicuspidization" of the tricuspid valve.[76] Any of these techniques can be effective in reducing regurgitation caused by isolated annular dilatation. If leaflet or chordal damage has occurred, other techniques described in the mitral section are necessary.

When leaflet or chordal damage is limited to the posterior leaflet, bicuspidization works well. Unfortunately, this is the exception, and most leaflet or chordal damage involves more than one leaflet, which requires more complex repair techniques. Because the right heart pressure is less than the left and because it should improve after mitral valve surgery, the use of prosthetic material for leaflet and chordal replacement is far more liberal than for mitral valve replacement. PTFE suture can be used for a best approximation of chordal properties. Various pericardial preparations have been used as leaflet substitutes, including fresh autologous, glutaraldehyde-treated autologous, and bovine pericardium. The tricuspid valve is remarkably forgiving, and the need for reduced regurgitation rather than total competency of the valve should encourage imaginative combinations of all the described techniques.

Algorithm for Tricuspid Valve Disease

The algorithm for treatment of tricuspid valve disease is shown in Figure 8–29. Unlike treatment for other valvular lesions, the option of deferring surgical intervention should be considered given the predictable change in right-sided physiology and hemodynamics after left-sided correction. However, surgical techniques have advanced enough that all but minimal disease (trivial or grade 1 to 2+) are usually corrected.

OPERATIVE FRONTIERS

Treatment of valvular heart disease remains a major area of innovation in cardiac surgery. No chapter on this topic would be complete without discussing the many new products and techniques on the horizon. Whether each of these will find a place in our armamentarium for treating valvular disease remains to be seen, but each addresses important issues of current care.

The perfect prosthesis for aortic or mitral valve replacement does not exist. The durability of all biologic valves, even homografts and possibly autografts, remains questionable and somewhat unpredictable. Mechanical valves, although durable, require anticoagulation, and even with stringent therapy, these patients continue to have thromboembolic and hemorrhagic complications.[77] For these reasons the search for a better prosthesis continues.

There are many options for aortic valve surgery, although none is without disadvantages. The most widely tested potential new aortic valve replacement is the stentless porcine valve. All major manufacturers have their own version in clinical trials or ready for release. The relative superiority of one over the other remains to be tested. However, all these new products are addressing the negative features of previously available products. Specifi-

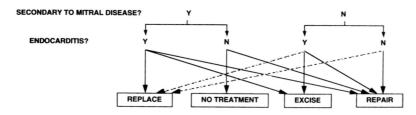

Figure 8·29 Algorithm for treating tricuspid valve disease.

cally, these new valves avoid anticoagulation, and are more physiologic because a sewing ring is not used, a feature that improves long-term ventricular function in association with a reduced transvalvular gradient.[78] In addition, this new design may have improved durability because of the more natural stress-strain configuration compared with the stented predecessor. We think this new generation of valve will prove beneficial in the older patient population (>65 years). To what extent it will be used in younger patients will be determined by its durability.

A couple of other aortic "prosthetics" are available but not widely used in this country. Both are combinations of technique and prosthetic material. The first is an innovative creation of an aortic prosthesis from autologous pericardium, using a template and mounting stent.[79] This design has not gained much popularity because of minimal clinical use and follow-up. It is appealing for cost containment and has some popularity outside the United States for this reason. If its intermediate and long-term durability are proved, this technique may find a place in the United States as cost issues increasingly influence medical care. Another potential cost-containment technique is cusp extension, a revisited older technique that is being revised with the creation of a template for accurate sizing to allow more reproducible creation of leaflet replacement using autologous pericardium (glutaraldehyde treated).[80, 81] This technique also is enjoying more popularity outside the United States than within. However, as greater pressure is brought to bear for cost containment, either of these techniques, if they have reasonable durability, may quickly find a place in the U.S. surgeons' range of therapeutic options for aortic valve disease.

Mitral valve innovations are primarily in the area of radical repair. However, there is no perfect replacement for the mitral valve, and few new types of replacement products are being tested. Most new prostheses use bovine pericardium as the replacement material, with various treatments and configurations, from bicuspid to quadricuspid, being used. Avoidance of anticoagulation in the patient with an irreparable valve is the common theme. The durability of any or all of these valves remains to be tested, because most are just entering clinical trials abroad.

A template concept for mitral valve replacement using autologous pericardium is also being developed. This technique has been advocated as a possibility for more than a decade and has had good experimental and some clinical support.[82, 83] The durability must be proved for these template replacements, but as cost issues become increasingly important, there may be a significant rebirth of interest.

Minimally Invasive Valve Surgery

In addition to innovations in prostheses and repair techniques, minimally invasive surgery has a potential role in valvular heart disease. Because of the rapid expansion and dissemination of this technology, it is difficult to provide data for comparison, and because of the great marketing appeal, there is little interest in conducting a prospective, randomized trial. Despite these drawbacks, we offer our perspective on this burgeoning technologic area of valvular intervention.

The motivation for minimally invasive valve surgery is less clear than the motivation for minimally invasive coronary surgery. Minimally invasive coronary surgery offers smaller incisions and avoids cardiopulmonary bypass, aortic crossclamping, cardioplegia, and cooling. Minimally invasive valve surgery usually changes the incision but still has all the attendant risks of cardiopulmonary bypass, crossclamping, cardioplegia, and cooling. The extensive use of peripheral vascular access may actually increase certain risks. However, early results show that it is technically feasible to do virtually all major valve procedures with minimally invasive techniques.[84, 85] The benefits of altered incisions are less postoperative restriction and earlier return to full activity.

Some caveats are worth mentioning. The disruption of the mammary artery to attain a "less invasive" approach should be avoided, because the potential need for arterial revascularization at a later date should not be compromised. Peripheral cannulation and endovascular occlusion must be used selectively to avoid increased risks of injury to the aorta, cerebral vessels, and the lower extremity vessels. Although popular as a marketing tool, the new technology needed to accomplish these minimally invasive techniques is quite costly. Whether the hoped for shortened hospital stay and more rapid return to full activity will warrant use of this technology or translate to increased cost-effectiveness for these procedures remains to be seen.

Minimally invasive valvular heart surgery is an exciting innovation that is finding its place. The opposing forces of market demand and cost constraint will probably be the determining factor in its use.

Needed Technology

A breakthrough in anticoagulation and biologic compatibility would completely alter the management of valvular heart disease. If anticoagulation were not the deterrent to using mechanical valves, we would suddenly have very durable prosthetics with no disadvantages. If biologic compatibility of cross-species tissue could be improved, we would have valves that require no anticoagulation and are not destroyed by the patient-host interaction. Unfortunately, after more than 50 years, warfarin remains the mainstay for anticoagulation, and after nearly 30 years, biologic valves have a relatively short half-life. A fundamental change in either area would radically alter the surgical treatment of valvular heart disease.

Valvular heart disease remains life threatening and lifestyle limiting for hundreds of thousands of persons worldwide. Innovation in this area of cardiac surgery has led much of the technology that has benefited all aspects of cardiac care. With increasing economic constraints, multiple medical options, and evolving surgical techniques, the challenge for surgeons and cardiologists is to continue to match the most appropriate intervention with each patient to ensure the greatest possibility of survival and improved quality of life.

References

1. McGiffin DC, O'Brien MF, Galbraith AH, et al: An analysis of risk factors for death and mode-specific death after aortic valve replacement with allograft, xenograft, and mechanical valves. J Thorac Cardiovasc Surg 1993;106:895–911.

2. Lahey SJ, Borlase BC, Lavin PT, Levitsky S: Preoperative risk factors that predict hospital length of stay in coronary artery bypass patients >60 years old. Circulation 1992;86(suppl II):II181–II185.

3. Higgins TL, Estafanous FG, Loop FD, Beck GJ, Blum JM, Paranandi L: Stratification of morbidity and mortality outcome by preoperative risk factors in coronary artery bypass patients: a clinical severity score. JAMA 1992;267:2344–2348.

4. Bolling SF, Deeb GM, Brunsting LA, Bach DS: Early outcome of mitral valve reconstruction in patients with end-stage cardiomyopathy. J Thorac Cardiovasc Surg 1995;109:676–682.

5. Ko W, Gold JP, Lazzaro R, et al: Survival analysis of octogenarian patients with coronary artery disease managed by elective coronary artery bypass surgery versus conventional medical treatment. Circulation 1992;86(suppl II):II91–II97.

6. Sahar G, Raanani E, Brauner R, Vidne BA: Cardiac surgery in octogenarians. J Cardiovasc Surg Torino 1994;35(6 suppl 1):201–205.

7. Freeman WK, Schaff HV, O'Brien PC, Orszulak A, Naessens JM, Tajik AJ: Cardiac surgery in the octogenarian: perioperative outcome and clinical follow-up. J Am Coll Cardiol 1991;18:29–35.

8. Glock Y, Faik M, Laghzauoui A, Moali I, Roux D, Fournial G: Cardiac surgery in the ninth decade of life. Cardiovasc Surg 1996;4:241–245.

9. Bashour T, Hanna E, Myler R, et al: Cardiac surgery in patients over the age of 80 years. Clin Cardiol 1990;13:267–270.

10. Estafanous FG, Higgins T, Loop F: A severity score for preoperative risk factors as related to morbidity and mortality in patients with coronary artery disease undergoing myocardial revascularization surgery. Curr Opin Cardiol 1992;7:950–958.

11. Higgins CB, Wagner S, Kondo C, Suzuki J, Caputo GR: Evaluation of valvular heart disease with cine gradient echo magnetic resonance imaging. Circulation 1991;84(3 suppl):II198–207.

12. Ross D, Jackson M, Davies J: The pulmonary autograft—a permanent aortic valve. Eur J Cardiothorac Surg 1992;6:113–117.

13. Ross D: Replacement of the aortic valve with a pulmonary autograft: the "switch" operation. Ann Thorac Surg 1991;52:1346–1350.

14. Oury JH, Angell WW, Eddy AC, Cleveland JC: Pulmonary autograft—past, present, and future. J Heart Valve Dis 1993;2:365–375.

15. Elkins RC, Santangelo K, Stelzer P, Randolph JD, Knott-Craig CJ: Pulmonary autograft replacement of the aortic valve: an evolution of technique. J Card Surg 1992;7:108–116.

16. Stelzer P, Elkins RC: Pulmonary autograft: An American experience. J Card Surg 1987;2:429–433.

17. Angell WW, Pupello DF, Bessone LN, Hiro SP: Universal method for insertion of unstented aortic autografts, homografts, and xenografts. J Thorac Cardiovasc Surg 1992;103:642–647.

18. Ross D: Homotransplantation of the aortic valve in the subcoronary position. J Thorac Cardiovasc Surg 1963;47:713–719.

19. O'Brien MF, McGiffin DC, Stafford EG, et al: Allograft aortic valve replacement: long-term comparative clinical analysis of the viable cryopreserved and

antibiotic 4C stored valves. J Card Surg 1991;6:534–543.

20. O'Brien MF, Stafford EG, Gardner MAH, Pohlner PG, McGiffin DC, Kirklin JW: A comparison of aortic valve replacement with viable cryopreserved and fresh allograft valves, with a note on chromosomal studies. J Thorac Cardiovasc Surg 1987;94:812–823.

21. Barratt-Boyes BG, Roche AHG: A review of aortic valve homografts over six and one-half year period. Ann Surg 1969;170:483–492.

22. Thompson R, Yacoub M, Ahmed M, Seabra-Gomes R, Rickards A, Towers M: Influence of preoperative left ventricular function on results of homograft replacement of the aortic valve for aortic stenosis. Am J Cardiol 1979;43:929–938.

23. Karp RB, Kirklin JW: Replacement of diseased aortic valves with homografts. Ann Surg 1969;169:921–926.

24. Karp R: The future of homografts. J Card Surg 1987;2(1 suppl):205–208.

25. Ross D: Application of homografts in clinical surgery. J Card Surg 1987;2(1 suppl):175–183.

26. Bailey W: Cryopreserved pulmonary homograft valved external conduits: early results. J Card Surg 1987;2(1 suppl):199–204.

27. Nicks R, Cartmill T, Bernstein L: Hypoplasia of the aortic root: the problem of aortic valve replacement. Thorax 1970;25:339–346.

28. Manouguian S, Seybold-Epting W: Patch enlargement of the aortic valve ring by extending the aortic incision into the anterior mitral leaflet: new operative technique. J Thorac Cardiovasc Surg 1979;78:402–412.

29. Konno S, Imai Y, Iida Y, Nakajima M, Tatsuno K: A new method for prosthetic valve replacement in congenital aortic stenosis associated with hypoplasia of the aortic valve ring. J Thorac Cardiovasc Surg 1975;70:909–917.

30. Rastan H, Koncz J: Aortoventriculoplasty: a new technique for the treatment of left ventricular outflow tract obstruction. J Thorac Cardiovasc Surg 1976;71:920–927.

31. Freeman WK, Schaff HV, Orszulak TA, Tajik AJ: Ultrasonic aortic valve decalcification: serial Doppler echocardiographic follow-up. J Am Coll Cardiol 1990;16:623–630.

32. McBride LR, Naunheim KS, Fiore AC, et al: Aortic valve decalcification. J Thorac Cardiovasc Surg 1990;100:36–42.

33. Cosgrove DM, Rosenkranz ER, Hendren WG, Bartlett JC, Stewart WJ: Valvuloplasty for aortic insufficiency. J Thorac Cardiovasc Surg 1991;102:571–576.

34. Miller D, Stinson E, Oyer P, et al: Operative treatment of aortic dissection. J Thorac Cardiovasc Surg 1979;78:365–382.

35. Miller DC: Surgical management of acute aortic dissection: new data. Semin Thorac Cardiovasc Surg 1991;3:225–237.

36. Ergin M, Griepp R: When, why and how should the native aortic valve be preserved in patients with annuloaortic ectasia or Marfan syndrome. Semin Thorac Cardiovasc Surg 1993;5:91–92.

37. David TE, Feindel CM, Bos J: Repair of the aortic valve in patients with aortic insufficiency and aortic root aneurysm. J Thorac Cardiovasc Surg 1995;109:345–351.

38. Sarsam MA, Yacoub M: Remodeling of the aortic valve anulus. J Thorac Cardiovasc Surg 1993;105:435–438.

39. David TE, Feindel CM: An aortic valve-sparing operation for patients with aortic incompetence and aneurysm of the ascending aorta. J Thorac Cardiovasc Surg 1992;103:617–621.

40. Cochran RP, Kunzelman KS, Eddy AC, Hofer BO, Verrier ED: Modified conduit preparation creates a pseudosinus in an aortic valve-sparing procedure for aneurysm of the ascending aorta. J Thorac Cardiovasc Surg 1995;109:1049–1057.

41. Bentall H, De Bono A: A technique for complete replacement of the ascending aorta. Thorax 1968;23:338–339.

42. Coselli JS, Crawford ES: Composite valve-graft replacement of aortic root using separate Dacron tube for coronary artery reattachment. Ann Thorac Surg 1989;47:558–565.

43. Carpentier A: La valvuloplastie: une nouvelle technique de valvuloplastie mitrale. Presse Med 1969;77:251–253.

44. Carpentier A, Deloche A, Dauptain J, et al: A new reconstructive operation for correction of mitral and tricuspid insufficiency. J Thorac Cardiovasc Surg 1971;61:1–13.

45. Carpentier A: Mitral valve repair: the "French correction." J Thorac Cardiovasc Surg 1983;86:323–337.

46. Carpentier A, Chauvaud S, Fabiani JN, et al: Reconstructive surgery of mitral valve incompetence: ten-year appraisal. J Thorac Cardiovasc Surg 1980;79:338–348.

47. Perier P, Deloche A, Chauvaud S, et al: Comparative evaluation of mitral valve repair and replacement with Starr, Bjork, and porcine valve prostheses. Circulation 1984;70(3 Pt 2):I187–192.

48. Murray G, Roschlau W, Lougheed W: Homologous aortic-valve-segment transplants as surgical treatment for aortic and mitral insufficiency. Angiology 1956;7:466–471.

49. Braunwald NS, Cooper T, Morrow AG: Complete replacement of the mitral valve. J Thorac Cardiovasc Surg 1960;40:1–11.

50. Starr A, Edwards L: Mitral replacement: clinical experience with a ball-valve prosthesis. Ann Surg 1961;154:726–740.

51. Goldman ME, Mora F, Guarino T, Fuster V, Mindich BP: Mitral valvuloplasty is superior to valve replacement for preservation of left ventricular function: an intraoperative two-dimensional echocardiographic study. J Am Coll Cardiol 1987;10:568–575.

52. David TE, Strauss HD, Mesher E, Anderson MJ, Macdonald IL, Buda AJ: Is it important to preserve the chordae tendineae and papillary muscles during mitral valve replacement? Can J Surg 1981;24:236–239.

53. David TE, Uden DE, Strauss HD: The importance of the mitral apparatus in left ventricular function after correction of mitral regurgitation. Circulation 1983;68(3 Pt 2):II76–82.

54. Sarris GE, Cahill PD, Hansen DE, Derby GC, Miller DC: Restoration of left ventricular systolic performance after reattachment of the mitral chordae tendineae: the importance of valvular-ventricular interaction. J Thorac Cardiovasc Surg 1988;95:969–979.

55. Sarris GE, Miller DC: Valvular-ventricular interaction: the importance of the mitral chordae tendineae in terms of global left ventricular systolic function. J Card Surg 1988;3:215–234.

56. Sarris GE, Fann JI, Niczyporuk MA, Derby GC, Handen CE, Miller DC: Global and regional left ventricular systolic performance in the in situ ejecting canine heart: importance of the mitral apparatus. Circulation 1989;80(3 Pt 1):I24–42.

57. Sousa Uva M, Grare P, Jebara V, et al: Transposition of chordae in mitral valve repair: mid-term results. Circulation 1993;88(5 Pt 2):II35–38.

58. Revuelta JM, Garcia Rinaldi R, Gaite L, Val F, Garijo F: Generation of chordae tendineae with polytetrafluoroethylene stents: results of mitral valve chordal replacement in sheep. J Thorac Cardiovasc Surg 1989;97:98–103.

59. David TE: Techniques and results of mitral valve repair for ischemic mitral regurgitation. J Card Surg 1994;9(2 suppl):274–277.

60. Cochran RP, Kunzelman KS: Comparison of viscoelastic properties of suture versus porcine mitral valve chordae tendineae. J Card Surg 1991;6:508–513.

61. Ghosh PK: Mitral annuloplasty: a ring-side view [review]. J Heart Valve Disease 1996;5:286–293.

62. Izumoto H, Kawazoe K, Kitahara H, et al: Can the maze procedure be combined safely with mitral valve repair? J Heart Valve Dis. 1997;6:166–170.

63. Frater RW, Gabbay S, Shore D, Factor S, Strom J: Reproducible replacement of elongated or ruptured mitral valve chordae. Ann Thorac Surg 1983;35:14–28.

64. Rittenhouse EA, Davis CC, Wood SJ, Sauvage LR: Replacement of ruptured chordae tendineae of the mitral valve with autologous pericardial chordae. J Thorac Cardiovasc Surg 1978;75:870–876.

65. David TE, Feindel CM: Reconstruction of the mitral anulus. Circulation 1987;76(3 Pt 2):III102–107.

66. Chauvaud S, Jebara V, Chachques JC, et al: Valve extension with glutaraldehyde-preserved autologous pericardium: results in mitral valve repair. J Thorac Cardiovasc Surg 1991;102:171–177.

67. Hvass U, Juliard JM, Assayag P, Laperche T, Pansard Y, Chatel D: Tricuspid autograft for mitral-valve repair. Lancet 1996;347:659–661.

68. Acar C, Tolan M, Berrebi A, et al: Homograft replacement of the mitral valve: graft selection, technique of implantation, and results in forty-three patients. J Thorac Cardiovasc Surg 1996;111:367–378.

69. Acar C, Gaer J, Chauvaud S, Carpentier A: Technique of homograft replacement of the mitral valve. J Heart Valve Dis 1995;4:31–34.

70. Acar C, Berrebi A, Tolan M, Chachques JC: Partial mitral homograft: a new technique for mitral valve repair. J Heart Valve Dis 1995;4:665–667.

71. Acar C, Iung B, Cormier B, et al: Double mitral homograft for recurrent bacterial endocarditis of the mitral and tricuspid valves [see comments]. J Heart Valve Dis 1994;3:470–472.

72. Acar C, Farge A, Ramsheyi A, et al: Mitral valve replacement using a cryopreserved mitral homograft. Ann Thorac Surg 1994;57:746–748.

73. Arbulu A, Asfaw I: Management of infective endocarditis: seventeen years' experience. Ann Thorac Surg 1987;43:144–149.

74. Allen MD, Slachman F, Eddy AC, Cohen D, Otto CM, Pearlman AS: Tricuspid valve repair for tricuspid valve endocarditis: tricuspid valve "recycling." Ann Thorac Surg 1991;51:593–598.

75. Grondin P, Meere C, Limet R, Lopez-Bescos L, Delcan JL, Rivera R: Carpentier's annulus and DeVega's annuloplasty, the end of the tricuspid challenge. J Thorac Cardiovasc Surg 1975;70:852–861.

76. Nakano S, Kawashima Y, Hirose H, et al: Evaluation of long-term results of bicuspidalization annuloplasty for functional tricuspid regurgitation: a seventeen-year experience with 133 consecutive patients. J Thorac Cardiovasc Surg 1988;95:340–345.

77. Ibrahim M, O'Kane H, Cleland J, Gladstone D, Sarsam M, Patterson C: The St. Jude Medical prosthesis. J Thorac Cardiovasc Surg 1994;108:221–230.

78. Jin XY, Gibson DG, Yacoub MH, Pepper JR: Perioperative assessment of aortic homograft, Toronto stentless valve, and stented valve in the aortic position. Ann Thorac Surg 1995;60(2 suppl):S395–401.

79. Love JW, Schoen FJ, Breznock EM, Shermer SP, Love CS: Experimental evaluation of an autologous tissue heart valve. J Heart Valve Dis 1992;1:232–41.

80. Duran CM, Gometza B, Kumar N, Gallo R, Martin-Duran R: Aortic valve replacement with freehand autologous pericardium. J Thorac Cardiovasc Surg 1995;110:511–516.

81. Duran CM, Gallo R, Kumar N: Aortic valve replacement with autologous pericardium: surgical technique. J Card Surg 1995;10:1–9.

82. Mickleborough LL, Ovil Y, Wilson GJ, et al: A simplified concept for a bileaflet atrioventricular valve that maintains annular-papillary muscle continuity. J Card Surg 1989;4:58–68.

83. Deac RF, Simionescu D, Deac D: New evolution in mitral physiology and surgery: mitral stentless pericardial valve. Ann Thorac Surg 1995;60(2 suppl):S433–438.

84. Chitwood WR Jr, Wixon CL, Elbeery JR, Moran JF, Chapman WH, Lust RM: Video-assisted minimally invasive mitral valve surgery. J Thorac Cardiovasc Surg 1997;114:773–780.

85. Cohn LH, Adams DH, Couper GS, et al: Minimally invasive cardiac valve surgery improves patient satisfaction while reducing costs of cardiac valve replacement and repair. Ann Surg 1997;226:421–426.

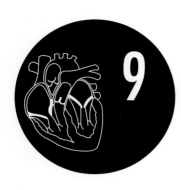

9 Aortic Stenosis

PATHOPHYSIOLOGY

The primary determinant of disease severity in patients with valvular aortic stenosis is the degree of obstruction to left ventricular outflow. Valve obstruction also has secondary effects on the left ventricle, peripheral vasculature, and coronary artery blood flow that influence the clinical presentation of disease and subsequent outcome.

Valvular Hemodynamics

Velocities and Pressure Gradients

Obstruction at the aortic valve level increases antegrade velocity across the narrowed valve corresponding to the systolic pressure gradient between the left ventricle and aorta (Fig. 9–1). For any given transvalvular volume flow rate, the antegrade velocity and transaortic pressure gradient increase with increasing degrees of valvular narrowing. However, for any given valve area, the magnitude of increase in jet velocity and pressure gradient varies with the volume flow rate across the valve. Thus, patients with severe stenosis and a low stroke volume (eg, left ventricular systolic dysfunction) have only a moderate increase in antegrade velocity and systolic pressure gradient, whereas those with moderate stenosis and a high transaortic flow rate (eg, coexisting aortic regurgitation) have a high jet velocity and systolic pressure gradient.

The rate of rise and fall of the antegrade

179

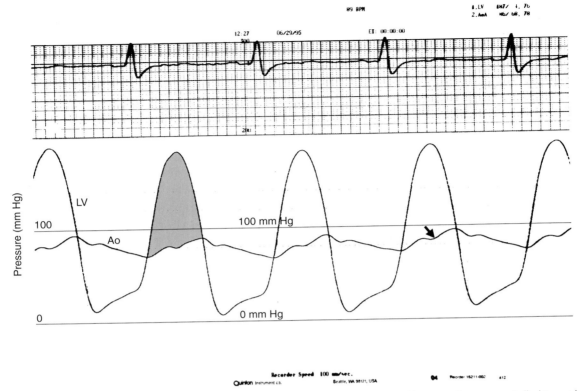

Figure 9·1   Left ventricular (LV) and aortic (Ao) pressure tracings for a 47-year-old man with a congenitally bicuspid valve and recent onset of congestive heart failure symptoms. The peak-to-peak pressure gradient is 100 mm Hg, with a mean transaortic pressure gradient of 62 mm Hg. The aortic valve area, calculated by the continuity equation, is 0.5 cm². Notice the marked delay and decrease in the aortic pressure waveform upstroke *(arrow)*.

velocity and the timing of the pressure gradient across the valve also are related to disease severity. With mild stenosis, the maximum velocity and maximum pressure difference across the valve occur in early systole, before the peak volume flow rate across the valve and at a time corresponding to the maximum rate of flow acceleration.[1, 2] As stenosis becomes more severe, the maximum velocity and pressure difference occur later in systole, eventually coinciding with the maximum volume flow rate across the valve. In addition to stenosis severity, the shape of the velocity curve and timing of the pressure gradient may be affected by other factors that alter left ventricular or aortic pressure, such as coexisting aortic regurgitation or an increased systemic vascular resistance.

The antegrade (or jet) velocity across the aortic valve usually is described in terms of the maximum instantaneous velocity, typically occurring in early to mid-systole. The maximum instantaneous velocity corresponds to the maximum instantaneous pressure gradient across the valve as stated in the Bernoulli equation; the pressure gradient is equal to the velocity squared multiplied by 4.[3–10] At cardiac catheterization, the difference between peak left ventricular and peak aortic pressures (ie, the peak-to-peak gradient) often is reported. Because the peak left ventricular and aortic pressures usually are not simultaneous, the difference between these two pressures is not a physiologic measurement and does not correspond to the maximum or any other instantaneous Doppler velocity. Imprecise reporting of the maximum Doppler gradient as the "peak" gradient may lead to confusion with the peak-to-peak gradient measured at catheterization (see Chapter 4).

Mean transaortic pressure gradients can be derived from Doppler data or invasive pressure recordings by averaging the instantaneous pressure gradients over the systolic ejection period. In adults with valvular aortic stenosis, maximum and mean pressure gradients are linearly related with a close correlation between these two gradients.[6, 11, 12] Although digitizing the pressure or velocity curve and calculation of the mean gradient is the most precise method, the mean transaortic gradient for native aortic valve stenosis can be estimated as the maximum velocity squared times 2.4.[6, 12, 13] Since the relationship between maximum and mean gradient depends on the shape of the velocity curve, this simplified approach cannot be used for other native or prosthetic valves.

The phenomenon of pressure recovery distal to the stenotic valve contributes to some of the confusion in comparisons of invasive and noninvasive transaortic gradients, because Doppler velocities reflect the pressure drop in the orifice itself, whereas catheter pressure data may include pressure recovery distal to the orifice, depending on the exact location of the catheter relative to the stenotic orifice.[14–17] Measuring the extent of pressure recovery may be of interest, because in vitro data indicate that the recovered pressure drop is directly related to the energy loss that determines ventricular pump work and may be a better measure of stenosis severity than the gradient across the orifice.[18]

Valve Area

Aortic valve area is defined as the extent of aortic valve opening in systole and provides a clinically useful measure of stenosis severity that depends less on volume flow rate than pressure gradients. Valve area can be calculated from Doppler data using the continuity equation, based on the principle that the volume flow rates just proximal to and in the stenotic orifice must be equal.[4, 19–23] Aortic valve area is calculated from determination of the stroke volume just proximal to the valve, based on measurement of left ventricular outflow tract diameter and velocity, and measurement of the velocity-time integral of maximum aortic jet velocity (Fig. 9–2). Valve area also can be calculated at cardiac catheterization using the Gorlin equation, based on measurement of transaortic volume flow rate and the systolic pressure gradient across the valve.[24–28]

There has been considerable controversy regarding the relative accuracy of Doppler continuity and catheterization Gorlin formula valve area calculations. In addition to technical differences between invasive and Doppler measures of valve area and the potential sources of error in each approach, these approaches differ in that Doppler valve areas represent the physiologic orifice area (ie, cross-sectional area of flow), whereas Gorlin formula valve areas

represent the anatomic orifice area (see Chapter 3).[29, 30] However, both valve area measurements reflect the same underlying physiologic parameter, and both provide reliable data for clinical decision making when performed correctly.

Although less flow dependent than pressure gradients, aortic valve area also varies with transaortic volume flow rate, especially in patients with calcific stenosis.[13, 31–33] The unfused commissures produce variable degrees of valve opening, depending on the interaction between the stiffness of the leaflets and the force directed against the valve in systole.[28, 34–39] The variable opening of stiff aortic valve leaflets is not surprising given the common echocardiographic observation in patients with dilated cardiomyopathy that changes in flow rate are associated with changes in the extent of aortic leaflet opening, even in the absence of leaflet thickening. With aortic valve stenosis, the increase in left ventricular outflow velocity with exercise may increase the extent of valve opening if the leaflets still have some degree of flexibility. Initial concerns that the observed increase was related to the mathematical assumptions of the calculations or to changes in the fluid dynamics across the valve have been resolved by direct observation of valve opening,[40] so that most investigators now concur that leaflet opening varies with flow rate. With disease progression, the gradual increase in the degree of leaflet thickening and calcification eventually reaches a point where valve area is fixed over the physiologic range of force that can be generated by the left ventricle.

Other Indices of Stenosis Severity

Some investigators have explored the concept of valve resistance as a measure of aortic stenosis severity.[39, 41, 42] Since valve resistance is calculated as the ratio of pressure gradient to flow across the valve, the assumption of this approach is that the relationship between pressure gradient and transvalvular flow rate is linear. This assumption is inconsistent with the Bernoulli equation, which assumes a quadratic relationship between pressure gradient and flow rate. While some disagreement persists as to the exact relationship between pressure and flow across a stenotic valve, in fact, careful fluid dynamic studies support the concept of a quadratic relationship.[43] The apparent observation of a linear relationship in earlier studies might have resulted from a narrow range of

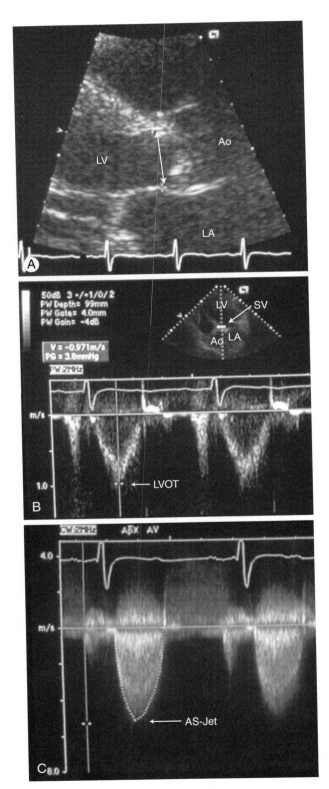

Figure 9·2 Echocardiographic measurements for calculation of valve area by the continuity equation. *A*, Parasternal long-axis view for measurement of the left ventricular outflow tract (LVOT) diameter *(arrow)*. Ao, aorta; LA, left atrium; LV, left ventricle. *B*, Left ventricular outflow velocity recorded from an apical view with the pulsed Doppler sample volume (SV) positioned just proximal to the stenotic aortic valve. *C*, Continuous wave Doppler recording of the aortic stenosis jet (AS-Jet) from an apical approach shows a maximum velocity of 5.2 m/s. Calculated by the continuity equation, the aortic valve area is 0.9 cm².

data, such that only a relatively linear segment of the curve was included in the analysis. In addition, the calculation of valve "resistance" has no clear advantages over jet velocities, pressure gradients, and valve areas in predicting clinical outcome.[44]

Compared with mitral stenosis, the fluid dynamics of aortic stenosis are more complex, because the pressure gradient and volume flow rate across the valve depend on the force of left ventricular contraction as well as the characteristics of the valve itself. Thus, another approach to describing aortic stenosis severity is to estimate the total work performed by the ventricle in opening the aortic valve. Total left ventricular stroke work is calculated as the integral of flow times pressure. Effective stroke work (calculated as aortic pressure times flow) then is subtracted to yield the stoke work "lost" across the valve.[45, 46] Even though left ventricular stroke work loss correlates with other measures of stenosis severity, it also varies with flow rate (even when normalized for stroke volume), is an unfamiliar concept for most physicians, and offers no obvious clinical advantages. Further, the calculation of stroke work loss mainly accounts for the potential energy components of total work, while kinetic energy losses, which are more difficult to estimate, may be even more important in valvular aortic stenosis.[38]

Since aortic valve hemodynamics depend on aortic valve anatomy, left ventricular mechanics, and the characteristics of the vascular system downstream from the valve, a complete description of aortic stenosis severity should include all three of these components. This type of descriptor is conceptually complex and may be difficult to derive in the clinical setting. A step toward an integrated descriptor of aortic stenosis severity is the concept of ventricular-vascular coupling with inclusion of components to describe the effect of the abnormal valve in the system.[47] Preliminary studies in this area are of interest but are not yet clinically applicable.

Left Ventricular Pressure Overload

The basic response of the left ventricle to the chronic and gradually progressive pressure overload of valvular aortic stenosis is concentric hypertrophy (Fig. 9–3). However, not all patients develop hypertrophy, even with severe stenosis, and there are significant gender differences in the degree and pattern of hypertrophy.[48–51] In pathophysiologic terms, left ventricular hypertrophy occurs as a mechanism to maintain normal wall stress by an increase in wall thickness as left ventricular pressure rises (see Chapter 6). Typically, contractility is normal, and ejection fraction is preserved until late in the disease course.

Even when contractility is normal, left ventricular systolic performance may appear to be impaired in patients with severe outflow obstruction for at least three reasons. First, ejection fraction may decline because of the excessive increase in afterload, often called *afterload mismatch*. Second, ventricular preload may be shifted to the left on the Starling curve given a small, hypertrophied, noncompliant ventricle. Third, the temporal sequence of myocardial contraction often is asynchronous in pressure overload hypertrophy, with an "uncoordinated" ventricular contraction. The resultant fall in the peak rate of circumferential shortening correlates with an increase in systolic wall stress.[52] This pattern of discordant contraction and the apparent decrease in ventricular function resolve after relief of aortic stenosis.

When left ventricular mass measurements are normalized for body size and gender, hypertrophy is seen in 54% of men and 81% of women with severe aortic stenosis.[49] The pattern of hypertrophy in women with aortic stenosis is characterized by a small ventricular chamber with increased wall thickness, normal or hypercontractile systolic function, and diastolic dysfunction.[48–51, 53] In men with aortic stenosis, the more common pattern is a dilated chamber with normal or only mildly increased wall thickness and impaired systolic function.

Diastolic dysfunction occurs early in the disease course of aortic stenosis[54] in association with an increase in the total collagen volume of the myocardium and an increase in the orthogonal collagen fiber network.[55] As with ventricular hypertrophy, significant gender differences in diastolic function are seen. Specifically, men have a higher constant of myocardial stiffness in association with a greater degree of endocardial fibrosis and an abnormal myocardial collagen pattern.[53] Age also affects the severity of diastolic dysfunction, with more severe left ventricular hypertrophy and diastolic dysfunction seen in elderly patients (>65 years).[56]

In addition, left ventricular diastolic filling is affected by factors other than diastolic function, producing heterogeneous patterns of ventricular filling in adults with aortic stenosis.[57–59] In those with left ventricular hypertro-

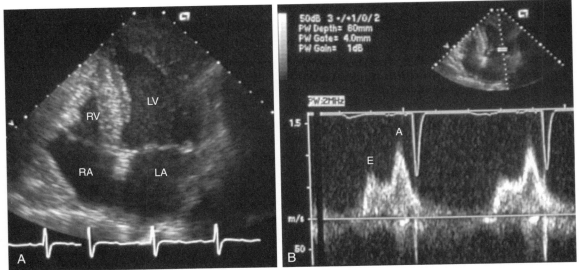

Figure 9·3 *A,* Apical four-chamber view shows marked left ventricular hypertrophy with preserved systolic function in the patient discussed in Figure 9–2. LA, left atrium; LV, left ventricle; RA, right atrium; RV, right ventricle. *B,* The Doppler recording of left ventricular diastolic inflow shows a reduced early velocity (E) and an increased atrial velocity (A) that is consistent with impaired relaxation.

phy and normal ejection performance, early diastolic filling typically is impaired because of impaired ventricular relaxation, whereas the atrial component in late diastole is more prominent. The Doppler velocity curve indicates a reduced early diastolic filling velocity (E-velocity), prolonged early diastolic deceleration time, increased time from flow onset to the E-velocity peak, and an increased late diastolic filling velocity after atrial contraction (A-velocity). With systolic dysfunction and an elevated end-diastolic pressure, the filling pattern reverses (increased E-velocity, rapid deceleration slope, and reduced A-velocity), reflecting reduced diastolic compliance and an elevated end-diastolic ventricular pressure.[57, 58]

Peripheral and Pulmonary Vasculature

In patients with aortic stenosis, the need to correct for peripheral amplification if femoral artery, rather than central aortic, pressures are used for invasive calculation of valve area has long been appreciated.[60] However, few data are available on the influence of systemic factors on valve or ventricular function in these patients. Although left ventricular afterload is predominantly affected by the severity of obstruction at the valvular level, both factors internal to the left ventricle and characteristics of the systemic vascular circuit also contribute to total afterload.[47] To date, few studies have

evaluated the impact of systemic vascular resistance (or impedance), wave reflections, or aortic elastance on the hemodynamics of valvular aortic stenosis.

Mild pulmonary hypertension is common in patients with isolated aortic stenosis when patients are followed prospectively.[44] A higher prevalence of moderate to severe pulmonary hypertension (up to 71% of patients) has been observed in some surgical series.[61] The presumed mechanism of mild to moderate pulmonary hypertension is a chronically elevated left ventricular end-diastolic pressure. More severe pulmonary hypertension may be related to concurrent pulmonary disease in some patients. In other patients, pulmonary hypertension is a marker of impaired ventricular systolic function.[62] Pulmonary hypertension is a risk factor for cardiac surgery,[63] but pulmonary pressure usually returns to normal after valve replacement for aortic stenosis even when severely elevated.[61, 62]

Coronary Blood Flow

Abnormalities in coronary blood flow, even without significant coronary atherosclerosis, contribute to the clinical presentation and long-term outcome of patients with valvular aortic stenosis. Although coronary artery size and therefore blood flow are increased in patients with aortic stenosis, the increase in coronary artery size often is inadequate for the increase in muscle mass, so that coronary flow reserve is limited (Fig. 9–4).[64–67] Left ventricular hypertrophy also is associated with decreased capillary density and increased diffusion distances.[68] Other factors that may affect coronary blood flow in patients with aortic stenosis include a decreased diastolic perfusion time, impaired early diastolic relaxation, and increased diastolic wall stresses, all of which lead to a reduction in subendocardial blood flow.[69]

Transthoracic echocardiographic evaluation of phasic coronary blood flow in adults with aortic stenosis shows reversal of early systolic flow and delayed forward flow in diastole, with resolution of both abnormalities after aortic valve replacement.[70] These findings were further elucidated by transthoracic and transesophageal echocardiographic studies that showed systolic coronary flow decreases in inverse relationship to the increase in left ventricular wall stress and diastolic flow increases in direct relationship to the transaortic pressure gradient, with these changes being most marked in symptomatic patients.[71, 72]

Coronary flow, measured by an intracoronary Doppler flow catheter, also shows retrograde systolic flow at rest, which correlates with the peak transaortic pressure gradient.[73] With stress induced by pacing or dobutamine, retrograde systolic flow increases, total systolic flow decreases, and forward diastolic flow increases compared with normal controls in whom systolic and diastolic flow increased proportionately.[73] These data suggest that an inadequate increase in total coronary blood flow in response to stress may contribute to the clinical presentation of aortic stenosis, specifically the symptom of angina in patients with normal coronary arteries.

Further imbalance in myocardial oxygen demand and supply occurs late in the disease course as left ventricular wall stress and oxygen demands increase out of proportion to the increase in coronary blood flow.[74] Angina, in the absence of coexisting coronary artery disease, is associated with an increased left ventricular wall stress because of inadequate hypertrophy in conjunction with increased ventricular systolic pressures.[68] This increase in wall stress leads to an increase in myocardial oxygen consumption. The combination of increased myocardial oxygen demand and limited coronary blood flow leads to myocardial ischemia and symptoms of coronary insufficiency.

Exercise Physiology

Even asymptomatic patients with aortic stenosis have slightly decreased exercise tolerance compared with normative age standards. The hemodynamic response to exercise is characterized by a normal increase in heart rate to age-predicted maximums, but only a 50% increase in cardiac output. The increase in cardiac output is mediated by an increase in heart rate as stroke volume remains unchanged or decreases slightly with upright exercise.[13, 33, 37, 38, 45, 75, 76] Although total stroke volume does not increase, the maximum instantaneous and mean systolic flow rates across the aortic valve increase because the systolic ejection period shortens due to the increased heart rate (Fig. 9–5). Transaortic velocity, maximum gradient, and mean gradient increase as the flow rate increases, although the degree of increase often is less than predicted by the resting valve area (Table 9–1).[13, 33, 37, 39, 76, 77]

Measures of left ventricular diastolic function also are abnormal with exercise in adults with aortic stenosis. Based on micromanometer pressure recordings, resting diastolic pressures are elevated, diastolic pressures increase further with exercise, and the rate of diastolic pressure decay and the isovolumic contraction interval fail to decrease with exercise compared with normal controls.[78]

With exercise, valve area increases by an

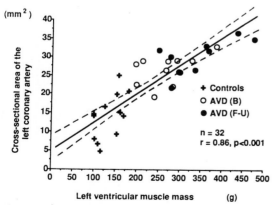

Figure 9·4 Correlation between left coronary artery cross-sectional area and left ventricular mass in 12 control subjects and 10 patients with aortic valve disease (AVD) at baseline (B) and follow-up (F-U). (From Villari B, Hess OM, Kaufman P, et al: Effect of progression of left ventricular hypertrophy on coronary artery dimensions in aortic valve disease. J Am Coll Cardiol 1992;20:1073; reprinted with permission from the American College of Cardiology.)

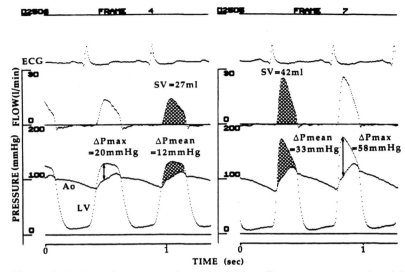

Figure 9·5 Hemodynamic recordings at two volume flow rates in an animal model of valvular aortic stenosis. The electrocardiographic (ECG) recording is displayed on top, the instantaneous volume flow rate in the middle, and the left ventricular (LV) and aortic (Ao) pressures at the bottom. ΔPmax, maximum instantaneous pressure gradient; ΔPmean, mean pressure gradient; and SV, stroke volume. (From Burwash IG, Thomas DD, Sadahiro M, et al: Dependence of Gorlin formula and continuity equation valve areas on transvalvular volume flow rate in valvular aortic stenosis. Circulation 1994;89:827–835; by permission of The American Heart Association.)

TABLE 9·1   PHYSIOLOGIC CHANGES WITH EXERCISE IN ADULTS WITH VALVULAR AORTIC STENOSIS

Characteristic	Bache, 1971[23]	Ettinger, 1972[77]	Otto, 1992[13]	Martin, 1992[76]	Burwash, 1994[37]
Number of patients	20	10	28	85	110
Measurements	Invasive	Invasive	Doppler echo	Invasive	Doppler echo
Type of exercise	Supine bicycle	Supine bicycle	Treadmill	Supine bicycle	Treadmill
Systolic BP (mm Hg)					
Rest	120 ± 3	118 ± 8	139 ± 15		143 ± 22
Exercise	136 ± 3	133 ± 8	155 ± 24		163 ± 29
HR (bpm)					
Rest	79 ± 3	87 ± 5	71 ± 17	71 ± 2	63 ± 14
Exercise	112 ± 5	109 ± 5	147 ± 28	98 ± 2	104 ± 23
SV (mL)					
Rest			98 ± 29		103 ± 30
Exercise			89 ± 32		96 ± 30
CO (L/min)					
Rest	5.4 ± 0.3	8.6 ± 1.1	6.5 ± 1.7	6.0 ± 0.2	6.3 ± 1.7
Exercise	8.5 ± 0.6	9.2 ± 0.9	10.7 ± 4.4	9.3 ± 0.2	9.9 ± 3.8
V_{max} (m/s)					
Rest			4.0 ± 0.9		3.6 ± 0.8
Exercise			4.6 ± 1.1		4.3 ± 0.8
ΔP_{mean} (mm Hg)					
Rest	59 ± 4	37 ± 9	39 ± 20	37 ± 2	30 ± 14
Exercise	74 ± 5	38 ± 11	52 ± 26	41 ± 2	41 ± 18
AVA (cm²)					
Rest	0.8 ± 0.1	1.8 ± 0.3	1.2 ± 0.5	1.1 ± 0.1	1.4 ± 0.5
Exercise	0.9 ± 0.1	1.9 ± 0.3	1.3 ± 0.7	1.3 ± 0.1	1.6 ± 0.7
LV-EDP (mm Hg)					
Rest	12 ± 6	15 ± 3			
Exercise	20 ± 2	15 ± 4			

BP, blood pressure; HR, heart rate; bpm, beats/min; AVA, aortic valve area; SV, stroke volume; CO, cardiac output; V_{max}, maximum aortic jet velocity; ΔP_{mean}, mean pressure gradient; LV-EDP, left ventricular end-diastolic pressure.

average of 0.2 cm^2, accounting for the smaller increase in jet velocity and gradient than expected for the resting valve area (Fig. 9–6).[13, 33, 37] The increase in valve area with exercise allows ejection of a relatively normal stroke volume across the valve and an appropriate increase in cardiac output. As the disease becomes more severe and the leaflets become more rigid and stiff, the degree of valve opening is progressively limited, resulting in a decrease in transaortic stroke volume and a failure of cardiac output to increase adequately with exercise.[13, 38] Some data suggest that this

point corresponds to symptom onset in adults with valvular aortic stenosis.

CLINICAL PRESENTATION

Clinical History

Valvular aortic stenosis is a gradually progressive disease in which patients remain asymptomatic for many years.[79–87] Aortic stenosis typically is first diagnosed based on detection of a systolic murmur on auscultation. Since the increase in hemodynamic severity

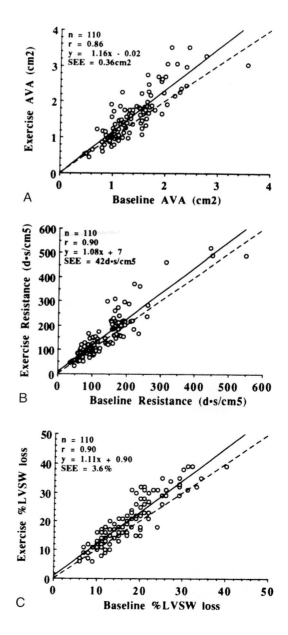

Figure 9·6   Relation of rest and continuity equation aortic valve area *(A)*, aortic valve resistance *(B)*, and percent left ventricular stroke work loss *(C)* in 110 exercise studies in adults with asymptomatic valvular aortic stenosis. The slopes of the regression lines *(solid lines)* are greater than the slopes of the lines of identity *(dashed lines)*, demonstrating an increase in all three indices with exercise. AVA, aortic valve area; LVSW, left ventricular stroke work. (From Burwash IG, Pearlman AS, Kraft CD, Miyake-Hull C, Healy NL, Otto CM: Flow dependence of measures of aortic stenosis severity during exercise. J Am Coll Cardiol 1994;24:1342–1350; reprinted with permission from the American College of Cardiology.)

occurs slowly, many patients fail to recognize early symptoms, and even when symptoms are appreciated, they often are ascribed to the "flu" or "stress," emphasizing the importance of patient education, including a discussion of the classic symptoms of aortic stenosis: heart failure, angina, and syncope. In addition, the clinician must carefully question the patient to elicit symptoms, specifically asking the patient to compare current activity levels with activities at a set time in the past.

The most common initial symptom of valvular aortic stenosis is decreased exercise tolerance due to exertional dyspnea or fatigue.[44, 88] The mechanism of this symptom most often is elevated left ventricular end-diastolic pressure due to a noncompliant, hypertrophied ventricle.[89] Exercise intolerance also may be related to left ventricular systolic dysfunction or coexisting coronary artery disease in some patients. Over time, exertional dyspnea may progress to frank heart failure with resting symptoms seen with long-standing severe valvular obstruction. Some patients present with the sudden onset of heart failure or pulmonary edema, often related to an acute infectious process, anemia, or other hemodynamic stress that leads to acute decompensation in a previously asymptomatic patient.

Exertional angina also is a common initial symptom in adults with valvular aortic stenosis due to an increased oxygen demand by the hypertrophied myocardium, even in the absence of coexisting epicardial coronary artery disease.[44, 88] Again, angina may be precipitated by other hemodynamic stresses, such as pregnancy, anemia, or a febrile disease.

The third classic symptom of aortic stenosis is exertional lightheadedness or syncope. Several potential mechanisms of syncope in aortic stenosis have been proposed, including ventricular arrhythmias and left ventricular systolic dysfunction, but most evidence supports an acute drop in blood pressure due to an inappropriate left ventricular baroreceptor response.[90–92] The elevated ventricular pressure activates baroreceptors that mediate peripheral vasodilation. In the setting of a restricted aortic orifice, cardiac output fails to rise so that blood pressure falls, and the patient loses consciousness.

Physical Examination

The key features in the physical examination of patients with suspected aortic stenosis are palpation of the carotid pulse contour and amplitude; auscultation of the location, loudness, timing, and radiation of the systolic murmur; assessment of splitting of the second heart sound; and examination for signs of heart failure (Fig. 9–7).[93–95]

The timing and amplitude of the carotid pulse contour reflect central aortic pressure. As aortic stenosis becomes more severe, the peak aortic pressure occurs later in systole (ie, pulsus tardus), and the pulse amplitude is decreased (ie, pulsus parvus). Both the timing and amplitude of the carotid pulse correlate with aortic stenosis severity.[96] However, the pulse contour is affected by factors other than stenosis severity, particularly in adult patients.[97] The pulse amplitude may be diminished with a reduced cardiac output and only mild to

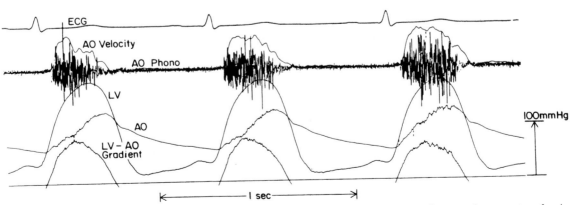

Figure 9·7 High-fidelity hemodynamic tracings in aortic stenosis. Shown from the top downward are tracings for the electrocardiogram (ECG); aortic (AO) root flow velocity and phonocardiogram (AO Phono); and left ventricular (LV) and aortic root pressures with their instantaneous point by point difference or "gradient." The murmur timing and intensity correspond to the time course of the pressure gradient across the valve. (From Pasipoularides A: Clinical assessment of ventricular ejection dynamics with and without outflow obstruction. J Am Coll Cardiol 1990;15:859–882; reprinted with permission from the American College of Cardiology.)

TABLE 9·2 PHYSICAL EXAMINATION IN AORTIC STENOSIS

Physical Examination Finding	Diagnosis of Severe Aortic Stenosis*	
	Sensitivity	*Specificity*
Murmur grade ≥3	29%	91%
Murmur grade ≥2	90%	22%
Late-peaking murmur	25%	86%
Carotid upstroke delay	32%	99%
Decreased carotid amplitude	32%	99%
Single S_2	76%	33%

*Defined as a maximum aortic jet velocity of more than 4.0 m/s. Data from reference 98.

moderate stenosis because of the low volume flow rate into the aorta, although the timing of the impulse typically is normal in this situation. Conversely, the pulse amplitude and timing may appear to be normal with coexisting atherosclerosis, because the stiff vessels cause a rapid and excessive rise in aortic pressure even when severe stenosis is present. Thus, a slowly rising, low-amplitude carotid pulse has a relatively high specificity for the diagnosis of severe valvular obstruction. However, sensitivity is poor, and severe stenosis cannot be excluded in adults with an apparently normal carotid upstroke (Table 9–2).

The systolic murmur of aortic stenosis most often is loudest at the base, over the right second intercostal space. In general, the loudness of the murmur correlates with jet velocity or pressure gradient (Fig. 9–8).[98–104] A systolic thrill in the aortic region (ie, grade IV murmur) is highly specific for severe valvular obstruction. Conversely, severe stenosis is un-

likely with a grade I murmur. Unfortunately, there is considerable overlap in disease severity with intermediate murmur grades and further evaluation often is needed, depending on the clinical setting.[88, 98] Besides the systolic pressure gradient across the valve, the loudness of the murmur is modulated by the volume flow rate across the valve, transmission of the murmur to the chest wall, and the direction of the turbulent jet. Even with severe stenosis, the murmur may be soft when cardiac output is low or if obesity or lung disease diminish transmission to the chest wall. In addition, there is considerable interobserver variability in detection and grading of cardiac murmurs, so that an experienced examiner is needed.

The murmur of aortic stenosis radiates to the carotids in the majority of patients as the turbulent jet is directed superiorly into the ascending aorta, allowing transmission of sound through the aorta to the carotids. In a minority of patients, the murmur radiates to the apex, a pattern referred to as the Gallavardin phenomenon.[105, 106] While the clinician should be aware of this atypical radiation pattern, there is no known correlation between murmur radiation and disease severity.

The murmur of aortic stenosis has a crescendo-decrescendo pattern of amplitude corresponding to the shape of the pressure difference between the left ventricle and aorta during the ejection period. As stenosis becomes more severe, the maximum instantaneous gradient occurs later in systole, so that a late-peaking murmur is appreciated on auscultation. While an early-peaking murmur typically represents mild stenosis, severe stenosis also may have an early-peaking murmur if co-

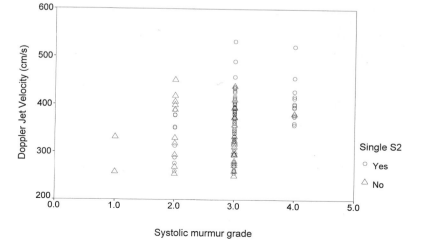

Figure 9·8 Doppler aortic jet velocity compared with systolic murmur grade for 123 adults with valvular aortic stenosis. A single second heart sound (S2) is indicated by the circles and a split-second heart sound by the triangles. Although the group differences are statistically significant (P = .003), substantial overlap in jet velocities is evident for different murmur grades. (Data from reference 98.)

existing regurgitation moves the peak gradient and murmur earlier in systole. Other conditions that are associated with a high transaortic volume flow rate also lead to early peaking of the murmur. Thus, even though a late-peaking murmur is specific for the presence of severe stenosis, sensitivity is low. In addition, accurate evaluation of murmur timing requires an experienced observer.[107]

Normal splitting of the second heart sound depends on flexible pulmonic and aortic valve leaflets that "snap" shut at end-systole and on normal timing of right and left ventricular ejection. The second heart sound in severe aortic stenosis typically is single as the aortic component is inaudible due to impaired motion of the thickened valve leaflets. Earlier in the disease course, the second heart sound may have reversed splitting with respiration because of a prolonged left ventricular ejection time. A single second heart sound is specific but not sensitive for the diagnosis of severe obstruction.[98]

An S_4 gallop may be appreciated in many patients with aortic stenosis and reflects an increased atrial contribution to ventricular filling.[108] Other physical examination findings in aortic stenosis patients depend on whether hemodynamic decompensation has occurred, leading to the typical signs of heart failure.

Chest Radiography and Electrocardiography

The chest radiograph may be entirely normal in patients with valvular aortic stenosis, although post-stenotic dilation of the ascending aorta may be appreciated in some cases, even early in the disease course (Fig. 9–9). The cardiac silhouette typically is normal since left ventricular hypertrophy due to an increased wall thickness with a normal chamber dimension is not evident on a standard chest radiograph. Calcification of the aortic valve rarely is evident on chest radiography but may be seen using fluoroscopy in a high percentage of patients with severe valvular obstruction.[109] Mitral annular calcification, which often accompanies degenerative aortic valve disease, also may be seen. With long-standing disease, left ventricular dilation and signs of heart failure are present. Radiographic find-

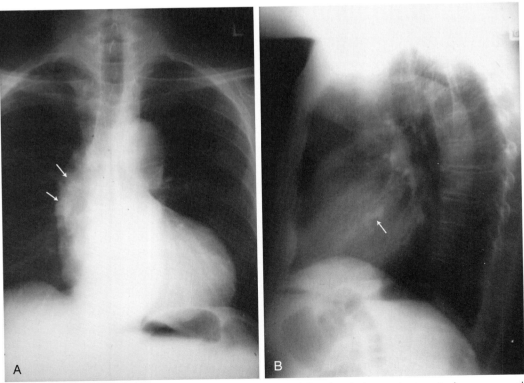

Figure 9·9 Posterior-anterior (PA) chest radiograph of an adult with valvular aortic stenosis shows a normal cardiac silhouette with mild dilation of the ascending aorta *(double arrows)*. In the lateral view *(right)* calcification of the aortic valve is seen *(arrow)*.

ings of pulmonary hypertension also may be evident late in the disease course.

The classic electrocardiographic finding in patients with aortic stenosis is left ventricular hypertrophy. However, many adults and children with severe aortic stenosis do not meet electrocardiographic criteria for left ventricular hypertrophy.[110, 111] Other nonspecific electrocardiographic changes in adults with aortic stenosis include left atrial enlargement, left axis deviation, and left bundle branch block. Although early studies suggested that T wave changes correlated with the degree of aortic stenosis, this finding has not been reliable in clinical practice.[112, 113]

Electrocardiographic changes with exercise, specifically ST depression, are common in adults with aortic stenosis. Significant (>1 mm) flat or downsloping ST depression is observed in about two thirds of patients, even those with only mild to moderate valve obstruction. Even when the resting electrocardiograph is normal, one half still have ST depression with exercise. The presence or severity of ST changes with exercise in adults with aortic stenosis does not correlate with the presence or absence of epicardial coronary artery disease.[44]

Echocardiography

The standard echocardiographic evaluation of a patient with known or suspected aortic stenosis includes assessment of stenosis severity, the degree of coexisting aortic regurgitation, left ventricular size and function, estimation of pulmonary pressures, and identification of any other cardiac abnormalities.[114] With an experienced examiner, diagnostic data are obtained by transthoracic examination of more than 99% of patients, even when ultrasound tissue penetration is poor. Transesophageal imaging rarely is needed and can be misleading because of the inability to align the Doppler beam parallel to the aortic jet. Although some investigators propose using two-dimensional (2D) planimetry of valve area determined on transesophageal images,[34, 115-118] other investigators question the validity of this approach given the nonplanar, irregular, stellate shape of the orifice and the reverberations and shadowing due to valve calcification.[119] Possibly, three-dimensional echocardiographic reconstructions of the stenotic orifice may avoid some of these limitations.[120]

The most clinically useful measures of stenosis severity are maximum aortic jet velocity and valve area determined with the continuity equation. Accurate Doppler data acquisition in patients with aortic stenosis requires trained and experienced sonographers and physicians, with meticulous attention to the technical details of imaging and Doppler flow recording (see Chapter 3). A suboptimal examination may underestimate stenosis severity because of failure to obtain a parallel intercept angle between the continuous wave Doppler beam and the high-velocity aortic jet. This limitation is evident on transesophageal imaging, where a parallel intercept angle is rarely achieved. Less often, stenosis severity is overestimated because of misidentification of the Doppler signal or due to errors in measurement of outflow tract diameter or velocity in the calculation of valve area. Despite these potential limitations, the validity and accuracy of Doppler measurements of aortic stenosis severity are well established both in comparison to catheterization data[8-10, 121-124] and in terms of clinical outcome.[6, 44]

Several other echocardiographic measures of stenosis severity have been proposed. Some of these measurements aim to more fully describe stenosis severity, including calculation of valve resistance and stroke work loss.[38, 45, 46, 125, 126] Others attempt to provide a simplified index such as the ratio of outflow tract to aortic jet velocity or the ratio of jet velocity to fractional shortening.[127-129] None of these proposed measures has gained widespread clinical acceptance, and none has demonstrated incremental diagnostic value in predicting patient outcome compared with measurement of jet velocity, pressure gradient, and aortic valve area.

Coexisting aortic regurgitation is present in between 70% and 80% of adults with predominant aortic stenosis.[11, 44] Regurgitant severity is evaluated using color flow imaging, with the parasternal short-axis view just proximal to the valve being particularly helpful. Evaluation also includes assessment of the signal strength and velocity curve of the continuous wave Doppler signal and the presence and degree of diastolic flow reversal in the descending aorta.

Left ventricular chamber dimensions and volumes, wall thickness, left ventricular mass, and ejection fraction are calculated using the standard techniques described in Chapter 3. Diastolic dysfunction may be evaluated on the basis of patterns of ventricular and atrial inflow and measurement of the isovolumic relaxation time. Left ventricular meridional and circumferential wall stress can be calculated from echocardiographic data in conjunction with a cuff blood pressure measurement as described in Chapters 3 and 7. However, while useful in clinical research studies, wall stress calculations are rarely performed routinely as these measurements are tedious to perform and clinical utility has not yet been convincingly demonstrated.

Other important information derived from the echocardiographic examination includes left atrial size, pulmonary artery systolic pressure, right ventricular size and systolic function, and mitral valve anatomy and function. Mitral annular calcification is seen in about 50% of adults with aortic stenosis.[44] About 90% of patients have mild coexisting mitral regurgitation, with a smaller number having moderate mitral regurgitation. In patients with rheumatic disease, evaluation of the severity of mitral stenosis or regurgitation also is needed for clinical decision making.

Stress Testing

Stress testing of adults with valvular aortic stenosis has illuminated several aspects of the pathophysiology and clinical presentation of this disease. However, the role of stress testing in the day-to-day management of adults with aortic stenosis remains unclear. Stress testing may be considered for an objective measure of exercise capacity in an asymptomatic patient, clarification of symptom status in a patient with an equivocal history, detection of coexisting coronary artery disease, or evaluation of the changes in valvular hemodynamics with stress.

Traditionally, valvular aortic stenosis has been considered to be a contraindication to stress testing. However, recent studies suggest that stress testing can be performed with a low likelihood of complications in selected patients if they are monitored closely during the stress test (Table 9–3). In several series of patients with minimal or no symptoms at the time of testing, no serious complications have been reported.[38, 44] However, even in this patient group, exertional hypotension occurs in about 10%, most have significant exertional ST segment depression, and ventricular ectopy is common.[38, 44, 130, 131]

Since these series have focused on asymptomatic patients, it is important to assess symptom status before stress testing, and the test should be deferred for patients with definite symptoms. In addition, evaluation of aortic stenosis severity and left ventricular function before stress testing improves safety, as the test can be canceled or more closely monitored if stenosis is very severe. In all patients with aortic stenosis, the stress test should be promptly stopped for any decline in blood pressure, symptom onset, or significant arrhythmia.

Probably the most common indication for stress testing of patients with valvular aortic stenosis is an objective measure of exercise capacity in the asymptomatic person to define the parameters of a safe exercise program. Although patients with aortic stenosis should

TABLE 9•3 SAFETY OF STRESS TESTING IN AORTIC STENOSIS

Study	Patients	Type of Stress	Max HR (bpm)	AS Severity	Reported Adverse Effects
Bache, 1971[33]	20	Supine bicycle	112 ± 5	AVA 0.76 ± 0.88 cm^2	None
Nylander, 1986[250]	76	Upright bicycle	NR	AVA 0.2–2.9 cm^2	↓ BP in 38%
Clyne, 1991[251]	14	Treadmill exercise	171 ± 19	Max ΔP 40–140 mm Hg	ST ↓ in 71% ↓ BP >10 mm Hg in 14%
Martin, 1992[76]	80	Supine bicycle	98 ± 2	AVA 1.1 ± 0.1 cm^2	None
Kupari, 1992[252]	44	Bicycle	126 ± 21	AVI 0.18–1.43 cm^2/m^2	None
Casale, 1992[39]	12	Dobutamine	86 ± 5	AVA 0.67 ± 0.05 cm^2	Ventricular ectopy in 17% Systolic hypertension in 17% Patient discomfort in 17%
deFilippi, 1995[253]	24	Dobutamine	99 ± 13	AVA ≤0.5 cm^2/m^2	Ventricular ectopy in 6%
Burwash, 1994[37]	110	Treadmill exercise	104 ± 23	AVA 1.38 ± 0.5 cm^2	↓ BP >10 mm Hg in 10% ST depression in 80%
Samuels, 1995[254]	35	Adenosine	90 ± 12	AVA 0.84 ± 0.16 cm^2	Transient 2° AV block in 9% Transient 3° AV block in 3%

AS, aortic stenosis; HR, heart rate; bpm, beats/min; NR, not reported; AVA, aortic valve area; AVI, aortic valve index (per body surface area); BP, blood pressure; ↓, decrease or depression; Max ΔP, maximum transaortic pressure gradient; 2°, second degree; 3°, third degree.

not participate in competitive sports or extremely vigorous activities, moderate levels of recreational activity are usually well tolerated by asymptomatic individuals.[132]

Exercise testing also may be used to clarify the status of patients with equivocal symptoms, denial of apparent symptoms, or decreased exercise tolerance that is perceived by other family members. Demonstrating symptom onset or hypotension with exercise shifts the balance toward earlier clinical intervention.

There has been considerable interest in the use of stress testing for detecting coexisting coronary artery disease in patients with valvular aortic stenosis. Exercise electrocardiography is not helpful, because most patients have significant ST depression with exertion, even in the absence of criteria for left ventricular hypertrophy on the resting electrocardiogram and in the absence of significant coronary artery disease.[44] Radionuclide stress imaging studies have shown much more promise (Table 9–4), with a fair sensitivity and specificity for detection of coronary artery disease. While there are little data on the utility of stress echocardiography for detection of coronary artery disease in adults with aortic stenosis, my experience is that it is insensitive, possibly because of diffuse subendocardial ischemia obscuring regional dysfunction. However, regional wall motion abnormalities appear to be specific for severe coronary obstruction in the rare positive cases.

Several investigators have suggested that the changes in hemodynamics during a stress study might provide a better index of stenosis severity than a single resting value. Specifically, it is hypothesized that impending symptom onset can be identified by a fixed valve area that fails to increase with an increase in transaortic volume flow rate. Although clinical studies comparing groups of patients support this hypothesis and provide insight into the pathophysiology of the disease process, stress testing to evaluate changes in valve area is rarely helpful in making clinical decisions about individual patients for several reasons.[38, 44] First, recording aortic stenosis jet and outflow tract velocities immediately after exercise is technically demanding and subject to considerable acquisition and measurement error, especially when performed by less experienced laboratories. Second, the magnitude of the hemodynamic changes seen with exercise or pharmacologic stress is similar to the expected measurement variability, even in the most experienced laboratories, limiting evaluation of individual patients, although group comparisons may be statistically valid. Third, the results do not affect clinical decision making, because the timing of surgical intervention is based on symptom status and resting measures of stenosis severity in most patients with valvular aortic stenosis.

However, evaluation of the change in valve area with changes in flow rate may be helpful for the subgroup of patients with aortic stenosis and coexisting significant left ventricular systolic dysfunction. It is difficult to separate patients in this subgroup with severe aortic stenosis and impaired ventricular function due to increased afterload from those with reduced aortic opening due to poor left ventricular function in the setting of only mild or moderate aortic valve obstruction. In both cases, the resting transaortic gradient is modest because of the low transaortic volume flow rate. In addition, valve area is reduced in both cases due to reduced opening of the valve leaflets. If the transaortic flow rate is increased using pharmacologic or exercise stress, the resultant

TABLE 9·4 ACCURACY OF STRESS TESTING FOR DIAGNOSIS OF CORONARY ARTERY DISEASE IN PATIENTS WITH VALVULAR AORTIC STENOSIS

Study	Type of Stress	Imaging Modality	Patients	Mean Age (Range) (y)	Mean AVA (Range) (cm²)	Sensitivity	Specificity
Kupari, 1992[252]	Bicycle exercise	[201]Thallium SPECT	44	63 (41–78)	0.5 (0.2–1.4)	90%	70%
Samuels, 1995[254]	Adenosine	[201]Thallium SPECT	35	76 (64–90)	0.8 (0.5–1.2)	92%	71%
Rask, 1995[255]	Dipyridamole	[201]Thallium SPECT	89	68 (44–79)	0.7 (0.4–1.3)	100%*	75%*
Kettunen, 1992[256]	Dipyridamole	MIBI-SPECT	22	61		61%† 91%	64%† 73%

AVA, aortic valve area; MIBI, ^{99m}Tc-sestamibi; SPECT, single photon emission computed tomography.
*Values for men.
†Values for women.

increase in volume flow rate increases the degree of aortic valve opening when the primary process is left ventricular dysfunction. In contrast, aortic valve area remains unchanged with an increased transaortic velocity and pressure gradient if severe valvular obstruction is present. When there is no increase in volume flow rate, it remains unclear whether the failure to increase flow rate results from an unresponsive myocardium or a stiff aortic valve restricting an increase in ventricular outflow.

Other approaches to the patient with aortic valve disease and concurrent left ventricular dysfunction include evaluation of the degree of leaflet thickening and calcification on echocardiography or fluoroscopy, reevaluation of hemodynamics after a trial of medical therapy for heart failure, and consideration of the impact of comorbid medical conditions on outcome. In theory, the patient with severe stenosis and poor ventricular function should benefit from valve replacement, and the patient with primary ventricular dysfunction and incidental mild to moderate valve disease should not. In fact, both subgroups have a poor clinical outcomes with or without surgery.[133, 134]

Cardiac Catheterization

In nearly all patients with valvular aortic stenosis, diagnostic data, including quantitation of stenosis severity, can be obtained noninvasively by Doppler echocardiography. Invasive measurement of the transaortic gradient and calculation of valve area using the Gorlin formula are needed only when echocardiographic data are nondiagnostic or are not congruent with other clinical data. As with any diagnostic modality, careful attention to technical details during cardiac catheterization is needed for accurate quantitation of aortic stenosis severity (see Chapter 4).

Coronary angiography often is indicated to ascertain whether anginal symptoms are due to coexisting coronary disease in patients with mild or moderate aortic stenosis. In cases of severe aortic stenosis, coronary angiography usually is needed before aortic valve surgery, unless the pretest likelihood of disease is extremely low, for example, in young women with congenital aortic stenosis.

DISEASE COURSE
Natural History
Asymptomatic Patients

In adults with valvular aortic stenosis, obstruction to left ventricular outflow develops gradually over many years (Table 9–5).[81, 87] Since a substantial decrease in valve area and increase in transaortic velocity occur prior to symptom onset, many patients are diagnosed by the finding of a systolic murmur on examination during this asymptomatic period. The average age at symptom onset for patients with secondary calcification of a congenitally bicuspid aortic valve is 50 to 60 years,[135, 136] whereas patients with degenerative calcification of a trileaflet valve present one to two decades later, typically at 70 to 80 years of age. Rheumatic aortic stenosis becomes symptomatic over a wider age range, with patients most often presenting between the ages of 20 and 50 years. Adults with congenital aortic stenosis or with restenosis after a prior surgical or balloon valvuloplasty in childhood or adolescence often become symptomatic at age 20 to 30 years.[137, 138]

Some data suggest that, on account of the insidious rate of disease progression, some adults fail to recognize the diminution in cardiac performance due to valvular obstruction. Exercise testing reveals a diminished exercise capacity in these apparently asymptomatic patients compared with age- and gender-matched normal subjects. In addition, some investigators suggest that irreversible changes of the ventricular myocardium occur even before symptom onset.[139] However, in the absence of overt symptoms, clinical outcome is excellent. Sudden death has not been observed among patients with no other symptoms of aortic stenosis,[44, 138, 140–142] although one study reported a single case of sudden death occurring shortly after the onset of anginal symptoms (Figs. 9–10 and 9–11).[143]

In initially asymptomatic patients, the rate of symptom onset is variable, with predictors of symptom onset including older age, male gender, aortic stenosis severity, and functional status. Although several measures of stenosis severity are univariate predictors of clinical outcome, the only baseline measures that remain predictive on multivariate analysis are Doppler aortic jet velocity and functional status score (Fig. 9–12). The rate of symptom onset is about 8% per year in those with a jet velocity less than 3.0 m/s, 17% per year in those with a jet velocity of 3 to 4 m/s, and 40% per year in those with a jet velocity greater than 4.0 m/s. In addition, the rate of increase in aortic jet velocity over time is a strong predictor of clinical outcome, emphasizing the importance of periodic evaluation in clinical management. There is no convincing

TABLE 9·5   NATURAL HISTORY OF VALVULAR AORTIC STENOSIS

Series	Entry Criteria	Patients	Age (y)	AS Severity	Mean Follow-Up	Survival*
Symptomatic Patients						
Frank, 1973[81]	$\Delta P_{peak} \geq 50$ mm Hg or AVI <0.7 cm²/m²	15	32–59	AVI 0.4 ± 0.1 cm²/m²	>2 y	50% at 5 y 10% at 9 y
Chizner, 1980[80]	Cardiac cath, no AVR	42	22–77	AVA 0.7 ± 0.3 (0.2–1.1) cm²	5.4 y	36% at 5 y 20% at 9 y
O'Keefe, 1987[145]	Severe AS, no AVR, age ≥60	50	60–89	V_{max} 4.5 m/s, AVA 0.6 cm²	1.7 y	37% at 2 y 25% at 3 y
Turina, 1987[140]	Cardiac cath, no AVR	125	43 (16–73)	Mean ΔP 60 mm Hg	6.6 y	12% at 5 y
Horstkotte, 1988[138]	Refused surgery	35		Severe AS (AVA <0.8 cm²)		18% at 5 y
Kelly, 1988[141]		39	72 ± 11	ΔP 68 ± 19 mm Hg		60% at 2 y
Asymptomatic Patients						
Turina, 1987[140]		65		Mean ΔP 57 mm Hg AVA 0.76 cm²		76% at 5 y
Horstkotte, 1988[138]	Cath for other reasons	142		Mild AS (AVA >1.5 cm²)		92% at 10 y
	Cath for other reasons	236		Mod AS (AVA 0.8–1.5 m²)		80% at 10 y
Kelly, 1988[141]	$V_{max} \geq 3.6$ m/s	51	63 ± 19	ΔP 68 ± 19 mm Hg	15 mo	90% at 2 y
Pellikka, 1990[142]	Doppler $V_{max} \geq 4$ m/s	143	72 (40–94)	V_{max} 4.4 (4–6.4) m/s	20 mo	62% at 2 y
Kennedy, 1991[146]	Moderate AS at cath, no AVR	66	67 ± 10 y	AVA 0.92 ± 0.13 (0.7–1.2)	35 mo	59% at 4 y
Otto, 1997[44]	Abnormal valve with V_{max} >2.6 m/s	123	63 ± 16 y	V_{max} < 3 m/s	2.5 ± 1.4 y	84 ± 16% at 2 y
				V_{max} 3–4 m/s		66 ± 13% at 2 y
				V_{max} > 4 m/s		21 ± 18% at 2 y

ΔP, pressure gradient; V_{max}, maximum aortic jet velocity; AVA, aortic valve area; AS, aortic stenosis; AVI, aortic valve index; AVR, aortic valve replacement; cath, catheterization.

*Actuarial survival is given for symptomatic patients, and event-free survival is given for asymptomatic patients.

evidence that clinical outcome in adults with asymptomatic aortic stenosis is related to the etiology of aortic stenosis.[44, 143]

Interestingly, a wide range of hemodynamic severity is found at symptom onset in adults with valvular aortic stenosis, contradicting the traditional view that a specific valve area, indexed for body size, indicates severe or "criti-

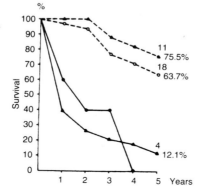
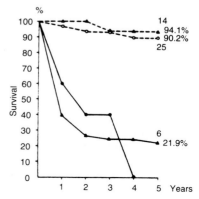

Figure 9·10 Life-table survival curves without death or aortic valve replacement (event-free survival, *left panel*) and effective survival (death is the only endpoint, *right panel*) in hemodynamically severe aortic stenosis and combined lesions *(triangles)* as well as aortic regurgitation *(circles)* in severely symptomatic *(closed symbols and solid lines)* and asymptomatic or mildly symptomatic patients *(open circles and dashed lines)*. (From Turina J, Hess O, Sepulcri F, Krayenbuehl HP: Spontaneous course of aortic valve disease. Eur Heart J 1987;8:471–483.)

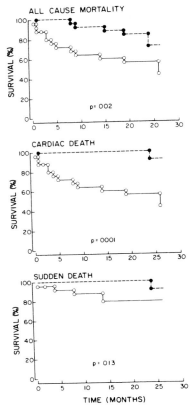

Figure 9·11 Cumulative life-table death rates for aortic stenosis patients. Asymptomatic patients *(closed circles)* had significantly better survival rates with respect to all causes of mortality, cardiac deaths, and sudden deaths than symptomatic patients *(open circles)*. (From Kelly TA, Rothbart RM, Cooper CM, Kaiser DL, Smucker ML, Gibson RS: Comparison of outcome of asymptomatic to symptomatic patients older than 20 years of age with valvular aortic stenosis. Am J Cardiol 1988;61:123–130.)

cal" stenosis.[44, 138, 140, 144] In the Balloon Valvuloplasty Registry, symptomatic patients had aortic jet velocities ranging from 2.3 to 6.6 m/s (mean, 4.4 ± 0.8 m/s), mean transaortic pressure gradients ranging from 13 to 120 mm Hg (mean, 48 ± 18 mm Hg), and aortic valve areas ranging from 0.1 to 1.4 cm² (mean, 0.6 ± 0.2 cm²).[11] In this study, there may have been bias toward overestimation of disease severity at symptom onset, because some patients might have been symptomatic for several months or years before study entry. However, a prospective study of initially asymptomatic adults with valvular aortic stenosis also found a wide range of hemodynamic severity at symptom onset, with an average jet velocity of 4.6 ± 0.8 m/s, a mean transaortic gradient of 49 ±18 mm Hg, and a valve area of 0.93 ± 0.31 cm² (Fig. 9–13).[44] The range of hemodynamic

severity at symptom onset is similar if indexed to body surface area, indicating that the differences between patients are not simply due to differences in body size. Other clinical series also show a substantial overlap in hemodynamic severity in symptomatic and asymptomatic patients (Fig. 9–14).[44, 138, 140]

These clinical observations support the hypothesis that symptom onset is due to the interaction of valve stiffness, left ventricular ejection force, and the metabolic requirements in each individual. Symptoms typically occur initially with conditions that increase total tissue oxygen demands, such as exertion, pregnancy, febrile illness, or anemia, related to the heart's inability to increase cardiac output across the narrowed valve. Thus, the specific degree of valve narrowing associated with clinical symptoms shows considerable individual variability. In addition, concurrent conditions, such as aortic regurgitation or coronary artery disease, modify the specific degree of hemodynamic perturbation associated with symptoms.

Symptomatic Patients

After definite symptoms of aortic stenosis are detected, outcome is very poor without surgical intervention (see Table 9–5). Autopsy studies performed before aortic valve replacement was available and more recent series of adults who refused surgical intervention indicate survival rates with severe symptomatic aortic stenosis of only 15% to 50% at 5 years (see Figs. 9–10 and 9–11).[80, 134, 138, 140, 141, 145, 146] Using data from earlier autopsy series, the average time from symptom onset to death was projected to be 2 years for patients with exertional syncope, 3 years for patients with heart failure symptoms, and 5 years for those with angina.[79, 81–85] Later studies do not support such clear distinctions in clinical outcome for patients with different symptoms and instead suggest that outcome is poor when any symptoms are present.

For adults with symptomatic aortic stenosis, predictors of survival are stenosis severity expressed as jet velocity or transaortic gradient, functional status, left ventricular systolic function, comorbid disease, and gender.[134] When symptoms of severe aortic stenosis are present, the prognosis is better with a higher gradient (or jet velocity), because a low gradient and transaortic velocity in the setting of severe valve narrowing indicate reduced forward cardiac output.

For symptomatic patients who refuse aortic

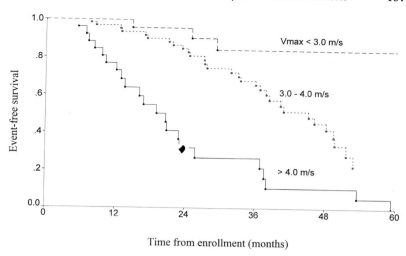

Figure 9·12 Cox regression analysis indicates event-free survival for 123 initially asymptomatic adults with valvular aortic stenosis, defined by aortic jet velocity at entry ($P < .001$ by log rank test). (From Otto CM, Burwash IG, Legget ME, et al: A prospective study of asymptomatic valvular aortic stenosis: clinical, echocardiographic, and exercise predictors of outcome. Circulation 1997;95:2262–2270; by permission of The American Heart Association.)

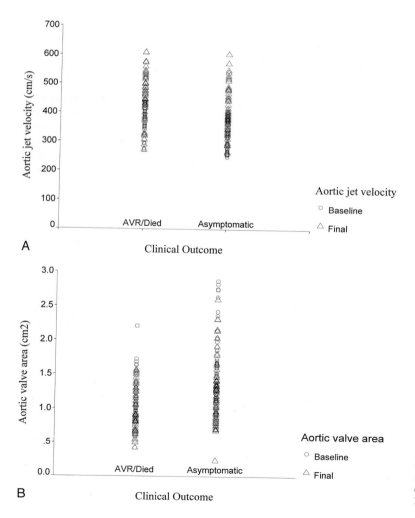

Figure 9·13 Clinical outcome, defined as the onset of symptoms requiring aortic valve replacement or producing death (AVR/Died) or as patients remaining free of symptoms (Asymptomatic), is plotted against two measures of aortic stenosis severity determined at the most recent echocardiographic examination: aortic jet velocity *(A)* and aortic valve area *(B)*. Although the group mean values are different, there is substantial overlap in jet velocity between symptomatic and asymptomatic patients. (Data from Otto CM, et al: Circulation 1997;95:2262–2270.)

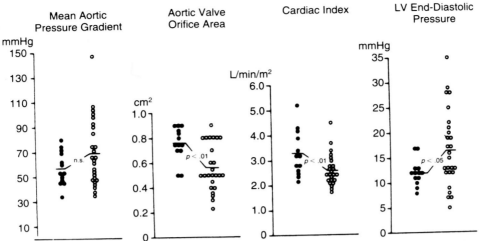

Figure 9·14 Hemodynamically severe aortic stenosis. Mean aortic pressure gradient, valve orifice area, cardiac index, and left ventricular (LV) end-diastolic pressure are plotted for severely symptomatic patients (open circle) and for asymptomatic or mildly symptomatic patients (solid circles). The mean value and statistical difference between groups are indicated (n.s., not significant). (From Turina J, Hess O, Sepulcri F, Krayenbuehl HP: Spontaneous course of aortic valve disease. Eur Heart J 1987;8:471–483.)

valve replacement, not only is survival short-ened, but quality of life is suboptimal. Often these patients have symptoms with minimal exertion or at rest, and many have recurrent hospital admissions for decompensated heart failure. Medical therapy, such as diuretics for acute pulmonary edema, may alleviate epi-sodes of acute decompensation but does not prevent recurrent episodes of decompensation or prolong life.

Rate of Hemodynamic Progression

Defining the rate of hemodynamic progres-sion of aortic stenosis during the phase before symptom onset offers the hope of predicting prognosis, identifying clinical factors associ-ated with disease progression, and increasing our understanding of the relationship between hemodynamic severity and symptom onset. Early studies were limited to describing the changes in hemodynamics observed between two clinically indicated cardiac catheteriza-tions. Despite concerns about sample size, potential selection bias, retrospective study design, and the availability of only two time points for these predominantly sympto-matic patients, these studies demonstrated that disease progression occurs slowly and varies considerably between individuals (Ta-ble 9–6).[147–152]

The availability of accurate, noninvasive Doppler measures of stenosis severity has ex-

panded our knowledge base with larger num-bers of patients. However, most of these stud-ies are retrospective, the patients' symptom status often is unclear, selection bias cannot be excluded, and only limited clinical data are available in published accounts of these studies.[57, 153–155] Even so, these studies show sim-ilar results, with an average decrease in valve area of about 0.1 cm²/year and an average increase in transaortic gradient of 6 to 7 mm Hg/year.

In a prospective study of 45 adults with aor-tic stenosis followed for a mean period of 1.5 years, aortic valve area decreased by 0.1 ± 0.13 cm²/year. The only clinical factor associ-ated with a faster rate of hemodynamic pro-gression was left ventricular systolic dysfunc-tion.[143] In a larger prospective study of 123 initially asymptomatic adults with valvular aor-tic stenosis (defined in both studies as a jet velocity ≥ 2.5 m/s) followed for 2.5 ± 1.4 years, jet velocity increased by 0.3 ± 0.3 m/s per year, mean gradient increased by 7 ± 7 mm Hg/year, and valve area decreased by 0.12 ± 0.19 cm²/year.[44] In general, the rate of he-modynamic progression is fairly linear, and the overall rate of change and the rate of change in the first year are not significantly different. However, it is possible that a more abrupt decrease in valve area occurs at the point where leaflet stiffness exceeds the capacity of ventricular ejection force to open the valve adequately, precipitating symptom onset, be-

TABLE 9·6 HEMODYNAMIC PROGRESS OF VALVULAR AORTIC STENOSIS FOR SELECTED STATES

Series	Clinical Status at Entry	Type of Study	Measurement Method	Patients	Mean Follow-Up Interval (y)	Increase in Mean ΔP* (mm Hg/y)	Increase in V_{max} (m/s/y)	Decrease in AVA* (cm²/y)
Bogart, 1979[147]	2 cardiac caths	Retrospective	Invasive	11	4.9	11.6 (1.2–24)		0.2 (0.02–0.6)
Cheitlin, 1979[148]	2 cardiac caths	Retrospective	Invasive	29	4	8.4 (−12–45)		
Wagner, 1982[149]	2 cardiac caths	Retrospective	Invasive	50	3.5			0.30 ± 0.08
Jonasson, 1983[150]	Calcific AS	Retrospective	Invasive	26	9			0.1
Nestico, 1983[151]	2 cardiac caths	Retrospective	Invasive	29	5.9	0.8 (−8–10.4)		0.05 (0–0.5)
Davies, 1991[152]	2 cardiac caths	Retrospective	Invasive	47		6.5 (−10–38)		
Otto, 1989[57]	Asymptomatic	Prospective	Doppler echo	42	1.7	7.9 ± 7.1	0.36 ± 0.31	0.1 (0–0.5)
Roger, 1990[153]	AS on echo	Retro cohort	Doppler echo	112	2.1		0.23 ± 0.37	
Faggiano, 1992[143]	AS on echo	Prospective	Doppler echo	45	1.5		0.4 ± 0.3	0.1 ± 0.13 (0.7–0.1)
Peter, 1993[154]	AS on echo	Retrospective	Doppler echo	49	2.7	7.2		
Brener, 1995[155]	AS on echo	Retrospective	Doppler echo	394	3.1	6.3		0.14
Otto, 1997[44]	Asymptomatic	Prospective	Doppler echo	123	2.5	7 ± 7	0.32 ± 0.34	0.12 ± 0.19

AS, aortic stenosis; ΔP, pressure gradient; V_{max}, maximum aortic jet velocity; AVA, aortic valve area; caths, catheterizations; echo, echocardiography; retro, retrospective.
*Mean (range).

cause there are no studies with periodic examinations that include repeat evaluation immediately before surgical intervention.

In all of these studies, despite a predictable and consistent average rate of hemodynamic progression, there is marked individual variability, with some persons showing little change over long periods and others having more rapid progression (Fig. 9–15). Despite individual variability, clinical factors that reliably predict the rate of hemodynamic progression have not been identified. A slight trend toward more rapid progression in patients with a trileaflet valve than in those with a bicuspid valve has been noted, but this observation may be confounded by the effect of patient age.[44] It is probable that the rate of disease progression is affected by other clinical factors, such as serum lipid levels and smoking, that would require a larger sample size to establish a relationship.[156]

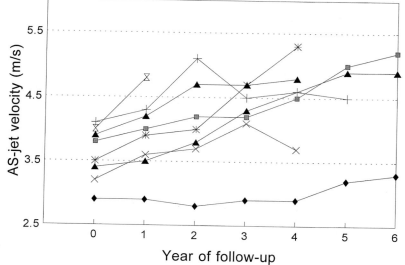

Figure 9·15 Examples of aortic stenosis (AS) jet velocity during prospective annual visits over a 6-year period for 8 patients with asymptomatic aortic stenosis demonstrate the marked individual variability in the rate of hemodynamic progression. (From Otto CM, Burwash IG, Legget ME, et al: A prospective study of asymptomatic valvular aortic stenosis: clinical, echocardiographic, and exercise predictors of outcome. Circulation 1997;95:2262–2270; by permission of The American Heart Association.)

Although aortic jet velocity alone is of great value in clinical decision making in adults with valvular aortic stenosis, calculation of valve area is essential for serial examinations. Typically, hemodynamic progression is manifested by an increase in jet velocity and a corresponding decrease in valve area. However, if there is an interim decrease in transaortic volume flow rate, there may be no interval change in jet velocity despite a substantial decrease in valve area. While significant systolic dysfunction of the left ventricle can be recognized in standard echocardiographic views, a reduction in transaortic volume flow rate caused by a slight reduction in ventricular volumes, diastolic dysfunction, or increased mitral regurgitation often is not evident on 2D imaging. Calculation of valve area with the continuity equation avoids this potential pitfall, allowing identification of a decrease in valve area associated with a decreased flow rate, an event that often shortly precedes symptom onset in my experience.

Coexisting Coronary Artery Disease

About 50% of adults undergoing valve replacement for aortic stenosis have significant coronary artery disease. The concurrence of valvular aortic stenosis and coronary artery disease complicates diagnosis and management of patients and complicates interpretation of outcome studies.

Clinical evaluation is hampered by the fact that angina may be caused by isolated aortic stenosis or by coexisting coronary artery disease. Only between 20% and 60% of patients with aortic stenosis and symptoms of angina have coronary disease, while 0% to 54% (mean, 16%) of those without angina also have significant coronary artery disease.[157] In the patient with previously asymptomatic aortic stenosis, it often is difficult to ascertain whether the onset of angina indicates severe valvular stenosis or is due to concurrent coronary artery disease. Noninvasive evaluation of aortic stenosis severity sometimes clarifies the issue, particularly if the degree of stenosis is severe, suggesting that valve replacement is needed, or only mild, suggesting that symptoms are not caused by valvular obstruction. When stenosis severity is intermediate, decision making is more difficult, especially given that symptoms can occur with a relatively wide range of stenosis severity. Coronary angiography often is needed to clarify the contribution

of coronary disease to symptoms in these patients.

In clinical studies of the natural history of aortic stenosis, it rarely is possible to separate outcomes due to coexisting coronary disease from those due to valvular obstruction because of the high rate of concordance for these diseases. Of the 4 cardiac deaths in a prospective study of 123 adults with asymptomatic aortic stenosis, 2 deaths were due to coexisting coronary artery disease, while the other 2 patients had severe aortic stenosis but refused valve replacement.[44]

Evaluation of coronary anatomy typically is performed just before planned surgical intervention. The operative mortality rate for patients with aortic stenosis and coexisting coronary artery disease ranges from 1.1% to 4.8% if coronary artery bypass grafting is performed at the time of valve replacement. If valve replacement alone is performed, operative mortality ranges from 4% to 13.2% in the setting of significant coronary disease, most likely related to inadequate myocardial blood flow immediately after cardiopulmonary bypass and in the early postoperative period.[139, 158] Thus, most clinicians perform coronary angiography before surgical intervention and perform coronary bypass grafting if significant coronary narrowings are present. Noninvasive tests generally are not helpful because the sensitivity is far less that 100% and since detailed coronary anatomy is needed for planning the surgical procedure when coronary disease is present.

MEDICAL THERAPY

In the asymptomatic patients with valvular aortic stenosis, medical therapy is directed toward prevention of complications, patient education, and prompt recognition of symptom onset. Once symptoms supervene, surgical intervention is needed to prolong life and relieve symptoms. Pharmacologic therapy alone is appropriate only for symptomatic patients who are not surgical candidates because of comorbid conditions or for those who refuse surgical intervention.

Noninvasive Follow-up

Echocardiographic evaluation is indicated at the time of diagnosis to confirm valvular stenosis, to quantitate disease severity, and to evaluate any coexisting lesions. Many patients with an aortic outflow murmur have no obstruction or only minimal sclerotic changes of the valve leaflets with only a minor increase in ante-grade velocity (<2.5 m/s). Because these patients do not have aortic stenosis, routine repeat examinations are unnecessary.

The differential diagnosis of a systolic murmur on physical examination includes hypertrophic cardiomyopathy and discrete subaortic stenosis, both of which are managed quite differently from valvular aortic stenosis. While the murmur of mitral regurgitation usually can be differentiated from aortic stenosis on auscultation, echocardiographic evaluation ensures that these lesions are not mistaken for each other.

After the initial diagnosis of aortic stenosis has been confirmed, the frequency of noninvasive follow-up is tailored to the disease severity and other clinical factors for each patient. Since the timing of surgical intervention is based on symptom onset, the most important parameters to follow are the patient's symptoms and functional status. Patient education regarding the typical symptoms of aortic stenosis allows prompt intervention as soon as symptoms occur. In addition, echocardiographic data can be used in conjunction with data on the average rate of hemodynamic progression to provide the patient with an estimated time window for symptom onset. Of course, the patient must be advised that individual variability occurs and that this estimate cannot provide a definite time point. Even so, the knowledge that symptom onset is likely within the next 2 to 3 years instead of 10 years, for example, is useful prognostic data.

Repeat echocardiographic examination is indicated for any change in clinical status and prior to major noncardiac procedures or events, such as pregnancy. In the absence of new symptoms, routine evaluation at annual intervals is appropriate for patients with moderate or severe stenosis (aortic jet velocity >3.0 m/s). With mild aortic stenosis (jet velocity 2.0 to 3.0 m/s), evaluation every 2 to 3 years is reasonable in the absence of any change in clinical status or physical examination findings. Because the rate of hemodynamic progression is relatively slow, echocardiography at less than 1-year intervals is rarely needed, unless there is reason to suspect underestimation of disease severity at the initial examination or the patient's clinical status changes substantially.

Prevention of Endocarditis

Patients with valvular aortic stenosis are at risk for endocarditis and should receive appro-priate antibiotic prophylaxis (see Chapter 6). The risk of endocarditis is especially high for patients with a bicuspid aortic valve, and extra efforts are needed to ensure these patients understand the risk of endocarditis and are provided with appropriate therapy.

Management During Periods of Hemodynamic Stress

Asymptomatic patients with severe valvular aortic stenosis undergoing noncardiac surgery are at risk for decompensation, with development of symptoms and potential hemodynamic instability. These concerns also apply to aortic stenosis patients with an intercurrent illness, particularly if accompanied by fever or anemia, and to the increased hemodynamic demands of pregnancy in a woman with aortic stenosis. Clinical decompensation in these situations is exacerbated by several factors, including changes in blood volume, fluid balance shifts, increased metabolic demands, decreased myocardial oxygen delivery, pain, and increased sympathetic system activity. Whenever possible, aortic stenosis severity should be evaluated prior to pregnancy or a surgical procedure. If stenosis is very severe, suggesting impending symptom onset, surgical relief of aortic stenosis before pregnancy or noncardiac surgery should be considered.

However, patients with asymptomatic, moderate aortic stenosis can successfully undergo noncardiac surgery or pregnancy if certain precautions are taken.[159, 160] First, echocardiographic evaluation of stenosis severity and left ventricular function is needed. Second, procedures are planned (eg, induction of labor rather than spontaneous labor) to allow invasive hemodynamic monitoring and to allow prevention or alleviation of pain (eg, using an epidural anesthetic for vaginal delivery). Third, invasive hemodynamic monitoring is used to optimize loading conditions during the procedure and in the postoperative period. It is especially important to continue monitoring postoperatively until fluid shifts have stabilized.

Using this approach, adults with aortic stenosis have undergone noncardiac surgery with an acceptable mortality and morbidity,[159] and women with aortic stenosis can undergo successful pregnancies with delivery of healthy infants, at a low maternal mortality and morbidity.[160, 161] The development of a second superimposed hemodynamic stress, such as a febrile illness during pregnancy in women with aortic stenosis, may tip the balance toward hemodynamic instability. In my experience, these patients usually can be managed with monitoring in the intensive care unit, but surgical intervention during pregnancy may be needed in extreme cases.[162, 163]

SURGICAL INTERVENTION AND POSTOPERATIVE OUTCOME

Operative Mortality and Long-Term Survival

Since the procedure became widely available in the 1960s, the operative mortality of valve replacement for aortic stenosis has decreased dramatically because of refinements in the operative procedure, improved myocardial preservation, earlier intervention, and better patient selection.[164] Contemporary series indicate an operative mortality rate ranging from 2.7% to 8.3% for adults younger than 70 years of age with isolated aortic stenosis (Table 9–7).[133, 165–169] Older adults have a higher operative mortality rate ranging from 2.7% to 16% for isolated aortic stenosis (Fig. 9–16).[133, 165, 167, 169–175]

Women tend to have a higher mortality rate for valve replacement for aortic stenosis. However, in one study, the difference in operative mortality rates for women and men (6% versus 2%) was not related to gender on multivariate analysis but instead was related to age, ejection fraction, coexisting coronary artery disease, and baseline functional class.[176]

When concurrent coronary artery bypass grafting is performed, operative mortality is higher, ranging from 4.4% to 12.8% for younger patients and from 8% to 21% for the elderly.[133, 165, 167, 169–175] However, operative mortality is doubled for patients with coexisting coronary disease who do not undergo concurrent bypass grafting,[133] most likely due to inadequate myocardial preservation of the hypertrophied ventricle. Thus, most surgeons perform concurrent coronary bypass grafting in adults with valvular aortic stenosis if angiography demonstrates significantly narrowed coronary arteries.

In a careful analysis separating the mortality related to aortic valve surgery from the expected "background" mortality based on age and gender, risk factors for excess mortality after aortic valve replacement are coronary artery disease, heart failure, atrial fibrillation, and previous myocardial infarction.[164] Risk factors for valve replacement identified in other clinical series of adults with aortic stenosis (Table 9–8) include age, previous coronary artery bypass grafting, emergency surgery, coronary

TABLE 9·7   AORTIC VALVE REPLACEMENT FOR AORTIC STENOSIS IN SELECTED STUDIES

Series	Age Group	Procedure	Patients	30-Day Op Mort	MI	Neurologic Events	Event-Free Survival
Craver, 1988[167]	Age <70 y	AVR	573	3.3%	2.6%	3.1%	
		AVR + CABG	251	5.2%	4.4%	2.8%	
	Age ≥70 y	AVR	188	10.1%	1.6%	5.3%	
		AVR + CABG	130	12.3%	7.7%	10.8%	
Fremes, 1989[133]	Age ≥70 y	AVR	110	2.7%			
		AVR + CABG	150	8.0%			
	Age <70 y	AVR	566	4.9%			
		AVR + CABG	212	3.3%			
Levinson, 1989[171]	Age ≥80 y	AVR ± CABG	64	9.4%			83 ± 5% at 1 y 67 ± 10% at 5 y
Freeman, 1991[170]	Age ≥80 y	AVR	45	11.1%			
		AVR + CABG	42	21.4%			
Culliford, 1991[172]	Age ≥80 y	AVR	35	5.7%	2.9%	0%	93.3% at 1 y
		AVR + CABG	36	19.4%	2.8%	2.8%	80.4% at 3 y
Azariades, 1991[173]	Age ≥80 y	AVR ± CABG	88	16%			64 ± 7% at 5 y
Olsson, 1992[169]	Age ≥80 y	AVR ± CABG	44	14%	7%	9%	73% at 2 y
	Age 65–75 y	AVR ± CABG	83	4%	5%	3%	90% at 2 y
Elayda, 1993[174]	Age ≥ 80 y	AVR	77	5.2%		11.1%	90.8% at 1 y
		AVR + CABG	75	24%			76% at 5 y
Logeais, 1994[175]	Age ≥75 y	AVR ± CABG	675	12.4%			
Connolly, 1997[208]	EF ≤ 35%	AVR ± CABG	154	9%			EF improved in 76%

AVR, aortic valve replacement; CABG, coronary artery bypass graft; MI, myocardial infarction; EF, ejection fraction; Op Mort, operative mortality.

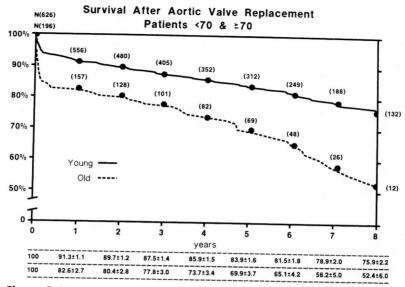

Figure 9·16 Survival curves for 1148 patients undergoing aortic valve replacement are provided for patients younger than 70 years of age *(solid line)* and for those 70 and older *(dashed line)*. (From Craver JM, Weintraub WS, Jones EL, Guyton RA, Hatcher CR Jr: Predictors of mortality, complications, and length of stay in aortic valve replacement for aortic stenosis. Circulation 1988;78(suppl I):85–90; by permission of The American Heart Association.)

artery disease, female gender, concurrent mitral valve surgery, hypertension, and left ventricular systolic dysfunction.[133, 167, 170, 174, 177, 178] In these series, older adults are variously identified as those older than 70, 75, or 80 years of age, and left ventricular systolic dysfunction typically is defined as an ejection fraction less than 45% or less than 50%.

In addition to a relatively high surgical mortality rate, aortic valve replacement in the elderly has a high rate of complications, including perioperative myocardial infarction in 3% to 8% and cerebrovascular events in up to 11% of patients.[133, 165, 167, 169–175] Complication rates are lower, but not negligible, for younger adults. Although some investigators suggest that elderly patients are more likely to have a prolonged hospitalization, require more extensive rehabilitation, and require interim or long-term skilled nursing care, a case-control study of younger and older adults found no difference in use of hospital resources between these age groups.[169]

Overall survival after valve replacement for aortic stenosis is excellent for younger and older adults, with event-free survival rates close to the expected survival rates for age (see Table 9–7). Factors contributing to a less-than-perfect postoperative clinical course include prosthetic valve–related complications (eg, anticoagulation, endocarditis), suboptimal prosthetic valve hemodynamics, and persistent systolic or diastolic left ventricular dysfunction.

TABLE 9·8   PREDICTORS OF OUTCOME AFTER AORTIC VALVE REPLACEMENT FOR AORTIC STENOSIS

Age[133, 167, 169, 175]
Female gender[133, 173]
Emergent surgery[133, 167, 170, 173, 175]
Coronary artery disease[133, 164, 178]
Previous coronary artery bypass grafting surgery[168, 178, 206]
Hypertension[174]
Left ventricular dysfunction (ejection fraction <45% or 50%)[133, 170, 174]
Heart failure[164, 170, 175]
Atrial fibrillation[164, 175]
Concurrent mitral valve replacement or repair[133, 170, 174]
Renal failure[178]

Changes in Left Ventricular Geometry, Function, and Hypertrophy

Postoperative Intracavitary Obstruction

In a subset of aortic stenosis patients, dynamic midventricular outflow obstruction occurs in the early postoperative period (Fig. 9–17). Intracavitary obstruction is most likely

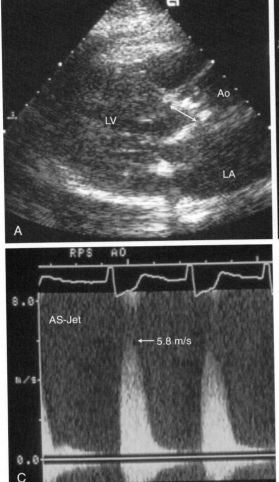

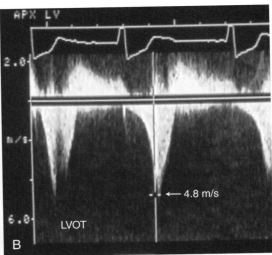

Figure 9·17 Echocardiographic examination of an elderly woman with calcific valvular aortic stenosis showing (A) outflow tract diameter (arrow) in a parasternal long-axis view. B, Concurrent severe left ventricular (LV) hypertrophy and hyperdynamic systolic function resulted in midcavity obliteration with a late peaking velocity (maximum, 4.8 m/s) at the midventricular level. C, The maximum jet velocity across the aortic valve, recorded from a right parasternal approach, was 5.8 m/s. Dynamic midcavity obstruction persisted in the early postoperative period but decreased as left ventricular hypertrophy regressed. Ao, aorta; LA, left atrium. LVOT, left ventricular outflow tract.

in patients with increased wall thickness, a small ventricular chamber, and preserved systolic function. With valve replacement, the acute decrease in left ventricular afterload results in hyperdynamic ventricular function with midcavity obliteration leading to obstruction on the basis of the ventricular walls being very close together. These patients do not have asymmetric septal hypertrophy, and systolic anterior motion of the mitral valve is seen only rarely. The late-peaking systolic velocity curve has a maximum velocity ranging from 1.8 to 6.8 m/s, corresponding to maximum gradients of 13 to 185 mm Hg.[179–181] The mean gradients corresponding to these maximum velocities are lower than those seen with valvular obstruction because of the late-peaking shape of the velocity curve with low velocities in early and mid-systole.

Dynamic outflow obstruction is more likely in the early postoperative period, being recognized in as many as 50% of patients when the study is performed immediately postoperatively, in as few as 14% of patients when echocardiography is performed within 10 days of surgery, and averaging about 25% of patients overall.[179–181] In patients without evidence for obstruction at rest, an intracavitary gradient can be induced in an additional 13% using nitroprusside or dobutamine infusion (or both) to decrease afterload and increase contractility.[181]

It is important to recognize dynamic intracavitary obstruction, as these patients often have significant hypotension and dyspnea due to impaired outflow from the small, hyperdynamic left ventricle. Prevention and treatment depend on maintaining an adequate preload and increasing (rather than decreasing as is common postoperatively) afterload. Patients with postoperative obstruction have a prolonged hospital course compared with patients without obstruction.[181] Some studies show no differences in 1-year survival rates,[181] while other studies suggest that excessive ventricular hypertrophy, specifically in women, is associated with increased postoperative mortality.[182]

Left Ventricular Systolic Function

Left ventricular ejection performance improves after aortic valve replacement because of the favorable effects of valve surgery on afterload. A small increase in ejection fraction occurs even in patients with a normal preoperative ejection fraction, and a dramatic increase in ejection fraction may be seen in patients with impaired systolic function at baseline.[183–186] Predictors of improvement in systolic function are female gender and less severe coronary artery disease.[176]

When preoperative ventricular function is normal, about 90% of patients have preserved systolic function postoperatively.[187] Ventricular ejection performance predictably improves after relief of aortic stenosis if the cause of impaired ventricular function was increased afterload due to valvular obstruction. Intraoperative transesophageal echocardiographic studies suggest that end-systolic wall stress decreases within 30 minutes of aortic valve replacement.[188] However, many adults with aortic stenosis have other reasons for ventricular dysfunction. Although some improvement still may be seen, the degree of improvement is minimal if changes in the myocardium are irreversible, for example, in patients with previous myocardial infarction or cardiomyopathy. In one study, predictors of the postoperative ejection fraction in patients with aortic stenosis were preoperative ejection fraction, history of myocardial infarction, lower aortic valve gradient, and incomplete coronary revascularization.[187] Of those with a preoperative ejection fraction less than 50%, two thirds still had left ventricular dysfunction postoperatively. In another study, women with an ejection fraction less than 45% preoperatively had greater improvement in ejection fraction after aortic valve replacement than men, with predictors of postoperative ejection fraction being gender and the extent of coronary artery disease.[176]

These data suggest that, despite pathophysiologic arguments that ventricular function should improve after surgery for aortic stenosis, it is preferable to operate before the onset of ventricular dysfunction.[139] While most aortic stenosis patients followed prospectively have definite symptoms before ventricular dysfunction is detected, rarely, the onset of left ventricular systolic dysfunction coincides with symptom onset. It is possible that more frequent evaluation may detect ventricular dysfunction before symptom onset, even though this sequence of events appears to be rare.

Regression of Left Ventricular Hypertrophy

Left ventricular hypertrophy gradually resolves after surgery for aortic stenosis, reaching a 43% total reduction in hypertrophy 8 years postoperatively, with two thirds of the regression occurring in the first 2 years.[53, 189–192] However, in most patients, some degree of left ventricular hypertrophy persists indefinitely after aortic valve replacement. The pathophysiology of persistent hypertrophy probably is multifactorial, with both permanent structural changes in the myocardium and the persistent, albeit less severe, outflow obstruction imposed by the prosthetic valve (Fig. 9–18). Some patients with baseline systolic dysfunction of the left ventricle (ejection fraction <50%) do not have regression of left ventricular hypertrophy postoperatively.[193] Gender differences in the rate and extent of regression of left ventricular hypertrophy after relief of aortic stenosis have not been fully elucidated, but it is likely that the marked gender difference in left ventricular geometry and function seen preoperatively will be reflected in the postoperative period.

Persistent Diastolic Dysfunction Postoperatively

The muscular component of left ventricular hypertrophy resolves more rapidly than the fibrous component, so that early and up to 2 years after valve replacement, the proportion of fibrous tissue in the myocardium increases compared with the cellular content. This relative increase in fibrous tissue is associated with an increase in myocardial stiffness early after valve replacement and a decrease in early diastolic relaxation rate, concurrent with a reduction in the degree of left ventricular hypertrophy.[53, 194–198]

The interstitial fibrosis component of ventricular hypertrophy regresses slowly, so that the balance between muscular and nonmuscular tissue does not normalize until 6 to 7 years

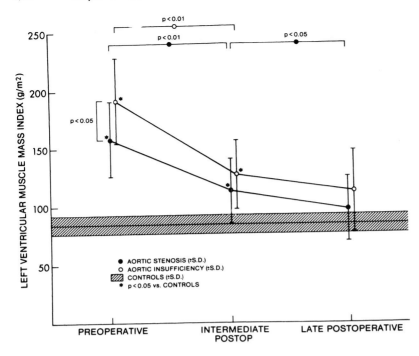

Figure 9·18 Left ventricular muscle mass index in patients with aortic stenosis preoperatively *(closed circles)* and in those with aortic insufficiency *(open circles)* preoperatively, at the intermediate postoperative study (1.6 ± 0.5 years), and late (8.1 ± 2 years) after aortic valve replacement. Although the greatest decrease in muscle mass index occurred 1 to 2 years after aortic valve surgery, significant further reductions continued to occur. (From Monrad ES, Hess OM, Murakami T, Nonogi H, Corin WJ, Krayenbuehl HP: Time course of regression of left ventricular hypertrophy after aortic valve replacement. Circulation 1988;77:1345–1355; by permission of The American Heart Association.)

after surgery. These ultrastructural changes of the myocardium are associated with a return toward normal of diastolic stiffness and relaxation.[53, 198] The prolonged persistence of diastolic dysfunction after surgery for aortic stenosis has significant clinical implications in terms of exercise capacity and functional status.[199] As surgical approaches to aortic stenosis improve in the future, the question as to whether surgery should be performed earlier in the disease course to prevent diastolic dysfunction will need to be addressed.

Exercise Capacity and Functional Status

There have been few comparisons of preoperative and postoperative functional status or exercise tolerance in adults with aortic stenosis. Nearly all patients have resolution of symptoms of angina, syncope, dizziness, or overt heart failure in the absence of coexisting left ventricular dysfunction or uncorrected coronary artery disease. Most patients also report an improvement in functional class, with all 6-month survivors in a series of patients older than 80 years being in New York Heart Association class I or II.[169, 200] In another series of patients older than 70 years, self-reported functional status improved significantly with predictors of improvement, including smoking, female gender, age, and the severity of comorbid disease.[201]

In a prospective study of 34 patients undergoing valve replacement for aortic stenosis, although left ventricular systolic function improved and left ventricular mass decreased, there was no objective improvement in treadmill exercise performance at 8 and 20 months after surgery.[183] Persistent diastolic dysfunction may account for the lack of improvement in exercise tolerance of these patients, as parameters of diastolic filling did not change. Results of another study suggest that exercise tolerance after aortic valve replacement is related to functional valve area.[202]

Timing of Surgical Intervention

Symptom Onset

Surgical intervention for aortic stenosis is indicated at symptom onset in adults given the dramatic improvement in survival with surgical intervention compared to medical therapy. Valve replacement can be deferred in asymptomatic adults, as survival and clinical outcome are excellent without surgical intervention. The only clinical difficulty with this approach is defining at what point the patient can be considered symptomatic.

Symptom onset in adults is so gradual that many patients fail to recognize early symptoms and first present for medical attention with a syncopal episode, frank congestive heart failure, or unstable angina. These patients clearly need surgical intervention. In contrast, patients followed prospectively who are educated about the possible symptoms tend to present with a history of gradually decreasing exercise tolerance and increasing exertional dyspnea that is elicited only by focused and detailed questions. Physical examination typically shows severe aortic stenosis but fails to reveal evidence of hemodynamic decompensation. Thus, it often is unclear whether these patients are truly symptomatic or whether these nonspecific symptoms result from age, intercurrent illness, or comorbid conditions.

In general, if severe aortic stenosis is detected by echocardiography or catheterization, even mild symptoms should be attributed to aortic stenosis, and the patient should be referred promptly for surgical intervention. Support for this approach includes natural history studies showing the high rate of symptom onset and death with Doppler evidence of severe stenosis such that, even if surgery is deferred initially, the patient is likely to develop more severe symptoms requiring surgical intervention within a relatively short time period.[44, 203, 204] Surgical intervention for mild symptoms is also supported by evidence that systolic dysfunction may be irreversible in some aortic stenosis patients and that nearly all patients have significant diastolic dysfunction that persists for several years after valve replacement. Some investigators suggest that even earlier intervention is needed (eg, in asymptomatic patients) to prevent the secondary left ventricular changes of this disease process.[139]

Surgical Intervention in the Elderly

As shown in Table 9–7, although surgical mortality is higher for elderly patients, life expectancy still is significantly prolonged after valve replacement. When considering surgical intervention in elderly patients, it is helpful to consult age-adjusted life tables so that expected survival after surgery (similar to age-matched adults without aortic stenosis) can be compared with the expected survival without surgical intervention. Since symptomatic aortic stenosis has such a high mortality rate without surgery, valve replacement remains the procedure of choice even in octogenarians. In an elegant decision-analysis model, Wong and colleagues[205] used the example of an 87-year-old women with severe symptomatic aortic stenosis, coronary artery disease, and depressed left ventricular systolic function to show that

life expectancy would be 5.1 years with valve replacement and bypass grafting versus 1.6 years with medical therapy.

Surgical intervention also improves quality of life, since elderly patients who refuse surgical intervention typically have recurrent hospital admissions for heart failure and have a very limited exercise tolerance and functional status between hospitalizations. The use of quality-adjusted life-years (QALYs) in the decision model described above highlights this point, showing a QALY of 5.0 years with surgery versus 1.1 years with medical therapy.[205]

Aortic Valve Replacement After Previous Coronary Artery Bypass Surgery

Given that many patients with aortic stenosis also have significant coronary artery disease, it is not surprising that surgical intervention sometimes is required for coronary disease before the development of severe valvular obstruction. Subsequent progression of stenosis severity then leads to the need for aortic valve surgery at a later date in many of these patients. Unfortunately, the operative mortality rate for aortic valve replacement in patients with previous cardiac surgery is very high (14% to 30%), although long-term outcome is more promising, with a 5-year survival rate of approximately 75%.[168, 178]

One study with a long interval (9 years) between the two surgical procedures reported there was no evidence of aortic stenosis at the time of the initial procedure.[178] However, in a study with a shorter interval (6 years) between surgeries, evidence of mild to moderate aortic stenosis was present at the time of the first procedure in many patients.[206] These observations have generated controversy about the role of aortic valve replacement for mild to moderate aortic stenosis in patients undergoing coronary bypass procedures. The rationale for not replacing the aortic valve is based on the hypothesis that disease progression is slow and does not occur in all patients so that valve surgery may never be needed or can be deferred to a much later date. The rationale for "prophylactic" replacement of the aortic valve is that disease progression is inevitable and that a second surgical intervention will be needed at a predictable time, depending on baseline stenosis severity. Studies on the natural history of mild to moderate aortic stenosis support the latter of these two rationales and suggest that prophylactic valve replacement be considered when the aortic valve is anatomically abnormal and the antegrade velocity is increased. The rate of hemodynamic progression in specific subgroups appears to be predictable, even though there is some variability in the individual rate of progression.[44, 143]

In asymptomatic patients with an anatomically abnormal aortic valve and an aortic jet velocity greater than 4.0 m/s, almost 80% need aortic valve replacement within 2 years, suggesting that valve surgery at the time of coronary artery surgery is appropriate to prevent early reoperation. In asymptomatic patients with a jet velocity of 3 to 4 m/s, the rate of valve replacement still is high, with about 40% requiring valve surgery by 2 years and nearly 80% needing surgery within 5 years. For this group, the decision about prophylactic valve replacement should be individualized, depending on the jet velocity within this range, the anatomic appearance of the valve on 2D echocardiography and on fluoroscopy, and other clinical factors, such as age, comorbid disease, and patient preference. When aortic sclerosis is present but the jet velocity is less than 3.0 m/s, it is appropriate to defer valvular intervention, as the rate of symptom development is considerably slower, being only 16% at 2 years.

This approach will need to be refined as additional data on the natural history of mild to moderate aortic stenosis become available and also will need to be modified as improved surgical procedures for aortic stenosis are developed. Since the major reasons to postpone valve replacement in a patient already undergoing cardiac surgery include the increased operative risk, the complications and inconvenience of long-term anticoagulation, suboptimal prosthetic valve hemodynamics, and the risk of prosthetic valve dysfunction or infection; improvements in any of these factors may tip the balance toward earlier intervention. Conversely, the use of minimally invasive surgical approaches may argue against performing valve surgery until it is absolutely necessary, because the coronary and valve procedures are performed from different approaches. In any case, a history of aortic valve disease or a pathologic murmur found on auscultation mandates careful evaluation of valve anatomy and function in the patient undergoing coronary artery surgery. When Doppler echocardiography shows moderate or severe disease, concurrent aortic valve surgery should be considered.

Aortic Valve Replacement in Patients With Left Ventricular Dysfunction

Left ventricular systolic dysfunction is a risk factor for operative mortality with valve replacement for aortic stenosis; elderly patients with an ejection fraction of less than 20% have a threefold higher mortality rate (15% versus 6%) than those with an ejection fraction of more than 60%.[133] However, clinical outcome is even worse without surgical intervention; the 12-month survival rate is only 20% to 50% for adults with aortic stenosis and severely reduced left ventricular systolic function (Fig. 9–19).[134] When left ventricular systolic dysfunction is caused by increased afterload with normal myocardial contractility, systolic function is expected to improve after relief of outflow obstruction. Even with superimposed myocardial dysfunction, ventricular ejection performance should improve because of the afterload-reducing effect of valve replacement.[207] In a recent series of 154 patients with severe aortic stenosis and an ejection fraction less than or equal to 35%, the operative mortality rate was only 9%. Even though over 50% of these patients had concurrent coronary artery bypass grafting, most had improved ejection fractions and decreased symptoms after surgical intervention.[208]

Type of Intervention
Valve Replacement

Aortic valve replacement with a mechanical or biologic valve remains the standard treat-

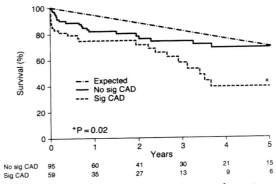

Figure 9·19 Kaplan-Meier survival curves for patients with aortic stenosis and reduced left ventricular function, with and without significant coronary artery disease (sig CAD; ie, two-vessel disease or greater or left main coronary disease) compared with expected survival. The number of patients alive at each point is shown on the x axis. (From Connolly HM, Oh JK, Orszulak TA, et al: Aortic valve replacement for aortic stenosis with severe left ventricular dysfunction: prognostic indicators. Circulation 1997; 95:2395–2400; by permission of The American Heart Association.)

ment for severe symptomatic aortic stenosis. The choice of valve substitute is based on durability of the valve compared with the patient's expected longevity, the risks of chronic anticoagulation, and the expected hemodynamics for the valve size in the patient (see Chapters 8 and 17).

In the young patient (<50 years), the pulmonic autograft procedure may be considered.[209] Another alternative is a homograft valve, particularly when there is evidence of active infection, in a young woman desiring a subsequent pregnancy, or in the patient with a definite contraindication to chronic anticoagulation. Children and young adults may benefit from percutaneous balloon aortic valvuloplasty, as discussed later. In other cases, mechanical valves are preferred because of their proven durability.

In the elderly patient, stented bioprosthetic valves were frequently used in the past based on the assumption that valve failure would not occur within the patient's expected lifespan and the risks of anticoagulation could be avoided. Some evidence suggests that bioprosthetic valve calcification occurs more slowly in older patients.[210–212] However, the life expectancy for many older patients now exceeds the expected durability of stented bioprosthetic valves. In addition, the smaller stented bioprosthetic valves have suboptimal hemodynamics, which is a particular problem in elderly women, who often have a small aortic root. The added risk of a root-enlarging procedure if a bioprosthetic valve is used may outweigh the risk of chronic anticoagulation with a mechanical valve.

Newer stentless bioprosthetic valves offer the possibility of improved hemodynamics and durability compared with conventional stented valves.[213–216] These valves may become the valve of choice in the elderly patient with aortic stenosis as we gain further experience with optimal surgical implantation and long-term outcome.

The relative risks and benefits of mechanical or bioprosthetic valves were evaluated in a series of elderly patients (>70 years) undergoing valve replacement for aortic stenosis.[217] The operative risks (6.6%) and 5-year survival rates (65%) are similar, and the rates of thromboembolic events, endocarditis, and hemorrhage were not different with the two valve types.[217] Although prosthetic valve failure required reoperation for 2% of bioprosthetic valves, there were no structural failures with the mechanical valves. These data suggest that mechanical

valve replacement should be considered, even in the elderly, although the final choice of valve type must be tailored to each patient.

Percutaneous Balloon Valvuloplasty

Despite initial enthusiasm in the late 1980s and early 1990s that balloon dilation of the aortic valve would relieve outflow obstruction, it has become clear that this procedure offers little benefit for adults with calcific aortic stenosis or with secondary calcification of a bicuspid valve. Even though randomized trials were not performed, in several large series of adults undergoing balloon aortic valvuloplasty, it was evident that the mortality rate was not different from that for untreated aortic stenosis, with 1-year actuarial mortality rates of 35% to 50%.[134, 218–228] In a study of 165 patents with 6-year follow-up after balloon aortic valvuloplasty, 93% had died or undergone aortic valve replacement, emphasizing the ineffectiveness of this procedure.[229] In those who underwent subsequent aortic valve replacement, survival was 84%, underlining the importance of valve replacement for treatment of symptomatic aortic stenosis in adults.

Balloon aortic valvuloplasty now is reserved for children and young adults with congenital aortic stenosis, and it may be the initial procedure of choice for this patient group. The success rate of balloon valvuloplasty in children is about 95%, with a procedural mortality rate less than 2% and an average reduction in transaortic gradient by 60%.[230, 231] Predictors of a suboptimal outcome include age younger than 3 months, coexisting unrepaired aortic coarctation, and a higher baseline transaortic gradient. In addition, results are optimal when the ratio of balloon to valve annulus diameter is 0.9 to 1.0.[231] Hemodynamic results after balloon valvotomy are similar to those for surgical valvotomy in children.[232] Long-term outcome is excellent, with a survival rate of 95% at 8 years after the procedure. However, because 25% to 50% of patients require repeat intervention for residual stenosis or progressive regurgitation at 8 to 9 years of follow-up,[233–235] continued noninvasive monitoring is needed after the procedure. In young adults, successful balloon valvotomy may allow deferral of surgical intervention to a later date, particularly in young women planning to have children.

Valve-Sparing Procedures for Aortic Stenosis

In children and young adults, surgical valvotomy can be used to open the commissures of a congenitally stenotic valve. The initial hemo-dynamic results and symptom relief are excel-lent with surgical valvotomy in children and young adults.[236–238] Only rare cases of aortic insufficiency are seen after careful surgical val-votomy in children.[239, 240] However, restenosis occurs in 20% to 35% of patients and requires reoperation at a mean interval of 15 to 20 years after the initial procedure.[137, 138, 238, 241, 242]

Approaches to valve preservation in adults with calcific stenosis of a trileaflet valve or calcification superimposed on a bicuspid valve have been less successful. Mechanical debride-ment of the valve at surgery results in an acute increase in leaflet flexibility, but rapid resteno-sis occurs within 4 years.[243–246] Ultrasonic de-bridement of the valve under direct vision also is promising in theory, and the degree of valve opening improves in the short term. How-ever, severe aortic regurgitation occurs in 26% and moderate aortic regurgitation in an addi-tional 37% by only 9 months after the proce-dure.[247, 248] Pathologic examination after ultra-sonic debridement shows leaflet fibrosis, thickening, and retraction with progressive central regurgitation.[249]

These results are not surprising in view of histologic studies of end-stage calcific aortic stenosis that demonstrate thinning and attenu-ation of the normal valve fibrosa in regions underlying the lipocalcific masses on the aor-tic side of the leaflet. After debridement, little normal tissue would be left. In view of the histopathology of calcific aortic stenosis, it is unlikely that valve-sparing procedures will ever be successful for end-stage calcific aortic valve disease.

References

1. Pasipoularides A: Clinical assessment of ventricular ejection dynamics with and without outflow obstruc-tion. J Am Coll Cardiol 1990;15:859–882.
2. Clark C: Relation between pressure difference across the aortic valve and left ventricular outflow. Cardiovasc Res 1978;12:276–287.
3. Hegrenaes L, Hatle L: Aortic stenosis in adults. Non-invasive estimation of pressure differences by continuous wave Doppler echocardiography. Br Heart J 1985;54:396–404.
4. Galan A, Zoghbi WA, Quinones MA: Determination of severity of valvular aortic stenosis by Doppler echocardiography and relation of findings to clini-cal outcome and agreement with hemodynamic measurements determined at cardiac catheteriza-tion. Am J Cardiol 1991;67:1007–1012.
5. Yeager M, Yock PG, Popp RL: Comparison of Dop-pler-derived pressure gradient to that determined at cardiac catheterization in adults with aortic valve ste-nosis: implications for management. Am J Cardiol 1986;57:644–648.
6. Otto CM, Pearlman AS: Doppler echocardiography in adults with symptomatic aortic stenosis: diagnos-tic utility and cost-effectiveness. Arch Intern Med 1988;148:2553–2560.
7. Harrison MR, Gurley JC, Smith MD, Grayburn PA, DeMaria AN: A practical application of Doppler echocardiography for the assessment of severity of aortic stenosis. Am Heart J 1988;115:622–628.
8. Hatle L, Angelsen A, Tromsdal A: Non-invasive as-sessment of aortic stenosis by Doppler ultrasound. Br Heart J 1980;43:284–292.
9. Currie PJ, Seward JB, Reeder GS, Vlietstra RE, Bres-nahan DR, Bresnahan JF, Smith HC, Hagler DJ, Tajik AJ: Continuous-wave Doppler echocardio-graphic assessment of severity of calcific aortic ste-nosis: a simultaneous Doppler-catheter correlative study in 100 adult patients. Circulation 1985;71:1162–1169.
10. Callahan MJ, Tajik AJ, Su-Fan Q, Bove AA: Valida-tion of instantaneous pressure gradients measured by continuous-wave Doppler in experimentally in-duced aortic stenosis. Am J Cardiol 1985;56:989–993.
11. Otto CM, Nishimura RA, Davis KB, Kisslo KB, Ba-shore TM, Balloon Valvuloplasty Registry Echocardi-ographers: Doppler echocardiographic findings in adults with severe symptomatic valvular aortic steno-sis. Am J Cardiol 1991;68:1477–1484.
12. Rozenman Y, Gotsman MS: Heart rate influence on the systolic gradient across the stenotic aortic valve: theoretical evaluation and implications. Cathet Cardiovasc Diagn 1985;11:533–538.
13. Otto CM, Pearlman AS, Kraft CD, Miyake-Hull CY, Burwash IG, Gardner CJ: Physiologic changes with maximal exercise in asymptomatic valvular aortic stenosis assessed by Doppler echocardiography. J Am Coll Cardiol 1992;20:1160–1167.
14. Levine RA, Cape EG, Yoganathan AP: Pressure re-covery distal to stenoses: expanding clinical applica-tions of engineering principles. J Am Coll Cardiol 1993;21:1026–1028.
15. Voelker W, Reul H, Stelzer T, Schmidt A, Karsch KR: Pressure recovery in aortic stenosis: an in vitro study in a pulsatile flow model. J Am Coll Cardiol 1992;20:1585–1593.
16. Laskey WK, Kussmaul WG: Pressure recovery in aor-tic valve stenosis. Circulation 1994;89:116–121.
17. Levine RA, Jimoh A, Cape EG, McMillan S, Yogana-than AP, Weyman AE: Pressure recovery distal to a stenosis: potential cause of gradient "overestima-tion" by Doppler echocardiography. J Am Coll Cardiol 1989;13:706–715.
18. Heinrich RS, Fontaine AA, Grimes RY, et al: Experi-mental analysis of fluid mechanical energy losses in aortic valve stenosis: importance of pressure recov-ery. Ann Biomed Eng 1996;24:685–694.
19. Otto CM, Pearlman AS, Comess KA, Reamer RP, Janko CL, Huntsman LL: Determination of the ste-notic aortic valve area in adults using Doppler echo-cardiography. J Am Coll Cardiol 1986;7:509–517.
20. Zoghbi WA, Farmer KL, Soto JG, Nelson JG, Qui-nones MA: Accurate noninvasive quantification of stenotic aortic valve area by Doppler echocardiogra-phy. Circulation 1986;73:452–459.
21. Grayburn PA, Smith MD, Harrison MR, Gurley JC, DeMaria AN: Pivotal role of aortic valve area calcula-tion by the continuity equation for Doppler assess-ment of aortic stenosis in patients with combined aortic stenosis and regurgitation. Am J Cardiol 1988;61:376–381.

22. Teirstein P, Yeager M, Yock PG, Popp RL: Doppler echocardiographic measurement of aortic valve area in aortic stenosis: a noninvasive application of the Gorlin formula. J Am Coll Cardiol 1986;8:1059–1065.

23. Ohlsson J, Wranne B: Noninvasive assessment of valve area in patients with aortic stenosis. J Am Coll Cardiol 1986;7:501–508.

24. Gorlin R, Gorlin SG: Hydraulic formula for calculation of the area of the stenotic mitral valve, other cardiac valves, and central circulatory shunts. Am Heart J 1951;41:1–29.

25. Cannon SR, Richards KL, Crawford MH, et al: Inadequacy of the Gorlin formula for predicting prosthetic valve area. Am J Cardiol 1988;62:113–116.

26. Cannon SR, Richards KL, Crawford MH: Hydraulic estimation of stenotic orifice area: a correction of the Gorlin formula. Circulation 1985;71:1170–1178.

27. Richards KL, Cannon SR, Miller JF, Crawford MH: Calculation of aortic valve area by Doppler echocardiography: a direct application of the continuity equation. Circulation 1986;73:964–969.

28. Segal J, Lerner DJ, Miller DC, Mitchell RS, Alderman EA, Popp RL: When should Doppler-determined valve area be better than the Gorlin formula? Variation in hydraulic constants in low flow states. J Am Coll Cardiol 1987;9:1294–1305.

29. Dumesnil JG, Yoganathan AP: Theoretical and practical differences between the Gorlin formula and the continuity equation for calculating aortic and mitral valve areas. Am J Cardiol 1991;67:1268–1272.

30. Gorlin R, Gorlin WB: Further reconciliation between pathoanatomy and pathophysiology of stenotic cardiac valves. J Am Coll Cardiol 1990;15:1181–1182.

31. Cochrane T, Kenyon CJ, Lawford PV, Black MM, Chambers JB, Springings DC: Validation of the orifice formula for estimating effective heart valve opening area. Clin Phys Physiol Meas 1991;12:21–37.

32. Montarello JK, Perakis AC, Rosenthal E, et al: Normal and stenotic human aortic valve opening: in vitro assessment of orifice area changes with flow. Eur Heart J 1990;11:484–491.

33. Bache RJ, Wang Y, Jorgensen CR: Hemodynamic effects of exercise in isolated valvular aortic stenosis. Circulation 1971;44:1003–1013.

34. Tardif JC, Rodrigues AG, Hardy JF, et al: Simultaneous determination of aortic valve area by the Gorlin formula and by transesophageal echocardiography under different transvalvular flow conditions. Evidence that anatomic aortic valve area does not change with variations in flow in aortic stenosis. J Am Coll Cardiol 1997;29:1296–1302.

35. Badano L, Cassottano P, Bertoli D, Carratino L, Lucatti A, Spirito P: Changes in effective aortic valve area during ejection in adults with aortic stenosis. Am J Cardiol 1996;78:1023–1028.

36. Bermejo J, Garcia Fernandez MA, Torrecilla EG, et al: Effects of dobutamine on Doppler echocardiographic indexes of aortic stenosis. J Am Coll Cardiol 1996;28:1206–1213.

37. Burwash IG, Thomas DD, Sadahiro M, et al: Dependence of Gorlin formula and continuity equation valve areas on transvalvular volume flow rate in valvular aortic stenosis. Circulation 1994;89:827–835.

38. Burwash IG, Pearlman AS, Kraft CD, Miyake-Hull C, Healy NL, Otto CM: Flow dependence of measures of aortic stenosis severity during exercise. J Am Coll Cardiol 1994;24:1342–1350.

39. Casale PN, Palacios IF, Abascal VM, et al: Effects of dobutamine on Gorlin and continuity equation valve areas and valve resistance in valvular aortic stenosis. Am J Cardiol 1992;70:1175–1179.

40. Chambers JB, Springings DC, Cochrane T, et al: Continuity equation and Gorlin formula compared with directly observed orifice area in native and prosthetic aortic valves. Br Heart J 1992;67:193–199.

41. Cannon JDJ, Zile MR, Crawford FAJ, Carabello BA: Aortic valve resistance as an adjunct to the Gorlin formula in assessing the severity of aortic stenosis in symptomatic patients. J Am Coll Cardiol 1992;20:1517–1523.

42. Ford LE, Feldman T, Chiu YC, Carroll JD: Hemodynamic resistance as a measure of functional impairment in aortic valvular stenosis. Circ Res 1990;66:1–7.

43. Voelker W, Reul H, Neinhaus G, et al: Comparison of valvular resistance, stroke work loss, and Gorlin valve area for quantification of aortic stenosis: an in vitro study in a pulsatile aortic flow model. Circulation 1995;91:1196–1204.

44. Otto CM, Burwash IG, Legget ME, et al: A prospective study of asymptomatic valvular aortic stenosis: clinical, echocardiographic, and exercise predictors of outcome. Circulation 1997;95:2262–2270.

45. Springings DC, Chambers JB, Cochrane T, Allen J, Jackson G: Ventricular stroke work loss: validation of a method of quantifying the severity of aortic stenosis and derivation of an orifice formula. J Am Coll Cardiol 1990;16:1608–1614.

46. Tobin JR, Rahimtoola SH, Blundell PE, Swan HJC: Percentage of left ventricular stoke work loss: a simple hemodynamic concept for estimation of severity in valvular aortic stenosis. Circulation 1967;35:868–874.

47. Laskey WK, Kussmaul WG, Noordergraaf A: Valvular and systemic arterial hemodynamics in aortic valve stenosis: a model-based approach. Circulation 1995;92:1473–1478.

48. Carroll JD, Carroll EP, Feldman T, et al: Sex-associated differences in left ventricular function in aortic stenosis of the elderly. Circulation 1992;86:1099–1107.

49. Douglas PS, Otto CM, Mickel MC, Labovitz A, Reid CL, Davis KB: Gender differences in left ventricular geometry and function in patients undergoing balloon dilation of the aortic valve for isolated aortic stenosis. Br Heart J 1995;73:548–554.

50. Aurigemma GP, Silver KH, McLaughlin M, Mauser J, Gaasch WH: Impact of chamber geometry and gender on left ventricular systolic function in patients >60 years of age with aortic stenosis. Am J Cardiol 1994;74:794–798.

51. Legget ME, Kuusisto J, Healy NL, Fujioka M, Schwaegler RG, Otto CM: Gender differences in left ventricular function at rest and with exercise in asymptomatic aortic stenosis. Am Heart J 1996;131:94–100.

52. Jin XY, Pepper JR, Gibson DG: Effects of incoordination on left ventricular force-velocity relation in aortic stenosis. Heart 1996;76:495–501.

53. Villari B, Campbell SE, Schneider J, Vassalli G, Chiariello M, Hess OM: Sex-dependent differences in left ventricular function and structure in chronic pressure overload. Eur Heart J 1995;16:1410–1419.

54. Douglas PS, Berko B, Lesh M, Reichek N: Alterations in diastolic function in response to progressive left ventricular hypertrophy. J Am Coll Cardiol 1989;13:461–467.

55. Villari B, Campbell SE, Hess OM, et al: Influence of collagen network on left ventricular systolic and diastolic function in aortic valve disease. J Am Coll Cardiol 1993;22:1477–1484.

56. Villari B, Vassalli G, Schneider J, Chiariello M, Hess OM: Age dependency of left ventricular diastolic function in pressure overload hypertrophy. J Am Coll Cardiol 1997;29:181–186.

57. Otto CM, Pearlman AS, Amsler LC: Doppler echocardiographic evaluation of left ventricular diastolic filling in isolated valvular aortic stenosis. Am J Cardiol 1989;63:313–316.

58. Vanoverschelde JL, Essamri B, Michel X, et al: Hemodynamic and volume correlates of left ventricular diastolic relaxation and filling in patients with aortic stenosis. J Am Coll Cardiol 1992;20:813–821.

59. Gallino RA, Milner MR, Goldstein SA, Pichard AD, Majchrzak C, Lindsay JJ: Left ventricular filling patterns in aortic stenosis in patients older than 65 years of age. Am J Cardiol 1989;63:1103–1106.

60. Folland ED, Parisi AF, Carbone C: Is peripheral arterial pressure a satisfactory substitute for ascending aortic pressure when measuring aortic valve gradients? J Am Coll Cardiol 1984;4:1207–1212.

61. Tracy GP, Proctor MS, Hizny CS: Reversibility of pulmonary artery hypertension in aortic stenosis after aortic valve replacement. Ann Thorac Surg 1990;50:89–93.

62. Snopek G, Pogorzelska H, Zielinski T, et al: Valve replacement for aortic stenosis with severe congestive heart failure and pulmonary hypertension. J Heart Valve Dis 1996;5:268–272.

63. Aragam JR, Folland ED, Lapsley D, Sharma S, Khuri SF, Sharma GV: Cause and impact of pulmonary hypertension in isolated aortic stenosis on operative mortality for aortic valve replacement in men. Am J Cardiol 1992;69:1365–1367.

64. Kaufmann P, Vassalli G, Lupi Wagner S, Jenni R, Hess OM: Coronary artery dimensions in primary and secondary left ventricular hypertrophy. J Am Coll Cardiol 1996;28:745–750.

65. Villari B, Hess OM, Kaufmann P, Krogmann ON, Grimm J, Krayenbuehl HP: Effect of aortic valve stenosis (pressure overload) and regurgitation (volume overload) on left ventricular systolic and diastolic function. Am J Cardiol 1992;69:927–934.

66. Marcus ML, Doty DB, Hiratzka LF, Wright CB, Eastham CL: Decreased coronary reserve: a mechanism for angina pectoris in patients with aortic stenosis and normal coronary arteries. N Engl J Med 1982;307:1362–1366.

67. Nadell R, DePace NL, Ren JF, Hakki AH, Iskandrian AS, Morganroth J: Myocardial oxygen supply/demand ratio in aortic stenosis: hemodynamic and echocardiographic evaluation of patients with and without angina pectoris. J Am Coll Cardiol 1983;2:258–262.

68. Julius BK, Spillmann M, Vassalli G, Villari B, Eberli FR, Hess OM: Angina pectoris in patients with aortic stenosis and normal coronary arteries: mechanisms and pathophysiological concepts. Circulation 1997;95:892–898.

69. Gould KL: Why angina pectoris in aortic stenosis? Circulation 1997;95:790–792.

70. Kenny A, Wisbey CR, Shapiro LM: Profiles of coronary blood flow velocity in patients with aortic stenosis and the effect of valve replacement: a transthoracic echocardiographic study. Br Heart J 1994;71:57–62.

71. Omran H, Fehske W, Rabahieh R, Hagendorff A, Luderitz B: Relation between symptoms and profiles of coronary artery blood flow velocities in patients with aortic valve stenosis: a study using transoesophageal Doppler echocardiography. Heart 1996;75:377–383.

72. Isaaz K, Bruntz JF, Paris D, Ethevenot G, Aliot E: Abnormal coronary flow velocity pattern in patients with left ventricular hypertrophy, angina pectoris, and normal coronary arteries: a transesophageal Doppler echocardiographic study. Am Heart J 1994;128:500–510.

73. Petropoulakis PN, Kyriakidis MK, Tentolouris CA, Kourouclis CV, Toutouzas PK: Changes in phasic coronary blood flow velocity profile in relation to changes in hemodynamic parameters during stress in patients with aortic valve stenosis. Circulation 1995;92:1437–1447.

74. Smucker ML, Tedesco CL, Manning SB, Owen RM, Feldman MD: Demonstration of an imbalance between coronary perfusion and excessive load as a mechanism of ischemia during stress in patients with aortic stenosis. Circulation 1988;78:573–582.

75. Anderson FL, Tsagaris TJ, Tikoff G, Thorne JL, Schmidt AM, Kuida H: Hemodynamic effects of exercise in patients with aortic stenosis. Am J Med 1969;46:872–885.

76. Martin TW, Moody JMJ, Bird JJ, Slife D, Murgo JP, Moody JM Jr: Effect of exercise on indices of valvular aortic stenosis. Cathet Cardiovasc Diagn 1992;25:265–271.

77. Ettinger PO, Frank MJ, Levison ME: Hemodynamic at rest and during exercise in combined aortic stenosis and insufficiency. Circulation 1972;45:267–276.

78. Movsowitz C, Kussmaul WG, Laskey WK: Left ventricular diastolic response to exercise in valvular aortic stenosis. Am J Cardiol 1996;77:275–280.

79. Bergerson J, Abelmann W, Vasquez-Milan H, Ellis L: Aortic stenosis: clinical manifestations and course of the disease. Arch Intern Med 1954;94:911–924.

80. Chizner MA, Pearle DL, deLeon JAC: The natural history of aortic stenosis in adults. Am Heart J 1980;99:419–424.

81. Frank S, Johnson A, Ross JJ: Natural history of valvular aortic stenosis. Br Heart J 1973;35:41–46.

82. Kumpe C, Bean W: Aortic stenosis: a study of the clinical and pathologic aspects of 107 proved cases. Medicine (Baltimore) 1949;27:139–185.

83. Mitchell A, Sackett C, Hunzicker W, Levine S: The clinical features of aortic stenosis. Am Heart J 1954;48:684–720.

84. Rapaport E: Natural history of aortic and mitral valve disease. Am J Cardiol 1975;35:221–227.

85. Ross J Jr, Braunwald E: Aortic stenosis. Circulation 1968;38(suppl 5):V61.

86. Wood P: Aortic stenosis. Am J Cardiol 1958;1:553.

87. Selzer A: Changing aspects of the natural history of valvular aortic stenosis. N Engl J Med 1987;317:91–98.

88. Lombard JT, Selzer A: Valvular aortic stenosis: a clinical and hemodynamic profile of patients. Ann Intern Med 1987;106:292–298.

89. Faggiano P, Sabatini T, Rusconi C, Ghizzoni G, Sorgato A: Abnormalities of left ventricular filling in valvular aortic stenosis: usefulness of combined evaluation of pulmonary veins and mitral flow by means of transthoracic Doppler echocardiography. Int J Cardiol 1995;49:77–85.

90. Schwartz LS, Goldfischer J, Sprague GJ, Schwartz SP: Syncope and sudden death in aortic stenosis. Am J Cardiol 1969;23:647–658.

91. Johnson AM: Aortic stenosis, sudden death, and the left ventricular baroceptors. Br Heart J 1971;33:1–5.

92. Richards AM, Nicholls MG, Ikram H, Hamilton EJ, Richards RD: Syncope in aortic valvular stenosis. Lancet 1984;2:1113–1116.

93. Shaver JA: Cardiac auscultation: a cost-effective diagnostic skill. Curr Probl Cardiol 1995;20:441–530.

94. Jaffe WM, Roche AHG, Coverdale HA, McAlister HF, Ormiston JA, Greene ER: Clinical evaluation versus Doppler echocardiography in the quantitative assessment of valvular heart disease. Circulation 1988;78:267–275.

95. Eddleman EE Jr, Frommeyer WB Jr, Lyle DP, Turner ME Jr, Bancroft WH Jr: Critical analysis of clinical factors in estimating severity of aortic valve disease. Am J Cardiol 1973;31:687–695.

96. Bonner AJ Jr, Sacks HN, Tavel ME: Assessing the severity of aortic stenosis by phonocardiography and external carotid pulse recordings. Circulation 1973;48:247–252.

97. Judge TP, Kennedy JW: Estimation of aortic regurgitation by diastolic pulse wave analysis. Circulation 1970;41:659–665.

98. Munt BI, Legget ME, Kraft CD, Miyake-Hull CY, Fujioka M, Otto CM: Physical examination in valvular aortic stenosis: correlation with stenosis severity and prediction of clinical outcome. Am Heart J 1998, in press.

99. Aronow WS, Kronzon I: Correlation of prevalence and severity of valvular aortic stenosis determined by continuous-wave Doppler echocardiography with physical signs of aortic stenosis in patients aged 62 to 100 years with aortic systolic ejection murmurs. Am J Cardiol 1987;60:399–401.

100. Forssell G, Jonasson R, Orinius E: Identifying severe aortic valvular stenosis by bedside examination. Acta Med Scand 1985;218:397–400.

101. Vigna C, Impagliatelli M, Russo A, et al: Systolic ejection murmurs in the elderly: aortic valve and carotid arteries echo-Doppler findings. Angiology 1991;42:455–461.

102. Wong M, Tei C, Shah PM: Degenerative calcific valvular disease and systolic murmurs in the elderly. J Am Geriatr Soc 1983;31:156–163.

103. Xu M, McHaffie DJ: Nonspecific systolic murmurs: an audit of the clinical value of echocardiography. N Z Med J 1993;106:54–56.

104. Aronow WS, Kronzon I: Prevalence and severity of valvular aortic stenosis determined by Doppler echocardiography and its association with echocardiographic and electrocardiographic left ventricular hypertrophy and physical signs of aortic stenosis in elderly patients. Am J Cardiol 1991;67:776–777.

105. Gallavardin L: La souffle du retrecissement aortique pent changer de timbre et devenir musical dans sa propagation apexienne. Lyon Med 1925;523.

106. Perloff JK: Physical examination of the heart and circulation. Philadelphia: WB Saunders, 1982.

107. St Clair EW, Oddone EZ, Waugh RA, Corey GR, Feussner JR: Assessing housestaff diagnostic skills using a cardiology patient simulator. Ann Intern Med 1992;117:751–756.

108. Caulfield WH, de Leon AC Jr, Perloff JK, Steelman RB: The clinical significance of the fourth heart sound in aortic stenosis. Am J Cardiol 1971;28:179–182.

109. Szamosi A, Wassberg B: Radiologic detection of aortic stenosis. Acta Radiol Diagn Stockh 1983;24:201–207.

110. Hugenholtz PG, Lees MN, Nadas AS: The scalar electrocardiogram, vectorcardiogram, and exercise electrocardiogram in the assessment of congenital aortic stenosis. Circulation 1962;26:79.

111. Braunwald E, Goldblatt A, Aygen MM, et al: Congenital aortic stenosis: I. Clinical and hemodynamic findings in 100 patients. Circulation 1963;27:426.

112. Abdin ZH: The electrocardiogram in aortic stenosis. Br Heart J 1957;195:31.

113. Fowler RS: Ventricular repolarization in congenital aortic stenosis. Am Heart J 1965;70:603.

114. Otto CM: Aortic stenosis: echocardiographic evaluation of disease severity, disease progression, and the role of echocardiography in clinical decision making. *In* Otto CM, ed. The Practice of Clinical Echocardiography. Philadelphia: WB Saunders, 1997.

115. Kim KS, Maxted W, Nanda NC, et al: Comparison of multiplane and biplane transesophageal echocardiography in the assessment of aortic stenosis. Am J Cardiol 1997;79:436–441.

116. Cormier B, Iung B, Porte JM, Barbant S, Vahanian A: Value of multiplane transesophageal echocardiography in determining aortic valve area in aortic stenosis. Am J Cardiol 1996;77:882–885.

117. Tribouilloy C, Shen WF, Peltier M, Mirode A, Rey JL, Lesbre JP: Quantitation of aortic valve area in aortic stenosis with multiplane transesophageal echocardiography: comparison with monoplane transesophageal approach. Am Heart J 1994;128:526–532.

118. Stoddard MF, Hammons RT, Longaker RA: Doppler transesophageal echocardiographic determination of aortic valve area in adults with aortic stenosis. Am Heart J 1996;132:337–342.

119. Bernard Y, Meneveau N, Vuillemenot A, et al: Is planimetry of aortic valve area using multiplane transesophageal echocardiography a reliable method for assessing severity of aortic stenosis? Heart 1997;78:68–73.

120. Menzel T, Mohr Kahaly S, Kolsch B, et al: Quantitative assessment of aortic stenosis by three-dimensional echocardiography. J Am Soc Echocardiogr 1997;10:215–223.

121. Smith MD, Dawson PL, Elion JL, et al: Correlation of continuous wave Doppler velocities with cardiac catheterization gradients: an experimental model of aortic stenosis. J Am Coll Cardiol 1985;6:1306–1314.

122. Smith MD, Kwan OL, DeMaria AN: Value and limitations of continuous-wave Doppler echocardiography in estimating severity of valvular stenosis. JAMA 1986;255:3145–3151.

123. Simpson IA, Houston AB, Sheldon CD, Hutton I, Lawrie TD: Clinical value of Doppler echocardiography in the assessment of adults with aortic stenosis. Br Heart J 1985;53:636–639.

124. Burwash IG, Forbes AD, Sadahiro M, et al: Echocardiographic volume flow and stenosis severity measures with changing flow rate in aortic stenosis. Am J Physiol 1993;265:H1734–1743.

125. Isaaz K, Munoz L, Ports T, Schiller NB: Demonstration of postvalvuloplasty improvement in aortic stenosis based on Doppler measurement of valvular resistance. J Am Coll Cardiol 1991;18:1661–1670.

126. Burwash IG, Pearlman AS, Sadahiro M, Thomas DD, Verrier ED, Otto CM: Ventricular stroke work loss as a measure of aortic stenosis severity [abstract]. Circulation 1992;86:I-539.

127. Otto CM, Pearlman AS, Gardner CL, Kraft CD, Fujioka MC: Simplification of the Doppler continuity equation for calculating stenotic aortic valve area. J Am Soc Echocardiogr 1988;1:155–157.

128. Raggi P, Vasavada BC, Rodney E, el Jandali A, Dogan O, Sacchi TJ: Doppler echocardiographic methods to estimate severity of aortic stenosis. Am J Cardiol 1995;76:615–618.

129. Mann DL, Usher BW, Hammerman S, Bell A, Gillam LD: The fractional shortening-velocity ratio: validation of a new echocardiographic Doppler method for identifying patients with significant aortic stenosis. J Am Coll Cardiol 1990;15:1578–1584.

130. Atwood JE, Kawanishi S, Myers J, Froelicher VF: Exercise testing in patients with aortic stenosis. Chest 1988;93:1083–1087.

131. Atterhog JH, Jonsson B, Samuelsson R: Exercise testing: a prospective study of complication rates. Am Heart J 1979;98:572–579.

132. Maron BJ, Thompson PD, Puffer JC, et al: Cardiovascular preparticipation screening of competitive athletes: a statement for health professionals from the Sudden Death Committee (clinical cardiology) and Congenital Cardiac Defects Committee (cardiovascular disease in the young), American Heart Association. Circulation 1996;94:850–856.

133. Fremes SE, Goldman BS, Ivanov J, Weisel RD, David TE, Salerno T: Valvular surgery in the elderly. Circulation 1989;80(suppl I):177–190.

134. Otto CM, Mickel MC, Kennedy JW, et al: Three-year outcome after balloon aortic valvuloplasty: insights into prognosis of valvular aortic stenosis. Circulation 1994;89:642–650.

135. Beppu S, Suzuki S, Matsuda H, Ohmori F, Nagata S, Miyatake K: Rapidity of progression of aortic stenosis in patients with congenital bicuspid aortic valves. Am J Cardiol 1993;71:322–327.

136. Pachulski RT, Chan KL: Progression of aortic valve dysfunction in 51 adult patients with congenital bicuspid aortic valve: assessment and follow-up by Doppler echocardiography. Br Heart J 1993;69:237–240.

137. Lao TT, Sermer M, MaGee L, Farine D, Colman JM: Congenital aortic stenosis and pregnancy—a reappraisal. Am J Obstet Gynecol 1993;169:540–545.

138. Horstkotte D, Loogen F: The natural history of aortic valve stenosis. Eur Heart J 1988;9(suppl E):57–64.

139. Lund O, Nielsen TT, Pilegaard HK, Magnussen K, Knudsen MA: The influence of coronary artery disease and bypass grafting on early and late survival after valve replacement for aortic stenosis. J Thorac Cardiovasc Surg 1990;100:327–337.

140. Turina J, Hess O, Sepulcri F, Krayenbuehl HP: Spontaneous course of aortic valve disease. Eur Heart J 1987;8:471–483.

141. Kelly TA, Rothbart RM, Cooper CM, Kaiser DL, Smucker ML, Gibson RS: Comparison of outcome of asymptomatic to symptomatic patients older than 20 years of age with valvular aortic stenosis. Am J Cardiol 1988;61:123–130.

142. Pellikka PA, Nishimura RA, Bailey KR, Tajik AJ: The natural history of adults with asymptomatic, hemodynamically significant aortic stenosis. J Am Coll Cardiol 1990;15:1012–1017.

143. Faggiano P, Ghizzoni G, Sorgato A, et al: Rate of progression of valvular aortic stenosis in adults. Am J Cardiol 1992;70:229–233.

144. Archer SL, Mike DK, Hetland MB, Kostamo KL, Shafer RB, Chesler E: Usefulness of mean aortic valve gradient and left ventricular diastolic filling pattern for distinguishing symptomatic from asymptomatic patients. Am J Cardiol 1994;73:275–281.

145. O'Keefe JHJ, Vlietstra RE, Bailey KR, Holmes DRJ: Natural history of candidates for balloon aortic valvuloplasty. Mayo Clin Proc 1987;62:986–991.

146. Kennedy KD, Nishimura RA, Holmes DRJ, Bailey KR: Natural history of moderate aortic stenosis. J Am Coll Cardiol 1991;17:313–319.

147. Bogart DB, Murphy BL, Wong BY, Pugh DM, Dunn MI: Progression of aortic stenosis. Chest 1979;76:391–396.

148. Cheitlin MD, Gertz EW, Brundage BH, Carlson CJ, Quash JA, Bode RSJ: Rate of progression of severity of valvular aortic stenosis in the adult. Am Heart J 1979;98:689–700.

149. Wagner S, Selzer A: Patterns of progression of aortic stenosis: a longitudinal hemodynamic study. Circulation 1982;65:709–712.

150. Jonasson R, Jonsson B, Nordlander R, Orinius E, Szamosi A: Rate of progression of severity of valvular aortic stenosis. Acta Med Scand 1983;213:51–54.

151. Nestico PF, DePace NL, Kimbiris D, et al: Progression of isolated aortic stenosis: analysis of 29 patients having more than 1 cardiac catheterization. Am J Cardiol 1983;52:1054–1058.

152. Davies SW, Gershlick AH, Balcon R: Progression of valvar aortic stenosis: a long-term retrospective study. Eur Heart J 1991;12:10–14.

153. Roger VL, Tajik AJ, Bailey KR, Oh JK, Taylor CL, Seward JB: Progression of aortic stenosis in adults: new appraisal using Doppler echocardiography. Am Heart J 1990;119:331–338.

154. Peter M, Hoffmann A, Parker C, Luscher T, Burckhardt D: Progression of aortic stenosis: role of age and concomitant coronary artery disease. Chest 1993;103:1715–1719.

155. Brener SJ, Duffy CI, Thomas JD, Stewart WJ: Progression of aortic stenosis in 394 patients: relation to changes in myocardial and mitral valve dysfunction. J Am Coll Cardiol 1995;25:305–310.

156. Stewart BF, Siscovick D, Lind BK, et al: Clinical factors associated with calcific aortic valve disease. J Am Coll Cardiol 1997;29:630–634.

157. Georgeson S, Meyer KB, Pauker SG: Decision analysis in clinical cardiology: when is coronary angiography required in aortic stenosis. J Am Coll Cardiol 1990;15:751–762.

158. Iung B, Drissi MF, Michel PL, et al: Prognosis of valve replacement for aortic stenosis with or without coexisting coronary heart disease: a comparative study. J Heart Valve Dis 1993;2:430–439.

159. O'Keefe JH Jr, Shub C, Rettke SR: Risk of noncardiac surgical procedures in patients with aortic stenosis. Mayo Clin Proc 1989;64:400.

160. Easterling TR, Chadwick HS, Otto CM, Benedetti TJ: Aortic stenosis in pregnancy. Obstet Gynecol 1988;72:113–118.

161. Brian JEJ, Seifen AB, Clark RB, Robertson DM, Quirk JG: Aortic stenosis, cesarean delivery, and epidural anesthesia. J Clin Anesth 1993;5:154–157.

162. Lao TT, Adelman AG, Sermer M, Colman JM: Balloon valvuloplasty for congenital aortic stenosis in pregnancy. Br J Obstet Gynaecol 1993;100:1141–1142.

163. Ben Ami M, Battino S, Rosenfeld T, Marin G, Shalev E: Aortic valve replacement during pregnancy: a case report and review of the literature. Acta Obstet Gynecol Scand 1990;69:651–653.

164. Verheul HA, van den Brink RB, Bouma BJ, et al: Analysis of risk factors for excess mortality after aortic valve replacement. J Am Coll Cardiol 1995;26:1280–1286.

165. Kirklin JK, Naftel DC, Blackstone EH, Kirklin JW, Brown RC: Risk factors for mortality after primary combined valvular and coronary artery surgery. Circulation 1989;79(suppl I):185–190.

166. Mullany CJ, Clarebrough JK, White AL, Wilson AC: Open heart surgery in the elderly. Aust N Z J Surg 1987;57:733–737.

167. Craver JM, Weintraub WS, Jones EL, Guyton RA, Hatcher CR Jr: Predictors of mortality, complications, and length of stay in aortic valve replacement for aortic stenosis. Circulation 1988;78(suppl I):85–90.

168. Sethi GK, Miller DC, Souchek J, et al: Clinical, hemodynamic, and angiographic predictors of operative mortality in patients undergoing single valve replacement. Veterans Administration Cooperative Study on Valvular Heart Disease. J Thorac Cardiovasc Surg 1987;93:884–897.

169. Olsson M, Granstrom L, Lindblom D, Rosenqvist M, Ryden L: Aortic valve replacement in octogenarians with aortic stenosis: a case-control study. J Am Coll Cardiol 1992;20:1512–1516.

170. Freeman WK, Schaff HV, O'Brien PC, Orszulak TA, Naessens JM, Tajik AJ: Cardiac surgery in the octogenarian: perioperative outcome and clinical follow-up. J Am Coll Cardiol 1991;18:29–35.

171. Levinson JR, Akins CW, Buckley MJ, et al: Octogenarians with aortic stenosis: outcome after aortic valve replacement. Circulation 1989;80(suppl I):49–56.

172. Culliford AT, Galloway AC, Colvin SB, et al: Aortic valve replacement for aortic stenosis in persons aged 80 years and over. Am J Cardiol 1991;67:1256–1260.

173. Azariades M, Fessler CL, Ahmad A, Starr A: Aortic valve replacement in patients over 80 years of age: a comparative standard for balloon valvuloplasty. Eur J Cardiothorac Surg 1991;5:373–377.

174. Elayda MA, Hall RJ, Reul RM, et al: Aortic valve replacement in patients 80 years and older: operative risks and long-term results. Circulation 1993;88(suppl II):11–16.

175. Logeais Y, Langanay T, Roussin R, et al: Surgery for aortic stenosis in elderly patients: a study of surgical risk and predictive factors. Circulation 1994;90:2891–2898.

176. Morris JJ, Schaff HV, Mullany CJ, Morris PB, Frye RL, Orszulak TA: Gender differences in left ventricular functional response to aortic valve replacement. Circulation 1994;90(suppl II):183–189.

177. Collins JJ, Aranki SF: Management of mild aortic stenosis during coronary artery bypass graft surgery. J Card Surg 1994;9:145–147.

178. Fighali SF, Avendano A, Elayda MA, et al: Early and late mortality of patients undergoing aortic valve replacement after previous coronary artery bypass graft surgery. Circulation 1995;92(suppl II):163–168.

179. Aurigemma G, Battista S, Orsinelli D, Sweeney A, Pape L, Cuenoud H: Abnormal left ventricular intracavitary flow acceleration in patients undergoing aortic valve replacement for aortic stenosis: a marker for high postoperative morbidity and mortality. Circulation 1992;86:926–936.

180. Wiseth R, Samstad S, Rossvoll O, Torp HG, Skjaerpe T, Hatle L: Cross-sectional left ventricular outflow tract velocities before and after aortic valve replacement: a comparative study with two-dimensional Doppler ultrasound. J Am Soc Echocardiogr 1993;6:279–285.

181. Bartunek J, Sys SU, Rodrigues AC, van Schuerbeeck E, Mortier L, de Bruyne B: Abnormal systolic intraventricular flow velocities after valve replacement for aortic stenosis: mechanisms, predictive factors, and prognostic significance. Circulation 1996;93:712–719.

182. Orsinelli DA, Aurigemma GP, Battista S, Krendel S, Gaasch WH: Left ventricular hypertrophy and mortality after aortic valve replacement for aortic stenosis: a high risk subgroup identified by preoperative relative wall thickness. J Am Coll Cardiol 1993;22:1679–1683.

183. Munt BI, Legget ME, Healy NL, Fujioka M, Schwaegler R, Otto CM: Effects of aortic valve replacement on exercise duration and functional status in adults with valvular aortic stenosis. Can J Cardiol 1997;13:346–350.

184. Smith N, McAnulty JH, Rahimtoola SH: Severe aortic stenosis with impaired left ventricular function and clinical heart failure: results of valve replacement. Circulation 1978;58:255–264.

185. Krayenbuehl HP, Turina M, Hess OM, Rothlin M, Senning A: Pre- and postoperative left ventricular contractile function in patients with aortic valve disease. Br Heart J 1979;41:204–213.

186. Harpole DH, Jones RH: Serial assessment of ventricular performance after valve replacement for aortic stenosis. J Thorac Cardiovasc Surg 1990;99:645–650.

187. Hwang MH, Hammermeister KE, Oprian C, et al: Pre-operative identification of patients likely to have left ventricular dysfunction after aortic valve replacement. Participants in the Veterans Administration Cooperative Study on Valvular Heart Disease. Circulation 1989;80(suppl I):65–76.

188. Jin XY, Pepper JR, Brecker SJ, Carey JA, Gibson DG: Early changes in left ventricular function after aortic valve replacement for isolated aortic stenosis. Am J Cardiol 1994;74:1142–1146.

189. Monrad ES, Hess OM, Murakami T, Nonogi H, Corin WJ, Krayenbuehl HP: Time course of regression of left ventricular hypertrophy after aortic valve replacement. Circulation 1988;77:1345–1355.

190. Pantely G, Morton M, Rahimtoola SH: Effects of successful, uncomplicated valve replacement on ventricular hypertrophy, volume, and performance in aortic stenosis and in aortic incompetence. J Thorac Cardiovasc Surg 1978;75:383–391.

191. Krayenbuehl HP, Hess OM, Monrad ES, Schneider J, Mall G, Turina M: Left ventricular myocardial structure in aortic valve disease before, intermediate, and late after aortic valve replacement. Circulation 1989;79:744–755.

192. Kennedy JW, Doces J, Stewart DK: Left ventricular function before and following aortic valve replacement. Circulation 1977;56:944–950.

193. Uwabe K, Kitamura M, Hachida M, Endo M, Hashimoto A, Koyanagi H: Long-term outcome of left ventricular dysfunction after surgery for severe aortic stenosis. J Heart Valve Dis 1995;4:503–507.

194. Diver DJ, Royal HD, Aroesty JM, et al: Diastolic function in patients with aortic stenosis: influence of left ventricular load reduction. J Am Coll Cardiol 1988;12:642–648.

195. Gilchrist IC, Waxman HL, Kurnik PB: Improvement

in early diastolic filling dynamics after aortic valve replacement. Am J Cardiol 1990;66:1124–1129.

196. Hess OM, Ritter M, Schneider J, Grimm J, Turina M, Krayenbuehl HP: Diastolic stiffness and myocardial structure in aortic valve disease before and after valve replacement. Circulation 1984;69:855–865.

197. Hess OM, Villari B, Krayenbuehl HP: Diastolic dysfunction in aortic stenosis. Circulation 1993;87(suppl IV):73–76.

198. Lorell BH, Grossman W: Cardiac hypertrophy: the consequences for diastole. J Am Coll Cardiol 1987;9:1189–1193.

199. Villari B, Vassalli G, Betocchi S, Briguori C, Chiariello M, Hess OM: Normalization of left ventricular nonuniformity late after valve replacement for aortic stenosis. Am J Cardiol 1996;78:66–71.

200. Driscoll DJ, Wolfe RR, Gersony WM, et al: Cardiorespiratory responses to exercise of patients with aortic stenosis, pulmonary stenosis, and ventricular septal defect. Circulation 1993;87(suppl I):102–113.

201. Jaeger AA, Hlatky MA, Paul SM, Gortner SR: Functional capacity after cardiac surgery in elderly patients. J Am Coll Cardiol 1994;24:104–108.

202. Hirooka K, Kawazoe K, Kosakai Y, et al: Prediction of postoperative exercise tolerance after aortic valve replacement. Ann Thorac Surg 1994;58:1626–1630.

203. Carabello BA: Timing of valve replacement in aortic stenosis: moving closer to perfection [editorial]. Circulation 1997;95:2241–2243.

204. Faggiano P, Aurigemma GP, Rusconi C, Gaasch WH: Progression of valvular aortic stenosis in adults: literature review and clinical implications. Am Heart J 1996;132:408–417.

205. Wong JB, Salem DN, Pauker SG: You're never too old. N Engl J Med 1993;328:971–975.

206. Collins JJ Jr, Aranki SF: Management of mild aortic stenosis during coronary artery bypass graft surgery. J Card Surg 1994;9:145–147.

207. Thibault GE: Too old for what? N Engl J Med 1993;328:946–950.

208. Connolly HM, Oh JK, Orszulak TA, et al: Aortic valve replacement for aortic stenosis with severe left ventricular dysfunction: prognostic indicators. Circulation 1997;95:2395–2400.

209. Elkins RC, Knott Craig CJ, McCue C, Lane MM: Congenital aortic valve disease: improved survival and quality of life. Ann Surg 1997;225:503–510.

210. Cohn LH, Collins JJ Jr, Disesa VJ, et al: Fifteen-year experience with 1678 Hancock porcine bioprosthetic heart valve replacements. Ann Surg 1989;210:435–442.

211. Pansini S, Ottino GM, Galloni M, Forsennati PG, Serpieri G, Morea M: Morphological comparison of primary tissue failure (PTF) in porcine mitral and aortic bioprostheses in the same patient. Eur J Cardiothorac Surg 1990;4:431–433.

212. al Khaja N, Belboul A, Rashid M, et al: The influence of age on the durability of Carpentier-Edwards biological valves: thirteen years follow-up. Eur J Cardiothorac Surg 1991;5:635–640.

213. David TE: Heart valve surgery in the '90s: a surgeon's perspective. Can J Cardiol 1990;6:175–179.

214. O'Brien MF: Composite stentless xenograft for aortic valve replacement: clinical evaluation of function. Ann Thorac Surg 1995;60(suppl 2):S406–409.

215. Westaby S, Amarasena N, Long V, et al: Time-related hemodynamic changes after aortic replacement with the freestyle stentless xenograft. Ann Thorac Surg 1995;60:1633–1638.

216. Konertz W, Hamann P, Schwammenthal E, Breithardt G, Scheld HH: Aortic valve replacement with stentless xenografts. J Heart Valve Dis 1992;1:249–252.

217. Davis EA, Greene PS, Cameron DE, et al: Bioprosthetic versus mechanical prostheses for aortic valve replacement in the elderly. Circulation 1996;94(suppl II):121–125.

218. Safian RD, Berman AD, Diver DJ, et al: Balloon aortic valvuloplasty in 170 consecutive patients. N Engl J Med 1988;319:125–130.

219. Litvack F, Jakubowski AT, Buchbinder NA, Eigler N: Lack of sustained clinical improvement in an elderly population after percutaneous aortic valvuloplasty. Am J Cardiol 1988;62:270–275.

220. Letac B, Cribier A, Koning R, Bellefleur JP: Results of percutaneous transluminal valvuloplasty in 218 adults with valvular aortic stenosis. Am J Cardiol 1988;62:598–605.

221. Block PC, Palacios IF: Clinical and hemodynamic follow-up after percutaneous aortic valvuloplasty in the elderly. Am J Cardiol 1988;62:1760–1763.

222. Sherman W, Hershman R, Lazzam C, Cohen M, Ambrose J, Gorlin R: Balloon valvuloplasty in adult aortic stenosis: determinants of clinical outcome. Ann Intern Med 1989;110:421–425.

223. Berland J, Cribier A, Savin T, Lefebvre E, Koning R, Letac B: Percutaneous balloon valvuloplasty in patients with severe aortic stenosis and low ejection fraction: immediate results and 1-year follow-up. Circulation 1989;79:1189–1196.

224. Lewin RF, Dorros G, King JF, Mathiak L: Percutaneous transluminal aortic valvuloplasty: acute outcome and follow-up of 125 patients. J Am Coll Cardiol 1989;14:1210–1217.

225. Holmes DR Jr, Nishimura RA, Reeder GS, Wagner PJ, Ilstrup DM: Clinical follow-up after percutaneous aortic balloon valvuloplasty. Arch Intern Med 1989;149:1405–1409.

226. O'Neill WW: Predictors of long-term survival after percutaneous aortic valvuloplasty: report of the Mansfield Scientific Balloon Aortic Valvuloplasty Registry. J Am Coll Cardiol 1991;17:193–198.

227. Davidson CJ, Harrison JK, Pieper KS, et al: Determinants of one-year outcome from balloon aortic valvuloplasty. Am J Cardiol 1991;68:75–80.

228. Kuntz RE, Tosteson AN, Berman AD, et al: Predictors of event-free survival after balloon aortic valvuloplasty. N Engl J Med 1991;325:17–23.

229. Lieberman EB, Bashore TM, Hermiller JB, et al: Balloon aortic valvuloplasty in adults: failure of procedure to improve long-term survival. J Am Coll Cardiol 1995;26:1522–1528.

230. Rocchini AP, Beekman RH, Ben Shachar G, Benson L, Schwartz D, Kan JS: Balloon aortic valvuloplasty: results of the Valvuloplasty and Angioplasty of Congenital Anomalies Registry. Am J Cardiol 1990;65:784–789.

231. McCrindle BW: Independent predictors of immediate results of percutaneous balloon aortic valvotomy in children. Valvuloplasty and Angioplasty of Congenital Anomalies (VACA) Registry Investigators. Am J Cardiol 1996;77:286–293.

232. Justo RN, McCrindle BW, Benson LN, Williams WG, Freedom RM, Smallhorn JF: Aortic valve regurgitation after surgical versus percutaneous balloon valvotomy for congenital aortic valve stenosis. Am J Cardiol 1996;77:1332–1338.

233. Moore P, Egito E, Mowrey H, Perry SB, Lock JE,

Keane JF: Midterm results of balloon dilation of congenital aortic stenosis: predictors of success. J Am Coll Cardiol 1996;27:1257–1263.

234. Kuhn MA, Latson LA, Cheatham JP, Fletcher SE, Foreman C: Management of pediatric patients with isolated valvar aortic stenosis by balloon aortic valvuloplasty. Cathet Cardiovasc Diagn 1996;39:55–61.

235. Galal O, Rao PS, Al Fadley F, Wilson AD: Follow-up results of balloon aortic valvuloplasty in children with special reference to causes of late aortic insufficiency. Am Heart J 1997;133:418–427.

236. Fisher RD, Mason DT, Morrow AG: Results of operative treatment in congenital aortic stenosis. Pre- and postoperative hemodynamic evaluations. J Thorac Cardiovasc Surg 1970;59:218–224.

237. Hsieh KS, Keane JF, Nadas AS, Bernhard WF, Castaneda AR: Long-term follow-up of valvotomy before 1968 for congenital aortic stenosis. Am J Cardiol 1986;58:338–341.

238. DeBoer DA, Robbins RC, Maron BJ, McIntosh CL, Clark RE: Late results of aortic valvotomy for congenital valvar aortic stenosis. Ann Thorac Surg 1990;50:69–73.

239. Johnson RG, Williams GR, Razook JD, Thompson WM, Lane MM, Elkins RC: Reoperation in congenital aortic stenosis. Ann Thorac Surg 1985;40:156–162.

240. Jones M, Barnhart GR, Morrow AG: Late results after operations for left ventricular outflow tract obstruction. Am J Cardiol 1982;50:569–579.

241. Keane JF, Driscoll DJ, Gersony WM, et al: Second natural history study of congenital heart defects: results of treatment of patients with aortic valvar stenosis. Circulation 1993;87(suppl I):16–27.

242. Gerosa G, McKay R, Davies J, Ross DN: Comparison of the aortic homograft and the pulmonary autograft for aortic valve or root replacement in children. J Thorac Cardiovasc Surg 1991;102:51–60.

243. Hurley PJ, Lowe JB, Barratt Boyes BG: Debridement-valvotomy for aortic stenosis in adults: a follow-up of 76 patients. Thorax 1967;22:314–319.

244. Enright LP, Hancock EW, Shumway NE: Aortic debridement—long-term follow-up. Circulation 1971;5(suppl I):68–72.

245. Hill DG: Long-term results of debridement valvotomy for calcific aortic stenosis. J Thorac Cardiovasc Surg 1973;65:708–711.

246. King RM, Pluth JR, Giuliani ER, Piehler JM: Mechanical decalcification of the aortic valve. Ann Thorac Surg 1986;42:269–272.

247. Scott WJ, Neumann AL, Karp RB: Ultrasonic debridement of the aortic valve with six-month echocardiographic follow-up. Am J Cardiol 1989;64:1206–1209.

248. Freeman WK, Hartzell HV, Schaff HV, Orszulak TA, Tajik AJ: Ultrasonic aortic valve decalcification: serial Doppler echocardiographic follow-up. J Am Coll Cardiol 1990;16:623–630.

249. Craver JM: Aortic valve debridement by ultrasonic surgical aspirator: a word of caution. Ann Thorac Surg 1990;49:746–52.

250. Nylander E, Ekman I, Marklund T, Sinnerstad B, Karlsson E, Wranne B: Severe aortic stenosis in elderly patients. Br Heart J 1986;55:480–487.

251. Clyne CA, Arrighi JA, Maron BJ, Dilsizian V, Bonow RO, Cannon RO III: Systemic and left ventricular responses to exercise stress in asymptomatic patients with valvular aortic stenosis. Am J Cardiol 1991;68:1469–1476.

252. Kupari M, Virtanen KS, Turto H, et al: Exclusion of coronary artery disease by exercise thallium-201 tomography in patients with aortic stenosis. Am J Cardiol 1992;70:635–640.

253. deFilippi CR, Willett DL, Brickner ME, et al: Usefulness of dobutamine echocardiography in distinguishing severe from non-severe valvular aortic stenosis in patients with depressed left ventricular function and low transvalvular gradients. Am J Cardiol 1995;75:191–194.

254. Samuels B, Kiat H, Friedman JD, Berman DS: Adenosine pharmacologic stress myocardial perfusion tomographic imaging in patients with significant aortic stenosis: diagnostic efficacy and comparison of clinical, hemodynamic and electrocardiographic variable with 100 age-matched control subjects. J Am Coll Cardiol 1995;25:99–106.

255. Rask P, Karp KL, Eriksson MP, Moore T: Dipyridamole thallium-201 single photon emission tomography in aortic stenosis: gender differences. Eur J Nucl Med 1995;22:1155–1162.

256. Kettunen R, Huikuri HV, Heikkila J, Takkunen JT: Preoperative diagnosis of coronary artery disease in patients with valvular heart disease using technetium-99m isonitrile tomographic imaging together with high-dose dipyridamole and handgrip exercise. Am J Cardiol 1992;69:1442–1445.

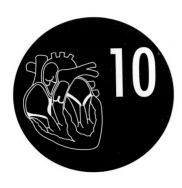

10 Mitral Stenosis

PATHOPHYSIOLOGY

The most characteristic anatomic finding for rheumatic mitral stenosis is fusion of the leaflet edges along the commissures between the anterior and posterior leaflets (Fig. 10–1). Additional features include fusion, thickening, and shortening of the mitral valve chordae; fibrosis and thickening of the valve leaflets; and superimposed calcific changes. Flow is obstructed by the combination of reduced leaflet opening caused by commissural fusion and increased rigidity of the leaflets and by obstruction at the subvalvular level (see Chapter 2).[1–3] Rarely, obstruction results from severe mitral annular calcification (Fig. 10–2). Determining the contribution of each of these components to overall stenosis severity in each patient is important in deciding on the optimal intervention after mitral stenosis has become severe (see Chapter 11).

The primary pathophysiologic abnormality in patients with mitral stenosis is mechanical obstruction at the mitral valve level. Secondary upstream consequences of mitral valve obstruction include the effects of an elevated transmitral pressure gradient on the left atrium and pulmonary vasculature. In isolated mitral stenosis, the downstream left ventricle is relatively spared and tends to be normal or small with normal contractile function unless aortic or mitral regurgitation also is present.

Mitral Valve Obstruction

Obstruction at the mitral valve level increases the diastolic pressure gradient between the left atrium and left ventricle. With sinus rhythm, the transmitral gradient increases further after atrial contraction. As obstruction becomes more severe, the pressure gradient increases, with mean transmitral pressure gradients at rest of 10 to 25 mm Hg in patients with severe mitral stenosis.[4–6]

In addition to the severity of valvular obstruction, transmitral pressure gradients also depend on the volume flow rate across the valve in diastole. For a given valve area, a higher transmitral gradient occurs with an elevated transmitral flow rate, for example, with fever, anemia, during exercise, or with coexisting mitral regurgitation. Conversely, a low transmitral flow rate may be associated with a

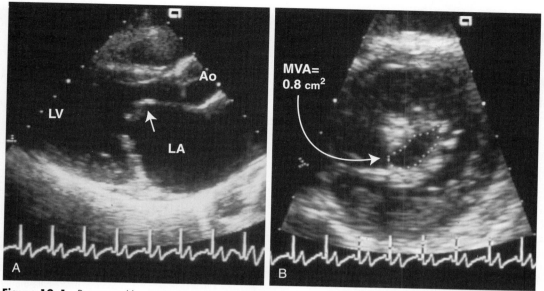

Figure 10·1   Parasternal long-axis *(A)* and short-axis *(B)* two-dimensional echocardiographic views in mid-diastole show the characteristic findings of rheumatic mitral stenosis. The commissural fusion results in doming of the leaflets in the long-axis view *(arrow)* and in a decreased width of the mitral orifice in the short-axis view. This patient has relatively thin, flexible leaflets with little subvalvular involvement. Ao, aorta; LA, left atrium; LV, left ventricle; MVA, mitral valve area.

relatively low gradient despite severe valvular obstruction.

Mitral valve obstruction is best described in terms of mitral valve area, defined as the anatomic or functional cross-sectional area of the mitral orifice in diastole. With significant rheumatic mitral stenosis, the mitral orifice is symmetric, elliptical, and reasonably constant in size and shape during the diastolic filling period with little contraction of the flowstream as it passes through the orifice. Thus, there is little discrepancy between anatomic and functional valve area. As in valvular aortic stenosis, the degree of valve opening varies with changes in flow rates. However, the magnitude of this effect is small due to the anatomy of

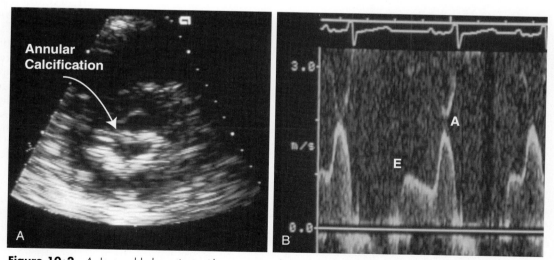

Figure 10·2   *A,* In an elderly patient with severe mitral annular calcification *(arrow),* involvement of the mitral leaflets by the calcific process is seen in the parasternal short-axis view. *B,* The Doppler velocity curve across the valve shows a prolonged pressure half-time of 227 ms, consistent with a functional mitral valve area of 1.0 cm². E, early velocity; A, atrial velocity.

rheumatic stenosis, so that any changes in valve area are unlikely to be clinically significant.[7, 8]

Effect of Mitral Stenosis on the Left Atrium

Chronic elevation of left atrial pressure leads to gradual chamber enlargement. To some extent, the degree of left atrial enlargement corresponds to the severity and chronicity of disease, but some patients with severe disease have only mild or moderate atrial enlargement, while other patients with less severe disease have marked atrial dilation. With long-standing, untreated disease, the atrium can become massively enlarged, leading to elevation of the left main stem bronchus and hoarseness from compression of the left recurrent laryngeal nerve.

Patterns of blood flow in the left atrium are altered by mitral valve obstruction. Flow proximal to the narrowed orifice accelerates as blood approaches the stenotic mitral orifice, forming a high-velocity jet in the orifice itself. Flow more distal to the valve orifice also is altered; pulmonary vein flow is decreased during systole, and atrial flow reversal is increased, with the magnitude of these changes corresponding to the degree of elevation in left atrial pressure.[9–12] Even with sinus rhythm, the

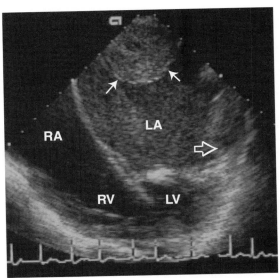

Figure 10·4   Spontaneous contrast in the left atrium (LA) seen on transesophageal echocardiography in a patient with severe rheumatic mitral stenosis and atrial fibrillation. This patient also had laminated thrombus in the body of the left atrium *(arrows)* and appendage *(open arrow)* despite long-term anticoagulation. RA, right atrium; RV, right ventricle; LV, left ventricle.

increased volume of the left atrium leads to low-velocity flow patterns, which predispose to development of atrial thrombi, particularly in the left atrial appendage.

When atrial fibrillation supervenes, blood flow in the atrial appendage and in the body of the atrium becomes even more disorganized, with low-velocity, multidirectional flow patterns, blood flow stasis, and development of atrial thrombi (Figs. 10–3 and 10–4). This swirling pattern of low-velocity flow often is evident as spontaneous contrast on echocardiography, particularly when using a high-frequency transducer from a transesophageal approach. About 17% of patients undergoing surgery for mitral stenosis have left atrial thrombus, and in about one third of these patients, the thrombus is restricted to the atrial appendage.[13]

Pulmonary Hypertension

Basic hydraulic principles indicate that elevated left atrial pressures must necessarily result in a passive rise in pulmonary venous and arterial pressures. However, most patients with mitral stenosis have pulmonary pressures that are increased more than expected for the degree of elevation in left atrial pressure. This component of the increase in pulmonary pres-

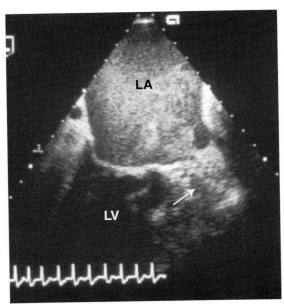

Figure 10·3   Left atrial thrombus *(arrow)* localized to the left atrial (LA) appendage in a patient with mitral stenosis and atrial fibrillation. LV, left ventricle.

sures can be estimated by subtracting mean left atrial pressure from mean pulmonary artery pressure (ie, expected passive component) to derive the pulmonary bed gradient. A normal pressure drop across the pulmonary bed is 10 to 15 mm Hg; gradients in excess of this value correspond to an increase in pulmonary vascular resistance. Pulmonary hypertension in excess of the passive rise caused by an elevated left atrial pressure is due to two components: reactive pulmonary arterial vasoconstriction and morphologic changes in the pulmonary vasculature.

The sequence of histologic changes in pulmonary hypertension due to mitral stenosis is characterized initially by medial thickening in muscular arteries and arterioles, followed by intimal thickening.[14] These changes probably are reversible with a decrease in intravascular pressures. More severe pulmonary hypertension is associated with fibrinoid necrosis and arteritis, loss of smooth muscle cell nuclei, fibrin deposition in the arterial wall, and the presence of inflammatory cells.

The pathologic hallmark of end-stage, irreversible pulmonary hypertension is the plexiform lesion. The plexiform lesion consists of aneurysmal dilation of the arterial wall with a plexus of glomus-like, thin-walled channels branching to join with adjacent capillaries. Nonspecific parenchymal changes in severe pulmonary hypertension include pulmonary hemosiderosis and cholesterol granuloma formation.

Despite the rough correlation between mitral stenosis severity and the degree of pulmonary hypertension, a wide range of pulmonary pressures exist for any degree of valve obstruction (Fig. 10–5).[15–18] Although an increase in pulmonary pressures greater than expected for the increase in left atrial pressure (ie, reactive pulmonary hypertension) rarely occurs with left atrial pressures less than 20 mm Hg, not all patients with pressures greater than 20 mm Hg develop pulmonary hypertension.[16] Factors predicting pulmonary hypertension in this study have not been identified, and the duration of symptoms does not correlate with the presence of pulmonary hypertension (Fig. 10–6).

In a different study of 744 patients with severe mitral stenosis, the factors that affected pulmonary vascular bed gradient on multivariate analysis were transmitral pressure gradient, left ventricular end-diastolic pressure, mitral valve area, and a history of chronic pulmonary disease.[18] In contrast, left atrial size, mitral regurgitation severity, cardiac output, and gender were not predictors of pulmonary artery pressures. These data suggest that, in addition to mitral stenosis severity, superimposed lung disease may play a role in the development of elevated pulmonary vascular resistance. The effect of duration of mitral stenosis on pulmonary vascular resistance could not be assessed in this study.

Another possible explanation for different degrees of pulmonary hypertension for a given severity of mitral stenosis is the role of vasoactive factors, such as endothelin, an endothelial tissue–derived peptide that has contractile and proliferative effects on vascular smooth

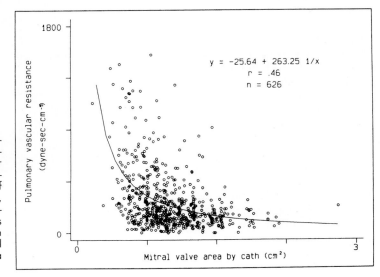

Figure 10·5 Mitral valve area at catheterization plotted against pulmonary vascular resistance with inverse curve fit for 637 patients before balloon mitral commissurotomy. (Reprinted by permission of the publisher from Otto CM, Davis KB, Reid CL, et al: Relation between pulmonary artery pressure and mitral stenosis severity in patients undergoing balloon mitral commissurotomy. Am J Cardiol 1993;71:874–878. © 1993 by Excerpta Medica, Inc.)

$$y = -25.64 + 263.25 \ 1/x$$
$$r = .46$$
$$n = 626$$

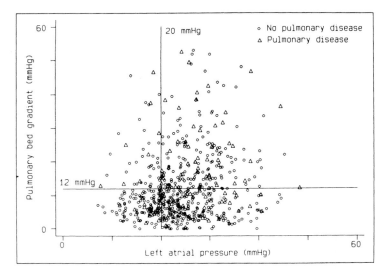

Figure 10·6 Left atrial mean pressure (x axis) plotted against the pulmonary bed gradient (y axis) for the same 637 patients with mitral stenosis shown in Figure 10·5. Lines indicate break points at a left atrial pressure of 20 mm Hg and at a pulmonary bed gradient of less than 12 mm Hg. Triangles indicate the presence and circles the absence of pulmonary disease. (Reprinted by permission of the publisher from Otto CM, Davis KB, Reid CL, et al: Relation between pulmonary artery pressure and mitral stenosis severity in patients undergoing balloon mitral commissurotomy. Am J Cardiol 1993;71: 874–878. © 1993 by Excerpta Medica, Inc.)

muscle cells.[19] In 10 patients with mitral stenosis undergoing balloon mitral valvuloplasty, levels of endothelin I were found to be higher in the left than the right atrium, suggesting increased endothelin I production in the pulmonary circulation. Endothelin I levels correlated directly with pulmonary artery mean and wedge pressures and inversely with mitral valve area, but they did not correlate with pulmonary vascular resistance. There were no differences between the right and left atrium in plasma levels of angiotensin II (ie, vasoconstrictor) or thrombomodulin (ie, thrombin receptor on vascular endothelial cells).

Right Heart Abnormalities

Chronic pulmonary hypertension leads to right ventricular hypertrophy, right ventricular dilation, and eventual right heart failure (Fig. 10–7). This process may be exacerbated by significant tricuspid regurgitation because of rheumatic involvement of the tricuspid valve or annular dilation secondary to right ventricular enlargement. Although pulmonary hypertension presumably is the cause of right heart dysfunction, pulmonary pressures correlate poorly with right ventricular failure in patients with mitral stenosis.[20–22]

To explain the apparent discrepancy between pulmonary pressures and right heart function, Kussmaul and colleagues[23] suggest that arterial wave reflections in the pulmonary artery (particularly the low-frequency components), increased pulmonary artery stiffness, and elevated small vessel resistance all contribute to the abnormal right ventricular hydraulic

load in patients with mitral stenosis. This hypothesis is supported by studies showing that characteristic impedance is not altered with pacing tachycardia and that relief of mitral stenosis results in an immediate improvement in the low-frequency components of impedance and in right ventricular hydraulic power requirements. Thus, ventricular-vascular coupling improves regardless of the distending pulmonary artery pressure. These data also

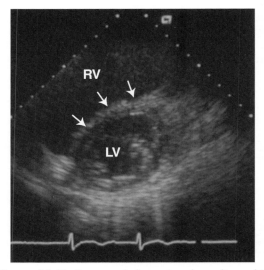

Figure 10·7 Parasternal short-axis echocardiographic view shows right ventricular (RV) enlargement caused by pulmonary hypertension in a patient with severe mitral stenosis. Notice the abnormal flattening of the septum *(arrows)* resulting from the combination of right ventricular pressure overload due to pulmonary hypertension and volume overload due to tricuspid regurgitation from annular dilation. LV, left ventricle.

suggest that the degree of improvement in the pulmonary vasculature after relief of mitral stenosis may be underestimated by conventional measures, such as pulmonary pressures and vascular resistance.

Effect of Mitral Stenosis on the Left Ventricle

The pattern of diastolic filling of the left ventricle in patients with mitral stenosis reflects the degree of obstruction at the mitral valve level. In contrast to normal subjects, early diastolic filling is prolonged, with the slow rate of increase in ventricular volumes evident on two-dimensional (2D) echocardiographic imaging and by Doppler flow recordings. Atrial fibrillation further alters diastolic filling through loss of effective atrial contraction with consequent loss of the atrial filling fraction. In addition, the diastolic left ventricular pressure volume curve is shifted to the left in patients with mitral stenosis due to low ventricular volumes.

Further impairment of diastolic filling is caused by abnormal left ventricular geometry associated with either volume overload (eg, tricuspid regurgitation) or pressure overload (eg, pulmonary hypertension) of the right ventricle.[24] Increased right ventricular diastolic filling pressure and volumes are associated with reversed septal curvature and altered septal motion, leading to impaired left ventricular diastolic filling (see Fig. 10–7).

Although left ventricular contractility typically is normal in isolated mitral stenosis, forward stroke volume may be reduced due to low filling volumes across the stenotic mitral valve. Scarring and shortening of the mitral valve chordae distort the normal papillary muscle and mitral annular relationships, which may further impair overall systolic function.

Exercise Physiology

The degree of change in valve area and valve resistance with exercise is heterogeneous in patients with mitral stenosis.[25] However, in general, an increase in mitral valve area with exercise is associated with flexible valve leaflets and mild to moderate stenosis. More severe valvular deformity and calcification is associated with little anatomic or physiologic change in valve area with exercise.[25, 26] This relatively fixed mitral orifice results in a blunted or absent increase in stroke volume with exercise

compared with normal controls. Therefore, it is not surprising that the initial symptoms in patients with mitral stenosis are typically exertional.[26]

Exercise also results in an increase in pulmonary artery pressures due to several other factors including an increased heart rate, decreased diastolic filling period, and increased left atrial pressure. In evaluating the increase in pulmonary pressures with exercise in a patient with mitral stenosis, it is important to reference this change against the expected changes for a normal individual, which vary with age and the extent of exercise (Fig. 10–8).[27] For example, pulmonary systolic pressure in a young individual normally rises from 15 mm Hg at rest to 30 mm Hg with exercise, whereas an increase from 20 to 50 mm Hg is normal in elderly subjects.

One study[28] of 60 adults with mitral stenosis showed little rise in the mean transmitral gradient with symptom-limited exercise when the resting valve area was larger than 1.4 cm² (from 5 ± 2 to 9 ± 3 mm Hg), a moderate increase when the resting valve area was 1.0 to 1.4 cm² (from 9 ± 5 to 15 ± 6 mm Hg), and a more significant rise when the mitral valve area was less than 1.0 cm² (from 12 ± 4 to 20 ± 6). The average tricuspid regurgitant jet velocity increased from 2.9 ± 0.5 to 3.6 ± 0.5 m/s, corresponding to a rise in pulmonary systolic pressures of 18 mm Hg.[28]

While the onset of atrial fibrillation may not adversely affect exercise performance, patients with atrial fibrillation have less improvement in exercise capacity after intervention compared with mitral stenosis subjects in sinus rhythm.[29]

CLINICAL PRESENTATION

History

In patients with mitral stenosis, the gradually increasing degree of obstruction corresponds to an insidious disease course with a slow, but progressive, decline in exercise capacity. In many cases, the disease process is so gradual that the patient may deny symptoms despite severe functional limitation, as expectations and lifestyle are gradually modified to accommodate decreased cardiac reserve.[30] Careful discussion with the patient and family members, including focused questions comparing current activity levels with activity levels 1, 5, and 10 years ago, often elicits evidence of decreased exercise capacity.

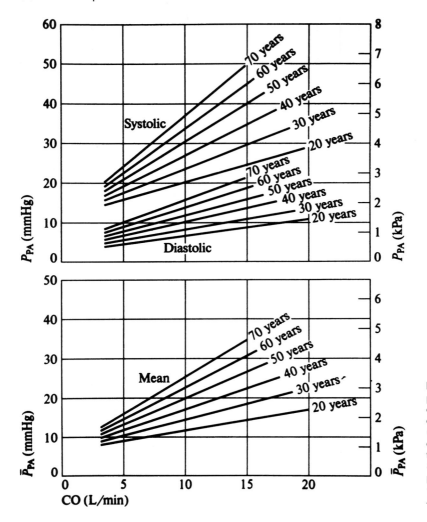

Figure 10·8 Relation between pulmonary artery pressure (PPA) and cardiac output (CO) at different ages in normal individuals. (From Lenter C, ed. Intracardiac and intravascular pressures section. *In* Heart and Circulation, ed 8. Copyright 1990. Novartis. Reprinted with permission from the *Geigy Scientific Tables, Volume 5*. All rights reserved.)

When symptoms are recognized, patients most often notice fatigue and decreased exercise tolerance related to a low forward cardiac output.[31–33] Elevated left atrial pressure commonly produces symptoms of pulmonary congestion, including dyspnea on exertion, shortness of breath, paroxysmal nocturnal dyspnea, and pulmonary edema. With severe mitral stenosis, hemoptysis may occur because of the chronic elevation in pulmonary venous pressures. Recurrent pulmonary infections also are a significant cause of comorbidity in patients with severe disease.[34] In patients with secondary pulmonary hypertension and right heart dysfunction, symptoms of right heart failure may predominate, including peripheral edema, abdominal distention, and decreased appetite. Less common symptoms include hoarseness from compression of the left recurrent laryngeal nerve by the enlarged left

atrium.[35] Hemoptysis, although considered a classic symptom of mitral stenosis, rarely occurs in patients receiving chronic medical care, because earlier intervention prevents severe pulmonary hypertension.[34, 36] The mechanism of hemoptysis appears to be rupture of dilated, high-pressure pulmonary veins but superimposed bronchitis also may lead to hemoptysis.[16]

In some patients with mitral stenosis, the first symptom may be the onset of atrial fibrillation or a systemic embolic event due to left atrial thrombus formation.[36, 37] Previously asymptomatic patients may develop symptoms during times of superimposed hemodynamic stress, such as acute infection or anemia. The increased cardiac demands of pregnancy in a previously asymptomatic patient also may lead to symptoms, so that mitral stenosis may be first diagnosed during pregnancy.[38, 39] Since the murmur of mitral stenosis may be difficult to appreciate in the pregnant patient, this possibility should always be considered in the pregnant patient with evidence of pulmonary congestion.

Physical Examination

Auscultatory Findings

The characteristic auscultatory findings in mitral stenosis are a diastolic murmur, an opening snap in early diastole, and a loud first heart sound (S$_1$) (Fig. 10–9). The diastolic murmur corresponds to the pressure gradient between the left atrium and ventricle in diastole and is best appreciated using the bell of the stethoscope positioned near the apex of the heart, with the patient in a left lateral decubitus position.[40] The murmur may be quite localized, requiring careful examination with the stethoscope positioned at several points between the apex and left sternal border for optimal detection. In addition, the low-pitched murmur, frequently described as

"rumbling," often is low intensity (or "soft"), making an auscultatory diagnosis difficult.

Although the loudness of the murmur does not correspond well with stenosis severity, more severe stenosis is associated with a longer duration of the murmur due to persistence of a significant pressure gradient throughout diastole. When sinus rhythm is present, late diastolic (or presystolic) accentuation of the murmur occurs as atrial contraction leads to an increased transmitral gradient. Some investigators have suggested that presystolic accentuation correlates with the absence of mitral regurgitation as well as the presence of sinus rhythm.[30, 41, 42]

The second characteristic finding in mitral stenosis is the opening snap, a crisp valve closure-like sound occurring in early diastole as the flexible but fused valve leaflets abruptly tense at their opening limit. With disease progression, higher transmitral pressure gradients correspond to a shorter interval between the second heart sound (S$_2$) and the opening snap (ie, S$_2$-OS interval), since left atrial pressure exceeds ventricular pressure earlier in diastole, resulting in earlier mitral valve opening. The opening snap may be diminished or absent with severe valve calcification because of limited motion of the stiffened leaflets. When audible, an S$_2$-OS interval less than 0.08 second indicates severe obstruction.[43, 44]

The third characteristic finding in mitral stenosis is a loud S$_1$ caused by increased amplitude of the mitral closing click as the flexible leaflets suddenly close at end-diastole. As with the opening snap, the loudness of S$_1$ may be blunted by severe valve calcification.

In isolated mitral stenosis, the left ventricle has normal to small internal dimensions, normal wall thickness, and normal contractility. A displaced left ventricular impulse on examination suggests coexisting volume overload of the ventricle due to mixed mitral stenosis and regurgitation or coexisting aortic valve involvement. Since early diastolic filling is impaired, an S$_3$ gallop is rare. Similarly, an S$_4$ is uncommon, as many patients are in atrial fibrillation.

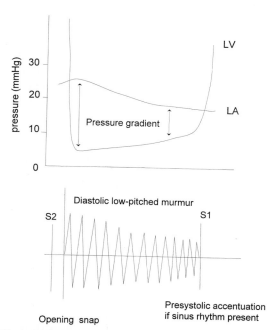

Figure 10·9 Key features of the physical examination for mitral stenosis. A diastolic rumbling murmur corresponding to the pressure gradient between the left atrium (LA) and left ventricle (LV) is best appreciated at the left ventricular apex with the patient in a left lateral decubitus position. With a sinus rhythm, presystolic accentuation of the murmur may be heard because of the increased pressure gradient with atrial contraction. The interval between the second heart sound (S2) and the opening snap decreases as mitral stenosis becomes more severe.

Signs of Pulmonary Hypertension

When secondary pulmonary hypertension is present, the pulmonic closure sound is prominent, a right ventricular lift is present, and signs of right heart failure (eg, elevated jugular venous pressure, peripheral edema, hepatosplenomegaly) may be seen. Tricuspid regurgitation may result from annular dilation in association with pulmonary hypertension or due to rheumatic involvement of the tricuspid valve. The holosystolic murmur of tricuspid regurgitation is differentiated from that of mitral regurgitation based on respiratory variation in the loudness of the murmur, systolic pulsation of the liver, and the presence of a v wave in the neck veins.

Classically, a pulmonic regurgitation murmur (ie, Graham-Steele murmur) has been described as accompanying pulmonary hypertension caused by mitral stenosis. However, echocardiographic evaluation has demonstrated a high prevalence of aortic valve involvement in patients with rheumatic mitral stenosis, raising the possibility that the blowing diastolic murmur at the left sternal border may represent aortic, rather than pulmonic, regurgitation in many of these patients.

Associated Findings

Other physical examination findings in patients with mitral stenosis depend on the presence or absence of concurrent lesions and complications of the disease process. For example, atrial fibrillation is a common complication of mitral stenosis and may be the initial manifestation of the disease. Most patients have some degree of coexisting mitral regurgitation. About 25% of patients also have rheumatic involvement of the aortic valve, and a murmur of aortic stenosis or regurgitation (or both) may be detected.

Patients with long-standing, severe mitral stenosis have been described as having a "mitral facies," characterized by patchy flushing of the cheeks due to the combination of a low cardiac output and peripheral vasoconstriction.[34] However, this sign is rarely seen in patients receiving regular medical care, as intervention is performed before this sign becomes evident.

Chest Radiography and Electrocardiography

The chest radiograph in a patient with mitral stenosis shows a normal-size cardiac silhouette early in the disease course. Later, evidence of left atrial enlargement may be present including prominence of the left atrial appendage contour, a left atrial double density, and elevation of the left main stem bronchus (Fig. 10–10). A barium swallow demonstrates posterior deviation of the esophagus adjacent to the enlarged left atrium (although rarely performed for this indication). Pulmonary vascular redistribution,

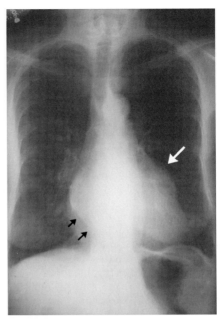

Figure 10·10   The chest radiograph of a patient with mitral stenosis shows mild left atrial enlargement with clear lung fields and a normal-size cardiac silhouette. The left atrial appendage bulge is indicated by the white arrow and the "double-density" due to an enlarged left atrium by the black arrows.

interstitial and alveolar edema may be seen if elevated left atrial pressures have led to hemodynamic decompensation. When pulmonary hypertension supervenes, the central pulmonary arteries are prominent and demonstrate a pattern of peripheral "pruning." Superimposed right heart dilation and failure lead to evidence of right ventricular and right atrial enlargement. Overall, the radiographic abnormalities correspond to the severity and chronicity of the disease process; findings are subtle early in the disease course.

Similarly, the classic electrocardiographic findings for patients with mitral stenosis include criteria for left atrial enlargement, right-axis deviation, and in severe cases, right ventricular hypertrophy. Notching of the P wave is a classic finding in mitral stenosis but also may be seen for patients with other cardiac diseases. Although early surgical series showed electrocardiographic evidence for right ventricular hypertrophy in 65% of patients,[45–47] right ventricular hypertrophy is less likely with earlier intervention. Electrocardiographic right-axis deviation and criteria for right ventricular hypertrophy indicate a mean pulmonary pressure of 40 mm Hg or higher, but the sensitivity of these criteria for detection of

TABLE 10·1	**ECHOCARDIOGRAPHIC EVALUATION OF THE PATIENT WITH MITRAL STENOSIS**

Mitral stenosis severity
   Mean pressure gradient
   Two-dimensional planimetered valve area
   Pressure half-time valve area
   Continuity equation valve area, if needed
Mitral valve morphology
Presence and severity of coexisting mitral
   regurgitation
Left atrial size and function
Evaluation for left atrial thrombus before balloon
   valvuloplasty (requires transesophageal
   echocardiography)
Pulmonary systolic pressures
Left ventricular size and function
Right ventricular size and function
Evaluation for rheumatic involvement of aortic or
   tricuspid valves

pulmonary hypertension in mitral stenosis have not been evaluated.[48, 49] Probably the most common electrocardiographic abnormality in patients with mitral stenosis is atrial fibrillation.

Echocardiography

Echocardiography is the cornerstone of the evaluation of the patient with suspected or known mitral stenosis (Table 10–1).[50] Echocardiographic evaluation includes quantitation of stenosis severity, description of valve morphology, evaluation of coexisting mitral regurgitation, and estimation of pulmonary systolic pressures (see Chapter 3). Left ventricular size and systolic function and the presence and severity of any associated valve lesions also can be evaluated. Evaluation of other valves is particularly important, as rheumatic mitral stenosis is associated with rheumatic aortic stenosis in 17% of cases, at least moderate aortic regurgitation in 8% of cases, tricuspid regurgitation in 38% of cases, and tricuspid stenosis in 4% of cases in a study of 205 consecutive patients.[51]

The severity of mitral stenosis ideally should be quantitated by 2D planimetry of valve area in a short-axis view and by the Doppler pressure half-time method (Fig. 10–11 and see Fig. 10–1). Although one or the other method may be more accurate in specific clinical situations, congruent results by both methods strengthen confidence in the data obtained. When the validity of one method is questioned, the other method should be used. For example, if 2D short-axis views are suboptimal, the pressure half-time method may be more accurate. Conversely, after balloon mitral valvuloplasty, the 2D approach is more accurate because of changing atrial and ventricular compliance im-

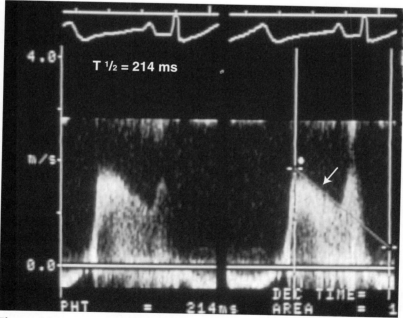

Figure 10·11 Mitral pressure half-time in a patient with mitral stenosis in sinus rhythm. The pressure half-time is measured from the early diastolic deceleration slope as shown by the line *(arrow)*. The pressure half-time of 214 ms in this patient corresponds to a valve area of 1.03 cm².

mediately after the procedure. Other methods for calculating mitral valve area, such as the continuity equation, are helpful when it is unclear why 2D and Doppler half-time valve areas are discrepant. Estimation of valve area from the size of the color flow vena contracta is not reliable.[52]

Mitral valve mean gradients can be calculated from the Doppler velocities. However, this information is less useful than valve area in the clinical setting due to the dependence of gradients on transvalvular volume flow rates.

Evaluation of mitral valve morphology is increasingly important as a prognostic indicator for hemodynamic progression and in choosing the optimal intervention for relief of mitral stenosis. Several approaches to describing mitral valve morphology have been proposed, but all focus on the degree of leaflet thickening and rigidity and on the extent of subvalvular deformity (see Tables 11–2 through 11–4). One method quantitates leaflet mobility by measurement of the height of the curve of the anterior leaflet relative to its base.[53] Another method classifies valve morphology into three groups based on flexibility of the valve leaflets and the degree of subvalvular involvement.[54] In this classification, Group 1 includes those patients with flexible leaflets with little chordal involvement, Group 2 includes those with flexible leaflets but extensive subvalvular disease, and Group 3 consists of those with calcified valves and rigid leaflets. Perhaps the most widely used approach is the Massachusetts General Hospital (MGH) morphology system, with a score of 0 to 4 assigned to each of four characteristics: leaflet thickening, calcification, mobility, and subvalvular involvement. These scores are summed to obtain a total morphology score ranging from 4 to 16.[55]

Whether one chooses to use one of these scoring systems or to use words to describe the morphology of the mitral valve apparatus, the key features are the degree of leaflet thickening, calcification, and mobility and the extent of subvalvular disease. In addition, the extent of commissural calcification may be important in predicting the results of valvuloplasty.[50, 56] Complications of the procedure may be predicted by the pattern of leaflet thickening and calcification (diffuse versus irregular). For example, severe mitral regurgitation after valvuloplasty appears to be caused by tearing of a relatively thin leaflet segment adjacent to an area of calcification.[57]

At least mild mitral regurgitation is present in 78% of patients with mitral stenosis.[51] Evaluation of mitral regurgitation typically includes color flow and continuous wave Doppler estimates of severity. However, when evaluating coexisting mitral regurgitation in patients with predominant mitral stenosis, potential underestimation due to shadowing of the left atrium by the abnormal valve must be considered. Transesophageal imaging may allow better definition of mitral regurgitant severity in this setting. Caution also is needed in using systolic blunting or reversal in the pulmonary venous flow pattern as a marker of mitral regurgitant severity. In patients with mitral stenosis, both the presence of atrial fibrillation and altered left atrial hemodynamics can result in abnormal systolic flow patterns, with blunting or reversal of the normal antegrade systolic flow pattern in the absence of significant mitral regurgitation.[10–12, 58] Systolic flow reversal associated with atrial fibrillation occurs early in systole, beginning an average of 58 ± 13 ms after the QRS, and is not related to the angiographic severity of mitral regurgitation. Late systolic flow reversal, beginning an average of 245 ± 46 ms after the QRS, is associated with higher left atrial v-wave pressures, but again does not correlate with mitral regurgitation severity.[58]

Although evaluation for left atrial thrombus is unnecessary for the routine management of the patient with mitral stenosis, left atrial thrombus is a contraindication to percutaneous valvuloplasty. Given the low sensitivity of transthoracic echocardiography for detection of atrial thrombus, transesophageal imaging is needed before valvuloplasty in patients who are otherwise appropriate candidates for this procedure (see Chapter 11).

Exercise Testing

Exercise testing is not a routine component in the evaluation of the patient with mitral stenosis, but it may be helpful in several specific situations. For example, in a patient with equivocal symptoms or an unclear history, exercise testing provides a quantitative and objective measure of exercise capacity. Conversely, in the patient with symptoms that appear to be out of proportion to resting hemodynamic severity, evaluation of exercise hemodynamics (noninvasively by Doppler echocardiography) may be invaluable in clinical decision making regarding the timing of intervention.[59] Exertional symptoms may be caused by an excessive rise in pulmonary pressures with exercise, which can be demonstrated by recording the tricuspid regurgitant jet at rest and immediately after exercise.[60] In some patients, resting systolic pressures of 40 to 60 mm Hg rise to more than 100 mm Hg with exercise, and in other patients, a much smaller increase (10 to 20 mm Hg) occurs (Table 10–2). Some investigators have suggested that an excessive rise in pulmonary pressures with exercise can be predicted from resting mitral valve resistance, but this hypothesis awaits further confirmation.[61]

Cardiac Catheterization

Echocardiography has largely replaced cardiac catheterization for the diagnosis and follow-up of patients with mitral stenosis. The major limitation of echocardiography is the lack of an accurate method for calculating pulmonary vascular resistance. While not all patients need pulmonary resistance measurement, particularly when pulmonary pressures are low, if the degree of elevation in pulmonary vascular resistance would alter clinical management, these data are optimally obtained at cardiac catheterization. In addition, cardiac catheterization should be considered in the occasional patient for whom echocardiographic data are nondiagnostic or when there is a discrepancy between the clinical presentation and echocardiographic findings.

In patients undergoing percutaneous mitral valvuloplasty, the hemodynamic results of the procedure can be optimized using the combined invasive and noninvasive approach for monitoring described in Chapter 11. In mitral stenosis patients undergoing surgical interven-

tion, coronary angiography may be needed, depending on clinical symptoms, age, gender, and other risk factors for coronary disease.

NATURAL HISTORY

Symptom Onset Relative to Acute Rheumatic Fever Episode

The interval between the episode of acute rheumatic fever and symptomatic mitral stenosis averaged 16.3 ± 5.2 years in a series of 159 European subjects (Fig. 10–12). This study found an additional interval of 9.2 ± 4.3 years from the onset of mild symptoms to progression to severe symptoms.[62] Typical European and North American patients undergoing intervention for mitral stenosis are 45 to 55 years of age.[5, 63] It remains unclear whether this long interval between acute rheumatic fever and symptomatic valve disease represents slow progression of the rheumatic process itself or reflects superimposed degenerative fibrosis and calcification due to abnormal blood flow through the damaged valve (see Chapter 2).

In contrast, there is a much shorter interval between the initial episode of acute rheumatic fever and symptomatic valve disease in developing countries. The mean age of patients undergoing mitral valvuloplasty in South Africa, India, and China is only 27 to 37 years.[6, 64, 65] In a series of 737 consecutive black patients undergoing mitral valve surgery in Soweto, South Africa, 39% had isolated mitral stenosis, 31% had isolated mitral regurgitation, and 30% had mixed stenosis and regurgitation (Fig. 10–13).[66] Mitral stenosis was caused by commissural fusion and chordal

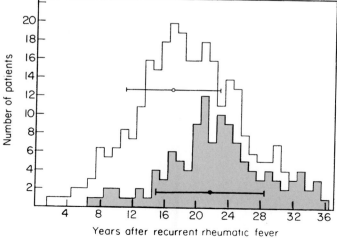

Figure 10·12 Interval between active rheumatic fever and clinical symptoms of valve disease in 177 patients with mitral stenosis *(open bars)* and 121 patients with aortic stenosis *(shaded bars)*. (From Horstkotte D, Niehues R, Strauer BE: Pathomorphological aspects, aetiology, and natural history of acquired mitral valve stenosis. Eur Heart J 1991;12(suppl):55–60.)

Years after recurrent rheumatic fever

TABLE 10·2 EXERCISE CHANGES IN MITRAL STENOSIS

Study	Patients		Mean Gradient (mm Hg)		Pulmonary Artery Systolic Pressure		Other Changes
			Rest	*Exercise*	*Rest*	*Exercise*	
Leavitt, 1991[60]	12		9 ± 7	17 ± 8	41 ± 19	70 ± 32	Exercise change in PA pressure, 24 mm Hg in symptomatic versus 15 mm Hg in asymptomatic patients (*P* = 0.04)
Tunick, 1992[59]	17						
Dahan, 1993[26]	27						Change in SV with exercise depends on change in MVA
Cheriex, 1994[28]	60	MVA >1.4 cm^2	5.2 ± 1.9	8.8 ± 3.0			⎰ TR jet increased from 2.9 ± 0.5 to 3.6 ± 0.5 m/s for entire study group
		MVA 1–1.4 cm^2	8.8 ± 4.9	14.8 ± 6.4			
		MVA <1.0 cm^2	11.8 ± 4.1	20.3 ± 5.8			
Tischler, 1995[93]	14		4.5 ± 1.4	12.7 ± 2.7	36 ± 5	63 ± 14	5 (35%) of 14 patients developed severe MR with exercise

MR, mitral regurgitation; MVA, mitral valve area; PA, pulmonary artery; SV, stroke volume; TR, tricuspid regurgitant.

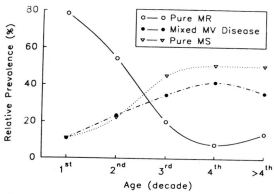

Figure 10·13 Analysis by decade of the relative prevalence of isolated mitral regurgitation, mixed mitral valve disease, and isolated mitral stenosis in a consecutive series of 714 black South Africans undergoing mitral valve surgery for rheumatic valve disease. (Reproduced with permission from Marcus RH, Sareli P, Pocock WA, Barlow JB: The spectrum of severe rheumatic mitral valve disease in a developing country: correlations among clinical presentation, surgical pathologic findings, and hemodynamic sequelae. Ann Intern Med 1994;120:177–183.)

shortening, as is seen in North American and European series; however, the patients undergoing surgery for mitral stenosis were only in the third or fourth decade of life. Evidence of active rheumatic disease was present in only 2% of those with mitral stenosis, suggesting that stenosis is caused by a slowly progressive form of the disease process.[66]

Clinical Outcome Without Surgical Intervention

Our knowledge of the natural history of mitral stenosis is largely based on clinical series compiled before the wide availability of surgical treatment and on smaller groups of subjects in the surgical era who refused intervention (Fig. 10–14). In these studies, even when a high proportion of the subjects were asymptomatic at entry, the 10-year mortality rate ranged from 33% to 70%, with a 20-year mortality rate of 80% to 87%.[31, 32] In these historical studies, the incidence of heart failure was about 60%, and about 20% of patients had embolic events.[31] A more recent series of patients who refused intervention for mitral stenosis had a 5-year survival rate of only 44% ± 6%, confirming the poor outcome associated with symptomatic mitral stenosis treated only with medical therapy (Fig. 10–15).[62]

Hemodynamic Progression

While clinical studies have provided considerable data on the rate of symptom develop-

ment and outcome for patients with mitral stenosis, data on the rate of hemodynamic progression have been scanty because catheterization usually was performed only before a planned intervention. One study with serial catheterization data for 42 mitral stenosis patients showed no progression in 15 subjects (mean age, 42 years) over a 1- to 10-year interval (mean, 3.7 years), whereas 27 patients (mean age, 45 years) followed for 1 to 8 years (mean, 2.6 years) had an average decrease in mitral valve area of 0.32 cm²/year (Table 10–3). However, no factors could be identified that predicted progression versus a stable valve area.[67]

Two recent observational studies used Doppler echocardiography to define the rate of hemodynamic progression of mitral stenosis. In a series of 50 patients with mitral stenosis (mean age, 56 years; 80% female), baseline Doppler hemodynamics included a mean transmitral gradient of 5 mm Hg, a mitral valve area of 1.7 ± 0.7 cm², and a left atrial dimension of 5.0 ± 0.9 cm.[68] Over a mean follow-up of 39 months, valve area decreased on average by 0.09 ± 0.21 cm²/year. In 68% of subjects, no significant progression occurred during the follow-up period. In the 32% of subjects with disease progression (ie, decrease in valve area of >0.1 cm²/year), the average rate of decrease in valve area was 0.3 cm²/year. Multivariate predictors of hemodynamic progression were a more deformed and calcified valve and a high transmitral gradient. A decrease in valve area of more than 0.1 cm²/year occurred in 80% of subjects with an MGH morphology score of 8 or higher and a peak transmitral gradient more than 10 mm Hg, compared with 5% of those with a score less than 8 and a peak gradient less than 10 mm Hg (Fig. 10–16).

A similar rate of hemodynamic progression was observed in a retrospective series of 103 patients for whom two echocardiographic studies had been performed at a mean interval of 3.3 ± 2 years. The average decrease in valve area was 0.09 ± 0.13 cm²/year.[69] Baseline characteristics were similar compared with the earlier series: the mean age was 61 ± 16 years, 74% were female, and the initial mitral valve area was 1.7 ± 0.6 cm². Again, marked heterogeneity in the rate of hemodynamic progression was observed, with 66% of patients having no or little (<0.1 cm²/year) decrease in valve area and 34% of patients having more rapid progression. No predictors of the rate of decrease in valve area could be identified in this

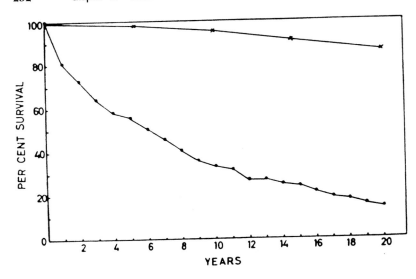

Figure 10·14 Survival of 271 mitral stenosis patients with medical therapy (no surgery) from the time of diagnosis *(lower curve)* compared with the normal survival of the population of Denmark *(upper curve)*. (From Olesen KH: The natural history of 271 patients with mitral stenosis under medical treatment. Br Heart J 1962;24:349–357. BMJ Publishing Group.)

study other than initial valve area (ie, more rapid progression in those with a larger mitral valve area). Of note, even with only mild to moderate mitral stenosis at baseline, increases

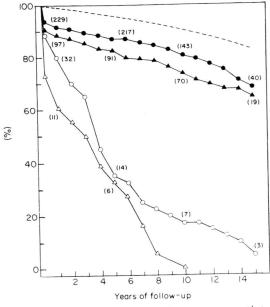

Figure 10·15 Natural history of 159 patients with isolated mitral stenosis *(open circles)* or mitral regurgitation *(open triangles)* who were not operated on (even though the operation was indicated) compared with patients treated with valve replacement for mitral stenosis *(solid circles)* or mitral regurgitation *(solid triangles)*. The expected survival in the absence of mitral valve disease is indicated by upper curve *(dashed line)*. (From Horstkotte D, Niehues R, Strauer BE: Pathomorphological aspects, aetiology, and natural history of acquired mitral valve stenosis. Eur Heart J 1991;12(suppl):55–60.)

in right ventricular diastolic area, tricuspid regurgitant severity, and pulmonary pressures were observed over the study interval.[69]

Both of these studies are limited by potential selection bias, because only subjects with two echocardiographic studies were included. Exclusion of patients with more rapid progression who were referred directly for valvuloplasty without an intervening noninvasive study would bias the results toward a slower mean rate of progression. Conversely, the absence of data from patients with a stable clinical course who were not referred for a second echocardiographic study would bias the results toward a more rapid rate of progression. Nevertheless, these data do provide a starting point for estimating the likelihood of disease progression in an individual patient in order to determine the appropriate timing of follow-up studies and for patient education.

Complications

The prevalence of atrial fibrillation among patients with mitral stenosis increases with age, affecting 17% of patients between 21 and 30 years, 45% of those between 31 and 40 years, 60% of those between 41 and 50 years, and 80% of those older than 51 years of age in one series.[37] The association of atrial fibrillation with age appears to be partly independent of the effect of disease severity, since recent series of patients undergoing valvuloplasty (all of whom have severe mitral stenosis) have a prevalence of atrial fibrillation ranging from 4% in younger patients in India to 45% in an older North American population (see Table

TABLE 10·3 RATE OF HEMODYNAMIC PROGRESSION OF MITRAL STENOSIS

Study	Patients	Mean Age (y)	Percent Female	MVA (cm²)	Follow-up Interval (y)	Rate of Progression	Predictors of Progression
Dubin, 1971[67]	Progressors = 27 Nonprogressors = 15	45 42			2.6 3.7	0.32 cm²/y No change	None
Gordon, 1992[68]	50	56	80%	1.7 ± 0.7 cm²	3.3	Overall 0.09 ± 0.21 cm²/y Rapid progression (>0.1 cm²/y) in 32%	Higher morphology score Higher transmitral gradient
Sagie, 1996[69]	103	61 ± 16	74%	1.7 ± 0.6 cm²	3.3 ± 2	Overall 0.09 ± 0.13 cm²/y Rapid progression (>0.1 cm²/y) in 34%	Larger initial valve area

MVA, mitral valve area.

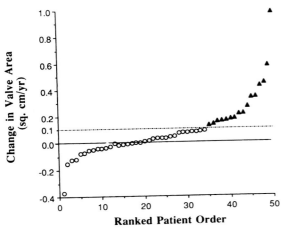

Figure 10·16 Individual rates of mitral valve narrowing in 50 mitral stenosis patients, in rank order. Patients were stratified into progression *(solid triangles)* or nonprogression *(open circles)* groups, defined on the basis of an annual rate of valve narrowing of less than 0.1 cm²/yr. (From Gordon SP, Douglas PS, Come PC, Manning WJ: Two-dimensional and Doppler echocardiographic determinants of the natural history of mitral valve narrowing in patients with rheumatic mitral stenosis: implications for follow-up. J Am Coll Cardiol 1992;19:968–973; reprinted with permission from the American College of Cardiology.)

11–4).[5] In a series of patients older than 65 years of age undergoing mitral valvuloplasty, the prevalence of atrial fibrillation was 74%.[70] A high prevalence of atrial fibrillation (60%) also was observed among mitral stenosis patients with pulmonary hypertension.[71]

The association between atrial fibrillation and left atrial thrombus formation is well known from autopsy studies showing a high prevalence of left atrial thrombus among patients with mitral stenosis.[72, 73] Most atrial thrombi occur in the atrial appendage, possibly related to the larger size of the left atrial appendage and less effective emptying in mitral stenosis patients compared with patients who have other reasons for atrial fibrillation.[74] In patients with mitral stenosis, atrial fibrillation is associated with a higher prevalence of embolic events compared with patients remaining in sinus rhythm. The incidence of systemic embolism in 737 patients with mitral stenosis was 32% in patients older than 35 years of age with atrial fibrillation versus 11% in those over age 35 years in sinus rhythm.[75]

The higher risk for embolic events in mitral stenosis patients with atrial fibrillation, compared to patients with atrial fibrillation without mitral valve disease, also is well documented.[76] The Framingham study estimated a 17-fold increase in the risk of stroke for patients with atrial fibrillation and mitral stenosis, compared with a 5-fold increased risk for atrial fibrillation without mitral valve disease.[77] A European series estimated the risk of embolic events in mitral stenosis with atrial fibrillation as 3.6 cases per 1000 patient-years for those with moderate stenosis and 5.7 cases per 1000 patient-years for those with severe mitral stenosis.[62] A study of 500 mitral stenosis patients identified atrial fibrillation and spontaneous left atrial contrast as risk factors for systemic embolism.[78]

In addition, mitral stenosis with atrial fibrillation is associated with excess mortality. A life insurance population showed a 5-year survival rate for mitral stenosis patients with atrial fibrillation of only 64%, compared with 85% in patients with atrial fibrillation but no mitral valve disease.[79]

Although the risk of left atrial thrombus formation and embolic events is thought to remain low for mitral stenosis patients in sinus rhythm, the high prevalence of spontaneous contrast observed on transesophageal echocardiography (up to 45% of patients) in this group raises the possibility of a higher embolic risk, even with sinus rhythm, in the presence of mitral stenosis.[78, 80] Some patients in sinus rhythm have demonstrable thrombus.[74, 80] Further, many patients with new-onset atrial fibrillation have left atrial thrombus, suggesting that thrombus formation occurred before the onset of the arrhythmia.[81] The possible mechanism of atrial thrombus formation with sinus rhythm is loss of the atrial appendage's mechanical function despite electrical evidence of sinus rhythm, leading to blood flow stasis.[74]

MEDICAL THERAPY

Since the time from diagnosis of mild mitral stenosis to severe stenosis requiring intervention can be quite long, medical therapy is the primary treatment modality in the management of these patients (Table 10–4). The goals of medical therapy include preventing complications of the disease process, treating symptoms, and defining the optimal timing of mechanical intervention (see Chapter 11). Other than prevention of recurrent episodes of rheumatic fever, there are no known therapies to decrease the rate of hemodynamic progression in patients with rheumatic mitral valve disease.

Noninvasive Follow-up

Once the diagnosis of mitral stenosis has been confirmed with a baseline Doppler echo-

TABLE 10·4 MEDICAL THERAPY FOR MITRAL STENOSIS

Noninvasive follow-up
  Symptoms and functional status
  Echocardiography at baseline and then as
    clinically indicated
  Exercise echocardiography if clinically indicated
Prevention of endocarditis
Prevention of recurrent rheumatic fever
Prevention of embolic events
Treatment of pulmonary congestive symptoms
Counseling about pregnancy and contraception

cardiographic examination, the timing of repeat studies should be tailored to the individual patient according to stenosis severity at baseline, coexisting cardiac abnormalities, and interim changes in symptoms or functional status. For example, echocardiography may be needed at only 2- to 3-year intervals for patients with mild stenosis (valve area >1.5 cm²), little mitral regurgitation, mild left atrial enlargement, and normal pulmonary pressures. More frequent examinations are needed for the patient with moderate stenosis, any evidence of pulmonary hypertension, or the onset of atrial fibrillation. Interim changes in symptoms or a change found on physical examination should prompt repeat evaluation.

Echocardiography should be repeated if there is a significant interim comorbid event for which accurate knowledge of disease severity is needed for patient management. For example, repeat evaluation of the pregnant patient with mitral stenosis allows adjustment of the frequency of prenatal visits, an assessment of the potential need for a planned delivery with invasive hemodynamic monitoring, and an opportunity for patient education about the need for prompt medical attention should cardiac symptoms occur. Of note, conditions associated with a high cardiac output, such as pregnancy, fever, or anemia, are associated with a higher transmitral pressure gradient, although valve area remains unchanged. The increased left atrial pressure associated with the increased cardiac output may lead to clinical decompensation with pulmonary edema, even though the severity of mitral stenosis has not changed in the interim.

Prevention of Recurrent Rheumatic Fever and Endocarditis

Primary prevention of rheumatic fever is based on treatment of streptococcal pharyngitis with appropriate antibiotics for a sufficient period. Patients with a history of rheumatic fever are at high risk for recurrent disease, leading to repeated episodes of valvulitis and increased damage to the valvular tissue. Since recurrent streptococcal infections may be asymptomatic, secondary prevention is achieved with continuous antibiotic therapy (see Table 6–3). The risk of recurrent disease is highest for those exposed to streptococcal infections (eg, contact with children, crowded situations) and economically disadvantaged persons. The recommended duration of secondary prevention is longer for patients with evidence of carditis or persistent valvular disease than for those with no evidence of valvular damage.

Patients with rheumatic mitral stenosis also should receive standard antibiotic prophylaxis for prevention of bacterial endocarditis (see Chapter 6), as the doses used for secondary prevention of rheumatic fever are inadequate for prevention of endocarditis.

Prevention of Embolic Events

Embolic events are best prevented by interventions to relieve mitral valve obstruction before the development of excessive left atrial enlargement and atrial fibrillation. When atrial fibrillation does occur, efforts should be directed toward restoration of sinus rhythm through mechanical intervention to increase mitral valve area, if appropriate, or through electrical cardioversion in conjunction with pharmacologic therapy, as in patients without mitral stenosis.[82] Both electrical cardioversion and pharmacologic therapy followed by valvuloplasty or surgery may be needed for maintenance of sinus rhythm.

If efforts to achieve and maintain sinus rhythm are unsuccessful, attention should be directed to pharmacologic rate control and long-term anticoagulation. Rapid ventricular rates are poorly tolerated in mitral stenosis due to impaired ventricular filling. Rate control, usually by pharmacologic depression of conduction and prolonged refractoriness in the atrioventricular node, allows an adequate period for diastolic filling of the left ventricle across the stenotic mitral valve. Standard approaches to rate control are appropriate in the patient with mitral stenosis, including treatment with a β blocker, a calcium channel blocker, or a combination of agents, depending on the clinical circumstances for each patient.[82] Rarely, rate control can only be achieved by surgical or catheter ablation of the atrioventricular node and implantation of a permanent pacemaker.

With persistent atrial fibrillation, anticoagulation with warfarin to achieve a therapeutic international normalized ratio (INR) is particularly important in patients with mitral stenosis given the high risk for embolic events. Most clinicians recommend an INR of 2.0 to 3.0 with careful monitoring of INR levels, especially in the elderly.[82]

Recent trials of alternate therapy for prevention of embolic events in patients with atrial fibrillation[83, 84] have excluded patients with mitral stenosis from the study population. Given that most patients with mitral stenosis and atrial fibrillation are at high risk for embolic events, therapy with aspirin is likely to be suboptimal and should be considered only if there is a definite contraindication to warfarin anticoagulation. Although there have been no randomized trials of warfarin versus aspirin therapy for mitral stenosis, one small observational study in Thailand found 3 of 56 patients taking aspirin had cardioembolic strokes, compared with none of the 17 on warfarin.[85]

Although transesophageal evaluation for left atrial thrombus has been proposed to allow earlier cardioversion in patients with atrial fibrillation, the risk of left atrial thrombus is so high among patients with mitral stenosis that it is prudent to consider therapeutic anticoagulation with warfarin for at least 2 weeks before cardioversion.[81] Similarly, all patients with mitral stenosis being considered for percutaneous mitral valvuloplasty should undergo transesophageal echocardiography shortly before the procedure given the high risk of embolic complications if a left atrial thrombus is present.[80]

In patients undergoing surgical intervention for mitral stenosis, another proposed approach to restoration of sinus rhythm is the Cox maze operation. This procedure attempts to surgically create a single electrical pathway from the sinus node to the atrioventricular node, while isolating the abnormal electrical activity of the left and right atrial tissue. In a series of 20 patients with atrial fibrillation and mitral valve disease, sinus rhythm was restored in 15 (75%) patients, 4 others showed an ectopic atrial rhythm, and only 1 had persistent atrial fibrillation. At 10-month follow-up, 18 (90%) of 20 did not require antiarrhythmic therapy.[86] A potential disadvantage of the maze procedure, in addition to the longer surgical time, is impaired atrial mechanical function,

despite restoration of sinus rhythm,[87] raising the possibility of continued risk for atrial thrombus formation after the procedure. Because atrial thrombus formation and embolic events remain a major cause of morbidity and mortality for mitral stenosis patients, further evaluation of surgical approaches to restoration of sinus rhythm is needed.

Treatment of Pulmonary Congestive Symptoms

The initial symptoms of patients with mitral stenosis most often are related to a low forward cardiac output, rather than to pulmonary congestion. Surgical or catheter balloon relief of mitral stenosis should be considered at the onset of definite symptoms or signs of pulmonary congestion. Possible precipitating factors, such as atrial fibrillation, anemia, or infection, should be sought and treated as appropriate. Symptoms include paroxysmal nocturnal dyspnea, orthopnea, shortness of breath, and at the extreme, pulmonary edema. Physical examination often reveals rales on auscultation of the lungs. Evidence of elevated pulmonary venous pressures and interstitial edema on chest radiography provides objective confirmation of the diagnosis.

If the patient has pulmonary congestion but disease severity does not warrant mechanical intervention or if comorbid disease prevents effective relief of mitral stenosis, pharmacologic therapy with diuretics may provide symptomatic improvement. β-blocking agents also may be beneficial, as the shortened diastolic filling pressure associated with an increased heart rate leads to elevated pulmonary venous pressure and pulmonary edema.[88, 89] Unfortunately, even though resting hemodynamics may be improved, β blockers do not appear to improve exercise tolerance in mitral stenosis patients.[90, 91]

Other Therapeutic Considerations

Women with mitral stenosis should receive appropriate counseling regarding contraception and pregnancy, particularly if they have atrial fibrillation and are on warfarin anticoagulation. Mild mitral stenosis may be well tolerated despite the increased hemodynamic load of pregnancy. However, patients with moderate stenosis may develop pulmonary congestion due to an increased flow rate in the setting of a fixed mitral orifice area, leading to elevations in left atrial and pulmonary venous pressures.

The normal increase in heart rate during pregnancy also may exacerbate symptoms as the diastolic filling time is shortened so that the use of β blockers to lengthen the diastolic filling period can be helpful.[89] For a patient with symptoms of severe stenosis, invasive hemodynamic monitoring at the time of induced labor may be necessary to maintain an adequate left atrial filling pressure while avoiding pulmonary edema. For pregnant patients with severe symptoms refractory to medical therapy, mitral valvuloplasty has been performed during pregnancy.[38, 39, 92]

References

1. Roberts WC, Virmani R: Aschoff bodies at necropsy in valvular heart disease: evidence from an analysis of 543 patients over 14 years of age that rheumatic heart disease, at least anatomically, is a disease of the mitral valve. Circulation 1978;57:803–807.
2. Virmani R, Roberts WC: Aschoff bodies in operatively excised atrial appendages and in papillary muscles: frequency and clinical significance. Circulation 1977;55:559–563.
3. Rusted IE, Scheiflay CH, Edwards JE: Studies of the mitral valve: certain anatomic features of the mitral valve and associated structures in mitral stenosis. Circulation 1956;14:398.
4. Pan M, Medina A, Suarez de Lezo J, et al: Factors determining late success after mitral balloon valvulotomy. Am J Cardiol 1993;71:1181–1185.
5. Balloon Valvuloplasty Registry: Multicenter experience with balloon mitral commissurotomy: NHLBI Balloon Valvuloplasty Registry Report on immediate and 30-day follow-up results. The National Heart, Lung, and Blood Institute Balloon Valvuloplasty Registry Participants. Circulation 1992;85:448–461.
6. Chen CR, Cheng TO: Percutaneous balloon mitral valvuloplasty by the Inoue technique: a multicenter study of 4832 patients in China. Am Heart J 1995;129:1197–1203.
7. Beyer RW, Olmos A, Bermudez RF, Noll HE: Mitral valve resistance as a hemodynamic indicator in mitral stenosis. Am J Cardiol 1992;69:775–779.
8. Braverman AC, Thomas JD, Lee RT: Doppler echocardiographic estimation of mitral valve area during changing hemodynamic conditions. Am J Cardiol 1991;68:1485–1490.
9. Stojnic BB, Radjen GS, Perisic NJ, Pavlovic PB, Stosic JJ, Prcovic M: Pulmonary venous flow pattern studied by transoesophageal pulsed Doppler echocardiography in mitral stenosis in sinus rhythm: effect of atrial systole. Eur Heart J 1993;14:1597–1601.
10. Lee MM, Park SW, Kim CH, et al: Relation of pulmonary venous flow to mean left atrial pressure in mitral stenosis with sinus rhythm. Am Heart J 1993;126:1401–1407.
11. Klein AL, Bailey AS, Cohen GI, et al: Importance of sampling both pulmonary veins in grading mitral regurgitation by transesophageal echocardiography. J Am Soc Echocardiogr 1993;6:115–123.
12. Jolly N, Arora R, Mohan JC, Khalilullah M: Pulmonary venous flow dynamics before and after balloon mitral valvuloplasty as determined by transesopha-geal Doppler echocardiography. Am J Cardiol 1992;70:780–784.
13. Waller BF: Etiology of mitral stenosis and pure mitral regurgitation. *In* Waller BF, ed. Pathology of the Heart and Great Vessels. New York: Churchill Livingstone; 1988:101–148.
14. Remetz MS, Cleman MW, Cabin HS: Pulmonary and pleural complications of cardiac disease. Clin Chest Med 1989;10:545–592.
15. Widimsky J: Pulmonary precapillary hypertension in mitral valve disease. Cor Vasa 1983;25:17–27.
16. Dalen JE: Mitral stenosis. *In* Dalen JE, Alpert JS, eds. Valvular Heart Disease. Boston: Little, Brown; 1987.
17. Tryka AF, Godleski JJ, Schoen FJ, Vandevanter SH: Pulmonary vascular disease and hypertension after valve surgery for mitral stenosis. Hum Pathol 1985;16:65–71.
18. Otto CM, Davis KB, Reid CL, et al: Relation between pulmonary artery pressure and mitral stenosis severity in patients undergoing balloon mitral commissurotomy. Am J Cardiol 1993;71:874–878.
19. Yamamoto K, Ikeda U, Mito H, Fujikawa H, Sekiguchi H, Shimada K: Endothelin production in pulmonary circulation of patients with mitral stenosis. Circulation 1994;89:2093–2098.
20. Iskandrian AS, Hakki AH, Ren JF, et al: Correlation among right ventricular preload, afterload and ejection fraction in mitral valve disease: radionuclide, echocardiographic and hemodynamic evaluation. J Am Coll Cardiol 1984;3:1403–1411.
21. Wroblewski E, James F, Spann JF, Bove AA: Right ventricular performance in mitral stenosis. Am J Cardiol 1981;47:51–55.
22. Morrison DA, Lancaster L, Henry R, Goldman S: Right ventricular function at rest and during exercise in aortic and mitral valve disease. J Am Coll Cardiol 1985;5:21–28.
23. Kussmaul WG, Noordergraaf A, Laskey WK: Right ventricular-pulmonary arterial interactions. Ann Biomed Eng 1992;20:63–80.
24. Gaasch WH, Folland ED: Left ventricular function in rheumatic mitral stenosis. Eur Heart J 1991;12(suppl B):66–69.
25. Voelker W, Berner A, Regele B, et al: Effect of exercise on valvular resistance in patients with mitral stenosis. J Am Coll Cardiol 1993;22:777–782.
26. Dahan M, Paillole C, Martin D, Gourgon R: Determinants of stroke volume response to exercise in patients with mitral stenosis: a Doppler echocardiographic study. J Am Coll Cardiol 1993;21:384–389.
27. Geigy Scientific Tables, vol 5: Heart and Circulation. Basel: Ciba-Geigy; 1990.
28. Cheriex EC, Pieters FA, Janssen JH, de Swart H, Palmans Meulemans A: Value of exercise Doppler-echocardiography in patients with mitral stenosis. Int J Cardiol 1994;45:219–226.
29. Triposkiadis F, Trikas A, Tentolouris K, et al: Effect of atrial fibrillation on exercise capacity in mitral stenosis. Am J Cardiol 1995;76:282–286.
30. Ravin A, Slonim NB, Balchum OJ, Dressler SH, Grow JB, et al: Diagnosis of tight mitral stenosis. JAMA 1952;149:1079–1084.
31. Rowe JC, Bland EF, Sprague HB, White PD: The course of mitral stenosis without surgery: ten and twenty year perspectives. Ann Intern Med 1960;52:741–749.
32. Olesen KH: The natural history of 271 patients with mitral stenosis under medical treatment. Br Heart J 1962;24:349–357.

33. Rapaport E: Natural history of aortic and mitral valve disease. Am J Cardiol 1975;35:221–227.
34. Wood P: An appreciation of mitral stenosis. Br Med J 1954;1:1054.
35. Camishion RC, Gibbon JH Jr, Pierucci L Jr: Paralysis of the left recurrent laryngeal nerve secondary to mitral valve disease: report of two cases and literature review. Ann Surg 1966;163:818–828.
36. Selzer A, Cohn KE: Natural history of mitral stenosis. Circulation 1972;45:878.
37. Deverall PB, Olley PM, Smith DR, Watson DA, Whitaker W: Incidence of systemic embolism before and after mitral valvotomy. Thorax 1968;23:530–536.
38. Patel JJ, Mitha AS, Hassen F, et al: Percutaneous balloon mitral valvotomy in pregnant patients with tight pliable mitral stenosis. Am Heart J 1993;125:1106–1109.
39. Ribeiro PA, Fawzy ME, Awad M, Dunn B, Duran CG: Balloon valvotomy for pregnant patients with severe pliable mitral stenosis using the Inoue technique with total abdominal and pelvic shielding. Am Heart J 1992;124:1558–1562.
40. Perloff JK: Physical Examination of the Heart and Circulation. Philadelphia: WB Saunders; 1982.
41. Criley JM, Feldman IM, Meredith T: Mitral valve closure and the crescendo presystolic murmur. Am J Med 1971;51:456–465.
42. Criley JM, Hermer AJ: The crescendo presystolic murmur of mitral stenosis with atrial fibrillation. N Engl J Med 1971;285:1284–1287.
43. Legler JF, Benchimol A, Dimond EG: The apex cardiogram in the study of the 2-OS interval. Br Heart J 1963;25:246.
44. Craige E: Phonocardiographic studies in mitral stenosis. N Engl J Med 1957;257:650.
45. Fraser HRL, Turner R: Electrocardiography in mitral valvular disease. Br Heart J 1955;17:459.
46. Cosby RS, Levinson DC, Dimitroff SP, et al: The electrocardiogram in congenital heart disease and mitral stenosis: a correlation of electrocardiographic pattern with right ventricular pressure, flow, and work. Am Heart J 1953;46:670.
47. Pruitt RD, Robinson JG: The electrocardiographic findings in patients undergoing surgical exploration of the mitral valve. Am Heart J 1956;52:881.
48. Fowler NO, Noble WJ, Giarratano SJ, et al: The clinical estimation of pulmonary hypertension accompanying mitral stenosis. Am Heart J 1955;49:237.
49. Semler HJ, Pruitt RD: An electrocardiographic estimation of the pulmonary vascular obstruction in 80 patients with mitral stenosis. Am Heart J 1960;59:541.
50. Reid CL: Echocardiography in the patient undergoing catheter balloon mitral commissurotomy. *In* Otto CM, ed. The Practice of Clinical Echocardiography. Philadelphia: WB Saunders; 1997:373–388.
51. Sagie A, Freitas N, Chen MH, Marshall JE, Weyman AE, Levine RA: Echocardiographic assessment of mitral stenosis and its associated valvular lesions in 205 patients and lack of association with mitral valve prolapse. J Am Soc Echocardiogr 1997;10:141–148.
52. Faletra F, Pezzano JA, Fusco R, et al: Measurement of mitral valve area in mitral stenosis: four echocardiographic methods compared with direct measurement of anatomic orifices. J Am Coll Cardiol 1996;28:1190–1197.
53. Reid CL, Chandraratna PA, Kawanishi DT, Kotlewski A, Rahimtoola SH: Influence of mitral valve morphology on double-balloon catheter balloon valvuloplasty in patients with mitral stenosis: analysis of factors predicting immediate and 3-month results. Circulation 1989;80:515–524.
54. Iung B, Cormier B, Ducimetiere P, et al: Functional results 5 years after successful percutaneous mitral commissurotomy in a series of 528 patients and analysis of predictive factors. J Am Coll Cardiol 1996;27:407–414.
55. Wilkins GT, Weyman AE, Abascal VM, Block PC, Palacios IF: Percutaneous balloon dilatation of the mitral valve: an analysis of echocardiographic variables related to outcome and the mechanism of dilatation. Br Heart J 1988;60:299–308.
56. Fatkin D, Roy P, Morgan JJ, Feneley MP: Percutaneous balloon mitral valvotomy with the Inoue single-balloon catheter: commissural morphology as a determinant of outcome. J Am Coll Cardiol 1993;21:390–397.
57. Padial LR, Freitas N, Sagie A, et al: Echocardiography can predict which patients will develop severe mitral regurgitation after percutaneous mitral valvulotomy. J Am Coll Cardiol 1996;27:1225–1231.
58. Tice FD, Heinle SK, Harrison JK, et al: Transesophageal echocardiographic assessment of reversal of systolic pulmonary venous flow in mitral stenosis. Am J Cardiol 1995;75:58–60.
59. Tunick PA, Freedberg RS, Gargiulo A, Kronzon I: Exercise Doppler echocardiography as an aid to clinical decision making in mitral valve disease. J Am Soc Echocardiogr 1992;5:225–230.
60. Leavitt JI, Coats MH, Falk RH: Effects of exercise on transmitral gradient and pulmonary artery pressure in patients with mitral stenosis or a prosthetic mitral valve: a Doppler echocardiographic study. J Am Coll Cardiol 1991;17:1520–1526.
61. Schwammenthal E, Rabinowitz B, Kaplinsky E, Vered Z, Feinberg MS: Mitral valve resistance: wrong physics, right physiology [abstract]? Circulation 1996;94(suppl I):617.
62. Horstkotte D, Niehues R, Strauer BE: Pathomorphological aspects, aetiology and natural history of acquired mitral valve stenosis. Eur Heart J 1991;12(suppl):55–60.
63. Vahanian A, Michel PL, Cormier B, et al: Immediate and mid-term results of percutaneous mitral commissurotomy. Eur Heart J 1991;12(suppl):84–89.
64. Rothlisberger C, Essop MR, Skudicky D, Skoularigis J, Wisenbaugh T, Sareli P: Results of percutaneous balloon mitral valvotomy in young adults. Am J Cardiol 1993;72:73–77.
65. Arora R, Kalra GS, Murty GS, et al: Percutaneous transatrial mitral commissurotomy: immediate and intermediate results. J Am Coll Cardiol 1994;23:1327–1332.
66. Marcus RH, Sareli P, Pocock WA, Barlow JB: The spectrum of severe rheumatic mitral valve disease in a developing country: correlations among clinical presentation, surgical pathologic findings, and hemodynamic sequelae. Ann Intern Med 1994;120:177–183.
67. Dubin AA, March HW, Cohn K, Selzer A: Longitudinal hemodynamic and clinical study of mitral stenosis. Circulation 1971;44:381–389.
68. Gordon SP, Douglas PS, Come PC, Manning WJ: Two-dimensional and Doppler echocardiographic determinants of the natural history of mitral valve narrowing in patients with rheumatic mitral stenosis: implications for follow-up. J Am Coll Cardiol 1992;19:968–973.

69. Sagie A, Freitas N, Padial LR, et al: Doppler echocardiographic assessment of long-term progression of mitral stenosis in 103 patients: valve area and right heart disease. J Am Coll Cardiol 1996;28:472–479.

70. Tuzcu EM, Block PC, Griffin BP, Newell JB, Palacios IF: Immediate and long-term outcome of percutaneous mitral valvotomy in patients 65 years and older. Circulation 1992;85:963–971.

71. Alfonso F, Macaya C, Hernandez R, et al: Percutaneous mitral valvuloplasty with severe pulmonary artery hypertension. Am J Cardiol 1993;72:325–330.

72. Aberg H: Atrial fibrillation. I. A study of atrial thrombosis and systemic embolism in a necropsy material. Acta Med Scand 1969;185:373–379.

73. Fatkin D, Feneley M: Stratification of thromboembolic risk of atrial fibrillation by transthoracic echocardiography and transesophageal echocardiography: the relative role of left atrial appendage function, mitral valve disease, and spontaneous echocardiographic contrast. Prog Cardiovasc Dis 1996;39:57–68.

74. Hwang JJ, Li YH, Lin JM, et al: Left atrial appendage function determined by transesophageal echocardiography in patients with rheumatic mitral valve disease. Cardiology 1994;85:121–128.

75. Coulshed N, Epstein EJ, McKendrick CS, Galloway RW, Walker E: Systemic embolism in mitral valve disease. Br Heart J 1970;32:26–34.

76. Hinton RC, Kistler JP, Fallon JT, Friedlich AL, Fisher CM: Influence of etiology of atrial fibrillation on incidence of systemic embolism. Am J Cardiol 1977;40:509–513.

77. Wolf PA, Dawber TR, Thomas HE Jr, Kannel WB: Epidemiologic assessment of chronic atrial fibrillation and risk of stroke: the Framingham study. Neurology 1978;28:973–977.

78. Chiang CW, Lo SK, Kuo CT, Cheng NJ, Hsu TS: Noninvasive predictors of systemic embolism in mitral stenosis: an echocardiographic and clinical study of 500 patients. Chest 1994;106:396–399.

79. Gajewski J, Singer RB: Mortality in an insured population with atrial fibrillation. JAMA 1981;245:1540–1544.

80. Rittoo D, Sutherland GR, Currie P, Starkey IR, Shaw TR: A prospective study of left atrial spontaneous echo contrast and thrombus in 100 consecutive patients referred for balloon dilation of the mitral valve. J Am Soc Echocardiogr 1994;7:516–527.

81. Stoddard MF, Dawkins PR, Prince CR, Longaker RA: Transesophageal echocardiographic guidance of cardioversion in patients with atrial fibrillation. Am Heart J 1995;129:1204–1215.

82. Prystowsky EN, Benson DW Jr, Fuster V, et al: Management of patients with atrial fibrillation: a Statement for Healthcare Professionals. From the Subcommittee on Electrocardiography and Electrophysiology, American Heart Association. Circulation 1996;93:1262–1277.

83. Stroke Prevention in Atrial Fibrillation Study: final results. Circulation 1991;84:527–539.

84. Risk factors for stroke and efficacy of antithrombotic therapy in atrial fibrillation: analysis of pooled data from five randomized controlled trials [published erratum appears in Arch Intern Med 1994;154:2254]. Arch Intern Med 1994;154:1449–1457.

85. Poungvarin N, Opartkiattikul N, Chaithiraphan S, Viriyavejakul A: A comparative study of Coumadin and aspirin for primary cardioembolic stroke and thromboembolic preventions of chronic rheumatic mitral stenosis with atrial fibrillation. J Med Assoc Thai 1994;77:1–6.

86. Gregori F Jr, Cordeiro CO, Couto WJ, da Silva SS, de Aquino WK, Nechar A Jr: Cox maze operation without cryoablation for the treatment of chronic atrial fibrillation. Ann Thorac Surg 1995;60:361–363.

87. Itoh T, Okamoto H, Nimi T, et al: Left atrial function after Cox's maze operation concomitant with mitral valve operation. Ann Thorac Surg 1995;60:354–359.

88. Ashcom TL, Johns JP, Bailey SR, Rubal BJ: Effects of chronic beta-blockade on rest and exercise hemodynamics in mitral stenosis. Cathet Cardiovasc Diagn 1995;35:110–115.

89. al Kasab SM, Sabag T, al Zaibag M, et al: Beta-adrenergic receptor blockade in the management of pregnant women with mitral stenosis. Am J Obstet Gynecol 1990;163:137–140.

90. Patel JJ, Dyer RB, Mitha AS: Beta adrenergic blockade does not improve effort tolerance in patients with mitral stenosis in sinus rhythm. Eur Heart J 1995;16:1264–1268.

91. Stoll BC, Ashcom TL, Johns JP, Johnson JE, Rubal BJ: Effects of atenolol on rest and exercise hemodynamics in patients with mitral stenosis. Am J Cardiol 1995;75:482–484.

92. Gangbar EW, Watson KR, Howard RJ, Chisholm RJ: Mitral balloon valvuloplasty in pregnancy: advantages of a unique balloon. Cathet Cardiovasc Diagn 1992;25:313–316.

93. Tischler MD, Plehn JF: Applications of stress echocardiography: beyond coronary disease. J Am Soc Echocardiogr 1995;8:185–197.

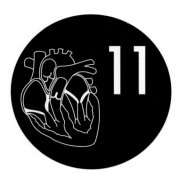

11 Surgical and Percutaneous Intervention for Mitral Stenosis

CLOSED SURGICAL COMMISSUROTOMY

Historically, the initial surgical approach to relieving mitral stenosis was "closed" commissurotomy (or valvuloplasty); specifically dilation of the stenotic valve through the left atrium, without direct visualization of the valve. This procedure has the advantage that it can be performed without cardiopulmonary bypass by using a left thoracotomy approach. Typically, after palpation of the fused commissures by the surgeon's finger, a transventricular dilator is inserted through the left atrial appendage and across the mitral valve. The dilator is opened one or more times to split the fused commissures. The disadvantages of this procedure are the risk of embolic events from dislodging atrial thrombi, incomplete relief of mitral stenosis, and induction of excessive mitral regurgitation from tearing of the leaflets rather than opening of the fused commissures.

Despite these limitations, after its introduction by Harken in Boston and Bailey in Philadelphia in 1948, this procedure became widely used and, although rarely performed now in the United States, it continues to be performed frequently in other countries.[1, 2] Closed mitral commissurotomy results in excellent relief of mitral stenosis symptoms and has an operative mortality rate averaging 3% to 4% (Fig. 11–1).[3] In a series of 1571 patients, operative mortality was found to be related to the severity of symptoms; the rate was only 1% to 2% for patients with exertional symptoms but 17% to 19% for those with heart failure at rest.[4]

Most patients have a significant improvement in symptoms after closed mitral commissurotomy and have an average increase of 1.0 cm^2 in valve area.[2, 5–7] Extensive calcification of the valve is associated with suboptimal hemodynamic results and a poor clinical outcome.

Long-term outcome after closed valvuloplasty is quite good, with only 31% of patients requiring reoperation within 15 years after the initial procedure.[8] Long-lasting hemodynamic relief has been documented by repeat catheterization up to 11 to 14 years after closed commissurotomy.[9, 10] Recurrent

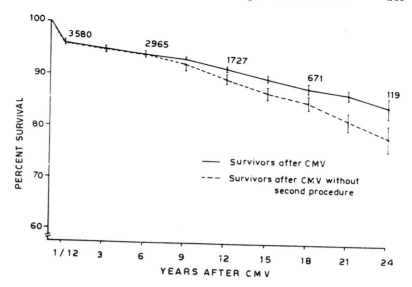

Figure 11·1 Actuarial survival curve after closed mitral valvotomy (CMV) in 3724 patients treated between 1956 and 1980 at the Christian Medical College Hospital in Vellore, India. (From John S, Bashi VV, Jairaj PS, et al: Closed mitral valvotomy: early results and long-term follow-up of 3724 consecutive patients. Circulation 1983;68:894; by permission of The American Heart Association.)

symptoms most often result from incomplete relief of mitral stenosis during the initial procedure (36%) or a combination of worsened mitral regurgitation and residual mitral stenosis (33%); restenosis after an initially successful procedure is the least common indication for reoperation (11%).[11] In 20% of these subjects, repeat cardiac surgery was performed for reasons other than mitral valve disease (eg, rheumatic involvement of the aortic valve).

In one report of long-term outcomes of 754 patients (mean age, 39 years; 71% female) undergoing closed mitral commissurotomy between 1958 and 1993, only 19% required subsequent mitral valve replacement at a mean of 17 years after closed commissurotomy.[1] In contrast to earlier series, the indication for surgery was restenosis in 59%, mixed stenosis and regurgitation in 30%, and severe mitral regurgitation in 11% of patients. It is possible that the higher rate of restenosis observed in this study was related to recurrent rheumatic fever in the study population, although data addressing this issue are not available. Multivariate predictors of the need for subsequent valve replacement were functional class, mitral valve calcification and subvalvular fusion, and the adequacy of the initial surgical procedure.

In another study of 267 patients followed for a mean of 14 years after closed commissurotomy,[12] 92% of the survivors had sustained symptomatic improvement. However, actuarial survival without repeat mitral valve surgery was only 57% at 10 years and 24% at 20 years (Fig. 11–2). Predictors of death were age, male gender, and the presence of atrial fibrillation.

Predictors of repeat mitral valve surgery were the extent of valvular calcification, cardiomegaly on chest radiography, and the presence of more than mild mitral regurgitation.

Closed mitral commissurotomy offers a simple surgical approach to relief of mitral stenosis in patients with flexible, noncalcified valve leaflets and little subvalvular involvement. The average increase in valve area is 1.0 cm² when the procedure is performed by an experienced surgeon. Complication rates are higher and hemodynamic results are poorer when the valve is calcified or deformed. For patients with good initial hemodynamic results, symptoms are improved, and repeat intervention typically is not needed until 10 to 15 years later. It is remarkable that the hemodynamic results, long-term outcome, and predictors of good results with closed mitral commissurotomy are similar to the results being reported with balloon mitral valvuloplasty. Use of the closed surgical procedure is decreasing in many countries due to the availability of an equivalent percutaneous approach, although experience with the surgical procedure and cost considerations suggest that closed commissurotomy will remain an option on a worldwide basis.

OPEN SURGICAL COMMISSUROTOMY

Open mitral commissurotomy is usually performed through a median sternotomy with the patient on full cardiopulmonary bypass. The mitral valve apparatus is directly visualized from the left atrium, with careful sharp dissec-

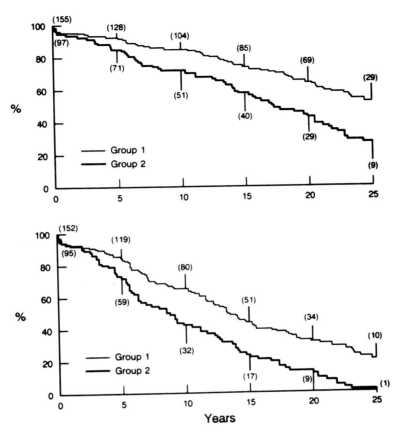

Figure 11·2 Outcome after closed transventricular mitral commissurotomy in 267 patients treated at the Mayo Clinic between 1960 and 1964. The 164 subjects without mitral anulus calcification determined by chest radiography or left atrial thrombi seen at operation (group 1) are compared with the 103 subjects with either of these characteristics (group 2). The Kaplan-Meier life tables show survival (*top*, P = .0002) and survival without repeat mitral valve operation by number of years after the procedure (*bottom*, P < .00001). The numbers within parentheses are the patients under observation, and error bars represent 2 SE. (From Rihal CD, Schaff HV, Frye RL, Bailey KR, Hammes LN, Holmes DR Jr: Long-term follow-up of patients undergoing closed transventricular mitral commissurotomy: a useful surrogate for percutaneous balloon mitral valvuloplasty? J Am Coll Cardiol 1992;20:784; reprinted with permission from the American College of Cardiology.)

tion of the fused commissures under direct vision. The degree of valve opening can be further improved by release of fused chordae or correction of chordal shortening.[13–15] If needed, an annuloplasty ring can be used to decrease the severity of coexisting mitral regurgitation.

Compared with closed commissurotomy, the advantages of the open procedure are the ability to visualize the valve structure in detail and to perform a more directed surgical repair. The left atrium also can be evaluated more fully, allowing detection and removal of left atrial thrombus. As with the closed approach, the best hemodynamic results and long-term outcomes are observed for patients with little valve calcification, flexible and mobile leaflets, and only minimal mitral regurgitation.

With appropriate patient selection and preoperative evaluation, open commissurotomy is feasible in 80% to 90% of referred subjects and has an operative mortality rate of about 1%.[13–15] The hemodynamic results of open commissurotomy are at least equivalent to the closed technique, with valve area increasing by about 1.0 cm² on average. One study showed a greater decrease in valve area over 3 years with open commissurotomy than with balloon valvuloplasty,[16] despite similar initial hemodynamic results. The average valve area was 2.4 ± 0.6 cm² in the balloon group versus 1.8 ± 0.4 cm² in the surgical group at the 3-year follow-up evaluation. Another study showed a similar rate of decrease in valve area (about 0.1 cm²/year) with both techniques.[17]

Long-term outcome after open surgical commissurotomy has been excellent. The rate of reoperation for mitral valve replacement is 0% to 16% at 36 to 53 months, and the 10-year actuarial survival rate is 81% to 100%.[13–15, 18–20]

MITRAL VALVE REPLACEMENT

Patient Selection

In many patients with rheumatic mitral stenosis, valve replacement is necessary because of extensive calcification and deformity of the valve apparatus, which precludes commissurotomy due to significant coexisting mitral regurgitation. If a prosthetic valve is used, a mechanical valve typically is preferable to a stented tissue valve because of its long-term durability and since most of these patients require long-term anticoagulation for atrial fibrillation in either case.

Operative Mortality, Morbidity, and Long-Term Outcome

Most studies reporting the operative mortality for mitral valve replacement include both patients with mitral stenosis and those with mitral regurgitation. In one study, the operative mortality rate for 81 elderly (>70 years) patients was 8.6%, compared with 3.2% for 744 younger (<70 years) patients undergoing isolated mitral valve replacement. The predominant valve lesion was mitral stenosis in 30% of the older and in 41% of the younger patients in this series.[21] Concurrent coronary bypass surgery was associated with a higher mortality rate: 19.6% in older patients and 12.1% in younger patients, but mortality was even higher if coronary artery disease was present and bypass grafting was not performed. The higher mortality associated with concurrent coronary disease also may be related to whether the valve lesion was regurgitation or stenosis, as ischemic mitral regurgitation is likely in many of these patients.

Long-term outcome after valve replacement for mitral stenosis depends on the durability, hemodynamics, and complications of the prosthetic valve (see Chapter 17); the risks of chronic anticoagulation; residual anatomic or hemodynamic abnormalities secondary to mitral stenosis, such as pulmonary hypertension, left atrial enlargement, atrial fibrillation, or right ventricular enlargement and dysfunction; and involvement of other valves by the rheumatic process.

Outcome of Patients With Pulmonary Hypertension

Mitral valve replacement carries a higher risk for patients with mitral stenosis and severe pulmonary hypertension. In a study of 42 patients with mitral stenosis and pulmonary systolic pressures of 60 mm Hg or higher, the surgical mortality rate was 11.6%, and an additional 16% of patients had major complications.[22] Of note, 42% of these patients had concurrent aortic valve procedures due to frequent involvement of the aortic valve by the rheumatic process. Univariate predictors of

perioperative death included an acute presentation, right heart failure, a reduced ejection fraction, and a high left ventricular end-diastolic pressure. On multivariate analysis, the primary predictor of death was acute presentation, while complications were predicted by electrocardiographic criteria for right ventricular hypertrophy.

Despite the higher risk of the surgical procedure itself, most patients had improved functional status. The overall 5-year actuarial survival rate was 80%, with a 10-year survival rate of 64% (Fig. 11–3).

Homograft Mitral Valve Replacement

Use of cryopreserved homografts in the mitral valve position[23] has recently been proposed. Potential advantages of this approach include maintenance of the normal left ventricular-annular attachments, normal valve function with a low antegrade gradient and little regurgitation, better longevity than standard tissue valves, and no absolute indication for chronic anticoagulation. In a series of 43 patients, 26 of whom had rheumatic mitral stenosis, the hospital mortality rate was 5%, and one additional patient required reoperation for dehiscence of a suture line.[23] The complexity of this procedure suggests that considerable expertise will be needed for optimal

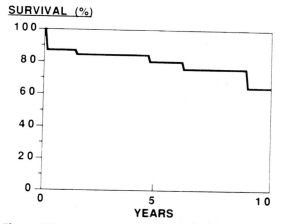

Figure 11·3 Kaplan-Meier actuarial survival after mitral valve surgery in 43 patients with mitral stenosis and severe pulmonary hypertension (pulmonary systolic pressure >60 mm Hg). The 5- and 10-year survival rates were 80% and 64%, respectively, with a mean follow-up period of 6.4 ± 3.7 years. (From Vincens JJ, Temizer D, Post JR, Edmunds LH Jr, Herrmann HC: Long-term outcome of cardiac surgery in patients with mitral stenosis and severe pulmonary hypertension. Circulation 1995;92(suppl II):139; by permission of The American Heart Association.)

results. In addition, issues such as the appropriate sizing and availability of valve tissue remain unresolved.

BALLOON MITRAL COMMISSUROTOMY
Patient Selection

In patients referred for an intervention for relief of mitral stenosis, several factors are important in selection of appropriate candidates for catheter balloon valvuloplasty. The first step in patient selection is to determine if the severity of valve obstruction warrants intervention. Second, the degree of coexisting mitral regurgitation is considered, since mixed stenosis and regurgitation do not benefit from the valvuloplasty procedure due to persistence or worsening of mitral regurgitation. Third, the presence and severity of other valve lesions or coronary artery disease are assessed, because if surgery is needed for other indications, it is logical to treat the stenotic mitral valve as part of the same surgical procedure. Fourth, any comorbid conditions or technical considerations that may affect the procedure are evaluated. Finally, the patient's preference for a catheter-based or surgical procedure is incorporated into the decision-making process.

After it has been determined that the patient is an appropriate candidate for balloon valvuloplasty on clinical and hemodynamic grounds, the probable short- and long-term outcomes with valvuloplasty are considered. Predictors of a poor initial result include older age, smaller baseline valve area, higher pulmonary pressures, and a smaller area of the dilating balloon.[24, 25]

In addition, the anatomy of the mitral valve significantly influences both the immediate hemodynamic results and long-term outcome. Detailed evaluation of mitral valve morphology allows exclusion of patients at high risk for complications or procedural death. There are several approaches to describing the morphology of the stenotic mitral valve, with key features in predicting outcome after balloon valvuloplasty being the degree of deformity and calcification of the valve apparatus. Patients with thin, flexible valve leaflets; little calcification of the leaflets or commissures; and minimal chordal involvement have the best hemodynamic results and long-term outcome. Patients with heavily calcified and deformed valves have a poor long-term outcome and also are at risk for procedural death and major complications (Fig. 11–4).

Perhaps the most widely used approach to evaluation of mitral valve morphology is the composite Massachusetts General Hospital (MGH) score (Table 11–1).[26] Initial data for

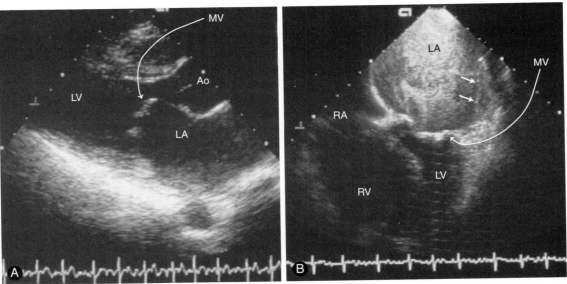

Figure 11·4   Echocardiographic evaluation before mitral valvuloplasty. *A,* A parasternal long-axis view shows favorable mitral valve morphology with thin, flexible valve leaflets and little calcification or subvalvular involvement. This patient underwent balloon valvuloplasty. *B,* A transesophageal view shows a different patient with extensively calcified and immobile leaflets and extensive subvalvular involvement. This image also shows left atrial spontaneous contrast and a laminated atrial thrombus *(arrows).* The patient was referred for surgical valve replacement. Ao, aorta; LA, left atrium; LV, left ventricle; MV, mitral valve; RA, right atrium.

TABLE 11·1   MASSACHUSETTS GENERAL HOSPITAL MITRAL VALVE MORPHOLOGY SCORE

Grade*	Mobility	Subvalvular Thickening	Valvular Thickening	Valvular Calcification
1	Highly mobile valve with only leaflet tips restricted	Minimal thickening just below the mitral leaflets	Leaflets near normal in thickness (4–5 mm)	A single area of increased echo brightness
2	Leaflet middle and base portions have normal mobility	Thickening of chordal structures extending up to one third of the chordal length	Mid-leaflets normal, considerable thickening of margins (5–8 mm)	Scattered areas of brightness confined to leaflet margins
3	Valve continues to move forward in diastole, mainly from the base	Thickening extending to the distal third of the chords	Thickening extending through the entire leaflet (5–8 mm)	Brightness extending into the midportion of the leaflets
4	No or minimal forward movement of the leaflets in diastole	Extensive thickening and shortening of all chordal structures extending down to the papillary muscles	Considerable thickening of all leaflet tissue (>8–10 mm)	Extensive brightness throughout much of the leaflet tissue

*The total echocardiographic score is derived from an analysis of mitral leaflet mobility, valvular and subvalvar thickening, and calcification. Each is graded from 0 to 4 according to the given criteria (with 0 indicating normal), producing a total score of 0 to 16.
From Wilkins GT, Weyman AE, Abascal VM, et al: Percutaneous balloon dilatation of the mitral valve: an analysis of echocardiographic variables related to outcome and the mechanism of dilatation. Br Heart J 1988;60:299–308. BMJ Publishing Group.

a small number of patients showed that this morphology score predicted both the immediate increase in valve area[26] and restenosis at the 6-month follow-up evaluation after valvuloplasty.[27] These observations were subsequently confirmed in a larger series from the same institution, and it was emphasized that a morphology score of more than 8 was associated with a suboptimal result (Fig. 11–5).[28] However, the data presented show considerable overlap of individual data points between groups with low and high morphology scores. Long-term follow-up also highlighted the im-

portance of the morphology score as a predictor of outcome, with event-free survival rates (at 20 ± 12 months) of 91% ± 4% for those with a score of 8 or less and 55% ± 13% for a score higher than 8.[29]

The MGH morphology score was used in the multicenter Balloon Valvuloplasty Registry and again was found to be a predictor of procedural mortality and complications,[30] the postvalvuloplasty valve area,[24, 31] and long-term outcome.[32] A similar association between mitral morphology and long-term outcome also was found in other series.[33, 34] In the Balloon

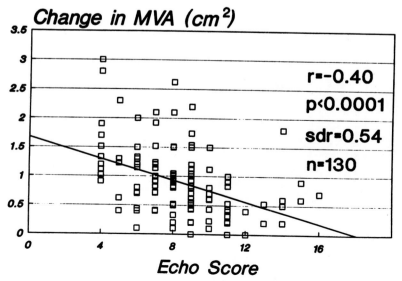

Figure 11·5 The Massachusetts General Hospital echocardiographic morphology score is plotted against the absolute change in mitral valve area (MVA) after mitral valvuloplasty in 130 patients from a single medical center. Despite the statistically significant correlation, the data are widely scattered. (From Abascal VM, Wilkins GT, O'Shea JP, et al: Prediction of successful outcome in 130 patients undergoing percutaneous balloon mitral valvotomy. Circulation 1990;82:448–456; by permission of The American Heart Association.)

Change in MVA (cm²)

r=-0.40
p<0.0001
sdr=0.54
n=130

Echo Score

Valvuloplasty Registry data, when the morphology score was considered as a dichotomous variable (score >8 or ≤8), a greater increase in valve area was seen in the low echocardiographic score group. However, when treated as a continuous variable, there was only a weak correlation between morphology score and increase in valve area ($r = -0.15$) or the post-valvuloplasty valve area ($r = -0.24$) (Fig. 11–6).[24, 31] Overall, the mitral valve morphology score is most useful clinically as a predictor of complications and a poor long-term outcome, rather than as a specific measure of the expected increase in valve area after the procedure. The score also appears to predict hospital costs, with higher total costs for those with deformed and calcified valves.[35]

Other approaches to evaluation of mitral valve morphology that also predict immediate hemodynamic results include quantitative analysis of the degree of leaflet motion[36] and a more focused evaluation of the extent and asymmetry of commissural fusion, fibrosis, and calcification.[37] In a study of 149 patients, commissural calcification alone was a stronger predictor of survival than morphology score.[38]

Another simple and effective approach to evaluation of mitral morphology is the three-group grading (Table 11–2), which is primarily based on the extent of subvalvular involvement and the extent of leaflet calcification.[39, 40] Using this classification for a series of 1512 patients, inadequate hemodynamic results were seen in only 2.2% of Group 1 and 7.4% of Group 2 patients but in 22.3% of Group 3 patients. Other important predictors of outcome were age, valve area, and the effective balloon dilating area.[40]

It is clear that groups of patients with heavily calcified and deformed valves have suboptimal hemodynamic results, a higher risk of procedural complications and death, and shorter event-free survival compared with groups of patients with flexible, noncalcified leaflets and little subvalvular disease. Several of these criteria have been combined by Reid[41] into overall criteria for assessment of mitral valve morphology (Table 11–3).

Although evaluation of mitral valve morphology is helpful in choosing alternate approaches for treating patients with the most

TABLE 11·2 THE THREE-GROUP GRADING OF MITRAL VALVE ANATOMY

Echocardiographic Group	Mitral Valve Anatomy
Group 1	Pliable, noncalcified anterior mitral leaflet and mild subvalvular disease (ie, thin chordae ≥10 mm long)
Group 2	Pliable, noncalcified anterior mitral leaflet and severe subvalvular disease (ie, thickened chordae <10 mm long)
Group 3	Calcification of mitral valve of any extent, as assessed by fluoroscopy, whatever the state of the subvalvular apparatus

From Iung B, Cormier B, Ducimetiere P, et al: Immediate results of percutaneous mitral commissurotomy: a predictive model on a series of 1514 patients. Circulation 1996;94:2124–2130.

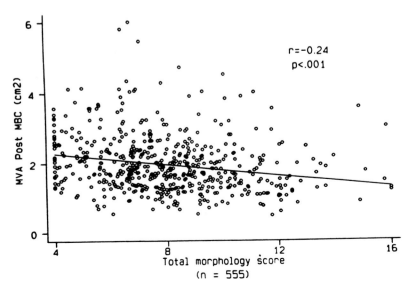

r=−0.24
p<.001

Figure 11·6 Plot of the correlation between the MGH morphology score and the mitral valve area (MVA) after balloon mitral valvuloplasty in 555 patients in the multicenter Balloon Valvuloplasty Registry. The correlation is statistically significant, but weak, and the data are widely scattered. (From Reid CL, Otto CM, Davis KB, Labovitz A, Kisslo KB, McKay CR: Influence of mitral valve morphology on mitral balloon commissurotomy: immediate and six-month results from the NHLBI Balloon Valvuloplasty Registry. Am Heart J 1992;124:657–665.)

TABLE 11·3 TWO-DIMENSIONAL ECHOCARDIOGRAPHIC ASSESSMENT OF MITRAL VALVE MORPHOLOGY

Variable	Predicted Results	
	Optimal	*Suboptimal*
Leaflet motion	Highly mobile with restriction only of leaflet tips, and H/L ratio ≥0.45	Minimal forward motion of leaflets in diastole, or H/L ratio ≤0.25
Leaflet thickening	Leaflets <4–5 mm or MV/PWAo ratio of 1.5–2.0	Leaflets >8.0 mm thick or a MV/PWAo ratio ≥5.0
Subvalvular disease	Thin, faintly visible chordae tendineae with only minimal thickening below valve	Thickening and shortening of chordae to papillary muscle; areas with echo density greater than endocardium
Commissural calcium	Homogeneous density of both commissures	Both commissures heavily calcified

H, height of doming of mitral valve; L, length of dome of mitral valve; MV, mitral valve; PWAo, posterior wall of aorta.
From Reid CL: Echocardiography in the patient undergoing catheter balloon mitral commissurotomy. *In* Otto CM, ed. The Clinical Practice of Echocardiography. Philadelphia: WB Saunders, 1997:376.

calcified and deformed valves and in proceeding with valvuloplasty in patients with favorable morphology, it remains somewhat hazardous to apply a rigid breakpoint to clinical decision making for patients with intermediate morphology scores. Some of these patients do have substantial hemodynamic improvement after valvuloplasty, while others have little increase in valve area. One problem with all of these scoring systems is that the continuous range of mitral valve anatomy is compressed into discrete categories, so that borderline cases may be classified inconsistently. Further, all of the proposed scoring systems are subject to interobserver variability between institutions and between physicians, limiting the reliability of a specific numerical breakpoint. In these cases, it is prudent for the echocardiographer, interventional cardiologist, and surgeon to review the mitral valve morphology together to determine the most appropriate therapy.

Technique

Both echocardiographic[36] and autopsy studies[42] suggest that the mechanism of the increase in mitral valve area with catheter balloon commissurotomy is splitting of the fused commissures, although fracturing of calcium in the leaflets may play a role in some cases. Many of the early reports on this technique used a single balloon with a circular cross-sectional area. Subsequently, interventionalists switched to using a double-balloon technique and then to the Inoue balloon as the improved hemodynamic results with these approaches quickly became evident.

The dilating balloon is advanced from the right femoral vein into the right atrium and then, through a transseptal approach, into the left atrium.[44-46] The transseptal approach is a potential cause of complications with this procedure and requires considerable expertise. Many interventionalists perform right atrial angiography to aid in correct positioning of the transseptal needle. Echocardiographic imaging for guidance also has been reported (Fig. 11–7).

Catheters also typically are placed in the pulmonary artery for measurement of pressures and calculation of cardiac output by the thermodilution method and in the left ventricle, retrograde across the aortic valve, for measurement of left ventricular pressure. Left atrial pressure is measured using the balloon dilating catheter before crossing the stenotic mitral valve. Measurement of the transmitral gradient from the left atrial and left ventricular catheters, in combination with cardiac output measurement, allows calculation of valve area using the Gorlin equation before and after the procedure.

The balloon dilating catheter then is advanced across the mitral valve. After correct positioning is ensured, the balloon is dilated briefly, with one to four inflations being needed to achieve an adequate increase in valve area. Using a double-balloon technique, one group of investigators suggests that an optimal increase in valve area without excessive regurgitation can be achieved by using balloons sized so that the sum of the inflated diameters equals the patient's mitral annulus diameter.[43] Other investigators use balloon sizes chosen empirically based on patient size, most often using a combination of 18- and 20-mm balloons, with the sum of balloon diameters ranging from 36 to 40 mm.[24] Many centers

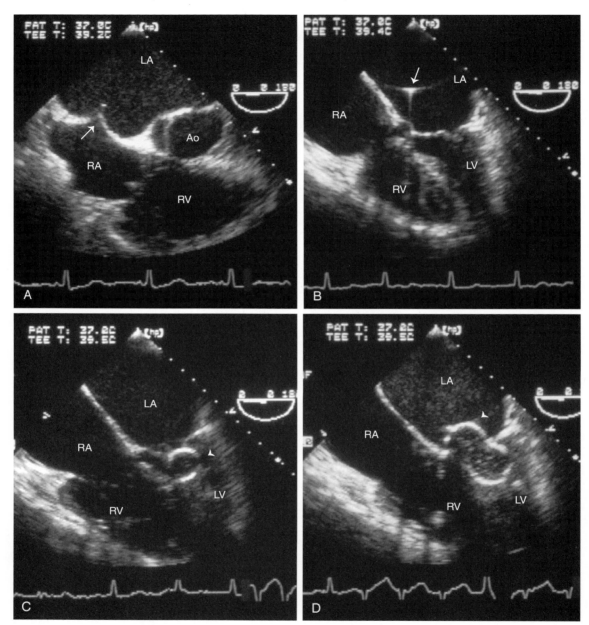

Figure 11·7 Transesophageal echocardiographic guidance of an Inoue balloon mitral valvuloplasty. The transseptal needle is seen indenting the atrial septum *(arrow)* just before puncture *(A)*, followed by positioning of the balloon catheter *(arrow)* in the left atrium *(B)*. After the balloon catheter is advanced across the mitral valve, first the distal segment of the balloon *(arrow)* is inflated *(C)*, followed by brief inflation *(arrow)* of the proximal and dilating segments *(D)*. Ao, aorta; LA, left atrium; LV, left ventricle; RV, right ventricle; RA, right atrium.

worldwide continue to use a double-balloon approach. One disadvantage of the double-balloon technique is the rare but serious complication of ejection of the balloons into the ventricular apex, causing ventricular rupture and tamponade. Another disadvantage is that it is more difficult to assess the degree of dilation achieved with each dilation sequence.

With the single Inoue balloon technique, balloon size is chosen based on the patient's height, with each balloon allowing inflation to several different final diameters, allowing a stepwise approach to valve dilation.[44-46] The Inoue balloon is unique in that, after the balloon is positioned across the mitral valve, the distal segment in the ventricle is dilated first, followed by the proximal segment in the left atrium (Fig. 11–8). This approach holds the balloon securely in position while the middle (dilating segment) is briefly inflated. The diameter of the dilating segment can be increased with each successive inflation in 1- to 2-mm increments to three different final diameters for each balloon. The diameter of the dilating segment of the Inoue balloon typically ranges from 20 to 30 mm. The Inoue balloon can be "stretched" for insertion into the vein and passage across the atrial septum, minimizing the cross-sectional area of the catheter and balloon assembly and thereby minimizing vascular damage at the insertion site and the size of the resultant atrial septal defect. Since the Inoue balloon is relatively simple to use and provides results at least equivalent to the double-balloon technique, most interventional cardiologists now use this approach. Optimal results are possible using transthoracic echocardiographic evaluation of valve area and the degree of mitral regurgitation after each balloon inflation so that the procedure can be stopped at the point where there is no further increase in valve area and

before there is a significant increase in mitral regurgitant severity.[47]

Even with improvements in technique and optimal balloons design, catheter mitral valvuloplasty remains a technically demanding procedure. The importance of operator experience and careful patient selection cannot be overemphasized.[24, 48]

Complications

Complications of catheter balloon valvuloplasty include the development of a small atrial septal defect at the site of passage of the catheter across the atrial septal in virtually all patients (Fig. 11–9; see also color insert). This defect can be detected by color flow Doppler echocardiography in more than 60% of cases, depending on the skill of the echocardiographer and the diligence of the search.[49] In most cases, this defect closes, with a detectable shunt visualized in 20% to 30% of patients at the 18-month follow-up evaluation.[39, 49] A significant shunt across the iatrogenic atrial septal defect is less common, occurring initially in only 4% to 20% of patients in different series. A signifi-

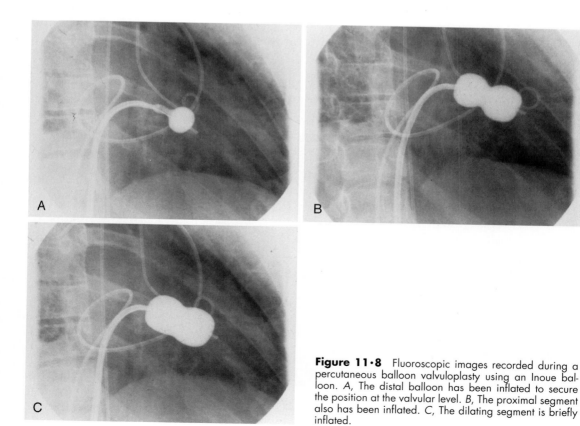

Figure 11·8 Fluoroscopic images recorded during a percutaneous balloon valvuloplasty using an Inoue balloon. *A,* The distal balloon has been inflated to secure the position at the valvular level. *B,* The proximal segment also has been inflated. *C,* The dilating segment is briefly inflated.

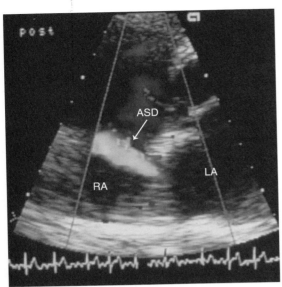

Figure 11·9 Parasternal short-axis echocardiographic image shows a small atrial septal defect (ASD) with left to right flow typically seen after balloon mitral valvuloplasty. LA, left atrium; RA, right atrium. (This illustration also occurs in the color insert section.)

cant and persistent atrial septal defect may reflect inadequate relief of mitral stenosis if persistently elevated left atrial pressures lead to tension on the atrial septum and flow from left to right across the stretched defect.

The most serious complication of balloon valvuloplasty is cardiac tamponade resulting from perforation by a guiding or dilating cath-

eter. This complication has been reported in 0.8% to 4% of cases, but appears to be decreasing with improvements in technique and with echocardiographic and fluoroscopic monitoring of the procedure (Table 11–4).

An increase in mitral regurgitation from none or mild at baseline to moderate or severe after the procedure is seen in 13% of patients,[24] with between 1% and 8% of patients developing severe mitral regurgitation after the procedure (Fig. 11–10; see also color insert). The incidence of severe mitral regurgitation is reported to be lower with the Inoue balloon, probably because the severity of regurgitation is reevaluated after each stepwise balloon inflation. Mitral regurgitation results from oversizing or overinflation of the dilating balloon in some cases. In other cases, mitral regurgitation appears to result from tearing of a thin, flexible region of the leaflet adjacent to a calcified nodule, presumably related to excessive force on the thin leaflet segment. This complication is more likely in patients with irregular (but not necessarily severe) leaflet thickening.[50]

Urgent surgical intervention for tamponade or regurgitation is needed in between 0.4% and 4.8% of patients undergoing balloon valvuloplasty, highlighting the need for prompt surgical back-up at centers performing this procedure.

Systemic embolization is a devastating complication that occurs in 0.5% to 3.3% of patients. Although there is always a small risk of embolic complications with any left heart

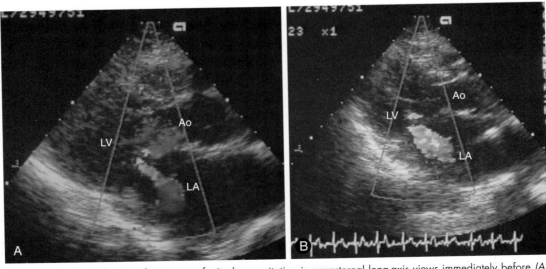

Figure 11·10 Color Doppler images of mitral regurgitation in parasternal long-axis views immediately before *(A)* and after *(B)* balloon mitral valvuloplasty. Little change in regurgitant severity is apparent in this patient. Ao, aorta; LA, left atrium; LV, left ventricle. (These illustrations also occur in the color insert section.)

TABLE 11·4 BALLOON MITRAL VALVULOPLASTY: COMPLICATIONS AND LONG-TERM OUTCOME

| Study | Procedural Mortality | Procedural Complications | | | | | Actuarial Survival | Event-free Survival* | Follow-up Interval |
		Systemic Embolism	Tamponade	Shunt	Severe MR	Immediate Surgery			
Arora, 1994[57]	0.5%	3.3%	0.8%	14%	3.8%	4.8%	87 ± 6%	81 ± 3%	15 ± 11 mo
Rothlisberger, 1993[56]	1% (3.2% 30 day)	2%	4%	9.9%	3%	4%	84 ± 1.6%	60 ± 2%	4 y
Chen, 1995[58]	2.3%	1.1%	2.9%	0.7%	6.7%	1.4%	94 ± 1%	85 ± 2%	5 y
Vahanian, 1991[39]	0.8%	1.1%	1.3%	10.6%	8%	0.4%			
Orrange, 1997[54]	4.5%	0%					95 ± 1%	65 ± 6%	7 y
Pan, 1993[55]	1%	0.5%	1.3%	4%	1%	1%	Restenosis in 2%		37 ± 8 mo
BVR, 1992–96[24,32]	0.1%	0.5%	0.8%		1.4%		Restenosis in 5.2%		32 ± 4 mo

BVR, Balloon Valvuloplasty Registry; MR, mitral regurgitation.
*Event-free survival is defined as alive without repeat valvuloplasty or mitral valve surgery.

catheterization procedure, the major cause of embolic events in patients undergoing mitral valvuloplasty is left atrial thrombus, which is dislodged by the catheters in the left atrium. The risk of this complication can be minimized by using transesophageal echocardiography to evaluate for atrial thrombus prior to the procedure.[51] If thrombus is present, the procedure should be postponed, anticoagulation instituted for at least 2 to 3 weeks, and the transesophageal study repeated to demonstrate resolution of the thrombus. If thrombus persists, some clinicians think balloon valvuloplasty is safe if the thrombus is confined to the atrial appendage[52]; however, most clinicians would recommend an open surgical procedure if the atrial thrombus does not resolve promptly with anticoagulant therapy. Note that atrial thrombus has been observed in mitral stenosis patients in sinus rhythm, so that transesophageal echocardiography is needed regardless of cardiac rhythm. Further, the transesophageal study should be performed within a few days of the procedure, as otherwise thrombus may have formed in the interim. For patients in atrial fibrillation on warfarin, anticoagulation is held for 4 to 5 days before the procedure to achieve an international normalized ratio (INR) of less than 1.5. After the transseptal procedure, all patients receive intravenous heparin in doses to maintain a therapeutic partial thromboplastin time for the remainder of the procedure. After the procedure, oral anticoagulation is resumed in patients in atrial fibrillation. For patients with a history of an embolic event, intravenous anticoagulation with heparin should be considered until the INR is therapeutic.

Univariate predictors of procedural death or complications in patients undergoing balloon mitral valvuloplasty include older age, a history of cardiac arrest, cerebrovascular disease, dementia, renal insufficiency, cachexia, heart failure symptoms at rest, use of an intraaortic balloon pump or sympathomimetic amines, a smaller valve area, and a higher echocardiographic morphology score.[30] On multivariate analysis of the Balloon Valvuloplasty Registry data, the only predictors of procedural death or complications were a higher echocardiographic morphology score and a smaller valve area before the procedure. Other series also have identified mitral valve anatomy and valve area as strong predictors of complications and procedural death, with other important factors including a history of previous commissurotomy.[39, 53]

Immediate Results

With appropriate patient selection, the balloon valvuloplasty procedure is successful in 90% to 95% of subjects.[34, 40, 54] Transmitral pressure gradient decreases, mitral valve area increases, and pulmonary pressures fall after successful balloon mitral valvuloplasty (Table 11–5). The average increase in mitral valve area is about 1.0 cm^2, as demonstrated in numerous clinical series.[24, 39, 54–58] Evaluation of the increase in mitral valve area immediately after balloon dilation may be limited in the catheterization laboratory by the presence of the atrial septal defect, which invalidates measurement of transmitral volume flow rate based on the forward cardiac output. In addition, a general decrease in all intracardiac pressures related to medications and contrast agents may decrease the apparent transmitral gradient and make accurate measurement more difficult (Fig. 11–11).

Echocardiographic assessment with short-axis two-dimensional (2D) planimetry of the orifice area remains valid after valvuloplasty if adequate image quality can be obtained (Fig. 11–12). The pressure half-time method may be misleading in the short term due to changing left atrial and left ventricular compliances as well as changes in chamber volumes and pressures immediately after the procedure,[59] although this method regains its accuracy within a few days. Despite the theoretical concerns with the accuracy of the pressure half-time method in the immediate postvalvuloplasty period, many clinicians continue to use this approach in the catheterization laboratory to monitor the procedure, particularly if 2D short-axis images are suboptimal for planimetry of valve area. When both methods are feasible, 2D and pressure half-time valve areas usually are similar.[60, 61]

Most clinicians use transthoracic imaging for calculation of 2D and pressure half-time mitral valve areas and evaluation of the degree of mitral regurgitation on color flow imaging after each balloon dilation to ensure an optimal increase in valve area without induction of excessive valvular regurgitation. Typically, a good result is defined as a final valve area of more than 1.5 cm^2 with a mitral regurgitation grade of 2+ or less. If image quality is inadequate or if more specific echocardiographic evaluation of the site of the atrial septal puncture and balloon position is needed, transesophageal imaging may be considered. The possible advantages of the transesophageal ap-

TABLE 11·5 BALLOON MITRAL VALVULOPLASTY: HEMODYNAMIC RESULTS

Study	Country	Patients	Mean Age (y)	Percent in AF	Percent Female	MVA (cm²)* Before	MVA (cm²)* After	Mean PA Pressures (mm Hg)* Before	Mean PA Pressures (mm Hg)* After
Arora, 1994[57]	India	600	27 ± 8	4.3%	77%	0.8 ± 0.2	2.2 ± 0.4	42 ± 16	23 ± 11
Rothlisberger, 1993[56]	South Africa	235	29 ± 11	7%	78%	0.8 ± 0.2	1.6 ± 0.6	40 ± 15	32 ± 13
Chen, 1995[58]	China	4832	37 ± 12	27%	70%	1.1 ± 0.3	2.1 ± 0.2	51 ± 15	34 ± 9
Vahanian, 1991[39]	France	600	43 ± 15	31%	79%	1.1 ± 0.3	2.2 ± 0.5	32 ± 12	21 ± 8
Orrange, 1997[54]	US	132	44 ± 14	49%	79%	1.0 ± 0.3	1.9 ± 0.6	40 ± 14	32 ± 11
Pan, 1993[55]	Spain	350	46 ± 12	52%	79%	1.0 ± 0.3	2.1 ± 0.7		
BVR, 1992–96[24,32]	US/Canada	738	54 ± 15	45%	81%	1.0 ± 0.3	2.0 ± 0.8	35 ± 13	29 ± 11

AF, atrial fibrillation; BVR, Balloon Valvuloplasty Registry; MVA, mitral valve area; PA, pulmonary artery.
*Values shown are group means ± SD. All changes from before to after balloon mitral valvuloplasty are statistically significant.

253

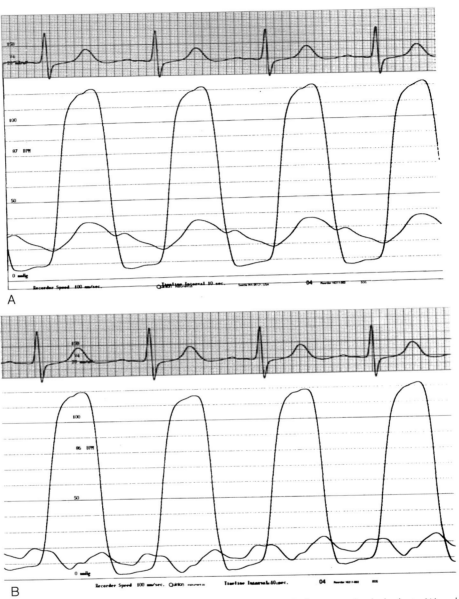

Figure 11·11 The transmitral gradient immediately before balloon mitral valvuloplasty *(A)* and immediately after the second inflation of a 23-mm Inoue balloon *(B)*. Notice that the mean gradient *(shaded areas)* has decreased from 10 to 6 mm Hg. Valve area increased from 1.1 to 2.1 cm².

proach must be balanced against the increased cost, risk, and patient discomfort of this approach. In addition, an increased level of sedation (sometimes general anesthesia) is needed for patient comfort given the duration of the valvuloplasty procedure.

Changes in Pulmonary Pressures

Mean pulmonary pressures fall by an average of 5 to 15 mm Hg immediately after bal-

loon valvuloplasty, corresponding to the acute decrease in left atrial pressure (see Table 11–5). Further decreases in pulmonary pressures are seen at the 6-month follow-up evaluation as the reactive component of the increased pulmonary resistance gradually resolves, while restenosis is associated with a return of pulmonary pressures to the preprocedure values.[62, 63] Even patients with severe pulmonary hypertension at baseline show improvement in pulmonary pressure after the procedure, with contin-

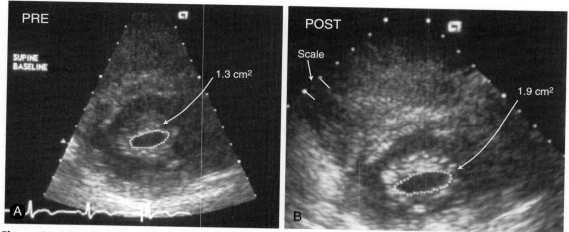

Figure 11·12 Short-axis, two-dimensional echocardiographic, planimetered mitral valve areas immediately before (A) and after (B) balloon mitral valvuloplasty. Mitral valve area increased from 1.2 to 1.9 cm² in this case.

ued decreases in pulmonary pressure observed up to 24 months later.[64, 65]

Long-Term Outcome

Long-term outcome after balloon mitral valvuloplasty is very encouraging, with overall event-free survival rates of 80% to 90% at 3 to 5 years in several large series (see Table 11–4).[29, 32, 39, 54, 55, 57, 58] Event-free survival (ie, survival without repeat valvuloplasty or mitral valve replacement) is 60% to 85% (Figs. 11–13 and 11–14). In European and North American

series, restenosis is rare, and most cases requiring a repeat procedure or surgical intervention either had incomplete relief of mitral stenosis at the initial procedure or developed significant mitral regurgitation.[49] In a series of 235 patients, the echocardiographic valve area was 2.0 ± 0.3 cm² immediately after the procedure and 1.9 ± 0.4 cm² at follow-up 18 ± 10 months after the procedure.[39] Restenosis caused by refusion of the commissure may be related to recurrent rheumatic fever, but even in the large series from China, the restenosis rate was only 5.2% at 32 ± 4 months of follow-

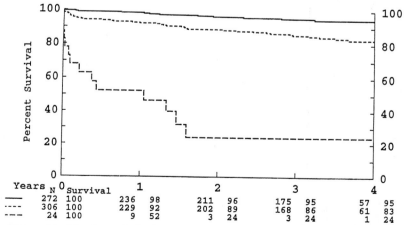

Years	N	Survival	1		2		3		4	
——	272	100	236	98	211	96	175	95	57	95
- - - -	306	100	229	92	202	89	168	86	61	83
– – –	24	100	9	52	3	24	3	24	1	24

Figure 11·13 Survival after balloon mitral valvuloplasty for 736 patients enrolled in the Balloon Valvuloplasty Registry who were stratified by baseline echocardiographic morphology score: less than 8 (solid line), 8 to 12 (short-dashed line), or more than 12 (long-dashed line); P < .0001. (From Dean LS, Mickel MC, Bonan R, et al: Four-year follow-up of patients undergoing percutaneous balloon mitral commissurotomy: a report form the National Heart, Lung, and Blood Institute Balloon Valvuloplasty Registry. J Am Coll Cardiol 1996;28:1452–1457; reprinted with permission from the American College of Cardiology.)

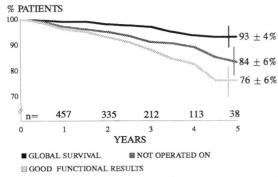

Figure 11·14 Actuarial results after percutaneous mitral valvuloplasty for 528 patients. The bars indicate 95% confidence intervals. The numbers along the x axis indicate the number of surviving patients with good functional results, defined as functional class I or II and no need for repeat valvuloplasty or mitral valve surgery. (From Iung B, Cormier B, Ducimetiere P, et al: Functional results 5 years after successful percutaneous mitral commissurotomy in a series of 528 patients and analysis of predictive factors. J Am Coll Cardiol 1996;27:407–414; reprinted with permission from the American College of Cardiology.)

up.[58] Another cause of restenosis may be superimposed degenerative fibrosis and calcification of the leaflets and chordae (without commissural fusion), but this process is likely to occur over a longer period than encompassed by current studies (Fig. 11–15).

The best long-term outcome with balloon mitral valvuloplasty is observed for patients with fewer symptoms before intervention,[24, 32, 34, 40] a lower MGH morphology score,[29, 32, 34] a successful valvuloplasty procedure,[32, 40] a lower left ventricular end-diastolic pressure,[32, 34] and lower pulmonary artery pressures after the procedure.[32]

Functional Outcome

Most clinical series report an improvement in symptoms and in New York Heart Association functional class after balloon valvuloplasty. However, few data are available on the overall impact of the procedure on activity level or the patient's perception of symptomatic improvement.

Although some studies suggested little improvement in maximum workload early after valvuloplasty despite good hemodynamic results,[66] other studies have shown improvement in both exercise tolerance and maximum oxygen consumption.[67, 68] The degree of improvement in exercise capacity does not correlate with the postprocedure valve area, suggesting persistent peripheral vasculature alterations also may be important.[68] Although no changes are seen in skeletal muscle histology, biochemistry, or function early (2 weeks) after the procedure, late changes in quadriceps cross-sectional area, torque production, and percentage of slow-twitch fibers have been documented at 4-month follow-up evaluation.[67] In patients with a postvalvuloplasty valve area of 1.5 cm[2] or larger, there is no increase in pulmonary vascular resistance with exercise.[69]

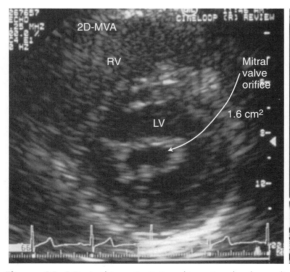

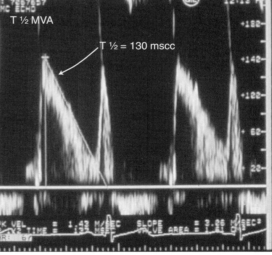

Figure 11·15 In this patient, two-dimensional echocardiographic *(left)* and pressure half-time (T½) mitral valve area *(right)* recorded 5 years after balloon mitral valvuloplasty shows no evidence of restenosis. The valve area is 1.6 to 1.7 cm[2], similar to her immediate postprocedure valve area. LV, left ventricle; RV, right ventricle.

Left Atrial Function

The prevalence of spontaneous contrast on transesophageal echocardiography decreases from 65% of patients before balloon valvuloplasty to 28% of patients at 6-month follow-up evaluation.[70] Resolution of spontaneous contrast on echocardiography occurred only in patients in sinus rhythm. At the 6-month follow-up assessment, only 4% of patients in sinus rhythm and 89% of those in atrial fibrillation continued to show spontaneous contrast in the left atrium on echocardiography. These data suggest that successful balloon valvuloplasty results in more effective atrial contraction in patients in sinus rhythm. None of the patients with long-standing atrial fibrillation (28% of the total) converted to sinus rhythm after the procedure.

Outcome for Specific Patient Groups

Given the overall effectiveness of balloon valvuloplasty, attention has focused on the value of this procedure in specific subgroups that may be at higher risk for complications or a worse outcome. In patients with a previous surgical commissurotomy, balloon mitral valvuloplasty can be performed successfully, with an increase in valve area only slightly less than that expected in those without a prior surgical procedure.[71] In patients with severe pulmonary hypertension, the success of balloon valvuloplasty is similar to that of patients with normal pulmonary pressures, although pulmonary pressures tend to remain higher after the procedure.[64]

Many asymptomatic patients with mitral stenosis develop symptoms during pregnancy due to a higher cardiac output and transmitral volume flow rate. Most of these patients can be managed medically, and mechanical intervention deferred until the postpartum period. However, balloon mitral valvuloplasty can be performed during pregnancy, if necessary. For 18 pregnant patients at 12 to 32 weeks' gestation, results of valvuloplasty were similar to nonpregnant patients.[57] Minor modifications of the procedure and shielding of the gravid uterus are appropriate to minimize fetal radiation exposure.

The elderly have slightly higher risks of mortality and complications with balloon valvuloplasty. Older patients are more likely to have deformed and calcified valves, which predict a suboptimal hemodynamic result just as for younger patients. Among 75 patients 70 years of age or older, procedural death occurred in 4%, and the procedure was unsuccessful due to technical failure in 2% of patients.[72] In the remainder, valve area increased from 1.0 ± 0.2 cm² to 1.6 ± 0.3 cm², as assessed by 2D echocardiography, despite the presence of significant valve calcification in 77% of these patients. Predictors of poor initial hemodynamic results were a previous commissurotomy and valve calcification. At 4 years after valvuloplasty, the actuarial survival rate was 59% ± 18%, but only 34% ± 16% were alive with no more than mild residual symptoms.

Another series of elderly (≥65 years) patients emphasizes the adverse baseline mitral valve anatomy in this patient group.[53] Of 99 patients, 26% had had previous surgical commissurotomy, 73% had calcification detectable on fluoroscopy, and 63% had an MGH morphology score higher than 8. The incidence of procedural death was 3%, while 5% suffered cardiac tamponade, and 3% had systemic embolic events. The procedure was successful in only 46%, with success defined as a valve area greater than or equal to 1.5 cm², a less than 2-grade increase in mitral regurgitation, and no significant atrial septal defect. Predictors of success were the MGH morphology score, functional class, and baseline mitral valve area. Actuarial survival at 3 years was better for those with good initial results than for those with suboptimal procedural results (79% ± 7% versus 62% ± 10%, P = .04).

Comparison With Surgical Intervention

Several studies have compared balloon mitral valvuloplasty with surgical commissurotomy (Table 11–6). In the largest, nonrandomized series, 230 patients with balloon mitral valvuloplasty were compared with 241 patients with surgical commissurotomy, of whom 130 had closed and 111 had open procedures. The improvement in valve area was similar in all three groups, and predictors of the rate of decrease in valve area after the procedure were time, mitral valve morphology, and subvalvular disease for both the surgical and balloon valvuloplasty groups.[17] Restenosis rates were 0.08 cm²/year for balloon valvuloplasty and 0.07 cm²/year for surgical commissurotomy.

In a study of 40 patients randomized to balloon mitral valvuloplasty or closed surgical commissurotomy, there was no difference in the degree of hemodynamic improvement at 1-week and 8-month follow-up evaluations in

TABLE 11·6   STUDIES COMPARING BALLOON MITRAL VALVULOPLASTY WITH SURGERY

| Study | Study Design | Groups | Patients | MVA (cm²) | | | |
				Before	1 Week	8 Weeks	3 Years
Turi, 1991[73]	Prospective, randomized	Balloon valvuloplasty	20	0.8 ± 0.2	1.6 ± 0.6	1.6 ± 0.6	
		Closed commissurotomy	20	0.9 ± 0.4, P = NS	1.6 ± 0.7, P = NS	1.8 ± 0.6, P = NS	
Reyes, 1994[16]	Prospective, randomized	Balloon valvuloplasty	30	0.9 ± 0.3	2.1 ± 0.6		2.4 ± 0.6
		Open commissurotomy	30	0.9 ± 0.3, P = NS	2.0 ± 0.6, P = NS		1.8 ± 0.4, P < .001

MVA, mitral valve area; NS, not significant.

the balloon valvuloplasty group compared with those undergoing closed commissurotomy. There were no deaths, and rate of complications was similar in both groups.[73] These researchers observed that in India the cost of balloon mitral valvuloplasty is higher than the cost of surgery due to the cost of the balloon catheter, whereas in the United States, the cost of surgery is higher due to surgeon and operating room fees. Of course, the comparative cost of the two procedures will vary temporally and geographically as the cost of the balloon catheter and surgical fees change. A major criticism of this study was that balloon valvuloplasty was compared with closed (not open) commissurotomy and thus the surgical technique was suboptimal.

A subsequent randomized trial in 60 patients with mitral stenosis and favorable valve anatomy compared balloon valvuloplasty to open surgical commissurotomy.[16] The initial increase in valve area was similar in both groups, with an average increase in valve area of 1.1 cm^2, but the surgical group had a smaller valve area at the 3-year follow-up evaluation compared with the balloon valvuloplasty group (1.8 ± 0.4 cm^2 versus 2.4 ± 0.6 cm^2, $P < .001$). The rates of restenosis were similar, occurring in 10% of the balloon valvuloplasty group and 13% of surgical group, with restenosis defined as a valve area less than 1.5 cm^2 and a loss of more than 50% of the initial gain after the procedure. Complication rates also were similar, with severe mitral regurgitation complicating two balloon valvuloplasty procedures and one surgical commissurotomy.

Taken together with the larger series of observational studies on the short- and long-term outcome after balloon valvuloplasty, these smaller, randomized trials offer convincing evidence that balloon mitral valvuloplasty is an effective procedure for relief of mitral stenosis in appropriately selected patients with a low complication rate and long-lasting hemodynamic results.

TIMING AND CHOICE OF INTERVENTION
Traditional Indications

Traditionally, patients with mitral stenosis were treated medically until the onset of heart failure symptoms refractory to medical therapy or symptoms elicited by only mild to moderate activity. Intervention was rarely performed before severe symptoms were experienced, since when the only mechanical intervention for relief of mitral stenosis was surgical, physicians hesitated in recommending the procedure unless a clear improvement in symptoms could be expected postoperatively. In addition, reasoning from basic fluid dynamic principles, mitral stenosis was not considered to be "severe" until the valve area was reduced to less than one fourth of the normal size (<1.0 cm^2 in adults), so that intervention was not thought to be beneficial in patients with larger valve areas. Using these traditional criteria, it is clear that surgical intervention prolongs the lives of patients with severe mitral stenosis based on comparisons of outcome of patients with mitral stenosis treated surgically and those treated medically.[3–6, 74]

However, rather than seeking only to prolong the lives of patients with severe symptoms, our efforts are increasingly directed toward earlier intervention to prevent the long-term, irreversible consequences of mitral valve obstruction, including left atrial enlargement, atrial fibrillation, and pulmonary hypertension. In addition, there is increasing recognition that patients with mitral stenosis develop symptoms gradually, and the decrease in exercise tolerance is insidious so that many patients have a substantial decline in functional status with valve areas larger than 1.0 cm^2. Further, the option of effective catheter-based approaches for mechanical relief of mitral stenosis helps tip the balance toward consideration of earlier intervention in many patients.

Newer Indications

The goals of earlier mechanical intervention for relief of mitral stenosis are: (1) improvement of symptoms due to mitral valve obstruction; (2) improved exercise tolerance and functional capacity; (3) prevention of left atrial enlargement, atrial fibrillation, and embolic events; and (4) prevention of irreversible pulmonary hypertension. The key factors that must be considered in each patient before recommending mechanical intervention include the degree to which the symptoms or decreased functional capacity are clearly due to mitral valve obstruction; the options available for relief of mitral stenosis in that patient, based on evaluation of mitral valve morphology and function; the expected risk and outcome of the procedure; patient preferences; and comorbid disease.

For patients with apparently normal exercise tolerance but a reported decrease from their own baseline exercise capacity, stress testing with Doppler echocardiographic evaluation of stenosis severity and pulmonary pressures often demonstrates hemodynamic exercise limitation. Although resting valve area may be larger than 1.0 cm², a disproportionate rise in pulmonary pressures is seen with exercise.[75, 76] These patients often show improvement in symptoms after relief of mitral stenosis, suggesting that earlier intervention may be appropriate, particularly if a catheter-based approach is possible.

Most patients with mitral stenosis eventually develop atrial fibrillation, and many clinicians consider intervention at the onset of paroxysmal or sustained atrial fibrillation in the hope of restoring normal sinus rhythm. While there is a paucity of data on the effect of even earlier intervention on the subsequent development of atrial fibrillation, it is plausible that avoidance of left atrial enlargement might prevent or delay the onset of atrial fibrillation. Few clinicians would consider intervention for the isolated finding of progressive left atrial enlargement; however, the size and rate of increase in left atrial size should be considered in the overall decision-making process.

Although pulmonary pressures decrease after relief of mitral stenosis, some patients are left with irreversible pulmonary hypertension and consequent right heart dysfunction. As for atrial fibrillation, data on the effect of earlier intervention on prevention of irreversible pulmonary hypertension are sparse. Physiologic considerations suggest that since the primary culprit in development of pulmonary hypertension is a prolonged elevation in left atrial pressure, earlier intervention to decrease left atrial pressure may be beneficial. The ability to follow pulmonary systolic pressures noninvasively with Doppler ultrasound allows serial evaluation of patients with mitral stenosis. Again, evidence of a progressive increase in pulmonary pressures is unlikely to be the sole indication for intervention, but it is one more factor to consider in the decision-making process.

Combining these factors, in the patient with mitral stenosis of sufficient severity to benefit from commissurotomy, intervention should be considered when there is evidence of decreased functional status or exercise capacity, progressive left atrial enlargement or the onset of atrial fibrillation, or evidence of a progressive increase in pulmonary pressures. When more than one of these factors are present, the justification for recommending earlier intervention is stronger. Patient preferences and

comorbid disease have a strong impact on the timing of intervention. If mitral valve anatomy is favorable, the informed younger patient may choose early balloon valvuloplasty to maintain as nearly normal cardiac anatomy and physiology as possible. Conversely, in the elderly patient with a calcified and deformed valve and significant comorbidity, intervention may be delayed until the development of severe symptoms refractory to medical therapy.

Choice of Procedure

The choice of which procedure to recommend for relief of mitral stenosis in an individual patient depends on several factors, including mitral valve morphology, the severity of coexisting mitral regurgitation, the presence and severity of other valve lesions, patient preferences, and comorbid disease (Tables 11–7 and 11–8).

In isolated mitral stenosis with favorable valve morphology, mitral regurgitation grade of 2 + or less, and no other contraindications, balloon mitral valvuloplasty is the procedure of choice. Transthoracic echocardiography is used to determine mitral stenosis severity, evaluate mitral morphology, and estimate the severity of coexisting mitral regurgitation. If the patient has severe mitral stenosis with only mild mitral regurgitation, the interventional cardiologist is consulted about the technical feasibility of the procedure and the likelihood of a good hemodynamic result. If balloon valvuloplasty is scheduled, transesophageal echocardiography is performed at a short interval before the procedure to evaluate for left atrial thrombus. When thrombus is detected, the procedure is deferred, and the patient is referred for surgical open commissurotomy or is treated with anticoagulation for several weeks, followed by repeat transesophageal echocardiography to ensure resolution of the atrial thrombus before valvuloplasty.

Closed mitral commissurotomy is rarely performed in Europe or North America but continues to be an appropriate therapeutic option worldwide. Patient selection, hemodynamic results, and long-term outcome can be similar to those for balloon valvuloplasty; however, considerable surgical expertise is needed for optimal results.

For isolated mitral stenosis with favorable anatomy and contraindications to balloon mitral valvuloplasty or with coexisting valve lesions requiring treatment, surgical open commissurotomy should be considered. Because

TABLE 11·7   APPROACHES TO MECHANICAL RELIEF OF MITRAL STENOSIS

Approach	Advantages	Disadvantages
Closed surgical commissurotomy	Inexpensive Relatively simple Good hemodynamic results in selected patients Good long-term outcome	No direct visualization of valve Only feasible with flexible, noncalcified valves Contraindicated if MR >2+ Surgical procedure with general anesthesia
Open surgical commissurotomy	Visualization of valve allows directed commissurotomy Concurrent annuloplasty for MR is feasible	Best results with flexible, noncalcified valves Surgical procedure with general anesthesia
Valve replacement	Feasible in all patients regardless of extent of valve calcification or severity of MR	Surgical procedure with general anesthesia Effect of loss of annular-papillary muscle continuity on LV function Prosthetic valve Chronic anticoagulation
Balloon mitral commissurotomy	Percutaneous approach Local anesthesia Good hemodynamic results in selected patients Good long-term outcome	No direct visualization of valve Only feasible with flexible, noncalcified valves Contraindicated if MR >2+

LV, left ventricular; MR, mitral regurgitation.

the basic anatomic mechanism of relief of mitral stenosis is similar for balloon and surgical commissurotomy, heavily calcified and deformed valves are unlikely to have an adequate increase in valve area with either type of commissurotomy. However, patients with favorable anatomy but a contraindication to the balloon procedure, such as a persistent atrial thrombus, prior atrial septal surgery, or difficult venous access, are appropriate candidates for a surgical commissurotomy. In patients with intermediate valve morphology (scores of 8 to 12), a better result may be obtained under direct vision at surgery, although there are no comparative studies in this specific subgroup.

Patients with coexisting aortic or tricuspid valve disease but favorable mitral valve anatomy may benefit from surgical commissurotomy. For example, mitral commissurotomy should be considered in the patient undergoing aortic valve replacement for rheumatic aortic valve disease with coexisting moderate to severe mitral stenosis. Although repeat surgery may be needed at a later date for mitral valve restenosis or regurgitation, the risks of two prosthetic valves are deferred. Combining mi-

TABLE 11·8   PATIENT SELECTION IN THE CHOICE OF INTERVENTION FOR RELIEF OF MITRAL STENOSIS

Procedure	MV Morphology Score	Severity of MR	Other Valve Lesions	Pulmonary Hypertension
Balloon mitral commissurotomy	<8 ideal <10 acceptable	≤2+	No other valve procedure needed	PA pressures improve after procedure, even when severely elevated
Open surgical commissurotomy	<8 ideal <10 acceptable	≤2+*	May have other valve procedures or CABG	
Mitral valve replacement	Valve may be calcified and deformed; score not predictive of outcome	MR may be severe	May have other valve procedures or CABG	Higher risk with PA systolic pressure >60 mm Hg

CABG, coronary artery bypass grafting; MR, mitral regurgitation; PA, pulmonary artery.
*Or annuloplasty ring if >2+.

tral commissurotomy with a valve-sparing aortic procedure or an aortic valve homograft allows avoidance of a mechanical valve in some of these patients.

Valve replacement is needed in patients with severely calcified and deformed mitral valves and in patients with mixed stenosis and regurgitation. Most often, a mechanical valve is used because of its long-term durability and the typical need for chronic anticoagulation due to the presence of atrial fibrillation in these patients. Some patients with mitral stenosis requiring valve replacement may be candidates for a mitral homograft valve, and the number of patients receiving this option is likely to increase as homograft valves become more available and more surgeons develop expertise with this procedure.[23]

References

1. Toumbouras M, Panagopoulos F, Papakonstantinou C, et al: Long-term surgical outcome of closed mitral commissurotomy. J Heart Valve Dis 1995;4:247–250.
2. Silverstein DM: Management of rheumatic mitral valve disease in Kenya. Personal communication, 1996.
3. John S, Bashi VV, Jairaj PS, et al: Closed mitral valvotomy: early results and long-term follow-up of 3724 consecutive patients. Circulation 1983;68:891–896.
4. Ellis LB, Harken DE: Closed valvuloplasty for mitral stenosis. N Engl J Med 1964;270:643.
5. Bruce RA, Merendino KA: Quantitative evaluation of mitral commissurotomy by means of a standardized exercise tolerance test. Surgery 1954;36:621.
6. Dexter L, Gorlin R, Lewis BM, Haynes FW, Harken DE: Physiologic evaluation of patients with mitral stenosis before and after mitral valvuloplasty. Trans Am Clin Climatol Assoc 1950;62:170–180.
7. Feigenbaum H, Linback RE, Nasser WK: Hemodynamic studies before and after instrumental mitral commissurotomy: a reappraisal of the pathophysiology of mitral stenosis and the efficacy of mitral valvotomy. Circulation 1968;38:261–276.
8. Ellis LB, Singh JB, Morales DD, Harken DE: Fifteen- to twenty-year study of one thousand patients undergoing closed mitral valvuloplasty. Circulation 1973;48:357–364.
9. Harrison DC, Dexter L: The evaluation of patients who develop recurrent cardiac symptoms after mitral valvuloplasty. Am Heart J 1963;65:583.
10. Heger JJ, Wann LS, Weyman AE, Dillon JC, Feigenbaum H: Long-term changes in mitral valve area after successful mitral commissurotomy. Circulation 1979;59:443–448.
11. Higgs LM, Glancy DL, O'Brien KP, Epstein SE, Morrow AG: Mitral restenosis: an uncommon cause of recurrent symptoms following mitral commissurotomy. Am J Cardiol 1970;26:34–37.
12. Rihal CS, Schaff HV, Frye RL, Bailey KR, Hammes LN, Holmes DR Jr: Long-term follow-up of patients undergoing closed transventricular mitral commissurotomy: a useful surrogate for percutaneous balloon mitral valvuloplasty? J Am Coll Cardiol 1992;20:781–786.
13. Smith WM, Neutze JM, Barratt Boyes BG, Lowe JB: Open mitral valvotomy: effect of preoperative factors on result. J Thorac Cardiovasc Surg 1981;82:738–751.
14. Halseth WL, Elliott DP, Walker EL, Smith EA: Open mitral commissurotomy: a modern re-evaluation. J Thorac Cardiovasc Surg 1980;80:842–848.
15. Cohn LH, Allred EN, Cohn LA, Disesa VJ, Shemin RJ, Collins JJ Jr: Long-term results of open mitral valve reconstruction for mitral stenosis. Am J Cardiol 1985;55:731–734.
16. Reyes VP, Raju BS, Wynne J, et al: Percutaneous balloon valvuloplasty compared with open surgical commissurotomy for mitral stenosis. N Engl J Med 1994;331:961–967.
17. Essop R, Rothlisberger C, Dullabh A, Sareli P: Can the long-term outcomes of percutaneous balloon mitral valvotomy and surgical commissurotomy be expected to be similar? J Heart Valve Dis 1995;4:446–452.
18. Vega JL, Fleitas M, Martinez R, et al: Open mitral commissurotomy. Ann Thorac Surg 1981;31:266–270.
19. Laschinger JC, Cunningham JN Jr, Baumann FG, et al: Early open radical commissurotomy: surgical treatment of choice for mitral stenosis. Ann Thorac Surg 1982;34:287–298.
20. Housman LB, Bonchek L, Lambert L, Grunkemeier G, Starr A: Prognosis of patients after open mitral commissurotomy: actuarial analysis of late results in 100 patients. J Thorac Cardiovasc Surg 1977;73:742–745.
21. Fremes SE, Goldman BS, Ivanov J, Weisel RD, David TE, Salerno T: Valvular surgery in the elderly. Circulation 1989;80(Suppl 1):I77–I90.
22. Vincens JJ, Temizer D, Post JR, Edmunds LH Jr, Herrmann HC: Long-term outcome of cardiac surgery in patients with mitral stenosis and severe pulmonary hypertension. Circulation 1995;92(suppl II):137–142.
23. Acar C, Tolan M, Berrebi A, et al: Homograft replacement of the mitral valve: graft selection, technique of implantation, and results in forty-three patients. J Thorac Cardiovasc Surg 1996;111:367–378.
24. Balloon Valvuloplasty Registry: Multicenter experience with balloon mitral commissurotomy. NHLBI Balloon Valvuloplasty Registry Report on immediate and 30-day follow-up results. The National Heart, Lung, and Blood Institute Balloon Valvuloplasty Registry participants. Circulation 1992;85:448–461.
25. Iung B, Cormier B, Ducimetiere P, et al: Immediate results of percutaneous mitral commissurotomy: a predictive model on a series of 1514 patients. Circulation 1996;94:2124–2130.
26. Wilkins GT, Weyman AE, Abascal VM, Block PC, Palacios IF: Percutaneous balloon dilatation of the mitral valve: an analysis of echocardiographic variables related to outcome and the mechanism of dilatation. Br Heart J 1988;60:299–308.
27. Abascal VM, Wilkins GT, Choong CY, et al: Echocardiographic evaluation of mitral valve structure and function in patients followed for at least 6 months after percutaneous balloon mitral valvuloplasty. J Am Coll Cardiol 1988;12:606–615.
28. Abascal VM, Wilkins GT, O'Shea JP, et al: Prediction of successful outcome in 130 patients undergoing percutaneous balloon mitral valvotomy. Circulation 1990;82:448–456.
29. Palacios IF, Tuzcu ME, Weyman AE, Newell JB, Block PC: Clinical follow-up of patients undergoing percutaneous mitral balloon valvotomy. Circulation 1995;91:671–676.

30. Balloon Valvuloplasty Registry: Complications and mortality of percutaneous balloon mitral commissurotomy: a report from the National Heart, Lung, and Blood Institute Balloon Valvuloplasty Registry. Circulation 1992;85:2014–2024.

31. Reid CL, Otto CM, Davis KB, Labovitz A, Kisslo KB, McKay CR: Influence of mitral valve morphology on mitral balloon commissurotomy: immediate and six-month results from the NHLBI Balloon Valvuloplasty Registry. Am Heart J 1992;124:657–665.

32. Dean LS, Mickel MC, Bonan R, et al: Four-year follow-up of patients undergoing percutaneous balloon mitral commissurotomy: a report from the National Heart, Lung, and Blood Institute Balloon Valvuloplasty Registry. J Am Coll Cardiol 1996;28:1452–1457.

33. Pavlides GS, Nahhas GT, London J, et al: Predictors of long-term event-free survival after percutaneous balloon mitral valvuloplasty. Am J Cardiol 1997;79:1370–1374.

34. Cohen DJ, Kuntz RE, Gordon SP, et al: Predictors of long-term outcome after percutaneous balloon mitral valvuloplasty. N Engl J Med 1992;327:1329–1335.

35. Eisenberg MJ, Ballal R, Heidenreich PA, et al: Echocardiographic score as a predictor of in-hospital cost in patients undergoing percutaneous balloon mitral valvuloplasty. Am J Cardiol 1996;78:790–794.

36. Reid CL, McKay CR, Chandraratna PA, Kawanishi DT, Rahimtoola SH: Mechanisms of increase in mitral valve area and influence of anatomic features in double-balloon, catheter balloon valvuloplasty in adults with rheumatic mitral stenosis: a Doppler and two-dimensional echocardiographic study. Circulation 1987;76:628–636.

37. Fatkin D, Roy P, Morgan JJ, Feneley MP: Percutaneous balloon mitral valvotomy with the Inoue single-balloon catheter: commissural morphology as a determinant of outcome. J Am Coll Cardiol 1993;21:390–397.

38. Cannan CR, Nishimura RA, Reeder GS, et al: Echocardiographic assessment of commissural calcium: a simple predictor of outcome after percutaneous mitral balloon valvotomy. J Am Coll Cardiol 1997;29:175–180.

39. Vahanian A, Michel PL, Cormier B, et al: Immediate and mid-term results of percutaneous mitral commissurotomy. Eur Heart J 1991;12(suppl):84–89.

40. Iung B, Cormier B, Ducimetiere P, et al: Functional results 5 years after successful percutaneous mitral commissurotomy in a series of 528 patients and analysis of predictive factors. J Am Coll Cardiol 1996;27:407–414.

41. Reid CL: Echocardiography in the patient undergoing catheter balloon mitral commissurotomy. In Otto CM, ed. The Practice of Clinical Echocardiography. Philadelphia: WB Saunders; 1997:373–388.

42. McKay RG, Lock JE, Safian RD, et al: Balloon dilation of mitral stenosis in adult patients: postmortem and percutaneous mitral valvuloplasty studies. J Am Coll Cardiol 1987;9:723–731.

43. Chen CG, Wang X, Wang Y, Lan YF: Value of two-dimensional echocardiography in selecting patients and balloon sizes for percutaneous balloon mitral valvuloplasty. J Am Coll Cardiol 1989;14:1651–1658.

44. Inoue K: Percutaneous transvenous mitral commissurotomy using the Inoue balloon. Eur Heart J 1991;12(suppl):99–108.

45. Inoue K, Feldman T: Percutaneous transvenous mitral commissurotomy using the Inoue balloon catheter. Cathet Cardiovasc Diagn 1993;28:119–125.

46. Feldman T, Herrmann HC, Inoue K: Technique of percutaneous transvenous mitral commissurotomy using the Inoue balloon catheter. Cathet Cardiovasc Diagn 1994;29(suppl):26–34.

47. Vahanian A, Cormier B, Iung B: Percutaneous transvenous mitral commissurotomy using the Inoue balloon: international experience. Cathet Cardiovasc Diagn 1994;30(suppl):8–15.

48. Tuzcu EM, Block PC, Palacios IF: Comparison of early versus late experience with percutaneous mitral balloon valvuloplasty. J Am Coll Cardiol 1991;17:1121–1124.

49. Desideri A, Vanderperren O, Serra A, et al: Long-term (9 to 33 months) echocardiographic follow-up after successful percutaneous mitral commissurotomy. Am J Cardiol 1992;69:1602–1606.

50. Padial LR, Freitas N, Sagie A, et al: Echocardiography can predict which patients will develop severe mitral regurgitation after percutaneous mitral valvulotomy. J Am Coll Cardiol 1996;27:1225–1231.

51. Cormier B, Vahanian A, Michel PL, et al: Transoesophageal echocardiography in the assessment of percutaneous mitral commissurotomy. Eur Heart J 1991;12(suppl):61–65.

52. Kamalesh M, Burger AJ, Shubrooks SJ Jr: The use of transesophageal echocardiography to avoid left atrial thrombus during percutaneous mitral valvuloplasty. Cathet Cardiovasc Diagn 1993;28:320–322.

53. Tuzcu EM, Block PC, Griffin BP, Newell JB, Palacios IF: Immediate and long-term outcome of percutaneous mitral valvotomy in patients 65 years and older. Circulation 1992;85:963–971.

54. Orrange SE, Kawanishi DT, Lopez BM, Curry SM, Rahimtoola SH: Actuarial outcome after catheter balloon commissurotomy in patients with mitral stenosis. Circulation 1997;95:382–389.

55. Pan M, Medina A, Suarez de Lezo J, et al: Factors determining late success after mitral balloon valvulotomy. Am J Cardiol 1993;71:1181–1185.

56. Rothlisberger C, Essop MR, Skudicky D, Skoularigis J, Wisenbaugh T, Sareli P: Results of percutaneous balloon mitral valvotomy in young adults. Am J Cardiol 1993;72:73–77.

57. Arora R, Kalra GS, Murty GS, et al: Percutaneous transatrial mitral commissurotomy: immediate and intermediate results. J Am Coll Cardiol 1994;23:1327–1332.

58. Chen CR, Cheng TO: Percutaneous balloon mitral valvuloplasty by the Inoue technique: a multicenter study of 4832 patients in China. Am Heart J 1995;129:1197–1203.

59. Thomas JD, Wilkins GT, Choong CY, et al: Inaccuracy of mitral pressure half-time immediately after percutaneous mitral valvotomy: dependence on transmitral gradient and left atrial and ventricular compliance. Circulation 1988;78:980–993.

60. Otto CM, Davis KB, Holmes DRJ, et al: Methodologic issues in clinical evaluation of stenosis severity in adults undergoing aortic or mitral balloon valvuloplasty. The NHLBI Balloon Valvuloplasty Registry. Am J Cardiol 1992;69:1607–1616.

61. Manga P, Singh S, Brandis S, Freidman B: Mitral valve area calculations immediately after percutaneous mitral balloon valvuloplasty. J Am Coll Cardiol 1993;21:1568–1573.

62. Schwammenthal E, Rabinowitz B, Kaplinsky E, Vered Z, Feinberg MS: Mitral valve resistance: wrong physics, right physiology [abstract]. Circulation 1996;94:I617.

63. Georgeson S, Panidis IP, Kleaveland JP, Heilbrunn S, Gonzales R: Effect of percutaneous balloon valvuloplasty on pulmonary hypertension in mitral stenosis. Am Heart J 1993;125:374–379.

64. Alfonso F, Macaya C, Hernandez R, et al: Percutaneous mitral valvuloplasty with severe pulmonary artery hypertension. Am J Cardiol 1993;72:325–330.

65. Fawzy ME, Mimish L, Sivanandam V, et al: Immediate and long-term effect of mitral balloon valvotomy on severe pulmonary hypertension in patients with mitral stenosis. Am Heart J 1996;131:89–93.

66. Martinez EE, Barros TL, Santos DV, et al: Cardiopulmonary exercise testing early after catheter-balloon mitral valvuloplasty in patients with mitral stenosis. Int J Cardiol 1992;37:7–13.

67. Barlow CW, Long JE, Brown G, Manga P, Meyer TE, Robbins PA: Exercise capacity and skeletal muscle structure and function before and after balloon mitral valvuloplasty. Am J Cardiol 1995;76:684–688.

68. Douard H, Gilles YM, Choussat A, Brousstet JP: Lack of correlation between haemodynamic and cardiopulmonary exercise capacity improvement after catheter-balloon mitral valvuloplasty. Eur Heart J 1995;16:1375–1379.

69. Ohshima M, Yamazoe M, Tamura Y, et al: Immediate effects of percutaneous transvenous mitral commissurotomy on pulmonary hemodynamics at rest and during exercise in mitral stenosis. Am J Cardiol 1992;70:641–644.

70. Cormier B, Vahanian A, Iung B, et al: Influence of percutaneous mitral commissurotomy on left atrial spontaneous contrast of mitral stenosis. Am J Cardiol 1993;71:842–847.

71. Davidson CJ, Bashore TM, Mickel M, Davis K: Balloon mitral commissurotomy after previous surgical commissurotomy. The National Heart, Lung, and Blood Institute Balloon Valvuloplasty Registry participants. Circulation 1992;86:91–99.

72. Iung B, Cormier B, Farah B, et al: Percutaneous mitral commissurotomy in the elderly. Eur Heart J 1995;16:1092–1099.

73. Turi ZG, Reyes VP, Raju BS, et al: Percutaneous balloon versus surgical closed commissurotomy for mitral stenosis: a prospective, randomized trial. Circulation 1991;83:1179–1185.

74. Olesen KH: The natural history of 271 patients with mitral stenosis under medical treatment. Br Heart J 1962;24:349–357.

75. Tunick PA, Freedberg RS, Gargiulo A, Kronzon I: Exercise Doppler echocardiography as an aid to clinical decision making in mitral valve disease. J Am Soc Echocardiogr 1992;5:225–230.

76. Schwammenthal E, Chen C, Giesler M, et al: New method for accurate calculation of regurgitant flow rate based on analysis of Doppler color flow maps of the proximal flow field: validation in a canine model of mitral regurgitation with initial application in patients. J Am Coll Cardiol 1996;27:161–172.

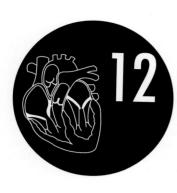

12 Aortic Regurgitation

PATHOPHYSIOLOGY

Understanding the pathophysiology of aortic regurgitation requires consideration of the three major components of the disease process: the left ventricle, the aortic valve, and the peripheral vasculature (Table 12–1).[1] Other factors relevant to the clinical presentation and disease course include coronary anatomy and blood flow, changes with exercise, and the differences between acute and chronic aortic regurgitation.

Left Ventricular Volume and Pressure Overload

The central hemodynamic feature of chronic aortic regurgitation is combined volume and pressure overload of the left ventricle.[2–4] Since total left ventricular stroke volume equals forward plus regurgitant stroke volume, normal forward cardiac output is maintained by an increase in total stroke volume corresponding to the severity of regurgitation (Fig. 12–1). This increase in total stroke volume is achieved by progressive ventricular dilation with increased end-diastolic and end-systolic volumes (Fig. 12–2). In this respect, both aortic and mitral regurgitation represent left ventricular "volume overload" leading to compensatory left ventricular dilation. However, aortic and mitral regurgitation differ in that forward stoke volume in the presence of aortic regurgitation is maintained predominantly by ventricular dilation with no change in ejection fraction, whereas the initial compensatory response to mitral regurgitation is an increased ejection fraction, with little ventricular dilation.[5]

In addition, unlike the physiology of mitral regurgitation, left ventricular afterload is increased in the presence of aortic regurgitation as the increased stroke volume is ejected into the high-impedance aorta. Although there are many potential descriptors of left ventricular afterload (see Chapter 7), one of the most robust and clinically relevant measures is end-systolic circumferential wall stress. In simplistic

TABLE 12·1	PHYSIOLOGIC FACTORS AFFECTING VENTRICULAR-VASCULAR COUPLING IN ACUTE AORTIC REGURGITATION

Anatomic Site	Physiologic Factors
Ventricle	Preload (ventricular volumes/venous return)
	Afterload (end-systolic circumferential wall stress)
	Systolic transaortic pressure gradient
	Contractility
	Heart rate
	Left ventricular geometry
	Coronary perfusion pressure
Valve	Regurgitant orifice area
	Regurgitant volume
	Diastolic transaortic pressure gradient
	Forward stroke volume
Vasculature	Systemic vascular resistance
	Vascular compliance and viscoelasticity
	Blood inertia
	Reflected pressure waves

terms, wall stress is the product of ventricular pressure and radius, divided by twice the wall thickness. Early in the disease course, end-systolic wall stress is maintained in the normal range, despite an increase in end-systolic dimension and pressure, by a compensatory increase in wall thickness. Thus, patients with compensated chronic aortic regurgitation have substantial increases in left ventricular mass as well as ventricular volumes. Ejection fraction and end-systolic elastance (E_{max}) tend to be normal (not increased) in compensated aortic regurgitation.

As the disease progresses and ventricular dimensions and systolic pressure increase further, the degree of wall thickening fails to keep pace so that end-systolic wall stress rises.[6] Hemodynamic decompensation ensues, with a decline in ejection performance related to the excessive afterload. At this point in the disease course, contractile function of the myocardium remains normal. Therefore, ejection performance should normalize after surgical correction of the regurgitant lesion. However, with continued volume and pressure overload of the left ventricle, depression of myocardial contractility supervenes, and both the ejection fraction and E_{max} are reduced. These patients may have irreversible systolic dysfunction of the left ventricle and are less likely to improve after surgical correction.

In the research setting, patients with a reduced ejection fraction due to increased afterload can be differentiated from those with impaired contractility by demonstration of a normal E_{max} (indicating normal myocardial contractility), despite a decrease in ejection fraction (Fig. 12–3).[7] While clinical evaluation of myocardial contractility is difficult in patients with aortic regurgitation and a decreased ejection fraction, particularly given the altered loading conditions associated with this lesion, measures of left ventricular function that predict outcome after valve replacement and provide guidance about the optimal timing of surgical intervention have been developed, as discussed below.

AORTIC REGURGITATION

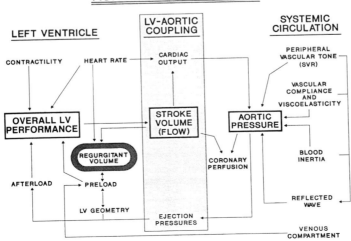

Figure 12·1 Physiologic framework for understanding the pathophysiology of chronic aortic regurgitation. LV, left ventricular; SVR, systemic vascular resistance. (From Borow KM, Marcus RH: Aortic regurgitation: the need for an integrated physiologic approach [editorial]. J Am Coll Cardiol 1991;17:898-900; reprinted with permission from the American College of Cardiology.)

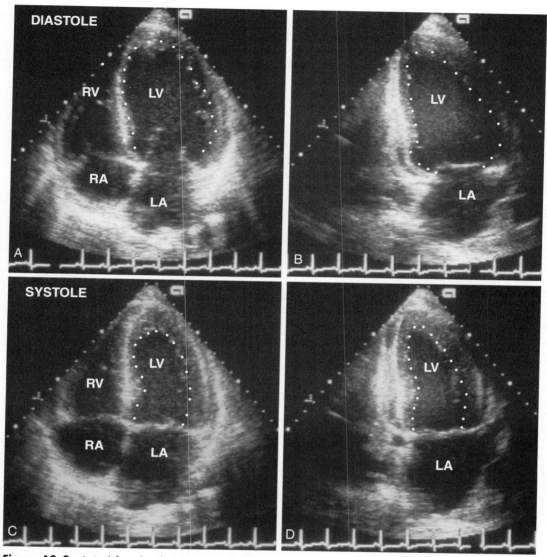

Figure 12·2 Apical four-chamber *(A)* and two-chamber *(B)* echocardiographic views at end-diastole and the same views at end-systole *(C, D)* in a patient with left ventricular dilation caused by chronic aortic regurgitation. Notice the more spherical shape of the left ventricle in the four-chamber views. LA, left atrium; LV, left ventricle; RA, right atrium; RV, right ventricle.

Valvular Hemodynamics

In systole, aortic regurgitation is associated with a small transaortic pressure gradient and increased antegrade flow velocity due to the increased volume flow rate across the valve. With isolated regurgitation, the maximum gradient typically is only 5 to 25 mm Hg corresponding to a Doppler flow velocity up to 2.5 m/s. However, many patients have some degree of associated stenosis so that substantially higher gradients are often seen in the clinical setting due to combined aortic stenosis and regurgitation.

In diastole, aortic pressure decreases more rapidly than normal, but left ventricular pressures typically remain low because of the increased compliance of the dilated ventricle. The time course of the difference between aortic and left ventricular pressures in diastole depends on both the severity of regurgitation and the degree of ventricular compensation. This diastolic pressure difference provides the basis for invasive and noninvasive measure-

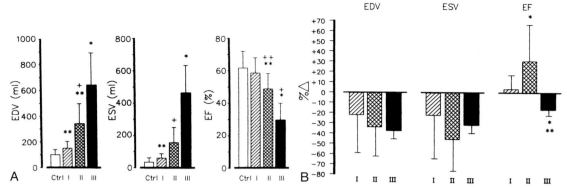

Figure 12·3 *A,* Average radionuclide left ventricular end-diastolic volume (EDV), end-systolic volume (ESV), and ejection fraction (EF) values are compared for control subjects (Ctrl) and patients with aortic regurgitation who were divided into group I (normal end-systolic elastance [E_{max}] and stress-shortening relations), group II (abnormal E_{max} but normal stress-shortening relations), and group III (abnormal E_{max} and stress-shortening relations). *B,* Postoperative changes in radionuclide ventricular volumes and ejection fraction values are shown as the percent change (%) from their corresponding preoperative values. There was a comparable reduction in left ventricular EDV in all three subgroups of patients with aortic regurgitation but a greater reduction in ESV in group II, which resulted in a proportionately greater increase in ejection fraction values for group II compared with groups I and III. Bars indicate mean values, and the lines indicate 1 SD. Symbols indicate statistically significant differences. (From Starling MR, Kirsh MM, Montgomery DG, Gross MD: Mechanisms for left ventricular systolic dysfunction in aortic regurgitation: importance for predicting the functional response to aortic valve replacement. J Am Coll Cardiol 1991;17:891, 893; reprinted with permission from the American College of Cardiology.)

ments of regurgitant severity (see Chapters 3 and 4). With chronic compensated aortic regurgitation, a large pressure difference between the aorta and left ventricle occurs throughout diastole, corresponding to the high-pitched murmur on examination and a continuous wave Doppler curve with high velocities and a flat deceleration slope (Fig. 12–4). With acute or decompensated aortic regurgitation, more rapid equilibration of aortic and ventricular pressures results in a low-

pitched murmur and in a continuous wave Doppler curve with a steep deceleration slope and low velocities at end-diastole.

Peripheral Vasculature

The hemodynamics of chronic aortic regurgitation are characterized by an increased pulse pressure in the aorta (ie, peak systolic minus end-diastolic pressure) because of the increased transaortic stroke volume leading to higher than normal systolic pressures and the rapid decline in diastolic pressures due to run-off across the incompetent valve from the aorta into the left ventricle.

The total load imposed on the left ventricle when the aortic valve is open includes ventricular afterload (ie, end-systolic wall stress) and the systemic vascular circuit. A simple measure of the load imposed by the systemic circuit is systemic vascular resistance, which tends to be decreased in patients with compensated aortic regurgitation.[8] However, standard vascular resistance calculations are based on mean flow and pressure data and do not adequately describe the effects of the pulsatile components of the peripheral circulation on total left ventricular afterload. In more complex terms, the interaction of the peripheral vasculature with ventricular ejection dynamics in patients with aortic regurgitation includes vascular compliance and viscoelasticity, blood inertia, and the

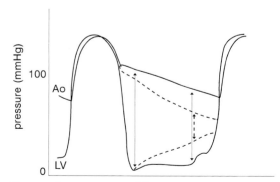

Figure 12·4 Diagram of the pressure curves in chronic *(solid lines)* and acute *(dashed lines)* aortic regurgitation. With chronic regurgitation, there is a large pressure difference between the left ventricle (LV) and aorta (Ao) throughout diastole. With acute regurgitation, aortic pressure falls rapidly, and left ventricular pressure is elevated at end-diastole such that there is rapid equilibration of aortic and ventricular pressures.

impact of reflected pressure waves and vascular resistance. Thus, the conventional calculation of systemic vascular resistance may underestimate the contribution of peripheral "load" in the pathophysiology of the aortic regurgitation. Some insight has been gained into ventricular-vascular coupling in aortic regurgitation using the concept of vascular impedance, a parameter with a modulus and a phase that accounts for pulsatile and steady components of the peripheral vascular circuit. Another approach is based on a "windkessel" model of the vasculature that includes additional components for the regurgitant orifice.[9, 10]

The potential importance of the peripheral vasculature in the disease process should not be underestimated. Experimental models show a strong correlation between total peripheral resistance and regurgitant volume.[11, 12] In addition, there is increasing evidence that altering peripheral vascular properties (eg, with pharmacologic afterload reduction) has a significant impact on disease progression.[1, 13, 14]

Coronary Blood Flow

Coronary blood flow in patients with aortic regurgitation is affected by two major factors: decreased diastolic coronary perfusion pressure, due to the low diastolic aortic pressure, and increased left ventricular oxygen demands, due to increased mass and wall stress. Coronary artery dimensions increase in patients with aortic valve disease in relation to the degree of ventricular hypertrophy.[15] However, with severe regurgitation and marked left ventricular dilation, the degree of coronary artery enlargement is inadequate for the increase in myocardial mass, leading to subendocardial ischemia when increased coronary blood flow is needed (eg, exercise, fever).[16] Resting coronary blood flow is increased in patients with aortic regurgitation, so that even though the maximal blood flow achieved with coronary vasodilation in response to dipyridamole is similar to that of controls, the increase in flow (or coronary flow reserve) is diminished.[17, 18]

Exercise Physiology

With isotonic exercise, regurgitant volume and fraction decrease in patients with aortic regurgitation by about 20%.[19] The decrease in regurgitant severity with exercise is related to both a relative decrease in the duration of diastole compared to systole as heart rate increases and to a decrease in systemic vascular resistance with exercise.[20, 21] In contrast, isometric exercise (eg, hand grip) results in an increase in the area of the color flow jet on Doppler imaging consistent with an increased regurgitant volume due to increased afterload.[22]

In patients with compensated aortic regurgitation, a normal increase in cardiac index occurs during supine exercise, with a decrease in left ventricular end-diastolic and end-systolic volumes and an increase in ejection fraction by 5 units or more.[19, 21, 23] In contrast, patients with impaired ventricular contractility have an increase in end-systolic volume with exercise associated with an increase in end-systolic wall stress and a *decrease* in ejection fraction by 5 units or more.[20, 21, 23] The change in ejection fraction is directly related to the change in systemic vascular resistance,[20] end-systolic volume, end-systolic wall stress, cardiac index, and the pulmonary capillary wedge pressure.[24, 25] In addition, the change in ejection fraction with exercise is affected by position (supine or upright),[26] the type of exercise (isometric or bicycle),[27] and systolic loading conditions.[28] Downregulation of β receptors also may contribute to a blunted cardiac response to exercise in chronic aortic regurgitation.[29]

In a study combining radionuclide angiography and cardiac catheterization during exercise in patients with chronic, severe aortic regurgitation, the major determinants of exercise ejection fraction were systolic chamber performance (ie, elastance), end-systolic volume, and stroke volume.[30] The primary determinant of the *change* in ejection fraction from rest to exercise was systemic vascular resistance.

A potential explanation for the common symptom of exertional dyspnea in patients with aortic regurgitation is elevated left ventricular end-diastolic pressure. Pulmonary wedge pressures are higher at rest and during exercise in patients with severe aortic regurgitation compared with patients with mild to moderate regurgitation.[20] Similarly higher rest and exercise pulmonary wedge pressures are seen in patients with a reduced ejection fraction with exercise compared with those with a normal increase in ejection fraction.[21] The possible role of subendocardial ischemia with exercise has not been evaluated.

Acute Aortic Regurgitation

The time course of acute aortic regurgitation precludes significant compensatory dilation of the left ventricle (Table 12–2).[31] Thus, the acute increase in diastolic flow into a nondilated left ventricle leads to a marked elevation in end-diastolic pressure due to a rightward shift along the normal diastolic pressure-volume curve. Compared with chronic compensated regurgitation, the increase in ventricular pressures in conjunction with a greater decrease in aortic pressures leads to more rapid equilibration of aortic and ventricular pressures over the diastolic filling period. In severe cases, aortic and left ventricular pressures equalize at end-diastole, such that diastolic blood pressure equals left ventricular end-diastolic pressure (Fig. 12–5).

With acute regurgitation, forward cardiac output is decreased, since the total stroke volume of the nondilated ventricle now includes both regurgitant and forward stroke volume. Compensatory tachycardia may partially correct this decline in forward stroke volume. Pulmonary edema results from the elevated left ventricular end-diastolic pressure and consequent elevated pulmonary venous pressure. In addition, coronary flow reserve is acutely diminished, which may lead to subendocardial ischemia.[32]

Thus, the patient with acute aortic regurgitation differs strikingly from the patient with chronic compensated disease. With acute regurgitation, the left ventricle is nondilated with an elevated end-diastolic pressure, the pulse pressure is narrow, aortic and ventricular pressures equalize at end-diastole, and the patient often has both pulmonary edema and a low forward cardiac output. These physiologic differences are reflected in the different clinical presentations and physical examination findings of acute versus chronic regurgitation (see Table 12–2).

CLINICAL PRESENTATION

Clinical History

Many patients with aortic regurgitation are diagnosed before symptom onset on the basis of finding a diastolic murmur on physical examination or an enlarged cardiac silhouette on chest radiography. After the initial diagnosis of significant aortic regurgitation, patients may remain asymptomatic for many years.

The most common initial symptom in patients with chronic aortic regurgitation is exertional dyspnea, most likely due to an elevated left ventricular end-diastolic pressure with exercise.[20] Angina may occur, even without atherosclerotic coronary artery disease, due to decreased myocardial perfusion pressure, increased myocardial oxygen demands, and a decreased ratio of coronary artery size to myocardial mass. Patients also may present with symptoms of heart failure, including dyspnea at rest, paroxysmal nocturnal dyspnea, and orthopnea. Syncope or sudden death, although rare, may occur in aortic regurgitation patients, even in the absence of prior symptoms. At least one study suggested that sudden death in previously asymptomatic patients is associated with marked left ventricular dilation.[6]

TABLE 12·2 CHRONIC COMPENSATED, DECOMPENSATED, AND ACUTE AORTIC REGURGITATION

Characteristic	Chronic Compensated	Decompensated	Acute
Etiology	Valvular or aortic root abnormalities		Dissection, endocarditis
Physiology			
LV volume	Increased (ESD < 55 mm)	Increased (ESD > 55 mm)	Normal
Ejection fraction	Normal (>55%)	Normal or decreased	Normal or decreased
LVEDP	Normal	Normal	Increased
Physical examination			
Diastolic murmur	High pitched, decrescendo, holodiastolic	High pitched, decrescendo, holodiastolic	Low pitched, harsh, early diastolic
Pulse pressure	Wide	Wide	Normal
LV impulse	Enlarged	Enlarged	Normal
Peripheral signs of AR	Present	Present	Absent
Clinical presentation	Asymptomatic	Gradual onset of symptoms, typically exertional	Sudden onset, pulmonary edema

AR, aortic regurgitation; ESD, end-systolic dimension; LV, left ventricular.

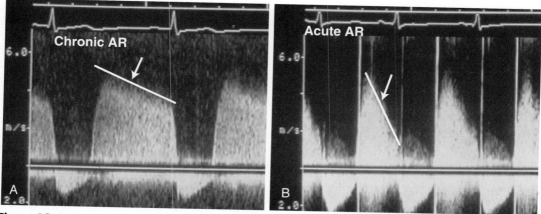

Figure 12·5 Continuous wave Doppler curves from a patient with chronic compensated aortic regurgitation (AR) due to a bicuspid aortic valve *(A)* and a patient with acute aortic regurgitation due to endocarditis *(B)*. Notice the steeper deceleration slope *(arrow)* in the acute case corresponding to the equalization of left ventricular and aortic pressures as shown in Figure 12–4. In addition, regurgitation is more severe in the acute case, as evidenced by the increased density of the diastolic signal relative to the antegrade velocity signal.

Chronic compensated aortic regurgitation has a slowly progressive course, so that a gradual decrease in exercise capacity may not be recognized as abnormal by the patient or family. Careful questioning is needed to elicit evidence of a subtle decrease in functional status. Some patients remain asymptomatic despite the onset of left ventricular systolic dysfunction, emphasizing the importance of periodic noninvasive diagnostic studies. Sudden symptom onset in a patient with chronic disease may be related to an acute increase in the severity of regurgitation, for example, due to infective endocarditis.

The possibility of aortic regurgitation should be considered in patients who have taken diet appetite suppressant medications, even in the absence of symptoms.[32a] Several studies support a relationship between appetite-suppressant medications and abnormal valvular regurgitation, especially of the aortic valve, but the magnitude of this risk remains unclear.[32a–d] Case control studies estimate odds ratio between 7.4 and 22.6, with some suggestion that risk is related to the dose and duration of therapy.[32b–c] In a randomized, placebo control trial of short duration therapy with dexfenfluramine, there was only a small increased risk of valvular regurgitation with most subjects having physiologic or mild aortic regurgitation.[32d] Currently, these drugs have been withdrawn from clinical use in the United States.

Physical Examination

On physical examination, patients with aortic regurgitation have a widened pulse pressure due to the increased forward systolic flow and retrograde diastolic flow in the ascending aorta. While the rate of diastolic pressure decline in the aorta, normalized for heart rate, correlates with regurgitant fraction, the pulse pressure itself is not a reliable predictor of hemodynamic severity.[33]

The carotid pulse typically is bounding, with a more rapid rate of pressure rise in early systole as well as an increase in the amplitude of the systolic pressure curve. There may be two palpable systolic impulses, often called a bisferiens pulse,[34] and a systolic thrill may be detected when regurgitation is severe.

The left ventricular apex typically is enlarged, hyperdynamic, and laterally displaced because of left ventricular dilation. An apical heave may be appreciated if significant left ventricular dilation is accompanied by systolic dysfunction.

The classic peripheral signs of aortic regurgitation are observed only with severe disease. The peripheral correlates of an increased pulse pressure include the "water-hammer" (Corrigan's) pulse,[35] systolic pulsations in the fingernail beds on gentle pressure (Quincke's pulse),[36] and synchronous movement of the patient's head with the arterial pulsation (head bob). Flow reversal in the descending aorta is recognized on physical examination as a systolic and diastolic bruit heard over the femoral arteries on gentle compression by the stethoscope (Duroziez's sign).

On auscultation, the first heart sound (S_1) most often is normal, but the aortic component of S_2 may be increased or decreased in intensity, depending on the cause of regurgitation. A loud aortic closure sound is associated with aortic root dilation, while a soft aortic component of S_2 occurs with abnormalities of the valve leaflets.[34] Ejection clicks are rare in adult patients but may be appreciated in a younger patient with a bicuspid aortic valve.

Classically, the murmur of aortic regurgitation is holodiastolic, high pitched, is loudest at the left sternal border, begins immediately after S_2, continues to S_1, and has a decrescendo intensity. Some experts suggest that aortic root disease is associated with selective radiation of the murmur to the right sternal border, whereas valve leaflet abnormalities are associated with radiation along the left sternal border.[34, 37] The murmur is best appreciated with the diaphragm of the stethoscope positioned at the lower left sternal border at held end-expiration with the patient sitting and leaning slightly forward. A systolic ejection-type murmur also may be heard, even in the absence of coexisting aortic stenosis, due to the high transaortic volume flow rate.

Compared with aortic angiography or Doppler echocardiography, physical examination often misses the murmur of aortic regurgitation; the reported sensitivity of auscultation for detection of aortic regurgitation is 37% to 73%, and the specificity is 85% to 92%.[38–40] The loudness of the murmur correlates with disease severity. In a series of 40 patients with chronic, isolated aortic regurgitation, a murmur grade of 3 or higher predicted severe regurgitation with a 71% accuracy, and a murmur grade of 1 or less predicted the absence of severe regurgitation with 100% accuracy.[41] However, the more common grade 2 murmur did not correlate with regurgitant severity.

Another classic finding in patients with severe, chronic aortic regurgitation is the Austin Flint murmur, a low-pitched mid-diastolic rumble that mimics the murmur of mitral stenosis.[42] Echocardiographic evaluation has shown no support for the theory that this murmur is associated with relative mitral stenosis caused by impingement of the aortic regurgitant jet on the anterior mitral leaflet, limiting the diastolic opening of the mitral valve. Instead, comparisons of Doppler echocardiographic with physical examination findings suggest that the diastolic rumble is related to the severity of aortic regurgitation,[43] with a jet directed toward the anterior mitral leaflet[44] or left ventricular free wall[45] causing the vibrations appreciated on auscultation as a low-pitched diastolic rumble.

The physical findings of acute aortic regurgitation differ from those of chronic regurgitation in parallel with the different hemodynamics of acute and chronic disease (see Table 12–2). Because of the acute hemodynamic deterioration, patients with acute regurgitation often are tachycardic and tachypneic and have pulmonary edema. However, the pulse pressure is narrow, so that carotid and peripheral pulse contours are not increased, and peripheral signs of aortic regurgitation are absent. While the precordium may appear hyperdynamic, the left ventricular apical impulse typically is not displaced or enlarged, as left ventricular dilation is absent. Although a diastolic murmur usually is present, the acoustic quality may lead to confusion unless the low-pitched, harsh, early diastolic murmur is recognized as aortic regurgitation. An accompanying systolic ejection murmur often leads to a "to and fro" sound of blood flow antegrade and retrograde across the aortic valve, with similar acoustic qualities of the antegrade and retrograde murmurs.

Electrocardiography and Chest Radiography

The electrocardiographic (ECG) findings in patients with aortic regurgitation include voltage criteria for left ventricular hypertrophy and associated repolarization abnormalities (ie, a "strain" pattern). A strain pattern on the resting ECG correlates strongly with abnormal left ventricular dimensions, mass, and wall stress.[46–48] A decrease in ECG voltage after aortic valve replacement is associated with regression of left ventricular hypertrophy.[49] However, some patients with severe aortic regurgitation and pathologic left ventricular hypertrophy do not meet ECG criteria for left ventricular hypertrophy.[50] When the resting ECG pattern is normal, with exercise flat, or downsloping, ST-segment depression may be seen even in the absence of coronary artery disease,[51] and is associated with an increased left ventricular systolic dimension.[47]

The chest radiograph shows an enlarged cardiac silhouette due to left ventricular dilation in chronic disease (Fig. 12–6). Aortic root dilation frequently is present, caused either by primary disease of the aorta or by dilation resulting from the increased aortic flow associated with the regurgitant lesion.[52] Since cardiac size on radiography and ECG evidence of left ventricular hypertrophy reflect the extent of left ventricular dilation, both parameters are predictors of outcome after valve replacement.[53–57] However, neither electrocardiography nor chest radiography offer sufficiently precise or accurate data for clinical decision making or sequential follow-up evaluation of patients with aortic regurgitation.

Echocardiography

Echocardiography provides reliable evaluation of aortic valve and root anatomy and allows identification of the mechanism of regurgitation in most cases. The specific cause of disease may be inferred when there are pathognomonic anatomic features (eg, bicuspid valve, Marfan's syndrome) (Figs. 12–7 and 12–8; see also Fig. 12–6).

Doppler and two-dimensional (2D) echocardiographic methods allow semiquantitative and quantitative evaluation of the severity of regurgitation (see Chapter 3). Although Doppler echocardiographic or angiographic evidence of severe regurgitation has been used as entry criteria for inclusion in most clinical series, no studies have correlated quantitative measures of regurgitant severity with disease progression or clinical outcome. Even so,

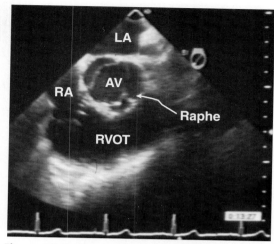

Figure 12·7 Transesophageal echocardiographic view of a bicuspid aortic valve (AV) in systole. Notice the raphe *(arrow)* in the anterior cusp. LA, left atrium; RA, right atrium; RVOT, right ventricular outflow tract.

echocardiographic evaluation of valve anatomy and regurgitant severity is key in deciding which patients have disease that merits further evaluation and may require medical or surgical intervention (Figs. 12–9 and 12–10; see also Fig. 12–8 and color insert).

Echocardiography also provides precise and reproducible measures of left ventricular dimensions, volumes, and systolic performance, which form the cornerstone for clinical decision making and follow-up evaluation of patients with chronic aortic regurgitation. Serial echocardiographic evaluation of ventricular size and function should take into account the potential confounding factors of interval changes in instrumentation, variability in recording and measuring the data, interim changes in loading condition, and physiologic variability (eg, changes in heart rate). One study estimated the 95% confidence limits that an apparent interval change represents in actual anatomic change as ±8 mm for ventricular dimensions and ±12% for fractional shortening.[58] Reliability is increased when the previous and current examinations are reviewed side by side and when a consistent directional change is seen on sequential examinations. When a change is detected, it often is prudent to repeat the examination after a shorter interval to confirm the magnitude and direction of the change.

Exercise Testing

Although patients with chronic aortic regurgitation have little exercise limitations until

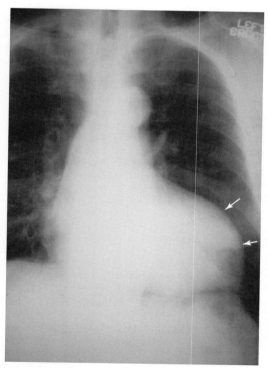

Figure 12·6 The chest radiograph of a patient with chronic compensated aortic regurgitation shows left ventricular enlargement *(arrows)* but no evidence of pulmonary congestion.

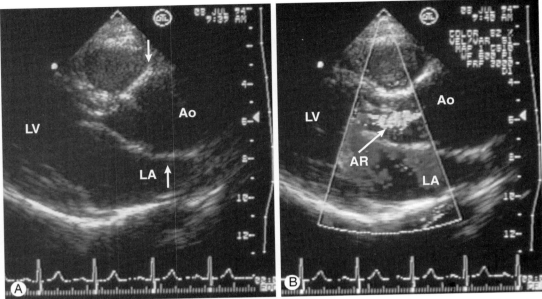

Figure 12·8 *A,* Parasternal, long-axis, two-dimensional echocardiographic image shows aortic root dilation in a patient with Marfan's syndrome with characteristic loss of the normal contour of the sinotubular junction *(arrows). B,* Central aortic regurgitation (AR), identified by color flow imaging, is caused by inadequate central coaptation of the stretched leaflets. Ao, aorta, LV, left ventricle; LA, left atrium. (See color plate.)

late in the disease course, several groups of investigators have suggested that exercise testing, with or without concurrent imaging, may help identify patients with early left ventricular systolic dysfunction.[59–65] On exercise electrocardiography, the finding of at least 0.1 mV of ST-segment depression is associated with a lower resting and exercise ejection fraction, a higher wall stress, and a greater end-systolic dimension compared with those with no ST-segment changes with exercise.[48, 59] Reduced maximal oxygen consumption and a reduced aerobic threshold also predict moderate to severe left ventricular dysfunction, suggesting

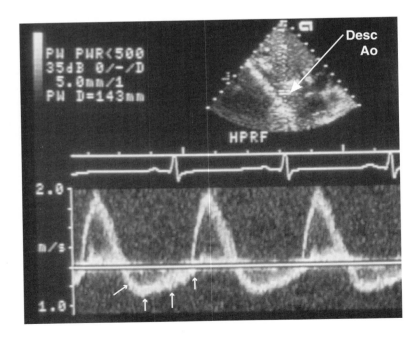

Figure 12·9 Holodiastolic flow reversal *(arrows)* in the proximal abdominal aorta in a patient with severe aortic regurgitation. Desc Ao, descending aorta.

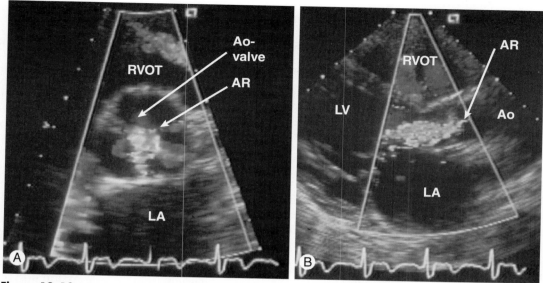

Figure 12·10 Parasternal short-axis *(A)* and long-axis *(B)* color flow images show aortic regurgitation (AR) in a patient with rheumatic valve disease. In short axis, the regurgitant jet is relatively small compared with the outflow tract, with the jet originating centrally and between the noncoronary and left coronary cusps of the aortic valve. In long axis, the narrow origin of the jet *(arrow)* can be appreciated even though the jet broadens as it extends into the left ventricular chamber. Ao, aorta; LA, left atrium; LV, left ventricle; RVOT, right ventricular outflow tract. (These illustrations also occur in the color insert section.)

that cardiopulmonary stress testing may be a useful adjunct for some patients.[60, 61]

Both echocardiography and radionuclide angiography can be used to measure the incremental change in ventricular dimensions and ejection fraction with exercise in patients with aortic regurgitation,[62, 63] but radionuclide measurements have been used most often in the clinical setting. Even though Doppler and echocardiographic measures have been used successfully by several centers,[20, 64] both depend on operator experience and show wide interobserver variability, particularly with exercise.[65] The intertest variability of radionuclide ejection fractions in patients with aortic regurgitation is relatively low, with a coefficient of variation of 5% to 10%.[66] This degree of variability should be taken into account in assessing the significance of an apparent change in ejection fraction in an individual patient. Several studies indicate that a rise in ejection fraction with exercise of at least 5 ejection fraction units correlates with preserved left ventricular systolic function and that a decrease or rise of less than 5 units indicates an elevated end-systolic wall stress, increased end-systolic dimension, and impaired systolic function.[19–21, 23, 24]

The role of exercise testing must be individualized for each patient with chronic aortic regurgitation. Resting echocardiographic or ra-

dionuclide measures of left ventricular size and systolic function are widely available, accurate, and predictive of clinical outcome, so that exercise testing adds little incremental data of value for clinical decision making.[6, 64, 67] Exercise testing may be helpful when there is a discrepancy between the clinical presentation and the resting echocardiographic findings, when echocardiographic data are nondiagnostic, and when indications for surgical intervention in an asymptomatic patient are borderline.

Other Imaging Modalities

Alternate imaging procedures for evaluation of valve anatomy and function include cardiac catheterization with measurement of intracardiac pressures, aortic root angiography, and calculation of regurgitant fraction (see Chapter 4). Although most patients can be managed based on noninvasive data alone, cardiac catheterization may be needed in some cases. For patients undergoing surgical intervention for aortic regurgitation, preoperative assessment of coronary anatomy may be needed, depending on the patient's age, gender, and other risk factors for coronary artery disease.

Velocity-coded cine magnetic resonance imaging provides a direct measurement of antegrade and retrograde flow across the aortic valve, and this method has been used to evaluate changes in regurgitant fraction and assess the forward and regurgitant stroke volumes in patients treated with angiotensin-converting enzyme inhibitors.[68] However, the specialized approaches to image processing needed to produce these magnetic resonance images are not widely available.

NATURAL HISTORY
Mild Aortic Regurgitation

Mild degrees of aortic regurgitation can be detected noninvasively by echocardiography, often on a study requested for unrelated clinical indications. The natural history of mild aortic regurgitation is unknown, but it is likely that most of these patients do not develop progressively more severe regurgitation. Careful evaluation of valve anatomy and consideration of the probable cause of regurgitation allows the physician to determine whether follow-up studies are needed and the appropriate frequency of evaluation. For example, mild aortic regurgitation in an elderly patient with a history of hypertension is unlikely to require further evaluation. Conversely, a young patient with mild insufficiency of a congenitally bicuspid valve requires close follow-up evaluation because progression to more severe regurgitation or stenosis is likely. It has been postulated that decreased aortic distensibility with age contributes to progressive aortic regurgitation due to the increase in left ventricular afterload.[69]

Moderate to Severe Aortic Regurgitation

Even with moderate or severe aortic regurgitation, many patients remain asymptomatic with no evidence of left ventricular dysfunction over a long time period.[70] A prospective study of the natural history of asymptomatic chronic severe aortic regurgitation and normal left ventricular function included 50 patients followed for a median of 44 months.[71] Entry criteria for this study were clinical evidence of aortic regurgitation, an end-diastolic volume of at least 100 mL/m², an ejection fraction of 50% or higher, and a stable clinical course. In this patient group, the rate of onset of significant symptoms or left ventricular dysfunction was only 4% ± 3% per year. Predictors of disease progression were left ventricular size (end-systolic volume index ≥60 mL/m², end-diastolic volume index ≥150 mL/m²), left ventricular systolic function (exercise ejection fraction <50%), and end-systolic wall stress (≥86 dynes/cm²). Of these measures, end-systolic size is most easily measured and depends least on loading conditions.

In another prospective study, 104 asymptomatic patients with chronic severe aortic regurgitation and normal left ventricular function were followed for an average of 8 years.[6] Of these 104 patients, 19 underwent valve replacement for symptom onset, 4 developed asymptomatic left ventricular systolic dysfunction, and 2 died suddenly (Figs. 12–11 and 12–12). The overall event rate was 5% per year (similar to the previous study), with a Kaplan Meier event-free survival at 11 years of 58% ±

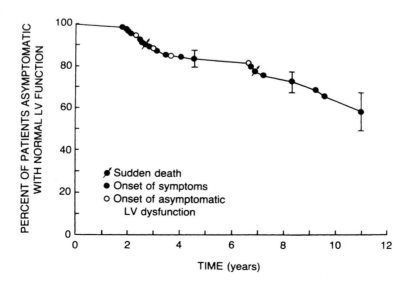

Figure 12·11 Life table depicting the clinical course of 104 initially asymptomatic patients with severe aortic regurgitation. At 11 years, 58.9% of the patients were alive and asymptomatic with normal left ventricular (LV) systolic function. Brackets indicate 1 SE. (From Bonow RO, Lakatos E, Maron BJ, Epstein SE: Serial long-term assessment of the natural history of asymptomatic patients with chronic aortic regurgitation and normal left ventricular systolic function. Circulation 1991;84:1628; by permission of The American Heart Association, Inc.)

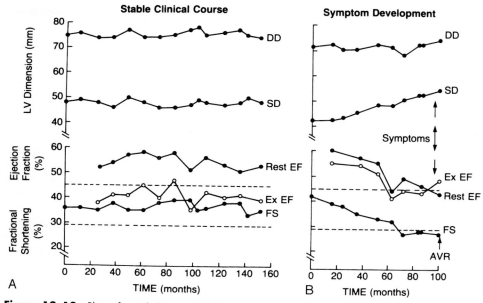

Figure 12·12 Plots of serial changes in left ventricular (LV) function in two patients. In each patient, the end-diastolic (DD) and end-systolic (SD) dimensions *(top)*, the fractional shortening (FS, *bottom*), and radionuclide angiographic ejection fraction (EF, *middle*) are plotted serially as functions of time. The exercise (Ex) ejection fraction data are shown as open circles. Dashed lines at 45% and 29% indicate the lower limit of normal for resting ejection fraction and fractional shortening, respectively. *A,* Despite ventricular dilation, this patient remained asymptomatic, with a normal resting ejection fraction and fractional shortening, for more than 12 years. *B,* This initially asymptomatic patient, who developed symptoms *(arrows)* and underwent an operation after 8 years, manifested consistent and progressive, although gradual, increases in the end-systolic dimension and decreases in the ejection fraction and fractional shortening preceding the development of symptoms. (From Bonow RO, Lakatos E, Maron BJ, Epstein SE. Serial long-term assessment of the natural history of asymptomatic patients with chronic aortic regurgitation and normal left ventricular systolic function. Circulation 1991;84:1630; by permission of The American Heart Association, Inc.)

9%. On multivariate Cox analysis, outcome was predicted by age, the initial and rate of change over time in echocardiographic end-systolic dimension, and the rate of change in the resting radionuclide ejection fraction. Other variables that were significant predictors of outcome on univariate analysis (ie, diastolic dimension, fractional shortening, and exercise ejection fraction) did not enter into the multivariate model. Risk stratification based on systolic dimension at entry showed that the likelihood of death, symptoms, or ventricular dysfunction was 19% per year for an end-systolic dimension larger than 50 mm, 6% per year for a dimension of 40 to 49 mm, and 0% per year for a dimension smaller than 40 mm. Sudden death, which occurred in two young asymptomatic men, was associated with excessive ventricular dilation (end-systolic dimension >55 mm, end-diastolic dimension >80 mm).

In another study[71a] of 104 asymptomatic patients with aortic regurgitation followed for 7.4

± 3.7 years, 28 (72%) developed symptoms warranting valve replacement, 7 (18%) developed asymptomatic excessive left ventricular dilation, and 4 (10%) experienced sudden death. The overall rate of endpoints of 6.2% per year is remarkably similar to that observed in earlier studies. In this study,[71a] the strongest multivariate predictor of clinical outcome was the change in left ventricular ejection fraction from rest to exercise, normalized for the exercise change in end-systolic wall stress. The major impediment to use of this approach in the clinical setting is that measurement of ejection fraction and end-systolic wall stress at rest and after exercise is cumbersome, requiring both radionuclide and echocardiographic data acquisition, in addition to exercise stress testing.

Although these studies used radionuclide measurements of ventricular volumes and ejection fraction[71] or M-mode echocardiography,[6] most clinicians now use 2D echocardiography in the initial and serial evaluation of patients with chronic aortic regurgitation. Clearly, 2D echocardiographic measures of ventricular volumes and ejection fraction are more reliable than M-mode data and are at least equivalent to radionuclide measures. Thus, it is reasonable to extrapolate these findings to 2D echocardiographic measurements and, in the future, to values measured on three-dimensional (3D) echocardiography.

Few studies have evaluated the rate of hemodynamic progression of aortic regurgitation in adults. In a study of 127 patients with aortic regurgitation and at least two echocardiographic studies, the severity of regurgitation increased in 30% of patients, mostly in those with baseline moderate to severe regurgitation. In addition, progressive left ventricular dilation was observed, with the greatest increases in left ventricular volume and mass seen in those with severe aortic regurgitation.[72]

Aortic Root Disease

For patients with aortic regurgitation secondary to enlargement of the aortic root, the natural history of the disease and thus the timing and choice of surgical intervention more often is based on the degree and rate of root dilation rather than the left ventricular response to chronic aortic regurgitation.[73]

A group of patients of particular concern are those with Marfan's syndrome.[74] Although this autosomal dominant inherited disease affects several organ systems through a defect in the gene encoding fibrillin (a major component of microtubules), aortic root aneurysmal dilation and dissection are the major cause of morbidity and mortality.[75–77] Echocardiographic evaluation is central to diagnosis of persons with Marfan's syndrome with the characteristic findings including dilation of the aortic root and ascending aorta, with loss of the normal tapering at the sinotubular junction. Aortic regurgitation results from incomplete central coaptation of the stretched leaflets due to annular dilation. The anterior mitral valve leaflet is elongated and redundant, often prolapsing into the left atrium in systole with some degree of mitral regurgitation.[78]

Periodic echocardiographic evaluation is critical for following the disease course and determining the appropriate timing of surgical intervention.[79, 80] The differing manifestations among individuals with Marfan's syndrome most likely are due to the different genetic alterations underlying this disease.[81] However, until a molecular approach is available that can identify patients at high risk, clinical and echocardiographic variables remain the most important prognostic indicators. Clinical risk factors for aortic dissection in Marfan's syndrome include a family history of cardiovascular events, generalized aortic root dilation, and most importantly, the degree of aortic root dilation.[80, 82, 83] Of note, the degree of root dilation is *not* primarily a function of age;[80, 84] some young patients have severe root dilation, while other patients have a stable root size for many years. Although previous recommendations have suggested that an aortic root dimension of more than 55 mm is an indication for surgical intervention,[85, 86] more recent data suggest that earlier surgical intervention might be warranted.[80, 87]

The rate of progression of aortic root dilation in Marfan's patients is variable, averaging 1.9 mm/year in one study[84] and averaging 0.7 ± 1 mm/year in those without a clinical end point and 5 ± 6 mm/year in those with an aortic complication in another study.[80] Because Marfan's patients typically are growing during the observation period, it is helpful to compare the patient's aortic root dimension to the expected dimension based on age and body surface area (BSA):[88]

Children (<18 years):
  Predicted sinus dimension (cm) =
  $1.02 + (0.98 \times BSA \ [m^2])$
Adults (18 to 40 years):
  Predicted sinus dimension (cm) =
  $0.97 + (1.12 \times BSA \ [m^2])$
Adults (>40 years):
  Predicted sinus dimension (cm) =
  $1.92 + (0.74 \times BSA \ [m^2])$
Aortic root ratio = Actual sinus dimension/Predicted sinus dimension

In a series of 89 consecutive Marfan's patients followed for a mean of 4 years, 5 patients died of aortic dissection, 4 patients survived surgery for ascending dissection, and 9 underwent root replacement for an ascending aneurysm, giving an actuarial event-free survival rate of 76% at 5 years. Using normalized aortic root dimensions, a low-risk subgroup could be defined as those with an aortic root ratio less than 1.3 and an annual change in the root ratio less than 5% (Figs. 12–13 and 12–14).[80] Although the decision to recommend prophylactic aortic root and valve replacement remains difficult and must be individualized, these data prompt consideration of intervention when progressive dilation occurs and di-

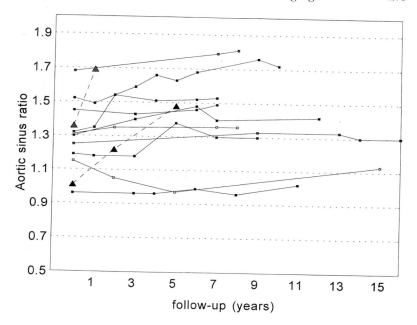

Figure 12·13 Examples of the rate of change in aortic sinus ratio over the follow-up period. In these 12 patients with Marfan's syndrome, two underwent surgery for ascending aortic aneurysm and increasing aortic regurgitation (Δ—) while the remaining 10 had no aortic complications (—). (From Legget ME, Unger TA, O'Sullivan CK, et al: Aortic root complications in Marfan's syndrome: identification of a lower risk group. Heart 1996;75:389–395. BMJ Publishing Group.)

mensions greatly exceed the expected values for body size.

MEDICAL THERAPY

After a patient has been diagnosed with significant aortic regurgitation, medical management is directed at slowing disease progression, identifying the optimal timing of surgical intervention, and preventing complications of the disease.

Noninvasive Follow-up

Since some patients with chronic asymptomatic aortic regurgitation develop irreversible left ventricular dysfunction without clinical symptoms, periodic noninvasive evaluation is central to optimal management. Most clinicians use 2D echocardiography with measurement of ventricular end-systolic and end-diastolic dimensions and volumes, with calculation of ejection fraction by the apical biplane method.

Based on the Doppler echocardiographic estimate of regurgitant severity and the degree of left ventricular dilation at the initial examination, the timing of follow-up can be tailored to each patient. A mild degree of regurgitation with normal ventricular dimensions does not warrant frequent examination and may require no further evaluation. However, this judgment must be tempered by consideration of the underlying cause of the valvular lesion

as deduced from the echocardiographic images and other clinical data. If the patient has a disease likely to progress (eg, Marfan's syndrome, bicuspid valve), leading to increasing degrees of valvular incompetence, periodic follow-up at intervals based on the natural history of the underlying disease process is appropriate. Any change in the patient's cardiac symptoms or signs also prompts repeat evaluation.

For the patient with moderate to severe regurgitation on Doppler echocardiography and mild ventricular dilation, annual echocardiographic evaluation is appropriate so long as cardiac dimensions and left ventricular function remain stable. When an interim change in ventricular dimensions or a decrease in systolic function is found, repeat examination at a shorter follow-up interval (3 to 6 months) is helpful in differentiating progressive disease from measurement variability.

Patients with moderate to severe regurgitation and evidence of left ventricular dilation that is significant but not severe enough to warrant immediate surgical intervention require more intense follow-up. These patients may have an enlarged but stable ventricular size or may have rapidly progressive disease. A second evaluation at 3 to 6 months can reassure the stable patient and allows prompt intervention in the patient with progressive ventricular dilation. The timing of subsequent examinations is based on the interval change observed between the initial two studies.

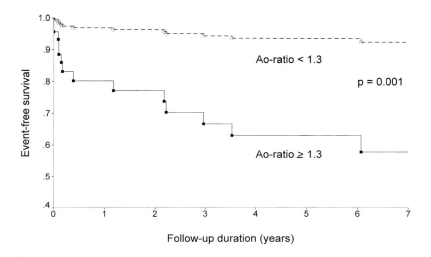

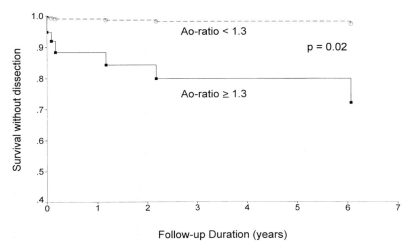

Figure 12·14 Cox proportional hazards model shows event-free survival *(top)* and survival without ascending aortic dissection *(bottom)* for 89 patients with Marfan's syndrome and an initial aortic sinus (Ao) ratio of less than 1.3 compared with those with a ratio 1.3 or higher. (From Legget ME, Unger TA, O'Sullivan CK, et al: Aortic root complications in Marfan's syndrome: identification of a lower risk group. Heart 1996;75: 393. BMJ Publishing Group.)

Although echocardiography is well suited for periodic evaluation of the patient with chronic aortic regurgitation, some clinicians prefer radionuclide measurements of ventricular volumes and ejection fraction. In selected cases, periodic evaluation of the exercise ejection fraction by using echocardiographic or radionuclide techniques may be helpful. Magnetic resonance imaging and computed tomography also can provide quantitative measures of ventricular size and (using cine techniques) function, but they are more expensive and less practical for clinical applications. As quantitative 3D echocardiography becomes more feasible and available, more accurate measures of ventricular size and function should become possible.

Prevention of Endocarditis

Endocarditis often affects a previously abnormal valve; persons with aortic regurgitation

are at particularly high risk for endocarditis. Approximately one third of all cases of aortic valve endocarditis involve a bicuspid valve (see Chapter 18). Given the continued high morbidity and mortality of infective endocarditis, even with aggressive medical and surgical therapy, it is important to take preventative measures when appropriate. Patients with aortic regurgitation should be instructed about the importance of good oral hygiene and regular dental cleanings and examinations. In addition, antibiotic therapy for prevention of endocarditis (see Table 6–6) is needed for (1) an audible aortic regurgitation murmur on cardiac auscultation, (2) a grade 2+ or higher regurgitation by Doppler criteria, (3) a bicuspid valve with any degree of aortic regurgitation, or (4) rheumatic valvular disease.

However, studies of the risk for endocarditis of patients with aortic regurgitation did not include the trivial amounts of regurgitation detectable by echocardiography. Therefore, the decision to recommend endocarditis prophylaxis must be individualized when the patient has only a minor degree of regurgitation. For example, a common clinical scenario is the elderly patient with minimal regurgitation, mild valve sclerosis, and mild root dilation. Whether these patients benefit from antibiotic therapy to prevent endocarditis is unknown. Thus, there are no absolute guidelines for antibiotic prophylaxis in this situation.

Afterload Reduction

Based on the concept that increased afterload is one of the primary pathophysiologic abnormalities in aortic regurgitation, there has long been interest in the potential benefit of pharmacologic afterload reduction therapy. In theory, afterload reduction might decrease end-systolic wall stress by a reduction in left ventricular systolic pressure and might decrease regurgitant fraction by a reduction in the driving pressure retrograde across the valve in diastole. These reductions in wall stress and regurgitant fraction then would decrease the pressure and volume overload of the left ventricle, preventing progressive left ventricular dilation or systolic dysfunction. Studies on the acute hemodynamic effects of nitroprusside (as an afterload reducing agent) in aortic regurgitation show that, although forward stroke volume is unchanged, systemic vascular resistance decreases, end-diastolic and end-systolic ventricular volumes decrease, ejection fraction increases, and regurgitant fraction decreases.[89–96]

Several studies have evaluated the long-term effects of afterload reduction therapy on left ventricular size and function (Table 12–3), including the use of hydralazine,[97–102] angiotensin-converting enzyme inhibitors,[101, 103–105] and nifedipine.[106] Although the study sizes are small, several different agents have been chosen for afterload reduction, and the reference standard has varied, these studies provide convincing evidence that afterload reduction therapy decreases the extent of left ventricular dilation and hypertrophy and prevents a decrease in ejection fraction.

Further, in a larger (143 patients), randomized trial of nifedipine versus digoxin in asymptomatic patients with chronic severe aortic regurgitation, vasodilator therapy reduced the rate of symptom onset and left ventricular dysfunction and was associated with a reduced rate of referral for aortic valve surgery (Fig. 12–15).[13] Severe aortic regurgitation in this study was defined based on the color Doppler jet width relative to the outflow tract diameter. At study entry, all these patients had left ventricular dilation with an end-diastolic volume index greater than 1.5 SD above the normal mean, and all had an ejection fraction of more than 50%. By actuarial analysis, 34% ± 6% of those receiving digoxin had undergone valve replacement by 6 years, compared with 15% ± 3% of those receiving nifedipine (P < .001). Note that the annual rate of valve replacement in the reference group was similar to that observed in the earlier natural history studies.[6, 71, 71a] The indications for aortic valve surgery were symptoms in 5 of 26 (19%, all in the digoxin group), and left ventricular systolic dysfunction in the remaining 21 of 26 (81%). The predetermined definition of left ventricular dysfunction was an ejection fraction less than 50% or an increase in the left ventricular end-diastolic volume index by at least 15%, with reconfirmation of the initial findings on repeat echocardiography within 1 month. The perioperative mortality rate was 4%, and left ventricular systolic function (mean preoperative ejection fraction of 48% ± 6%) improved in all subjects after valve replacement (mean postoperative ejection fraction of 58% ± 9%).

Given these data, afterload reduction therapy is appropriate in the patient with chronic severe aortic regurgitation to prevent progressive increases in left ventricular size and mass and to delay the onset of symptoms or left ventricular dysfunction. The choice of pharmacologic agent, nifedipine or an angiotensin-converting enzyme inhibitor, depends on comorbid conditions (eg, coronary artery disease) as well as patient tolerance. Periodic echocardiographic monitoring continues during medical therapy as these patients remain at risk for the eventual onset of left ventricular systolic dysfunction, albeit with a lower likelihood than those not on afterload reduction therapy.

Primary Aortic Root Disease With Secondary Aortic Regurgitation

Management of the patient with aortic regurgitation due to aortic root disease differs somewhat from that for the patient with a primary leaflet abnormality. First, the timing of surgical intervention may depend more on the rate and extent of root dilation rather than on the left ventricular response to chronic

TABLE 12•3 EFFECT OF AFTERLOAD REDUCTION THERAPY FOR CHRONIC, ASYMPTOMATIC AORTIC REGURGITATION

Study	Patients	Study Design	Follow-up	Treatment Groups	LV EDV (mL/m²)	Mean Wall Stress (kdyne/cm²)	LV ESV (mL/m²)	EF (%)	LV Mass Index (g/m²)
Scognamiglio, 1990[106]	72	Randomized, double-blind	1 y	Nifedipine	110 ± 19	360 ± 27		72 ± 8	115 ± 19
				Placebo	113 ± 22	479 ± 26		60 ± 6	142 ± 16
				P value	<.01	<.001		<.05	<.01
Schon, 1994[104]	12	Baseline values compared with values after 1 y of Rx	1 y	Quinapril	128 ± 30		44 ± 28	67 ± 11	
				Baseline	150 ± 33		55 ± 27	64 ± 11	
				P value	.0001		.005	NS	
Lin, 1994[101]	76	Randomized, double-blind	1 y	Enalapril	108 ± 17		45 ± 14		113 ± 19
				Hydralazine	124 ± 15		50 ± 12		131 ± 16
				P value	<.01		<.01		<.01

EDV, end-diastolic volume; ESV, end-systolic volume; EF, ejection fraction; LV, left ventricular; Rx, treatment.

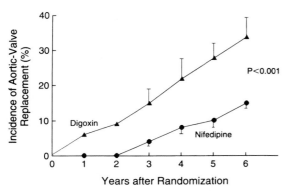

Figure 12·15 Cumulative actuarial incidence of progression to aortic valve replacement for 143 initially asymptomatic patients with severe aortic regurgitation randomized to treatment with 0.25 mg of digoxin daily or 20 mg of nifedipine twice each day. (From Scognamiglio R, Rahimtoola SH, Fasoli G, Nistri S, Dalla Volta S: Nifedipine in asymptomatic patients with severe aortic regurgitation and normal left ventricular function. N Engl J Med 1994;331:691; copyright 1994, Massachusetts Medical Society. All rights reserved.)

pressure or volume overload. For example, patients with Marfan's syndrome with a measured aortic root dimension greater than 1.3 times that expected for age and body size have a higher likelihood of an adverse clinical event than those with lesser degrees of root dilation.[80]

Second, optimal medical therapy may differ based on the pathophysiology of the disease processes. For a patient with Marfan's syndrome, β-blocker therapy may be preferred over afterload reduction, because β-blocker therapy decreases the stress on the aortic wall through a reduction in blood pressure and, more importantly, a reduction in the rate of rise of pressure (dP/dt) in systole.[79]

Management of Acute Aortic Regurgitation

Acute aortic regurgitation leads to rapid hemodynamic deterioration as the sudden increase in left ventricular filling retrograde across the aortic valve in diastole results in a markedly elevated end-diastolic pressure and acute pulmonary edema. These patients require emergency or urgent surgery for correction of the underlying disease process and relief of the acute hemodynamic load. While diagnostic evaluation is in progress to define the cause of the acute decompensation and to prepare for surgical intervention, the patient is treated with aggressive pharmacologic afterload reduction therapy. The use of intraaortic balloon counterpulsation is relatively

contraindicated due to the concern that balloon inflation in diastole may increase the volume of flow retrograde across the valve. In patients with acute aortic regurgitation due to infective endocarditis, prompt initiation of antibiotic therapy and valve replacement may be lifesaving.[31] In patients with acute aortic regurgitation due to an ascending aortic dissection, prompt pharmacologic therapy and surgical intervention are needed.

TIMING AND CHOICE OF SURGICAL INTERVENTION

The optimal timing of surgical intervention in the patient with chronic aortic regurgitation remains controversial. Clearly, surgical intervention is appropriate in the patient with severe valvular disease and significant symptoms or functional limitation that is attributable to the valvular pathology. In the asymptomatic patient, the risks of surgery, the expected hemodynamics after surgical intervention, the longevity of the prosthetic valve or surgical repair, and the risks of long-term anticoagulation (with a mechanical valve prosthesis) must be weighed against the risk of a poor outcome after surgery if intervention is delayed. The clinical challenge is to identify the time point *just before* the onset of irreversible left ventricular systolic dysfunction in the patient with chronic asymptomatic aortic regurgitation.

Predictors of Outcome After Surgery

Several groups of investigators have attempted to identify predictors of outcome and left ventricular function after aortic valve surgery for chronic regurgitation.[107–117] Although the number of subjects in any one study is small, the aggregate number is large (Table 12–4). Most of these studies included symptomatic patients who underwent valve replacement for severe aortic regurgitation.[108–117] Preoperative clinical variables were compared based on groups defined by postoperative ventricular function. Baseline predictors of postoperative left ventricular dysfunction included (1) increased left ventricular size at end-systole (defined as end-systolic dimension[108, 113] or end-systolic volume index[115, 116]), (2) the duration of left ventricular dysfunction,[110] (3) end-systolic wall stress,[115, 116] and (4) ejection fraction.[117] The predictors identified in these surgical studies of symptomatic patients have been extrapolated to clinical decision making

TABLE 12·4 TIMING OF VALVE REPLACEMENT IN CHRONIC AORTIC REGURGITATION

Study	Patients	Symptoms	Mean Age (Range)	Percent Male	Study Design*	Conclusions	LV Dysfunction at Entry
Henry, 1980[108]	49	Yes	46 (19–68)	82%	AVR	Preop ESD >55 mm and FS <25% were associated with poor outcome after AVR.	
Henry, 1980[118]	37	No	35 (17–64)	54%	Prospt	ESD and FS predicted which patients became symptomatic and required AVR.	
Bonow, 1983[119]	77	No	37 (16–67)		Prospt	AVR is not needed until symptoms or LV dysfunction occurs.	Normal LV systolic function in all.
Fioretti, 1983[109]	47	Yes	47 (22–75)	62%	AVR	Preop ESD ≥55 mm does not preclude AVR.	
Bonow, 1984[110]	37	Yes	41 (20–46)	89%	AVR	Duration of preop LV dysfunction is an important predictor of reversibility of LV function.	Entry criteria included FS <29%.
Daniel, 1985[111]	84	Yes	46 (18–71)	77%	AVR	Preop ESD >55 mm or FS <25% does not reliably predict outcome after AVR.	
Taniguchi, 1987[112]	62	Yes	43 (18–64)	77%	AVR	Preop LV-ES volume index was most important predictor of subsequent cardiac death.	
Carabello, 1987[113]	14	Yes	49 ± 6		AVR	Preop ESD correlated best with postop EF.	Entry criteria included EF <55%.
Bonow, 1988[114]	61	Yes	43 (19–72)	84%	AVR	Long-term improvement in LV function is related to early reduction in EDD postop.	
Siemienczuk, 1989[71]	50	No	48 ± 16		Prospt	Patients can be risk stratified for "early progression to AVR" based on measurement of LV size and function.	
Taniguchi, 1990[116]	35	Yes	43 (15–60)	86%	AVR	The postop increase in EF correlated with the decrease in ESS. Contractile dysfunction persisted.	

Bonow, 1991[6]	104	No	36 (17–67)	86%	Prospt	Multivariate predictors of outcome (death, ventricular dysfunction, or symptoms) were age, initial ESD and rate of change in ESD and rest EF.
Pirwitz, 1994[115]	27	Yes	(18–72)	78%	AVR	The peak systolic pressure to ESV ratio was the strongest predictor of postop functional class.
Klodas, 1996[117]	31	Yes	50 ± 15	100%	AVR	Preop EF (not EDD) predicted late survival and postop EF. Severe LV dilation is not a contraindication to surgery.

AVR, aortic valve replacement; AR, aortic regurgitation; FS, percent fractional shortening by echocardiography; ESD, end-systolic dimension; ESS, end-systolic stress; EDD, end-diastolic dimension; EF, ejection fraction; LV, left ventricular.

*Study design AVR: all patients underwent AVR, subgroups defined preoperative baseline variables, and outcome after AVR was compared. Study design Prospt: patients with chronic asymptomatic AR were followed prospectively for development of symptoms and onset of LV dysfunction. All studies included only patients with severe AR and excluded patients with coexisting cardiac conditions (eg, aortic stenosis, other valvular disease, coronary artery disease).

for the patient with asymptomatic disease (Figs. 12–16 and 12–17).

A smaller number of studies have followed asymptomatic patients with chronic aortic regurgitation prospectively to identify predictors of symptom onset or left ventricular dysfunction.[6, 71, 118, 119] These series established the principle that valve replacement is not needed until symptoms supervene or there is evidence of left ventricular systolic dysfunction.[119] In addition, the same factors that predict outcome after valve replacement in symptomatic patients were found to predict the onset of symptoms or left ventricular dysfunction in asymptomatic patients, specifically ventricular size and contractile function.[6, 71, 108] Further, the rate of change over time in measures of left ventricular size and function were found to predict clinical progression.[6]

Other predictors of outcome after valve replacement for aortic regurgitation include age,[54, 120] severity of symptoms,[121] exercise tolerance,[122, 123] evidence of left ventricular hypertrophy on electrocardiography,[56] an elevated left ventricular end-diastolic pressure,[54] and the ratio of wall thickness to chamber dimensions.[124, 125]

A recent study suggested that long-term outcome is worse for women than men after valve replacement for aortic regurgitation. Predictors of late mortality for women included age and the need for concurrent coronary artery bypass grafting surgery.[126] However, the women in this series had a very high preva-

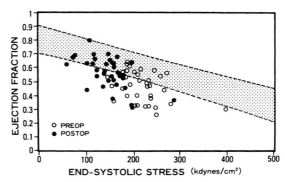

Figure 12·17 Relationship between ejection fraction and end-systolic wall stress before *(open circles)* and after *(solid circles)* aortic valve replacement in 35 patients with severe aortic regurgitation. (From Taniguchi K, Nakano S, Kawashima Y, et al: Left ventricular ejection performance, wall stress, and contractile state in aortic regurgitation before and after aortic valve replacement. Circulation 1990;82:802; by permission of The American Heart Association, Inc.)

lence (about 50%) of aortic aneurysm requiring aortic root replacement in addition to valve surgery. It also is noteworthy that many of the women had significant symptoms attributed to aortic regurgitation without excessive left ventricular dilation or evidence for systolic dysfunction, suggesting that the left ventricular dimension criteria developed for predominantly male subjects may not apply to women. Alternatively, diastolic dysfunction and concurrent coronary artery disease may play a role in the different clinical presentation of women with aortic regurgitation.[127]

Surgical Options, Mortality, and Postoperative Course

In addition to valve replacement with a mechanical or tissue prosthetic valve, several other surgical options are available for the patient with aortic regurgitation. In some cases, repair is possible, particularly with a congenital fenestration or an acquired perforation of the leaflet. With aortic root dilation and central regurgitation, the native valve may be preserved by resuspension of the valve in a prosthetic conduit (ie, David procedure).[128, 129] In younger patients, the pulmonic autograft procedure (ie, Ross procedure) offers excellent hemodynamics, the absence of anticoagulation, and reasonable durability when there is an appropriate size match between the aorta and pulmonary artery.[130, 131] Homograft valve replacement and stentless prosthetic tissue valves offer improved hemodynamics and du-

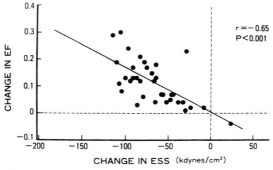

Figure 12·16 Plot of the relation between postoperative changes in ejection fraction (EF) and postoperative changes in end-systolic wall stress (ESS) in 35 patients undergoing aortic valve replacement for severe aortic regurgitation. The strong inverse correlation suggests that improvement in pump function mostly results from a long-term decrease in afterload. (From Taniguchi K, Nakano S, Kawashima Y, et al: Left ventricular ejection performance, wall stress, and contractile state in aortic regurgitation before and after aortic valve replacement. Circulation 1990;82:802; by permission of The American Heart Association, Inc.)

rability compared with conventional tissue valves (see Chapter 17).[132-135]

The operative mortality rate for elective aortic valve replacement in patients with chronic aortic regurgitation is 4% to 10%, with 5-year survival rates of 70% to 85% in recent series.[54, 112, 136-139] Operative mortality is similar in women and men.[126] Most patients experience a decrease in cardiac symptoms and an improved functional capacity postoperatively.[138, 140, 141] Predictors of operative mortality include severe symptoms, renal failure, and atrial fibrillation.[142]

If surgery is performed before the onset of irreversible left ventricular dysfunction, relief of the chronic volume overload leads to decreased ventricular volumes and mass.[78, 143-150] Ventricular volumes and myocardial mass decrease postoperatively by 30% to 35%, but this decrease occurs over a prolonged period. Ventricular volumes decrease to near-normal values within 1 to 2 years, but ventricular mass continues to decrease up to 8 years postoperatively.[144] Therefore, after valve replacement for aortic regurgitation, left ventricular geometry is characterized by concentric hypertrophy due to the differing rates of decrease in ventricular volumes and mass. The excess afterload imposed by the prosthetic valve may be an additional factor contributing to a persistent increase in left ventricular mass postoperatively. The early postoperative decrease in muscle mass reflects regression of myocardial cell hypertrophy and a decrease in myocardial fibrous content, with the later decrease in myocardial mass caused by a continued decrease in fibrous tissue content.[151]

When the left ventricular ejection fraction is abnormal preoperatively because of increased afterload with preserved contractile function, the decrease in afterload and wall stress still leads to an improvement in ejection performance postoperatively. However, when a reduced ejection fraction is caused by contractile dysfunction, impaired ventricular systolic function persists postoperatively.[108, 114, 124, 138] The ejection fraction also continues to improve over a long period postoperatively, reaching a stable value only after 4 to 6 years.[152]

Optimal Timing of Surgery

Several approaches have been proposed for defining the optimal timing of surgical intervention in the asymptomatic patient with aortic regurgitation. These approaches have been derived empirically based on outcome after surgery in symptomatic patients, from basic physiologic principles, or from decision-analysis models. Despite their different origins, all converge on the same basic parameters for clinical decision making.

Asymptomatic Aortic Regurgitation With Normal Left Ventricular Function

Data on the natural history of patients with asymptomatic aortic regurgitation and predictors of ventricular function postoperatively have been extrapolated to form guidelines for the optimal timing of intervention in adults with asymptomatic aortic regurgitation. The underlying assumption of this empirical approach is that intervention just before or soon after the onset of left ventricular systolic dysfunction will prevent irreversible changes in ventricular contractility. The difficulty with this approach is identifying the time point just before irreversible changes occur. This difficulty is compounded by the load dependence of standard measures of ventricular function and the altered loading conditions in patients with aortic regurgitation due to the regurgitant lesion itself.

Despite these potential limitations, it is clear that excessive ventricular dilation, particularly at end-systole, is a marker of incipient systolic dysfunction. When ventricular end-systolic dimension exceeds 55 mm or the end-systolic volume index exceeds 60 mL/m^2, surgical intervention should be considered.[14] Again, the importance of verifying accuracy of these measurements and repeating the study after some interval to confirm the degree and progression of dilation must be emphasized.

Other clinical markers indicating the need for surgery include overt evidence of systolic dysfunction (ejection fraction <50%),[153] diastolic ventricular dilation (end-diastolic dimension >80 mm),[108, 124] or an elevated end-diastolic pressure (>20 mm Hg).[54] More sophisticated load-independent parameters of ventricular function, including end-systolic wall stress and elastance, provide useful insights into the pathophysiology of the disease process but are not practical for routine clinical application.[7, 154]

Although most clinicians concur that surgical intervention is indicated even in the asymptomatic patient to prevent irreversible left ventricular dysfunction, no randomized trial has been conducted on the timing of surgical intervention for aortic regurgitation. Such a trial would be difficult logistically and financially

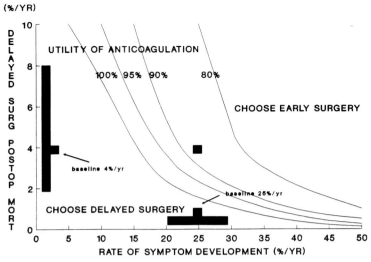

Figure 12·18   Decision analysis model for the timing of surgery for chronic aortic regurgitation. Three-way sensitivity analysis of the three important variables in the choice of surgery only at symptom onset (delayed surgery) is compared with surgery for asymptomatic left ventricular systolic dysfunction (early surgery) for a patient with chronic aortic regurgitation. To evaluate a decision with three-way sensitivity analysis, the derived probabilities for the rate of symptom development and delayed-surgery postoperative mortality are plotted along with threshold curves corresponding to the utility of anticoagulation. If the point of intersection lies above the threshold curve, early surgery is chosen. If it lies below it, delayed surgery is chosen. Baseline values are plotted. (From Biem HJ, Detsky AS, Armstrong PW: Management of asymptomatic chronic aortic regurgitation with left ventricular dysfunction: a decision analysis. J Gen Intern Med 1990;5:398.)

given the number of subjects needed to demonstrate a significant difference. Further, few clinicians would agree to randomize patients because of the strength of the published observational data.

The clinical decision-analysis model by Biem, Detsky, and Armstrong[155] of early and late interventions for chronic aortic regurgitation is of particular importance. In this decision-analysis model, *early surgery* is defined as valve replacement at the first sign of left ventricular dysfunction, and *late surgery* is defined as intervention after symptom onset. The criteria used for onset of left ventricular dysfunction in this model were an end-systolic dimension greater than 55 mm, a fractional shortening of less than 29%, or a fall in the ejection fraction on serial studies. These values were chosen to reflect the criteria most commonly cited in the previous literature. For a typical case of chronic aortic regurgitation, the rate of symptom development per year and the probabilities of mortality, nonfatal stroke, and congestive heart failure with early or late surgery were derived from published values. In addition, a quality of life measure was used

in the analysis. Using one-way sensitivity analysis for each major variable (ie, rate of symptom development, outcome after surgery, and quality of life) and using three-way sensitivity analysis (Fig. 12–18), this model convincingly demonstrates the value of early surgical intervention.

An algorithm for the timing of surgery in asymptomatic patients with aortic regurgitation has been proposed by Donovan and Starling,[156] using a point system that incorporates clinical variables, measures of left ventricular size and systolic function, and exercise capacity as shown in Table 12–5. This algorithm provides a useful guideline for making clinical decisions in patients with asymptomatic aortic regurgitation, although other clinical data may affect the final decision in a specific patient.

Surgical Intervention With Preexisting Left Ventricular Dysfunction

Evidence of left ventricular systolic dysfunction, manifested as excessive left ventricular dilation or a reduced ejection fraction, at the time of the initial diagnosis of aortic regurgita-

TABLE 12·5   PROPOSED ALGORITHM FOR THE TIMING OF SURGERY IN ASYMPTOMATIC PATIENTS WITH AORTIC REGURGITATION

Part A

Points	Clinical Factors*	Ejection Fraction (%)	End-Systolic Dimension (mm)	Exercise Capacity†
0	None	>60	<45	Preserved
1	1	50–60	45–55	
2	2 or more	<50	>55	Decreased

*Age >65, cardiothoracic ratio ≥ 0.58; left ventricular (LV) hypertrophy on electrocardiogram; cardiac index ≤2.5 L/m/m²; LV end-diastolic pressure >20 mm Hg.

†Preserved, ability to complete at least 8 METs on graded exercise treadmill testing or stable exercise performance; decreased, inability to complete 8 METs on graded exercise treadmill testing or a decline in exercise performance from an established baseline.

Part B

Total Points	Decision Regarding Surgical Intervention
0–1	Delay surgery; clinical and echocardiographic follow-up at 12 mo
2	Borderline; recommend clinical and echocardiographic follow-up at 6 mo
≥3	Proceed with surgery

Part C

Additional Predictors of Adverse Outcome in Aortic Regurgitation*

Percentage fractional shortening	<29%
End-systolic volume index	>60 mL/m²
End-systolic wall stress	>235 mm Hg
End-diastolic dimension	>80 mm
End-diastolic dimension (radius) (R)	≥3.2
End-diastolic wall thickness (T)	

*Add two points for each additional predictor present.

Algorithm for the timing of surgical intervention in aortic regurgitation:

(A) Assign a point score for each of the four designated categories.

(B) Based on the total point score, follow suggested guidelines regarding timing of surgery.

(C) Although not a requisite part of the algorithm, these additional predictors of adverse outcome can also be used in decision analysis.

From Donovan CL, Starling MR: Role of echocardiography in the timing of surgical intervention for chronic mitral and aortic regurgitation. *In* Otto CM, ed. The Practice of Clinical Echocardiography. Philadelphia: WB Saunders, 1997:349.

tion raises the concern that irreversible left ventricular contractile dysfunction might have already occurred, limiting the benefit and possibly increasing the risk of surgical intervention. However, since aortic regurgitation results in both pressure and volume overload of the left ventricle, the decrease in afterload following valve replacement is associated with an improvement in ventricular function in most patients. In one study, 20 patients with an end-systolic dimension of 55 mm or larger had the same operative mortality rate (0%) as the 27 patients with an end-systolic dimension of less than 55 mm. Further, left ventricular dimensions decreased substantially in both groups.[109] Another study of 31 patients with

chronic aortic regurgitation and a preoperative end-diastolic dimension of 80 mm or larger found a low operative mortality rate and improvement in the ejection fraction postoperatively (from 43% ± 12% to 53% ± 11%, P < .0001).[117]

The duration of left ventricular dysfunction has a significant impact on outcome; a greater increase in ejection fraction and decrease in ventricular dimensions are found in patients with "brief" (<14 months) than in those with "prolonged" (>18 months) or an unknown duration of left ventricular dysfunction.[110] In this study, even those with prolonged left ventricular dysfunction had a decrease in ventricular dimensions postoperatively, and only 2 of

11 (18%) had reductions in ejection fraction; the remainder showed no change or improvement. Persistent postoperative left ventricular dilation (>60 mm) was associated with an increased risk of death (4 of 7 [57%]), most often from heart failure.

Taken together, these data suggest that, although the overall benefit of surgical intervention is greatest when performed before the onset of ventricular dysfunction, surgery still is beneficial for most patients with chronic aortic regurgitation and evidence of systolic dysfunction. Of course, clinical decision making includes evaluation of comorbid cardiac and noncardiac diseases. The risk of the surgical procedure must be weighed against the potential benefit for each patient.

Special Considerations for the Patient With Aortic Root Dilation

Surgical intervention in the patient with aortic root dilation and aortic regurgitation typically includes replacement of the ascending aorta with a valved prosthetic conduit or a homograft valve and ascending aorta. If the cause of aortic regurgitation is annular dilation with normal valve leaflets, it may be possible to preserve the native aortic valve by resuspension of the leaflets in a prosthetic graft.

In patients with Marfan's syndrome, standard surgical management includes a composite valve and graft with reimplantation of the coronary arteries.[157-159] This procedure, known as the Bentall technique,[160] has become standard because of dilation and rupture of the residual aortic sinus tissue in Marfan patients treated with separate valve and root procedures in the past. Some surgeons are proposing valve-sparing operations in Marfan's patients,[161] but the long-term outcome of the aortic valve tissue is these patients is unknown.

Although the initial surgical procedure in patients with Marfan's syndrome most often is ascending aortic graft for dissection or aneurysm, 53% also require subsequent surgical intervention at other aortic sites with aggressive surgical management needed to correct these abnormalities.[157, 158] Predictors of the need for a second intervention are the presence of dissection at the first surgical procedure, hypertension, and a history of smoking.[159]

References

1. Borow KM, Marcus RH: Aortic regurgitation: the need for an integrated physiologic approach [editorial]. J Am Coll Cardiol 1991;17:898–900.
2. Carabello BA: Aortic regurgitation. A lesion with similarities to both aortic stenosis and mitral regurgitation. Circulation 1990;82:1051–1053.
3. Ross J Jr: Afterload mismatch in aortic and mitral valve disease: implications for surgical therapy. J Am Coll Cardiol 1985;5:811–826.
4. Borow KM: Surgical outcome in chronic aortic regurgitation: a physiologic framework for assessing preoperative predictors. J Am Coll Cardiol 1987;10:1165–1170.
5. Ross J Jr: Left ventricular function and the timing of surgical treatment in valvular heart disease. Ann Intern Med 1981;94:498–504.
6. Bonow RO, Lakatos E, Maron BJ, Epstein SE: Serial long-term assessment of the natural history of asymptomatic patients with chronic aortic regurgitation and normal left ventricular systolic function. Circulation 1991;84:1625–1635.
7. Starling MR, Kirsh MM, Montgomery DG, Gross MD: Mechanisms for left ventricular systolic dysfunction in aortic regurgitation: importance for predicting the functional response to aortic valve replacement. J Am Coll Cardiol 1991;17:887–897.
8. Razzolini R, Zennaro M, Ramondo A, et al: Measurement of systemic resistances in aortic regurgitation. Jpn Heart J 1994;35:733–743.
9. Slordahl SA, Piene H, Solbakken JE, Rossvoll O, Samstad SO, Angelsen BA: Estimation of arterial compliance in aortic regurgitation: three methods evaluated in pigs. Med Biol Eng Comput 1990;28:293–299.
10. Cochrane T: Simple model of circulatory system dynamics including heart valve mechanics. J Biomed Eng 1991;13:335–340.
11. Slordahl SA, Piene H: Haemodynamic effects of arterial compliance, total peripheral resistance, and glyceryl trinitrate on regurgitant volume in aortic regurgitation. Cardiovasc Res 1991;25:869–874.
12. Griffin BP, Flachskampf FA, Siu S, Weyman AE, Thomas JD: The effects of regurgitant orifice size, chamber compliance, and systemic vascular resistance on aortic regurgitant velocity slope and pressure half-time. Am Heart J 1991;122:1049–1056.
13. Scognamiglio R, Rahimtoola SH, Fasoli G, Nistri S, Dalla Volta S: Nifedipine in asymptomatic patients with severe aortic regurgitation and normal left ventricular function. N Engl J Med 1994;331:689–694.
14. Bonow RO: Asymptomatic aortic regurgitation: indications for operation. J Card Surg 1994;9:170–173.
15. Kaufmann P, Vassalli G, Lupi-Wagner S, Jenni R, Hess OM: Coronary artery dimensions in primary and secondary left ventricular hypertrophy. J Am Coll Cardiol 1996;28:745–750.
16. Miyahara K, Sonoda M, Kukihara T, et al: Relationships between left ventricular mass, left ventricular work and coronary artery size in aortic regurgitation—possible mechanism of myocardial ischemia. Jpn Circ J 1993;57:263–271.
17. Nitenberg A, Foult JM, Antony I, Blanchet F, Rahali M: Coronary flow and resistance reserve in patients with chronic aortic regurgitation, angina pectoris and normal coronary arteries. J Am Coll Cardiol 1988;11:478–486.
18. Eberli FR, Ritter M, Schwitter J, et al: Coronary reserve in patients with aortic valve disease before and after successful aortic valve replacement. Eur Heart J 1991;12:127–138.
19. Thompson R, Ross I, Leslie P, Easthope R: Haemodynamic adaptation to exercise in asymptomatic pa-

tients with severe aortic regurgitation. Cardiovasc Res 1985;19:212–218.

20. Kawanishi DT, McKay CR, Chandraratna PA, et al: Cardiovascular response to dynamic exercise in patients with chronic symptomatic mild to moderate and severe aortic regurgitation. Circulation 1986;73:62–72.

21. Massie BM, Kramer BL, Loge D, et al: Ejection fraction response to supine exercise in asymptomatic aortic regurgitation: relation to simultaneous hemodynamic measurements. J Am Coll Cardiol 1985;5:847–855.

22. Spain MG, Smith MD, Kwan OL, DeMaria AN: Effect of isometric exercise on mitral and aortic regurgitation as assessed by color Doppler flow imaging. Am J Cardiol 1990;65:78–83.

23. Greenberg B, Massie B, Thomas D, et al: Association between the exercise ejection fraction response and systolic wall stress in patients with chronic aortic insufficiency. Circulation 1985;71:458–465.

24. Bassand JP, Faivre R, Berthout P, et al: Factors influencing the variations of ejection fraction during exercise in chronic aortic regurgitation. Eur J Nucl Med 1987;13:419–424.

25. Iskandrian AS, Heo J: Radionuclide angiographic evaluation of left ventricular performance at rest and during exercise in patients with aortic regurgitation. Am Heart J 1986;111:1143–1149.

26. Shen WF, Roubin GS, Fletcher PJ, et al: Effects of upright and supine position on cardiac rest and exercise response in aortic regurgitation. Am J Cardiol 1985;55:428–431.

27. Shen WF, Fletcher PJ, Roubin GS, et al: Comparison of effects of isometric and supine bicycle exercise on left ventricular performance in patients with aortic regurgitation and normal ejection fraction at rest. Am Heart J 1985;109:1300–1305.

28. Shen WF, Fletcher PJ, Roubin GS, Harris PJ, Kelly DT: Relation between left ventricular functional reserve during exercise and resting systolic loading conditions in chronic aortic regurgitation. Am J Cardiol 1986;58:757–761.

29. Matsuyama T, Sato H, Kitabatake A, et al: Blunted cardiac responses to exercise-induced sympathetic stimulation in non-failing aortic regurgitation: insight into role of cardiac dilation in hyporesponse of failing hearts. Jpn Circ J 1992;56:117–127.

30. Stewart RE, Gross MD, Starling MR: Mechanisms for an abnormal radionuclide left ventricular ejection fraction response to exercise in patients with chronic, severe aortic regurgitation. Am Heart J 1992;123:453–461.

31. Dervan J, Goldberg S: Acute aortic regurgitation: pathophysiology and management. Cardiovasc Clin 1986;16:281–288.

32. Ardehali A, Segal J, Cheitlin MD: Coronary blood flow reserve in acute aortic regurgitation. J Am Coll Cardiol 1995;25:1387–1392.

32a. Connolly HM, Crary JL, McGoon MD, et al: Valvular heart disease associated with fenfluramine-phentermine. N Engl J Med 1997;337:581–588.

32b. Khan MA, Herzog CA, St Peter JV, et al: The prevalence of cardiac valvular insufficiency assessed by transthoracic echocardiography in obese patients treated with appetite-suppressant drugs. New Engl J Med 1998;339:713–718.

32c. Jick J, Vasilakis C, Weinrauch LA, et al: A population-based study of appetite-suppressant drugs and the risk of cardiac-valve regurgitation. New Engl J Med 1998;339:719–724.

32d. Weissman NJ, Tighe JF, Gottdiener JS, Gwynne JT, for the Sustained Release Dexfenfluramine Study Group: An assessment of heart valve abnormalities in obese patients taking dexfenfluramine, sustained-release dexfenfluramine, or placebo. New Engl J Med 1998;339:725–732.

33. Judge TP, Kennedy JW: Estimation of aortic regurgitation by diastolic pulse wave analysis. Circulation 1970;41:659–665.

34. Perloff JK: Physical examination of the heart and circulation. Philadelphia: WB Saunders; 1982.

35. Corrigan DJ: On permanent patency of the mouth of the aorta, or inadequacy of the aortic valve. Edinburgh Med Surg J 1832;37:225.

36. Quincke H: Observations on capillary and venous pulse. Berlin Klin Wochenschr 1868;5:357 (Translated in Willius FA, Keys TE, eds. Classics of Cardiology. New York: Dover Publications; 1961).

37. Harvey WP, Corrado MA, Perloff JK: "Right-sided" murmurs of aortic insufficiency (diastolic murmurs better heard to the right of the sternum than to the left). Am J Med Sci 1963;245:533.

38. Grayburn PA, Smith MD, Handshoe R, Friedman BJ, DeMaria AN: Detection of aortic insufficiency by standard echocardiography, pulsed Doppler echocardiography, and auscultation: a comparison of accuracies. Ann Intern Med 1986;104:599–605.

39. Kinney EL: Causes of false-negative auscultation of regurgitant lesions: a Doppler echocardiographic study of 294 patients. J Gen Intern Med 1988;3:429–434.

40. Aronow WS, Kronzon I: Correlation of prevalence and severity of aortic regurgitation detected by pulsed Doppler echocardiography with the murmur of aortic regurgitation in elderly patients in a long-term health care facility. Am J Cardiol 1989;63:128–129.

41. Desjardins VA, Enriquez Sarano M, Tajik AJ, Bailey KR, Seward JB: Intensity of murmurs correlates with severity of valvular regurgitation. Am J Med 1996;100:149–156.

42. Flint A: On cardiac murmurs. Am J Med Sci 1862;44:23.

43. Emi S, Fukuda N, Oki T, et al: Genesis of the Austin Flint murmur: relation to mitral inflow and aortic regurgitant flow dynamics. J Am Coll Cardiol 1993;21:1399–1405.

44. Rahko PS: Doppler and echocardiographic characteristics of patients having an Austin Flint murmur. Circulation 1991;83:1940–1950.

45. Landzberg JS, Pflugfelder PW, Cassidy MM, Schiller NB, Higgins CB, Cheitlin MD: Etiology of the Austin Flint murmur. J Am Coll Cardiol 1992;20:408–413.

46. Roman MJ, Kligfield P, Devereux RB, et al: Geometric and functional correlates of electrocardiographic repolarization and voltage abnormalities in aortic regurgitation. J Am Coll Cardiol 1987;9:500.

47. Chen J, Okin PM, Roman MJ, et al: Combined rest and exercise electrocardiographic repolarization findings in relation to structural and functional abnormalities in asymptomatic aortic regurgitation. Am Heart J 1996;132:343–347.

48. Kligfield P, Ameisen O, Okin PM, et al: Relationship of the electrocardiographic response to exercise to geometric and functional findings in aortic regurgitation. Am Heart J 1987;113:1097–1102.

49. Carroll JD, Gaasch WH, Naimi S, Levine HJ: Regression of myocardial hypertrophy: electrocardio-

graphic-echocardiographic correlations after aortic valve replacement in patients with chronic aortic regurgitation. Circulation 1982;65:980.

50. Reichek N, Devereux RB: Left ventricular hypertrophy: relationship of anatomic, echocardiographic and electrocardiographic findings. Circulation 1981;63:1391.

51. Bishop N, Boyle RM, Watson DA, Stoker JB, Mary DA: Aortic valve disease and the ST segment/heart rate relationship: a longitudinal study before and after aortic valve replacement. J Electrocardiol 1988;21:31–37.

52. Hahn RT, Roman MJ, Mogtader AH, Devereux RB: Association of aortic dilation with regurgitant, stenotic and functionally normal bicuspid aortic valves. J Am Coll Cardiol 1992;19:283–288.

53. Samuels DA, Curfman GD, Friedlich AL, Buckley MJ, Austen WG: Valve replacement for aortic regurgitation: long-term follow-up with factors influencing the results. Circulation 1979;60:647–654.

54. Acar J, Luxereau P, Ducimetiere P, Cadilhac M, Jallut H, Vahanian A: Prognosis of surgically treated chronic aortic valve disease: predictive indicators of early postoperative risk and long-term survival, based on 439 cases. J Thorac Cardiovasc Surg 1981;82:114–126.

55. Isom OW, Dembrow JM, Glassman E, Pasternack BS, Sackler JP, Spencer FC: Factors influencing long-term survival after isolated aortic valve replacement. Circulation 1974;50 (Suppl II):154–162.

56. Hirshfeld JW Jr, Epstein SE, Roberts AJ, Glancy DL, Morrow AG: Indices predicting long-term survival after valve replacement in patients with aortic regurgitation and patients with aortic stenosis. Circulation 1974;50:1190–1199.

57. Spagnuolo M, Kloth H, Taranta A, Doyle E, Pasternack B: Natural history of rheumatic aortic regurgitation. Criteria predictive of death, congestive heart failure, and angina in young patients. Circulation 1971;44:368–380.

58. Szlachcic J, Massie BM, Greenberg B, Thomas D, Cheitlin M, Bristow JD: Intertest variability of echocardiographic and chest x-ray measurements: implications for decision making in patients with aortic regurgitation. J Am Coll Cardiol 1986;7:1310–1317.

59. Misra M, Thakur R, Bhandari K, Puri VK: Value of the treadmill exercise test in asymptomatic and minimally symptomatic patients with chronic severe aortic regurgitation. Int J Cardiol 1987;15:309–316.

60. Scriven AJ, Lipkin DP, Fox KM, Poole Wilson PA: Maximal oxygen uptake in severe aortic regurgitation: a different view of left ventricular function. Am Heart J 1990;120:902–909.

61. Weber KT, Janicki JS, McElroy PA: Cardiopulmonary exercise testing in the evaluation of mitral and aortic valve incompetence. Herz 1986;11:88–96.

62. Groundstroem K, Huikuri H, Korhonen U, et al: Left ventricular dimensions during isometric exercise in aortic valve incompetence assessed by M-mode echocardiography and gated equilibrium radionuclide angiography. Eur J Nucl Med 1989;15:204–206.

63. Wilson RA, Greenberg BH, Massie BM, et al: Left ventricular response to submaximal and maximal exercise in asymptomatic aortic regurgitation. Am J Cardiol 1988;62:606–610.

64. Yousof A, Khan N, Askhar M, Simo M, Hayat N: Echocardiographic studies during stress testing using cold pressor test combined with hand grip exercise in asymptomatic patients with severe aortic regurgitation. Can J Cardiol 1986;2:200–205.

65. Wong M, Matsumura M, Omoto R: Left and right ventricular flows by Doppler echocardiography: serial measurements in patients with aortic regurgitation during exercise, cold pressor stimulation, and vasodilation. J Am Soc Echocardiogr 1990;3:285–293.

66. Cornyn JW, Massie BM, Greenberg B, et al: Reproducibility of rest and exercise left ventricular ejection fraction and volumes in chronic aortic regurgitation. Am J Cardiol 1987;59:1361–1365.

67. van den Brink RB, Verheul HA, Hoedemaker G, et al: The value of Doppler echocardiography in the management of patients with valvular heart disease: analysis of one year of clinical practice. J Am Soc Echocardiogr 1991;4:109–120.

68. Globits S, Blake L, Bourne M, et al: Assessment of hemodynamic effects of angiotensin-converting enzyme inhibitor therapy in chronic aortic regurgitation by using velocity-encoded cine magnetic resonance imaging. Am Heart J 1996;131:289–293.

69. Wilson RA, McDonald RW, Bristow JD, et al: Correlates of aortic distensibility in chronic aortic regurgitation and relation to progression to surgery. J Am Coll Cardiol 1992;19:733–738.

70. Turina J, Hess O, Sepulcri F, Krayenbuehl HP: Spontaneous course of aortic valve disease. Eur Heart J 1987;8:471–483.

71. Siemienczuk D, Greenberg B, Morris C, et al: Chronic aortic insufficiency: factors associated with progression to aortic valve replacement. Ann Intern Med 1989;110:587–592.

71a. Borer JS, Hochreiter C, Herrold EM, et al: Prediction of indications for valve replacement among asymptomatic or minimally symptomatic patients with chronic aortic regurgitation and normal left ventricular performance. Circulation 1998;97:525–534.

72. Padial LR, Oliver A, Vivaldi M, et al: Doppler echocardiographic assessment of progression of aortic regurgitation. Am J Cardiol 1997;80:306–314.

73. Marsalese DL, Moodie DS, Lytle BW, et al: Cystic medial necrosis of the aorta in patients without Marfan's syndrome: surgical outcome and long-term follow-up. J Am Coll Cardiol 1990;16:68–73.

74. Pyeritz RE, McKusick VA: The Marfan syndrome: diagnosis and management. N Engl J Med 1979;300:772–777.

75. Kielty CM, Phillips JE, Child AH, Pope FM, Shuttleworth CA: Fibrillin secretion and microfibril assembly by Marfan dermal fibroblasts. Matrix Biol 1994;14:191–199.

76. Silverman DI, Burton KJ, Gray J, et al: Life expectancy in the Marfan syndrome. Am J Cardiol 1995;75:157–160.

77. Marsalese DL, Moodie DS, Vacante M, et al: Marfan's syndrome: natural history and long-term follow-up of cardiovascular involvement. J Am Coll Cardiol 1989;14:422–428.

78. Roman MJ, Devereux RB, Kramer-Fox R, Spitzer MC: Comparison of cardiovascular and skeletal features of primary mitral valve prolapse and Marfan syndrome. Am J Cardiol 1989;63:317–321.

79. Shores J, Berger KR, Murphy EA, Pyeritz RE: Progression of aortic dilatation and the benefit of long-term beta-adrenergic blockade in Marfan's syndrome. N Eng J Med 1994;330:1335–1341.

80. Legget ME, Unger TA, O'Sullivan CK, et al: Aortic

root complications in Marfan's syndrome: identification of a lower risk group. Heart 1996;75:389–395.

81. Pereira L, Levran O, Ramirez F, et al: A molecular approach to the stratification of cardiovascular risk in families with Marfan's syndrome. N Engl J Med 1994;331:148–153.

82. Roman MJ, Rosen SE, Kramer Fox R, Devereux RB: Prognostic significance of the pattern of aortic root dilation in the Marfan syndrome. J Am Coll Cardiol 1993;22:1470–1476.

83. Silverman DI, Gray J, Roman MJ, et al: Family history of severe cardiovascular disease in Marfan syndrome is associated with increased aortic diameter and decreased survival. J Am Coll Cardiol 1995;26:1062–1067.

84. Hwa J, Richards JG, Huang H, McKay D, Pressley L, Hughes CF, Jeremy RW: The natural history of aortic dilatation in Marfan syndrome. Med J Aust 1993;158:558–562.

85. Gott VL, Pyeritz RE, Cameron DE, Greene PS, McKusick VA: Composite graft repair of Marfan aneurysm of the ascending aorta: results in 100 patients. Ann Thorac Surg 1991;52:38–44.

86. Simpson IA, de Belder MA, Treasure T, Camm AJ, Pumphrey CW: Cardiovascular manifestations of Marfan's syndrome: improved evaluation by transoesophageal echocardiography. Br Heart J 1993;69:104–108.

87. Treasure T: Elective replacement of the aortic root in Marfan's syndrome [editorial]. Br Heart J 1993;69:101–103.

88. Roman MJ, Devereaux RB, Kramer-Fox R, O'Loughlin J: Two dimensional echocardiographic aortic root dimensions in normal children and adults. Am J Cardiol 1989;64:507–512.

89. Miller RR, Vismara LA, DeMaria AN, Salel AF, Mason DT: Afterload reduction therapy with nitroprusside in severe aortic regurgitation: improved cardiac performance and reduced regurgitant volume. Am J Cardiol 1976;38:564–567.

90. Sasayama S, Ohyagi A, Lee JD, et al: Effect of the vasodilator therapy in regurgitant valvular disease. Jpn Circ J 1982;46:433–441.

91. Greenberg BH, DeMots H, Murphy E, Rahimtoola SH: Mechanism for improved cardiac performance with arteriolar dilators in aortic insufficiency. Circulation 1981;63:263–268.

92. Reske SN, Heck I, Kropp J, et al: Captopril mediated decrease of aortic regurgitation. Br Heart J 1985;54:415–419.

93. Rothlisberger C, Sareli P, Wisenbaugh T: Comparison of single-dose nifedipine and captopril for chronic severe aortic regurgitation. Am J Cardiol 1993;72:799–804.

94. Fioretti P, Benussi B, Scardi S, Klugmann S, Brower RW, Camerini F: Afterload reduction with nifedipine in aortic insufficiency. Am J Cardiol 1982;49:1728–1732.

95. Shen WF, Roubin GS, Hirasawa K, et al: Noninvasive assessment of acute effects of nifedipine on rest and exercise hemodynamics and cardiac function in patients with aortic regurgitation. J Am Coll Cardiol 1984;4:902–907.

96. Levine HJ, Gaasch WH: Vasoactive drugs in chronic regurgitant lesions of the mitral and aortic valves. J Am Coll Cardiol 1996;28:1083–1091.

97. Jensen T, Kornerup HJ, Lederballe O, Videbaek J, Henningsen P: Treatment with hydralazine in mild to moderate mitral or aortic incompetence. Eur Heart J 1983;4:306–312.

98. Kleaveland JP, Reichek N, McCarthy DM, et al: Effects of six-month afterload reduction therapy with hydralazine in chronic aortic regurgitation. Am J Cardiol 1986;57:1109–1116.

99. Greenberg B, Massie B, Bristow JD, et al: Long-term vasodilator therapy of chronic aortic insufficiency: a randomized double-blinded, placebo-controlled clinical trial. Circulation 1988;78:92–103.

100. Dumesnil JG, Tran K, Dagenais GR: Beneficial long-term effect of hydralazine in aortic regurgitation. Arch Int Med 1990;150:757–760.

101. Lin M, Chiang HT, Lin SL, et al: Vasodilator therapy in chronic asymptomatic aortic regurgitation: enalapril versus hydralazine therapy. J Am Coll Cardiol 1994;24:1046–1053.

102. Crawford MH, Wilson RS, O'Rourke RA, Vittitoe JA: Effect of digoxin and vasodilators on left ventricular function in aortic regurgitation. Int J Cardiol 1989;23:385–393.

103. Heck I, Schmidt J, Mattern H, Fricke G, Kropp J, Reske S: Reduction of regurgitation in aortic and mitral insufficiency by captopril in acute and long-term trials [in German]. Schweiz Med Wochenschr 1985;115:1615–1618.

104. Schon HR: Hemodynamic and morphologic changes after long-term angiotensin converting enzyme inhibition in patients with chronic valvular regurgitation. J Hypertens Suppl 1994;12:S95–104.

105. Wisenbaugh T, Sinovich V, Dullabh A, Sareli P: Six month pilot study of captopril for mildly symptomatic, severe isolated mitral and isolated aortic regurgitation. J Heart Valve Dis 1994;3:197–204.

106. Scognamiglio R, Fasoli G, Ponchia A, Dalla Volta S: Long-term nifedipine unloading therapy in asymptomatic patients with chronic severe aortic regurgitation. J Am Coll Cardiol 1990;16:424–429.

107. Roman MJ, Klein L, Devereux RB, et al: Reversal of left ventricular dilatation, hypertrophy and dysfunction by valve replacement in aortic regurgitation. Am Heart J 1989;118:553–563.

108. Henry WL, Bonow RO, Borer JS, et al: Observations on the optimal time for operative intervention for aortic regurgitation. I. Evaluation of the results of aortic valve replacement in symptomatic patients. Circulation 1980;61:471–483.

109. Fioretti P, Roelandt J, Bos RJ, et al: Echocardiography in chronic aortic insufficiency. Is valve replacement too late when left ventricular end-systolic dimension reaches 55 mm? Circulation 1983;67:216–221.

110. Bonow RO, Rosing DR, Maron BJ, et al: Reversal of left ventricular dysfunction after aortic valve replacement for chronic aortic regurgitation: influence of duration of preoperative left ventricular dysfunction. Circulation 1984;70:570–579.

111. Daniel WG, Hood WP Jr, Siart A, et al: Chronic aortic regurgitation: reassessment of the prognostic value of preoperative left ventricular end-systolic dimension and fractional shortening. Circulation 1985;71:669–680.

112. Taniguchi K, Nakano S, Hirose H, et al: Preoperative left ventricular function: minimal requirement for successful late results of valve replacement for aortic regurgitation. J Am Coll Cardiol 1987;10:510–518.

113. Carabello BA, Usher BW, Hendrix GH, Assey ME, Crawford FA, Leman RB: Predictors of outcome for

aortic valve replacement in patients with aortic regurgitation and left ventricular dysfunction: a change in the measuring stick. J Am Coll Cardiol 1987;10:991–997.

114. Bonow RO, Dodd JT, Maron BJ, et al: Long-term serial changes in left ventricular function and reversal of ventricular dilatation after valve replacement for chronic aortic regurgitation. Circulation 1988;78:11108–11120.

115. Pirwitz MJ, Lange RA, Willard JE, Landau C, Glamann DB, Hillis LD: Use of the left ventricular peak systolic pressure/end-systolic volume ratio to predict symptomatic improvement with valve replacement in patients with aortic regurgitation and enlarged end-systolic volume. J Am Coll Cardiol 1994;24:1672–1677.

116. Taniguchi K, Nakano S, Kawashima Y, et al: Left ventricular ejection performance, wall stress, and contractile state in aortic regurgitation before and after aortic valve replacement. Circulation 1990;82:798–807.

117. Klodas E, Enriquez Sarano M, Tajik AJ, Mullany CJ, Bailey KR, Seward JB: Aortic regurgitation complicated by extreme left ventricular dilation: long-term outcome after surgical correction. J Am Coll Cardiol 1996;27:670–677.

118. Henry WL, Bonow RO, Rosing DR, Epstein SE: Observations on the optimum time for operative intervention for aortic regurgitation. II. Serial echocardiographic evaluation of asymptomatic patients. Circulation 1980;61:484–492.

119. Bonow RO, Rosing DR, McIntosh CL, et al: The natural history of asymptomatic patients with aortic regurgitation and normal left ventricular function. Circulation 1983;68:509–517.

120. Copeland JG, Griepp RB, Stinson EB, Shumway NE: Long-term follow-up after isolated aortic valve replacement. J Thorac Cardiovasc Surg 1977;74:875–889.

121. Klodas E, Enriquez SM, Tajik AJ, Mullany CJ, Bailey KR, Seward JB: Optimizing timing of surgical correction in patients with severe aortic regurgitation: role of symptoms. J Am Coll Cardiol 1997;30:746–752.

122. Bonow RO, Borer JS, Rosing DR, et al: Preoperative exercise capacity in symptomatic patients with aortic regurgitation as a predictor of postoperative left ventricular function and long-term prognosis. Circulation 1980;62:1280–1290.

123. Bonow RO, Rosing DR, Kent KM, Epstein SE: Timing of operation for chronic aortic regurgitation. Am J Cardiol 1982;50:325–336.

124. Gaasch WH, Carroll JD, Levine HJ, Criscitiello MG: Chronic aortic regurgitation: prognostic value of left ventricular end-systolic dimension and end-diastolic radius/thickness ratio. J Am Coll Cardiol 1983;1:775–782.

125. Kumpuris AG, Quinones MA, Waggoner AD, Kanon DJ, Nelson JG, Miller RR: Importance of preoperative hypertrophy, wall stress and end-systolic dimension as echocardiographic predictors of normalization of left ventricular dilatation after valve replacement in chronic aortic insufficiency. Am J Cardiol 1982;49:1091–1100.

126. Klodas E, Enriquez Sarano M, Tajik AJ, Mullany CJ, Bailey KR, Seward JB: Surgery for aortic regurgitation in women: contrasting indications and outcomes compared with men. Circulation 1996;94:2472–2478.

127. Carabello BA: Aortic regurgitation in women: does the measuring stick need a change? Circulation 1996;94:2355–2357.

128. David TE, Feindel CM, Bos J: Repair of the aortic valve in patients with aortic insufficiency and aortic root aneurysm. J Thorac Cardiovasc Surg 1995;109:345–351.

129. Kunzelman KS, Grande KJ, David TE, Cochran RP, Verrier ED: Aortic root and valve relationships. Impact on surgical repair [published erratum appears in J Thorac Cardiovasc Surg 1994;107:1402]. J Thorac Cardiovasc Surg 1994;107:162–170.

130. Elkins RC, Knott Craig CJ, Razook JD, Ward KE, Overholt ED, Lane MM: Pulmonary autograft replacement of the aortic valve in the potential parent. J Card Surg 1994;9:198–203.

131. Sievers HH, Leyh R, Loose R, Guha M, Petry A, Bernhard A: Time course of dimension and function of the autologous pulmonary root in the aortic position. J Thorac Cardiovasc Surg 1993;105:775–780.

132. Knott Craig CJ, Elkins RC, Stelzer PL, et al: Homograft replacement of the aortic valve and root as a functional unit. Ann Thorac Surg 1994;57:1501–1505.

133. Daly RC, Orszulak TA, Schaff HV, McGovern E, Wallace RB: Long-term results of aortic valve replacement with nonviable homografts. Circulation 1991;84 (suppl III):81–88.

134. Del Rizzo DF, Goldman BS, David TE: Aortic valve replacement with a stentless porcine bioprosthesis: multicentre trial. Canadian Investigators of the Toronto SPV Valve Trial. Can J Cardiol 1995;11:597–603.

135. David TE, Bos J, Rakowski H: Aortic valve replacement with the Toronto SPV bioprosthesis. J Heart Valve Dis 1992;1:244–248.

136. Greves J, Rahimtoola SH, McAnulty JH, et al: Preoperative criteria predictive of late survival following valve replacement for severe aortic regurgitation. Am Heart J 1981;101:300–308.

137. Louagie Y, Brohet C, Lopez E, et al: Early surgery for severe aortic regurgitation. J Cardiovasc Surg (Torino) 1984;25:304–312.

138. Bonow RO, Picone AL, McIntosh CL, et al: Survival and functional results after valve replacement for aortic regurgitation from 1976 to 1983: impact of preoperative left ventricular function. Circulation 1985;72:1244–1256.

139. Lytle BW, Cosgrove DM, Loop FD, et al: Replacement of aortic valve combined with myocardial revascularization: determinants of early and late risk for 500 patients, 1967–1981. Circulation 1983;68:1149–1162.

140. Stone PH, Clark RD, Goldschlager N, Selzer A, Cohn K: Determinants of prognosis of patients with aortic regurgitation who undergo aortic valve replacement. J Am Coll Cardiol 1984;3:1118–1126.

141. McGoon MD, Fuster V, McGoon DC, Pumphrey CW, Pluth JR, Elveback LR: Aortic and mitral valve incompetence: long-term follow-up (10 to 19 years) of patients treated with the Starr-Edwards prosthesis. J Am Coll Cardiol 1984;3:930–938.

142. Scott WC, Miller DC, Haverich A, et al: Determinants of operative mortality for patients undergoing aortic valve replacement: discriminant analysis of 1,479 operations. J Thorac Cardiovasc Surg 1985;89:400–413.

143. Boucher CA, Bingham JB, Osbakken MD, et al:

Early changes in left ventricular size and function after correction of left ventricular volume overload. Am J Cardiol 1981;47:991–1004.

144. Monrad ES, Hess OM, Murakami T, Nonogi H, Corin WJ, Krayenbuehl HP: Time course of regression of left ventricular hypertrophy after aortic valve replacement. Circulation 1988;77:1345–1355.

145. Carroll JD, Gaasch WH, Zile MR, Levine HJ: Serial changes in left ventricular function after correction of chronic aortic regurgitation: dependence on early changes in preload and subsequent regression of hypertrophy. Am J Cardiol 1983;51:476–482.

146. Gaasch WH, Andrias CW, Levine HJ: Chronic aortic regurgitation: the effect of aortic valve replacement on left ventricular volume, mass and function. Circulation 1978;58:825–836.

147. Zile MR, Gaasch WH, Levine HJ: Left ventricular stress—dimension-shortening relations before and after correction of chronic aortic and mitral regurgitation. Am J Cardiol 1985;56:99–105.

148. Schuler G, Peterson KL, Johnson AD, et al: Serial noninvasive assessment of left ventricular hypertrophy and function after surgical correction of aortic regurgitation. Am J Cardiol 1979;44:585–594.

149. Herreman F, Ameur A, de Vernejoul F, et al: Pre- and postoperative hemodynamic and cineangiocardiographic assessment of left ventricular function in patients with aortic regurgitation. Am Heart J 1979;98:63–72.

150. Clark RD, Korcuska K, Cohn K: Serial echocardiographic evaluation of left ventricular function in valvular disease, including reproducibility guidelines for serial studies. Circulation 1980;62:564–575.

151. Krayenbuehl HP, Hess OM, Monrad ES, Schneider J, Mall G, Turina M: Left ventricular myocardial structure in aortic valve disease before, intermediate, and late after aortic valve replacement. Circulation 1989;79:744–755.

152. Borer JS, Herrold EM, Hochreiter C, et al: Natural history of left ventricular performance at rest and during exercise after aortic valve replacement for aortic regurgitation. Circulation 1991;84(suppl III):133–139.

153. Forman R, Firth BG, Barnard MS: Prognostic significance of preoperative left ventricular ejection fraction and valve lesion in patients with aortic valve replacement. Am J Cardiol 1980;45:1120–1125.

154. Percy RF, Miller AB, Conetta DA: Usefulness of left ventricular wall stress at rest and after exercise for outcome prediction in asymptomatic aortic regurgitation. Am Heart J 1993;125:151–155.

155. Biem HJ, Detsky AS, Armstrong PW: Management of asymptomatic chronic aortic regurgitation with left ventricular dysfunction: a decision analysis. J Gen Intern Med 1990;5:394–401.

156. Donovan CL, Starling MR: Role of echocardiography in the timing of surgical intervention for chronic mitral and aortic regurgitation. *In* Otto CM, ed. The Practice of Clinical Echocardiography. Philadelphia: WB Saunders; 1997:327–354.

157. Svensson LG, Crawford ES, Coselli JS, Safi HJ, Hess KR: Impact of cardiovascular operation on survival in the Marfan patient. Circulation 1989;80(suppl I):233–242.

158. Smith JA, Fann JI, Miller DC, et al: Surgical management of aortic dissection in patients with the Marfan syndrome. Circulation 1994;90:(suppl II)235–242.

159. Finkbohner R, Johnston D, Crawford ES, Coselli J, Milewicz DM: Marfan syndrome: long-term survival and complications after aortic aneurysm repair. Circulation 1995;91:728–733.

160. Bentall H, De Bono A: A technique for complete replacement of the ascending aorta. Thorax 1968;23:338–339.

161. David TE: Aortic valve repair in patients with Marfan syndrome and ascending aorta aneurysms due to degenerative disease. J Card Surg 1994;9:182–187.

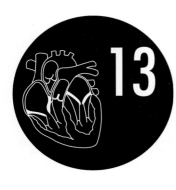

13 Mitral Regurgitation

ANATOMIC MECHANISMS OF MITRAL REGURGITATION

Normal mitral valve closure, which prevents systolic backflow of blood into the left atrium, depends on the complex interaction of each of the components of the valve apparatus—the left atrial wall, the annulus, the mitral valve leaflets, the chordae, the papillary muscles, and the left ventricular wall (Fig. 13–1).[1, 2] Abnormalities in the anatomy and function of any one of these components leads to valvular regurgitation, so that an understanding of normal valve anatomy and closure is needed to understand the mechanisms of regurgitation.[3, 4]

Normal mitral valve closure is thought to be a passive process mediated by flow deceleration through the valve with generation of vortices on the ventricular side of the leaflets in conjunction with an adverse pressure gradient between the left ventricle and atrium.[5–7] In addition, other factors such as papillary muscle traction also may be important for maintaining valve competence during systole.

The term mitral "annulus" refers to the elliptical region of valve leaflet attachment

contiguous with the base of the left atrium. Anteriorly, there is fibrous continuity between the mitral valve leaflet and posterior aortic root, without histologic evidence of a discrete annular structure. Posteriorly, the presence of a discrete fibrous annulus shows considerable individual variability; a C-shaped annulus is most common. In three dimensions, the mitral annulus is saddle-shaped with the basal points of the saddle located medially and laterally, and the apical points located anteriorly and posteriorly (Fig. 13–2, see also color insert).[8] The normal diameter of the mitral annulus is 3.1 ± 0.4 cm, with a circumference of 8 to 9 cm.[9–12] In systole, the mitral annulus moves toward the left ventricular apex, while contraction of the left ventricular myocardium underlying the posterior annulus decreases the annular area by about 25%.[13] The normal motion and contraction of the annulus appear to be important factors in maintaining valve competence.[14–18]

Although left atrial dilation typically is the result, rather than the cause, of mitral regurgitation, the shape of the left atrial wall may distort mitral annular shape and dimensions,

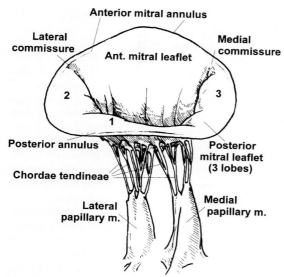

Figure 13·1 The mitral valve apparatus consists of the mitral annulus, anterior and posterior leaflets, chordae tendineae, and the papillary muscles. Abnormal function of any one these components results in mitral regurgitation. The three scallops of the posterior leaflet are indicated by 1 = central, 2 = lateral, 3 = medial. (Illustration by Starr Kaplan.)

posterior leaflet typically has three distinct scallops: medial, central, and lateral. When the leaflets are closed in systole, the line of contact between the leaflets is termed coaptation, and the region of leaflet overlap is called the zone of apposition. Excess leaflet tissue, inadequate tissue, or restricted motion of the leaflets can lead to mitral regurgitation.

There are approximately 12 primary chordae arising from each papillary muscle, which subdivide into secondary and then numerous tertiary branches that attach to the leaflets, mainly at their free margins. In addition, a substantial number of basal (or rough) chordae attach to the ventricular surface of the leaflets and to the commissures (ie, commissural chordae). Often, two large "strut" chordae attach to the anterior leaflet near its margin.[21] Because the papillary muscles are located anterolaterally and posteromedially, both papillary muscles supply chordae to both leaflets; the anterolateral papillary muscle supplies the lateral aspects, and the posteromedial papillary muscle supplies the medial aspects of both leaflets. Rupture, fusion, or redun-

which may increase the severity of valvular regurgitation. In contrast, while the pattern of blood flow across the mitral valve in diastole and the pattern of pulmonary venous inflow into the left atrium are affected by left atrial contraction and relaxation, left atrial mechanical function appears to have little effect on mitral valve closure. A prospective study of patients with atrial fibrillation and initially normal left atrial size suggests that atrial fibrillation may lead to atrial enlargement,[19] which in turn is associated with mitral annular dilation and progressive mitral regurgitation.[20]

The mitral valve is composed of two leaflets, each about 1 mm thick. The regions where the anterior and posterior leaflets meet are termed the medial and lateral commissures. The U-shaped anterior leaflet is longer than it is wide, with an average height of 1.8 to 2.0 cm, an annular length of 3.0 ± 0.5 cm, and an area of 4.3 ± 1.0 cm². The posterior leaflet is wider and shorter than the anterior leaflet, with a height of about 1.1 to 1.2 cm, annular length of 5.2 ± 0.5 cm, and an area averaging 1.7 ± 0.5 cm².[10, 12] The posterior leaflet occupies about two thirds of the annular circumference, with the anterior leaflet occupying the remaining one third. The combined area of the two leaflets is adequate to cover about 2.5 times the area of the mitral annulus. The

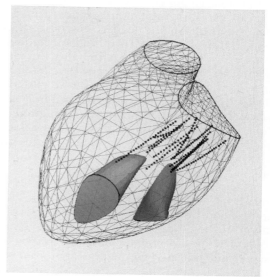

Figure 13·2 Three-dimensional reconstruction of the left ventricle *(wire frame)*, papillary muscles *(blue)*, and mitral chordae *(dashed lines)*. This reconstruction was made from tracings of echocardiographic images acquired using a magnetic locator system. The left ventricular reconstruction was performed with the piece-wise smooth subdivision method. The mitral annulus was reconstructed in 3D using Fourier series approximations. The 3D reconstruction demonstrates the normal saddle shape of the mitral annulus and the nearly orthogonal relationship of the chordae to the plane of the mitral annulus. (Courtesy of Florence H. Sheehan, MD.) (This figure also occurs in the color insert section.)

dancy of the chordae can lead to valvular regurgitation, with the severity of regurgitation related to the number and location of the affected chordae.

The systolic tension provided by the papillary muscles opposes the pressure load on the leaflets, helping to maintain normal leaflet closure. The bases of the papillary muscles are positioned about two thirds of the distance from the mitral annulus to the apex, with a relatively perpendicular angle between the plane of the annulus and the long axis of the papillary muscles. The posteromedial papillary muscle is predisposed to ischemic dysfunction and infarction because it is supplied by a single branch of the posterior descending artery and tends to have few collaterals. Since the anterolateral papillary muscle typically receives blood from branches of both the left anterior descending and circumflex arteries, it is less susceptible to ischemic injury. In addition to ischemia, abnormal papillary muscle function may be caused by fibrosis or infiltrative processes.

The function of the left ventricle affects mitral valve closure in several ways. First, segmental wall motion abnormalities of the myocardium underlying the papillary muscles can lead to mitral regurgitation because of inadequate tension on the leaflets in systole. Second, diffuse left ventricular dilation and increased sphericity may alter the normal alignment of the papillary muscle, resulting in systolic traction that opposes valve closure. Third, ventricular dilation leads to mitral annular dilation and resultant mitral regurgitation. These mechanisms can create a vicious cycle in which mitral regurgitation leads to ventricular dilation, which leads to more mitral regurgitation, and so forth.

As discussed in Chapters 1 and 2, a wide variety of disease processes lead to mitral regurgitation by affecting one or more components of the mitral valve apparatus (see Table 2–2). The most common conditions leading to significant mitral regurgitation are myxomatous mitral valve disease, rheumatic disease, coronary artery disease, and dilated cardiomyopathy. Mitral valve prolapse and myxomatous valve disease are discussed in Chapter 14. The natural history of the other causes of mitral regurgitation is presented in this chapter.

PATHOPHYSIOLOGY
Valvular Hemodynamics

The regurgitant mitral valve has an orifice that allows passage of blood from the left ven-

tricle to the left atrium in systole (Fig. 13–3). Although this regurgitant orifice may have a complex shape and may be dynamic in terms of shape and size during the cardiac cycle,[22] the flow volume and pressure drop across this orifice depend on basic hydraulic principles.[23] Regurgitant volume is the product of regurgitant orifice area and the mean velocity of flow through the orifice, with blood flow velocity related to the ventricular-atrial systolic pressure difference stated in the Bernoulli equation ($\Delta P = 4v^2$). These relationships can be used to derive regurgitant orifice area from Doppler measurements of regurgitant volume and flow velocity or using invasive measurements of the regurgitant volume and pressure gradient. Although earlier angiographic studies suggested that a substantial portion of the mitral regurgitant volume occurs during the preejection period,[24] it now is clear that mitral regurgitant flow occurs predominantly during the systolic ejection period.[25]

Left ventricular systolic pressures in patients with mitral regurgitation typically are normal, with a rapid rate of rise in pressure during "isovolumic" contraction (ie, high dP/dt). Of course, when mitral regurgitation is present, this phase of the cardiac cycle is not truly isovolumic since blood exits the ventricle across the incompetent mitral valve into the left atrium. Higher left ventricular systolic pressures (eg, with hypertension) lead to in-

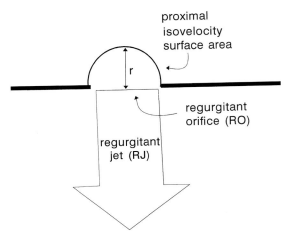

regurg. volume = PISA x velocity

RO area = regurg. volume/VTI$_{RJ}$

Figure 13·3 Schematic diagram illustrating the concept of regurgitant orifice (RO) area and the relationships of regurgitant volume, velocity, and orifice area. PISA, proximal isovelocity surface area; VTI, velocity-time integral.

creasing degrees of mitral regurgitation. Lower left ventricular pressures result in decreased regurgitant volume as the pressure gradient across the valve declines.[26]

Unlike the situation in aortic regurgitation, the force of left ventricular contraction may affect regurgitant severity as kinetic energy, in addition to the potential energy described by the pressure gradient, drives blood flow across the regurgitant valve. The clinical implications of the kinetic and potential energy components of mitral regurgitation have not been fully explored.

Left atrial pressures in patients with acute mitral regurgitation are elevated, with a v wave in late systole, due to the increased volume and velocity of blood entering the left atrium across the regurgitant valve. With chronic mitral regurgitation, an increase in the size and compliance of the left atrium tends to compensate for the volume and velocity overload of the left atrium, so that pressures are only moderately elevated, and a v wave may or may not be present (Fig. 13–4). Thus, the absence of a v wave on the left atrial or pulmonary wedge pressure tracing does not exclude a diagnosis of severe mitral regurgitation (see Chapter 4). In addition, while left atrial size correlates with regurgitant severity, there is no relationship between left atrial size and the presence of a v wave.[27, 28]

Two factors contribute to an increased antegrade diastolic flow velocity across the mitral valve in patients with mitral regurgitation. First, the pressure difference between the left atrium and ventricle at mitral valve opening is increased due to the elevated left atrial pressure at end-systole. This increased antegrade velocity across the mitral valve in diastole is followed by a steep deceleration slope as left atrial and left ventricular diastolic pressures rapidly equilibrate. Second, antegrade velocities are elevated compared with normal values as a result of the increased flow volume across the valve in diastole, reflecting the sum of forward and regurgitant stroke volumes.

Mitral regurgitation often is a dynamic lesion in that the size of the regurgitant orifice and thus regurgitant volume may vary with the pressure gradient across the valve and with changes in left ventricular volume or geometry. The dynamic nature of the lesion leads to a complex interplay of physiologic factors such that as mitral regurgitation leads to left ventricular dilation, the regurgitant orifice increases because of abnormal ventricular geometry, which then leads to more mitral regurgitation. Therefore, the use of medical therapy to decrease left ventricular volumes may reduce regurgitant severity through a favorable effect on the left ventricular to left atrial pressure difference and may lead to a smaller regurgitant orifice as the leaflets close more completely due to a smaller annular area or improved alignment of the papillary muscles relative to the annulus.[29]

Left Ventricular Volume Overload

The pathophysiology of mitral regurgitation is different from the combined pressure and volume overload seen in aortic regurgitation. Mitral regurgitation results in isolated volume overload of the left ventricle, with the increased volume pumped by the ventricle ejected into the low-impedance left atrium. Overall, the volume of blood flow exiting the left ventricle retrograde across the incompetent mitral valve compared with antegrade flow across the aortic valve depends on the relative impedance of the left atrium compared with the systemic circuit.

In chronic compensated mitral regurgitation, the backflow of blood across the mitral valve in systole provides the physiologic equivalent of afterload reduction, and a normal for-

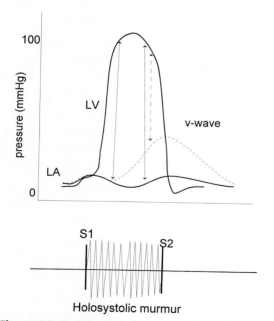

Figure 13·4 Schematic diagram of left ventricular (LV) and left atrial (LA) pressures in chronic *(solid line)* and acute *(dashed line)* mitral regurgitation. The systolic murmur of chronic mitral regurgitation corresponds to the time course of the difference between the LV and LA pressures.

ward cardiac output is maintained by the combination of an increase in the ejection fraction and a higher preload (or end-diastolic volume). The consequent decreased ventricular pressure and end-systolic radius allow an increase in the extent and velocity of fiber shortening without an increase in wall stress and only a mild increase in myocardial oxygen consumption.[30] In an animal model, the lesser degree of ventricular hypertrophy seen with isolated volume, compared with pressure overload of the ventricle was associated with a lower rate of myosin heavy chain synthesis.[31]

The intrinsic afterload-reducing effect of chronic mitral regurgitation makes detection of contractile dysfunction difficult, as a normal ejection fraction may be observed even with a significant decline in left ventricular contractility (Fig. 13–5).[32] If contractile dysfunction is not recognized early, ventricular ejection performance may deteriorate after surgical intervention due to the increased afterload present after correction of the mitral regurgitation, although other factors, such as maintenance of annular-papillary muscle continuity, also affect the postoperative outcome (see Chapter 15).[33]

Evaluation of left ventricular chamber elastance (E_{max}) in patients with mitral regurgitation supports the concept that contractile dysfunction may exist despite a normal ejection fraction and, further, that contractile dysfunction may be reversible in some cases (Fig. 13–6). Patients with chronic mitral regurgitation can be divided into three groups based on ventricular ejection fraction and determination of E_{max}. The first group includes patients with compensated left ventricular volume overload, increased left ventricular volumes, eccentric hypertrophy, a normal ejection fraction, and a normal E_{max}. These patients maintain a normal ejection fraction and have regression of left ventricular dilation after successful intervention for mitral regurgitation. The second group includes patients with a normal ejection fraction but a reduced E_{max}, suggesting contractile dysfunction. These patients tend to have clinical improvement and an improvement in ejection fraction observed at the 1-year follow-up evaluation. The third group includes patients with a reduced ejection fraction and E_{max}. These patients are likely to show no improvement in ejection fraction at 3 months and 1 year postoperatively.[34, 35]

Left Atrial Changes

Left atrial dilation occurs in patients with chronic mitral regurgitation as a compensatory response to the increased volume flow entering the left atrium in systole.[27, 28] Other factors that may contribute to atrial enlargement include transmission of the kinetic energy of the mitral regurgitant jet to the left atrial wall and atrial fibrillation.[19] Along with increased atrial size, atrial compliance increases with chronic regurgitation.[27, 36–38] Both factors tend to buffer the effect of the regurgitant flow on left atrial pressure, such that normal left atrial pressures commonly are present in compensated patients. A subgroup of mitral regurgitation patients develop massive left atrial enlargement with fibrosis of the atrial wall and a low atrial pressure, due to a large, compliant chamber.[36, 37] These patients typically have only mild pulmonary hypertension but do have atrial fibrillation and a low cardiac output.

Due to the rapid motion of blood in the enlarged atrium, patients with mitral regurgitation are thought to be at lower risk of atrial thrombus formation than patients with other causes of left atrial enlargement.[39, 40] This hypothesis is supported by studies showing that the prevalence of atrial thrombi in patients with rheumatic and nonrheumatic mitral valve disease is inversely related to mitral regurgitant severity.[39–41] In one study, left atrial throm-

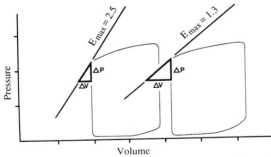

Figure 13·5 Pressure-volume loops and end-systolic pressure-volume relations in a mildly depressed and a myopathic ventricle. In the pressure-volume loop on the left, the ejection fraction is 50%, and the slope of the end-systolic pressure-volume relation (E_{max}) is 2.5. In the pressure-volume loop on the right, the ejection fraction is 30%, and E_{max} is only 1.3. In the case of the myopathic ventricle, a given reduction in end-systolic pressure (P) effects a greater reduction in end-systolic volume (V) than in the mildly depressed ventricle. In patients with chronic mitral regurgitation, the salutary hemodynamic effects of vasodilators are most marked in the most symptomatic patients with the largest hearts and the most depressed systolic function. (From Levine HJ, Gaasch WH: Vasoactive drugs in the chronic regurgitant lesions of the mitral and aortic valves. J Am Coll Cardiol 1996;28:1083–1091; reprinted with permission from the American College of Cardiology.)

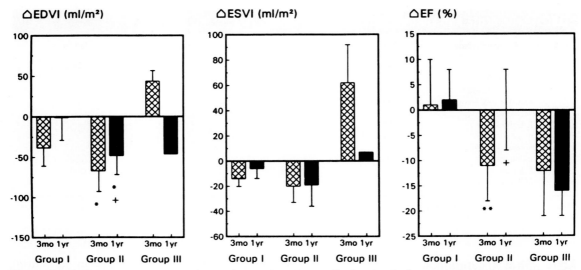

Figure 13·6 Preoperative to postoperative changes in patients with chronic mitral regurgitation with normal baseline contractile function (Group I), with impaired left ventricular contractile function (E_{max}) but normal ejection fraction (Group II), and with a reduced E_{max} and reduced systolic myocardial stiffness (Group III). Changes in radionuclide left ventricular end-diastolic volume indices (EDVI), end-systolic volume indices (ESVI), and ejection fractions (EF) are shown as the absolute change from their corresponding preoperative values. This format eliminates the preoperative differences in these variables between subgroups so that comparisons between subgroups can be made. There was a greater decrease in the left ventricular end-diastolic volume index at 3 months than at 1 year in Group II, which resulted in a greater reduction in left ventricular ejection fraction at 3 months and a subsequent increase in left ventricular ejection fraction at 1 year after mitral valve surgery compared with Group I. The left ventricular size and ejection fraction responses to mitral valve surgery in Group III were poor. *, $P \le .05$ compared with Group I; **, $P < .01$ compared with Group I; +, $P < .01$ compared with 3 months. (Starling MR, Kirsh MM, Montgomery DG, Gross MD: Impaired left ventricular contractile function in patients with long-term mitral regurgitation and normal ejection fraction. J Am Coll Cardiol 1993;22:239–250; reprinted with permission from the American College of Cardiology.)

bus was found in 39% of patients with no mitral regurgitation, 33% with mild regurgitation, 9% with moderate regurgitation, and 0% with severe regurgitation.[42] In a transesophageal study, atrial thrombus in patients with mitral valve disease was associated with little mitral regurgitation and the presence of atrial fibrillation.[43, 44] Even with atrial fibrillation, the risk of atrial thrombus is low (<1%) for patients with severe regurgitation and only intermediate for patients with moderate regurgitation.[40]

The Right Heart

Chronic mitral regurgitation leads to elevated pulmonary pressures due to the passive elevation in pulmonary venous pressure. With long-standing disease, some patients develop superimposed reactive pulmonary hypertension that becomes irreversible because of progressive histologic changes in the pulmonary vasculature, as described for mitral stenosis in Chapter 10.

Pulmonary hypertension leads to right ventricular dilation and systolic dysfunction, often

in association with tricuspid regurgitation due to the dilated tricuspid annulus. In a study using electron beam tomography, a negative association between regurgitant fraction and right ventricular ejection fraction was found for a series of 35 patients with mitral regurgitation.[45] Since these changes in right ventricular function occurred without left ventricular systolic dysfunction, serial evaluation of right heart function may be a more sensitive approach for following disease progression in patients with mitral regurgitation.

Exercise Physiology

In patients with chronic mitral regurgitation, the left ventricular ejection fraction increases by 15% to 20% with exercise. Although some studies suggest that forward stroke volume increases and regurgitant stroke volume decreases with exercise,[46] other studies suggest that regurgitant volume increases with exercise.[47, 48] The response to exercise is similar in patients on afterload reduction therapy and those not on therapy.[46, 48]

TABLE 13·1   ACUTE AND CHRONIC MITRAL REGURGITATION

Characteristic	Chronic Compensated	Chronic Decompensated	Acute
Symptom onset	None	Gradual DOE	Abrupt CHF
Physical examination			
Blood pressure	Normal	Normal	↓
Pulmonary congestion	None	Variable	↑ ↑ ↑ ↑
Hemodynamics			
LA pressure	Normal	↑	↑ ↑
v wave	Absent	Variable	↑
Echocardiography			
LV size	↑	↑ ↑	Normal
LA size	↑	↑	Normal
MR jet v wave	Absent	Variable	↑

DOE, dyspnea on exertion; CHF, congestive heart failure; LA, left atrium; LV, left ventricle; MR, mitral regurgitation; arrows indicate relative increase (↑) or decrease (↓) compared with normal.

Acute Mitral Regurgitation

In patients with the acute onset of mitral regurgitation or sudden worsening of chronic disease, the abrupt increase in the volume of regurgitant flow into the left atrium causes severe elevation of left atrial pressure and consequent pulmonary edema (Table 13–1). Left atrial and left ventricular dimensions may be normal in patients with acute regurgitation, although some degree of enlargement may be seen if chronic, milder disease has been present. Typically, acute regurgitation is associated with a left atrial v wave due to the late systolic rise in left atrial pressure, which is reflected in the continuous wave Doppler waveform as a rapid decline in velocity in late systole (Fig. 13–7). Unlike chronic regurgitation, left atrial compliance is low with acute regurgitation,

leading to an abrupt increase in left atrial pressure.[1, 49] Over 6 to 12 months, a marked increase in the thickness of the left atrial wall occurs in conjunction with an increase in pulmonary vascular resistance.[36]

Although left ventricular afterload is markedly reduced in acute and chronic mitral regurgitation, these beneficial compensatory mechanisms may not be evident as the clinical picture is dominated by an acute increase in left atrial pressure, which leads to pulmonary edema.

CLINICAL PRESENTATION
Clinical History

The clinical history of patients with mitral regurgitation depends on the cause of valve

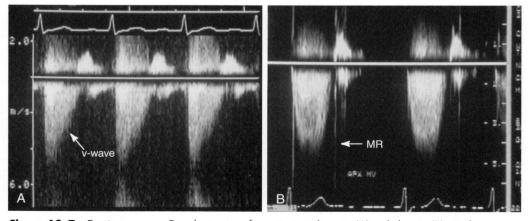

Figure 13·7   Continuous wave Doppler tracings for patients with acute *(A)* and chronic *(B)* mitral regurgitation (MR). Notice the more rapid rate of decline in velocity in late systole, with acute regurgitation as the left ventricular to atrial pressure difference decreases. The hemodynamic correlate of this Doppler finding is a left atrial v wave.

dysfunction. For example, patients with secondary mitral regurgitation from ischemic disease or dilated cardiomyopathy typically present with symptoms related to the underlying disease process. Patients with primary disease of the mitral leaflets (eg, rheumatic, myxomatous) may remain asymptomatic for many years. The timing of intervention to prevent irreversible systolic dysfunction of the left ventricle in patients with asymptomatic mitral regurgitation remains a difficult clinical problem (see Chapter 15).

When symptoms supervene, patients initially notice the gradual onset of exertional dyspnea or decreased exercise tolerance, followed by overt symptoms and signs of pulmonary congestion and heart failure. However, symptom onset may be more acute if there is a sudden change in disease severity, such as chordal rupture or bacterial endocarditis, so that the initial presentation of some patients is frank congestive heart failure. In other patients, mitral regurgitation is recognized during a time of increased hemodynamic stress, such as pregnancy or an infectious disease, with symptom onset caused by the increased hemodynamic

demands of the superimposed condition. Occasionally, mitral regurgitation is initially diagnosed in a patient with new onset of atrial fibrillation.

Physical Examination

Unlike aortic regurgitation, mitral regurgitation has few peripheral vasculature manifestations. If forward cardiac output is impaired, as with acute regurgitation or decompensated chronic disease, the carotid upstroke is brisk, but with a low total amplitude, and has an early peak and rapid decline in late systole because of ejection of blood backward across the mitral valve instead of forward across the aortic valve. Blood pressure is normal to low, and the pulse pressure is normal. The jugular venous pressure and waveform typically are normal unless the patient has right heart failure. Atrial fibrillation with an irregular pulse may be detected in patients with chronic disease. Evidence of pulmonary congestion is seen only in patients with decompensated disease (Table 13–2).

Precordial palpation reveals a normal left

TABLE 13·2   DIAGNOSTIC EVALUATION OF THE PATIENT WITH MITRAL REGURGITATION

Evaluation	Findings
Physical examination	Brisk carotid upstroke
	Holosystolic murmur at apex
	Mitral systolic click
Electrocardiogram	Atrial fibrillation
	Left ventricular hypertrophy
	Left atrial enlargement
Chest radiography	Left atrial enlargement
	Pulmonary congestion
Echocardiography	Mitral valve anatomy
	Cause of regurgitation
	Normal, excessive, or restrictive leaflet motion
	Reparability of valve
	Left ventricular size and systolic function
	Dimensions or volumes
	Ejection fraction
	Regional wall motion
	Left atrial size
	Pulmonary artery pressures
	Regurgitant severity
	Color flow Doppler
	Continuous wave Doppler signal strength and shape
	Regurgitant volume
	Regurgitant orifice area
Cardiac catheterization*	Mitral regurgitant severity on left ventricular angiography
	Hemodynamics
	Left atrial v wave
	Pulmonary hypertension
	Coronary angiography

*Often only needed preoperatively for coronary anatomy.

ventricular apical impulse early in the disease course, with a diffuse or displaced apical impulse when left ventricular dilatation is present. If chronic mitral regurgitation has led to pulmonary hypertension, a right ventricular heave caused by compensatory right ventricular hypertrophy may be appreciated, although a right parasternal heave also may be due to systolic expansion of the left atrium with anterior displacement of the right heart when severe regurgitation is present.[50]

On cardiac auscultation, the patient with mitral regurgitation classically has a soft S_1 with a holosystolic murmur that is loudest at the apex and radiates to the axilla. A midsystolic click and late systolic murmur occur with mitral valve prolapse (see Chapter 14). The second heart sound is normal early in the disease course, but the loudness of the pulmonic component is increased compared with normal when pulmonary hypertension is present. Respiratory splitting of the second heart sound usually is normal, but persistent splitting due to early aortic valve closure may occur in severe cases. An S_3 may be present due to the increased rate and velocity of early diastolic filling. With severe regurgitation, a mid-diastolic murmur may be appreciated at the apex because of the increased transmitral flow in diastole.[51]

In chronic mitral regurgitation, the loudness of the murmur correlates somewhat with regurgitant severity in that a systolic thrill (grade 4 or greater murmur) is associated with severe regurgitation, whereas a murmur less than grade 2 indicates mild disease. However, the severity of regurgitation varies widely in patients with a grade 2 or 3 murmur, which is present in the majority of patients (Fig. 13–8).[52] With acute regurgitation, mitral regurgitation may be severe despite a soft murmur. In fact, as many as 50% of patients with acute mitral regurgitation have no audible murmur.[53]

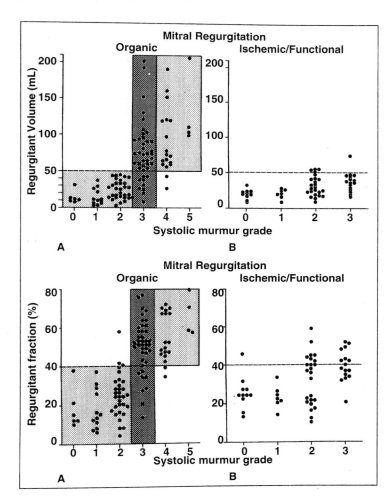

Figure 13·8 Murmur intensity is plotted against regurgitant volume *(upper panels)* and against regurgitant fraction *(lower panels)* by Doppler echocardiography in mitral regurgitation of organic *(A)* and ischemic or functional *(B)* cause. The light-shaded area on the left of each graph is the low-intensity, low-severity area, and that on the right is the high-intensity, high-severity area. The dark-shaded central area is the uncertainty zone. Horizontal lines are threshold values for severe regurgitation. (From Desjardins VA, Enriquez Sarano M, Tajik AJ, Bailey KR, Seward JB: Intensity of murmurs correlates with severity of valvular regurgitation. Am J Med 1996;100:149–156.)

The radiation of the murmur in mitral regurgitation depends on the direction of the regurgitant jet. A posterolaterally directed jet, as with ischemic disease, anterior leaflet abnormalities, and dilated cardiomyopathy, radiates from the apex to the axilla. Sometimes, this murmur even radiates to the back and can be appreciated with the stethoscope placed in the left infrascapular region.[54] In contrast, a jet that is directed anteriorly or superiorly in the left atrium (eg, with posterior leaflet prolapse) radiates to the cardiac base and may be heard in the carotids, mimicking the murmur of aortic stenosis.[55] Sometimes, the murmur of mitral regurgitation can be appreciated on top of the head.[56]

The murmur of mitral regurgitation can be differentiated from aortic stenosis by changes in the loudness of the murmur with maneuvers to alter preload or afterload. A decrease in left ventricular preload, induced by having the patient stand from a squatting position or by the strain phase of the Valsalva maneuver, typically augments a mitral regurgitant murmur, especially when caused by mitral valve prolapse, while the murmur of aortic stenosis diminishes with this maneuver. An increase in afterload induced by a hand grip also increases the murmur of mitral regurgitation. Conversely, the murmur of aortic stenosis decreases or is unchanged with an increase in afterload. Note that with dynamic subaortic obstruction, the systolic murmur increases with a decrease in preload but decreases with an increase in afterload (Table 13–3).

Chest Radiography and Electrocardiography

The chest radiograph may be relatively normal with the earliest abnormality typically being left atrial enlargement. With left ventricular dilation, the cardiac silhouette increases (Fig. 13–9). Decompensated disease is associated with evidence of pulmonary interstitial edema, alveolar fluid, and pleural effusions.

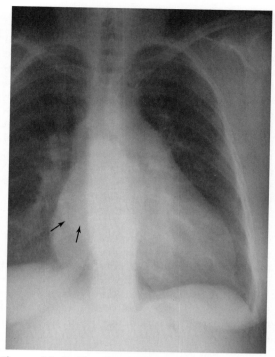

Figure 13·9 The chest radiograph of a patient with chronic compensated mitral regurgitation. Shows left atrial enlargement *(arrows)* and left ventricular enlargement but no pulmonary congestion.

Pulmonary hypertension is manifested as increased size of the central pulmonary arteries with peripheral attenuation of pulmonary vessels. Right heart enlargement is seen late in the disease course.

The electrocardiographic findings in mitral regurgitation are nonspecific, including left atrial enlargement, atrial fibrillation, and left ventricular hypertrophy in patients with severe mitral regurgitation. However, the correlation between mitral regurgitant severity and electrocardiographic findings is poor.[57] Right-axis deviation and criteria for right ventricular hypertrophy may be observed in patients with secondary pulmonary hypertension.

TABLE 13·3 RESPONSE OF THE SYSTOLIC MURMUR ON PHYSICAL EXAMINATION

Cause of Murmur	Respiratory Variation	Decreased Preload	Increased Afterload
Mitral regurgitation	No	↑ (MVP)	↑
Aortic stenosis	No	↓	No change
Ventricular septal defect	No	Variable	Variable
Hypertrophic obstructive cardiomyopathy	No	↑ ↑	↓ ↓
Tricuspid regurgitation	Yes		

MVP, mitral valve prolapse; arrows indicate relative increase (↑, ↑ ↑) or decrease (↓, ↓ ↓) compared with baseline.

Echocardiography

The echocardiographic evaluation of mitral regurgitation includes evaluation of the cause and severity of mitral regurgitation, left ventricular size and systolic function, left atrial size, pulmonary artery pressures, and any associated abnormalities (see Chapter 3). Increasingly, echocardiography plays a key role in defining the anatomic mechanism of mitral regurgitation, following disease progression, defining the optimal timing for surgical intervention (see Chapter 15), and assessing the results of medical or surgical therapy.

In the initial echocardiographic evaluation of the patient with mitral regurgitation, the first goal is to define the cause and anatomic mechanism of mitral regurgitation, because this information affects clinical management and overall prognosis (Figs. 13–10 through 13–13, see also color insert). For example, the treatment and expected outcome for mitral regurgitation due to a dilated cardiomyopathy differ substantially from those for mitral regurgitation due to rheumatic valve disease. Even within a disease category, prognosis depends on mitral valve anatomy and regurgitant severity; a young woman with mitral valve prolapse, thin leaflets, and mild regurgitation has a markedly different prognosis from that of an older man with thickened leaflets, a partial flail segment, and severe mitral regurgitation. Echocardiographic imaging provides detailed data on leaflet size, shape and function, annular size, chordal anatomy, and papillary muscle function. When transthoracic images are nondiagnostic, transesophageal imaging should be considered.

For surgical planning, mitral leaflet motion often is classified as normal, excessive, or restrictive. Excessive leaflet motion is characterized by movement of the leaflets beyond the mitral annulus plane (into the left atrium) in systole, as occurs with myxomatous mitral valve disease. In contrast, with restrictive leaflet motion there is inadequate excursion of the valve leaflets due to annular and left ventricular dilation, abnormal papillary muscle function, or scarred and shortened leaflets. Restrictive leaflet motion is characterized by closure of the valve on the left ventricular side of the annulus, with incomplete closure and decreased leaflet apposition. The area under the tented leaflets sometimes is used as a descriptor of the degree of restricted motion.[3, 4] In the future, three-dimensional (3D) reconstruction of the mitral valve apparatus may allow even more precise evaluation of anatomy and function.[58]

In the clinical setting, regurgitation severity is estimated on the basis of color flow imaging of the regurgitant jet from multiple acoustic windows, comparison of antegrade velocities across mitral and aortic valves, the signal strength and shape of the continuous wave Doppler velocity curve, evidence for systolic

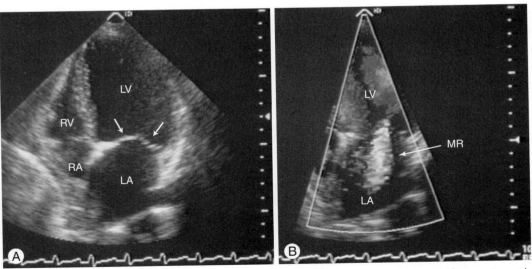

Figure 13·10 Apical four-chamber echocardiography *(A)* and color flow Doppler images *(B)* for a patient with ischemic mitral regurgitation (MR). Notice the inadequate coaptation, or tenting, of the mitral leaflets in systole *(arrows)* and the centrally directed regurgitant jet. LA, left atrium; LV, left ventricle; RA, right atrium; RV, right ventricle. *(B also occurs in the color insert section.)*

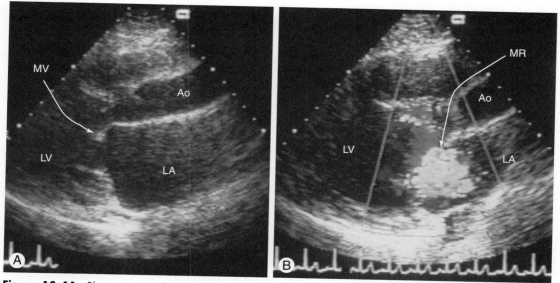

Figure 13·11 Rheumatic mitral regurgitation (MR) is caused by thickening and increased rigidity of the leaflets, especially at the leaflet tips. *A,* In diastole, characteristic diastolic doming is seen *(arrow)* with mild mitral stenosis. *B,* In systole, coaptation appears normal, but severe mitral regurgitation is caused by inadequate leaflet apposition and decreased leaflet flexibility. Ao, aorta; LA, left atrium; LV, left ventricle; MV, mitral valve. (*B* also occurs in the color insert section.)

flow reversal in the pulmonary veins, and the degree of left atrial and ventricular enlargement. When transthoracic image quality is suboptimal, transesophageal imaging should be considered for evaluation of valve morphology and regurgitant severity. In the candidate for valve repair, transesophageal imaging assists in defining the type of valve repair needed and

the likelihood of a good surgical outcome. In patients with acute mitral regurgitation, transesophageal assessment of regurgitant severity may be more accurate than transthoracic imaging.[59]

Although a quantitative measurement of regurgitant severity can be based on measurement of volume flow at two intracardiac sites

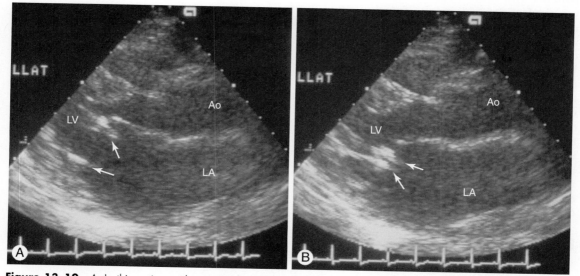

Figure 13·12 *A,* In this patient with systemic lupus erythematosus, the mitral leaflets show irregular thickening at the leaflet tips *(arrows)*, but without diastolic doming. *B,* In systole, these masses *(arrows)* prevent normal leaflet closure, resulting in significant mitral regurgitation. Ao, aorta; LA, left atrium; LV, left ventricle.

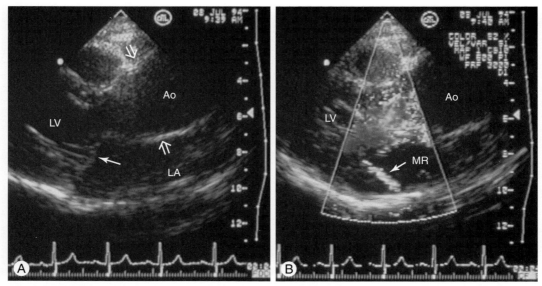

Figure 13·13 *A,* With Marfan's syndrome, the classic findings of aortic root dilation and effacement of the sinotubular junction *(open arrows)* often are accompanied by elongation and redundancy of the anterior mitral leaflet. In the parasternal long-axis view at end-systole, the elongated anterior leaflet sags into the left atrium *(small arrow). B,* Color flow imaging shows only mild mitral regurgitation (MR). Ao, aorta; LA, left atrium; LV, left ventricle. *(B* also occurs in the color insert section.)

or on the proximal isovelocity surface area approach,[60] precise measurement of regurgitant severity rarely is needed in clinical practice. Instead, grading regurgitant severity as mild, moderate, or severe usually is adequate for determining which patients merit periodic evaluation. Currently, the echocardiographic parameters used in making decisions about patients with mitral regurgitation include left ventricular size and systolic function, pulmonary artery pressures, and left atrial size, all of which can be measured accurately and reproducibly by echocardiography (see Chapter 3). When surgical intervention is contemplated, the echocardiographic assessment of whether the valve anatomy allows valve repair, rather than replacement, is a key factor in the clinical decision-making process. Inclusion of quantitative noninvasive measures of regurgitant severity in prospective studies of the natural history of patients with mitral regurgitation is needed to determine whether more precise measures of regurgitant severity are better predictors of clinical outcome.

Exercise Testing

Exercise testing may be performed for patients with chronic mitral regurgitation as an objective measure of exercise tolerance or to evaluate whether a patient with an equivocal history of decreased exercise capacity has symptoms. Exercise testing also may be helpful in eliciting the mechanism of exertional limitation in patients with mitral valve prolapse and little mitral regurgitation at rest, since many of these patients develop significant regurgitation with exercise.[61] In addition, exercise-induced mitral regurgitation occurs in about one third of patients with rheumatic mitral disease.[62]

Patients with mitral regurgitation achieve a lower maximum oxygen consumption with exercise than normal controls, but the exercise changes in forward stroke volume and regurgitant volume vary, with some patients showing little change in regurgitant volume and others showing a substantial increase in the degree of regurgitation.[63] In patients with mitral regurgitation, the primary determinants of maximum oxygen consumption are the forward cardiac output with exercise, age, and gender.[63]

Exercise testing also may be helpful in predicting clinical prognosis and outcome after mitral valve surgery. In one study of patients with severe mitral regurgitation due to mitral prolapse, only the change in the right ventricular ejection fraction with exercise predicted disease progression.[64]

Although most investigators have found that measurements of resting left ventricular size and systolic function predict outcome after valve surgery, in a series of 74 patients with severe mitral regurgitation, the change in left ventricular end-systolic volume index with exercise was the best predictor of postoperative outcome.[65] Routine exercise testing is not yet part of the basic evaluation of patients with chronic mitral regurgitation, but these data suggest that it is helpful for selected patients, and it may become routine if additional studies support its clinical value.

Cardiac Catheterization

Left ventricular angiography rarely is needed for evaluation of chronic mitral regurgitation but may be helpful when the clinical picture and noninvasive findings are discrepant.[66] Measurement of left ventricular volumes and ejection fraction may be needed if noninvasive assessment of ventricular size and function is limited by technical factors.

Coronary angiography is needed in patients with ischemic mitral regurgitation. When the cause of regurgitation is unclear, coronary angiography helps to define the contribution of ischemia to the abnormal function of the mitral valve apparatus. In the patient scheduled for mitral valve surgery for regurgitation of any cause, coronary angiography typically is performed unless the pretest likelihood of coronary disease is extremely low.

Although the classic hemodynamic finding in acute mitral regurgitation is a v wave on the pulmonary artery wedge pressure tracing, this finding is neither sensitive nor specific for the diagnosis of significant mitral regurgitation.[67] A v wave may be absent even with severe mitral regurgitation if left atrial pressures are low or if the compliance of the pulmonary venous bed is high. Conversely, a v wave may be present without severe mitral regurgitation in conditions associated with impaired left atrial emptying, including mitral stenosis, a prosthetic mitral valve, coronary artery disease, or a ventricular septal defect. In the patient with a new systolic murmur after myocardial infarction, comparison of oxygen saturation in the right atrium and ventricle is a more accurate way to differentiate acute mitral regurgitation from a ventricular septal defect.[67]

More sophisticated measurements at cardiac catheterization, such as measurement of left ventricular elastance, have provided important insights into the pathophysiology of this disease but are rarely needed for routine patient management.[34, 35]

NATURAL HISTORY

Patients with mitral regurgitation may remain asymptomatic for many years[26] with an average time from diagnosis to symptom onset of 16 years in one study.[68] After symptoms occur, outcome is improved with surgical intervention compared with medical therapy, with a reported survival of only 45% at 5 years without surgical intervention.[69] Even recent series show an actuarial survival of only 33% at 8 years for unoperated patients with symptomatic mitral regurgitation.[68] Further, it is well established that some patients with asymptomatic severe mitral regurgitation develop irreversible contractile dysfunction of the left ventricle, which often is masked by the afterload-reducing effect of the regurgitant lesion itself.[65, 70–78] Careful, periodic, noninvasive evaluation of left ventricular size and function is essential for optimizing the timing of surgical intervention in these patients (see Chapter 15).

Scanty data are available on the rate of hemodynamic progression of regurgitant severity, the rate of left ventricular dilation, or on the natural history of patients with only mild to moderate regurgitation. Moreover, the available data on the natural history of patients with mitral regurgitation is problematic for several reasons. First, most series have included only patients with severe mitral regurgitation and excluded those with lesser degrees of valvular incompetence. Second, the criteria for evaluating regurgitant severity have varied and were not always clearly defined. Third, patients with mitral regurgitation of different causes are often included in the same study. Since outcome of patients with mitral regurgitation may be primarily influenced by the underlying disease process, rather than regurgitant severity, interpretation of data from these mixed series is difficult. For example, the outcome of patients with mitral regurgitation due to ischemic cardiac disease may be predominantly affected by the severity of coronary artery disease, whereas in patients with a dilated cardiomyopathy, left ventricular systolic function may be the primary determinant of outcome.

Despite these limitations, studies suggest that patients with severe mitral regurgitation have an annual mortality rate of approximately 5% to 6% per year.[68, 79] Most deaths are related to heart failure, but sudden death in up to 5% of patients has been reported, even in the absence of significant left ventricular systolic dysfunction, suggesting that arrhythmias may be an important feature of the disease process.[80, 81] Other adverse outcomes of patients with mitral regurgitation include congestive heart failure, atrial fibrillation, cerebral ischemic events, and endocarditis.

Patients with mild to moderate mitral regurgitation have a much lower rate of cardiac events, with a 5-year event-free survival of more than 95% for those with mild regurgitation, 85% for those with moderate regurgitation, and 70% for those with severe regurgitation in a study of 229 patients with mitral valve prolapse.[82] In another study of mitral valve prolapse, patients with asymptomatic severe mitral regurgitation had a 10.3% annual risk of developing surgical indications.[64]

Myxomatous Mitral Valve Disease

Myxomatous mitral valve disease encompasses a wide spectrum of disease severity, ranging from young women with mitral valve prolapse and little mitral regurgitation to middle-aged men with severe leaflet prolapse or a flail leaflet and severe mitral regurgitation. This disease spectrum is reflected in the different clinical outcomes reported in series of patients with a flail leaflet and severe mitral regurgitation,[79] those with severe asymptomatic mitral regurgitation due to mitral valve prolapse,[64] and those with a range of mitral regurgitant severity (Table 13–4).[82, 83] Disease progression may be slow and insidious due to gradually more severe leaflet prolapse or may be more abrupt due to rupture of the valve chordae, resulting in a flail segment and an increase in the severity of mitral regurgitation.[84] These data are discussed in more detail in Chapter 14.

Rheumatic Disease

The relative frequency of rheumatic mitral regurgitation leading to valve replacement has decreased in Europe and North America, paralleling the declining prevalence of rheumatic heart disease in these countries (see Chapter 1). However, rheumatic disease continues to be a major cause of mitral regurgitation worldwide.

In acute rheumatic fever, left ventricular dilation and clinical heart failure probably are caused by the regurgitant lesion, not myocardial contractile dysfunction.[85–87] In a series of patients undergoing surgery for rheumatic mitral regurgitation, annular dilation, lengthen-

ing, and rupture of chordae with prolapse of the anterior leaflet leading to mitral regurgitation were associated with evidence of an active rheumatic process.[88] However, most other series report that acute rheumatic carditis is associated with valvular thickening, focal nodules, and restriction of leaflet mobility. Mitral regurgitation due to ventricular dilation is associated with restriction of leaflet motion, and prolapse and annular dilation are seen only rarely in other series.[85–87]

Chronically, scarring of the valve leaflets leads to mitral regurgitation because of shortening and increased rigidity of the valve leaflets in combination with shortening and fusion of the valve chordae; these changes lead to inadequate leaflet coaptation and apposition.[84] As with rheumatic mitral stenosis, the interval between acute rheumatic fever and the onset of symptoms due to chronic rheumatic valvular disease shows wide geographic variation.

Many patients with rheumatic mitral regurgitation have some degree of mitral stenosis and many have involvement of the aortic valve, tricuspid valve, or both valves. The natural history of the disease in an individual patient depends on the presence and severity of coexisting valve lesions as well as on the severity of mitral regurgitation. Rheumatic mitral regurgitation currently is most common in Africa, Asia, and South America, accounting for only 15% of cases in a European series of patients with mitral regurgitation.[68] In this study, the prognosis for rheumatic mitral regurgitation was better than for ischemic mitral regurgitation.[68]

Ischemic Mitral Regurgitation

The natural history of ischemic mitral regurgitation depends on the specific clinical setting and mechanism of mitral regurgitation. Ischemic mitral regurgitation can be divided into four general categories: papillary muscle rupture, mitral regurgitation in the setting of an acute myocardial infarction, mitral regurgitation due to reversible ischemia with preserved overall left ventricular systolic function, and mitral regurgitation associated with end-stage ischemic disease and severely reduced left ventricular systolic function (Fig. 13–14).[89]

Ischemic mitral regurgitation accounts for about one third of patients undergoing mitral valve replacement,[84] but the prevalence of ischemic mitral regurgitation probably is much higher than this estimate suggests, because

TABLE 13-4 NATURAL HISTORY OF SEVERE MITRAL REGURGITATION

Study	Patients	Cause of MR	Percent Male	Age (y)	Symptoms at Entry	LV-EF (%)	ESD	Long-Term Outcome	Predictors of Outcome
Ling, 1996[79]	229	Flail leaflet	70%	66 ± 13	53% Severe MR in 87%	65 ± 9	19 ± 4 mm/m²	Surgery or death: 90 ± 3% at 10 y CHF: 63 ± 8% 10 y AF: 30 ± 12% 10 y Annual mortality rate = 6.3%	Age, NYHA class, ejection fraction, LA size
Rosen, 1994[64]	31	MVP	61%	51 ± 13	Asymptomatic severe MR in all	57 ± 6	40 ± 5 mm	Surgery 28% at 5 y (for symptom onset)	Exercise change in RV-EF
Delahaye, 1991[68]	54	Ischemic 13%, MVP 44%, Rheumatic 15%, Endocarditis 9%	70%	59 ± 19	Severe MR in 91%	56 ± 17	42 ± 9 mm	Actuarial survival: 52 ± 7% at 5 y 33 ± 9% at 8 y	Ischemic MR LV-EF

MR, mitral regurgitation; CHF, congestive heart failure; AF, atrial fibrillation; EF, ejection fraction; LA, left atrial; NYHA, New York Heart Association; RV, right ventricular; MVP, mitral valve prolapse; ESD, end-systolic dimension.

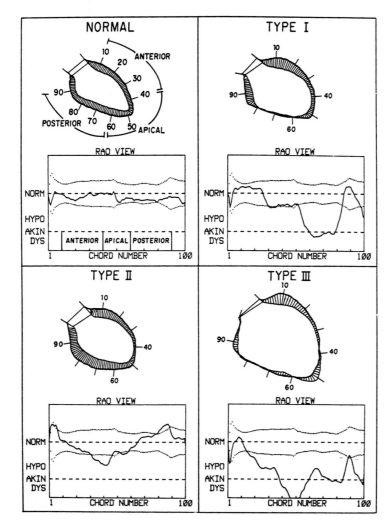

Figure 13·14 Schematic right anterior oblique (RAO) left ventriculograms allow categorization of ischemic mitral regurgitation into three types: type I, posterior papillary-annular dysfunction; type II, papillary muscle rupture; and type III, severe left ventricular dysfunction. A modified center-line regional wall motion analysis was used where the circumference of the right anterior oblique projection was divided into 100 equidistant chords, constructed perpendicular to a center line drawn midway between the end-diastolic and end-systolic contours. The shortening fraction for each chord was normalized by defining the average shortening observed for each chord in a normal group of 50 patients as 100% wall motion and by defining akinesis as 0%. Average chordal shortening was computed for the anterior wall (chords 11 through 40), the apical region (chords 41 through 60), and the posterior wall (chords 61 through 90). Chords 1 through 10 and 91 through 100 were omitted from the analysis because of greater variability in defining normal wall motion in the paravalvular regions. (From Rankin JS, Livesey SA, Smith LR, et al: Trends in the surgical treatment of ischemic mitral regurgitation: effects of mitral valve repair on hospital mortality. Semin Thorac Cardiovasc Surg 1989;1:149–163.)

most patients with ischemic regurgitation do not undergo mitral valve surgery. In addition, apparent differences in estimates of disease prevalence, treatment, and prognosis reflect the inclusion of several distinct mechanisms of valve dysfunction in the category of ischemic mitral regurgitation.

Patients with coronary artery disease and coexisting myxomatous mitral valve disease should not be classified as having ischemic mitral regurgitation, as there are substantial differences in both the overall prognosis and optimal treatment of myxomatous compared with ischemic mitral regurgitation.

Papillary Muscle Rupture

Localized transmural infarction can lead to partial or complete rupture of the papillary muscle or one of its heads, with consequent catastrophic acute mitral regurgitation. Papillary muscle rupture is a rare (<0.1%) complication of acute myocardial infarction, typically occurring several days after infarction.[89–92] Papillary muscle rupture can occur with small localized infarctions so that the regional wall motion abnormality is small and may be missed on a cursory examination. Complete papillary muscle rupture results in acute, massive mitral regurgitation and is rapidly fatal. Incomplete rupture or rupture of one head of a papillary muscle results in severe mitral regurgitation, pulmonary edema, and cardiogenic shock, but the patient is likely to survive to reach medical assistance.[37, 93]

Without surgical intervention, the mortality rate for papillary muscle rupture is extremely high; 75% of these patients die within 24 hours, and 95% die within 2 weeks.[94] Surgical mitral valve replacement usually is needed, as repair of the necrotic papillary muscle head rarely is feasible in the acute setting.[95–99] The mortality rate for emergent surgery for partial papillary muscle rupture is extremely high, averaging 50% in several series.[100–103] However, outcome is even worse with medical therapy, and the risk of surgical intervention varies depending on coronary anatomy, left ventricular function, comorbid diseases, and clinical status. Thus, surgical intervention can be lifesaving in appropriately selected patients.[89]

With improved imaging techniques there is increasing recognition of previously unsuspected partial papillary muscle rupture.[104–106] Some of these patients have less acute and less severe symptoms than patients described in earlier series of patients with papillary muscle rupture (Fig. 13–15).

Acute Myocardial Infarction

In addition to papillary muscle rupture, significant mitral regurgitation complicates 3% to 16% of acute myocardial infarctions by ischemic dysfunction of the papillary muscle or the underlying left ventricular wall.[107–109] Ischemic mitral regurgitation is primarily caused by

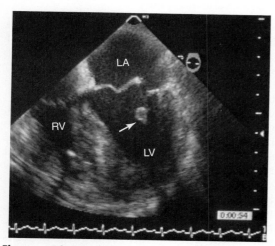

Figure 13·15 Transesophageal echocardiography shows partial papillary muscle rupture with a mobile mass (the papillary muscle head) in the left ventricle, attached to the mitral chordae, and prolapse of the mitral leaflet into the left atrium in systole. This 64-year-old man, who presented with symptoms of congestive heart failure, was found to have severe mitral regurgitation. He also was found to have two-vessel coronary disease at catheterization. The cause of the mitral regurgitation at surgery was partial papillary muscle rupture. LA, left atrium; LV, left ventricle; RV, right ventricle.

alterations in left ventricular regional function and shape, with normal valve leaflets and annular dimensions.[110] While most patients with acute ischemic mitral regurgitation present as an acute myocardial infarction with a subsequent diagnosis of mitral regurgitation, in as many as 22% of patients, the myocardial infarction itself is asymptomatic, and the initial presentation is cardiogenic shock.[106]

Mitral regurgitation caused by acute myocardial infarction most often (in 80% of patients) complicates right coronary or circumflex artery disease. Although overall left ventricular systolic function is normal or only mildly reduced, regurgitation typically (in 86%) is associated with an inferior wall motion abnormality.[106] Mitral regurgitation severity is not related to infarct size but often results from localized ischemia or infarction of the posteromedial papillary muscle, with resultant loss of support of the medial aspects of anterior and posterior leaflets. On 2D echocardiography, the posterior leaflet appears to slide under the anterior leaflet in association with a posterolaterally directed mitral regurgitant jet. Mitral regurgitation is not diagnosed on physical examination for up to 50% of these patients, although whether this truly represents silent regurgitation or a failure to consider the diagnosis remains unclear.[107, 111]

Mitral regurgitation is a poor prognostic factor for patients with acute myocardial infarction; the mortality rate is 24% at 30 days and 52% at 1 year for patients with moderate to severe regurgitation.[107, 109, 111] Patients with mitral regurgitation tend to be older, female, have diabetes, cerebrovascular disease, and prior symptomatic coronary artery disease.[107] In patients receiving thrombolytic therapy, resolution of mitral regurgitation at follow-up is not predicted by coronary reperfusion.[107, 108] However, the effect of reperfusion on ischemic mitral regurgitation remains controversial, because other studies have suggested that surgical or percutaneous coronary revascularization restores valve competence.[112–116]

Chronic Ischemic Disease With Normal Resting Ventricular Function

In the setting of normal overall left ventricular systolic function, ischemic mitral regurgitation may result from a regional wall motion abnormality affecting a papillary muscle or underlying ventricular myocardium.[117] Most often, the medial papillary muscle or inferior ventricular wall is affected, producing a laterally directed mitral regurgitant jet. Patients with normal regional function at rest may develop ischemia with exercise, leading to intermittent mitral regurgitation. Intermittent ischemic mitral regurgitation may account for "atypical" exertional symptoms in patients with coronary artery disease. In some cases, the intermittent regurgitation may be so severe that episodes of "flash" pulmonary edema dominate the clinical picture.

The diagnosis of ischemic mitral regurgitation is based on the clinical presentation and auscultatory findings, with confirmation by echocardiography showing mitral regurgitation in association with a regional wall motion abnormality at rest or with stress. Although one small study showed that about one third of patients with inducible ischemia on dobutamine stress also have inducible mitral regurgitation,[118] a larger study found only rare cases of increased mitral regurgitation with dobutamine stress.[119]

The prognosis for a patient with mitral regurgitation due to a focal wall motion abnormality or intermittent ischemia is partially determined by the extent and severity of coronary artery disease. However, mitral regurgitation may lead to pulmonary congestion symptoms superimposed on anginal symptoms. Mitral regurgitation is associated with a poorer overall prognosis when coronary patients are stratified according to regurgitant severity.[89]

The medical treatment of ischemic mitral regurgitation focuses on prevention of ischemia with anti-anginal agents. Afterload reduction therapy may be helpful in selected patients. Surgical intervention remains controversial. Some investigators suggest that regurgitation may resolve with reperfusion of the ischemic areas, but others suggest that mitral valve repair with placement of an annuloplasty ring is needed to decrease regurgitant severity. It is probable that both points of view are correct, with some patients having regurgitation caused by intermittent ischemia and others having annular dilation associated with an inferior wall motion abnormality.[89, 113, 117, 120]

End-Stage Ischemic Disease and Ventricular Systolic Dysfunction

Mitral regurgitation commonly occurs in patients with left ventricular dilation and systolic dysfunction resulting from end-stage ischemic disease with the degree of regurgitation ranging from mild to severe. Typically, the valve

leaflets and chordae are structurally normal, so that the regurgitation is considered to be functional rather than anatomic, a concept that is supported by the sometimes dramatic decrease in regurgitant severity in response to changes in loading conditions. However, the concept of functional regurgitation is not strictly correct, since the 3D anatomic relationships of the valve apparatus are distorted.

There are several possible mechanisms of mitral regurgitation in patients with end-stage ischemic disease, including annular dilation,[121, 122] inadequate papillary muscle traction caused by myocardial ischemia, an obtuse angle between the papillary muscle and mitral annular plane,[123, 124] and altered left ventricular geometry[125] in association with dilation and systolic dysfunction. In addition, an occasional patient has combined end-stage ischemic disease and a primary anatomic abnormality of the mitral valve, such as rheumatic disease or myxomatous mitral valve disease.

Mitral regurgitation caused by end-stage ischemic disease may decrease in response to vasodilator therapy. This decrease in mitral regurgitation is due to a combination of factors including reduced preload, normalization of left ventricular geometry, and reduced afterload.

Dilated Cardiomyopathy

Significant mitral regurgitation often occurs in patients with a dilated cardiomyopathy of any cause and may contribute to heart failure symptoms.[126] As in end-stage ischemic disease, there appear to be diverse mechanisms of mitral regurgitation in this patient group, including annular dilation, left ventricular systolic dysfunction and dilation, and altered ventricular geometry with distortion of the normal subvalvular relationships (Fig. 13–16).[127] Mitral regurgitation due to dilated cardiomyopathy can be differentiated from end-stage left ventricular dilation and dysfunction due to severe mitral regurgitation based on whether the mitral leaflets and chordae are anatomically abnormal or whether mitral regurgitation is functional due to annular and ventricular dilation. The clinical history often is useful in this differentiation, although occasionally, a patient initially presents with severe mitral regurgitation and severe ventricular dysfunction with few clues about which is the primary abnormality.

In general, dilated cardiomyopathy patients with significant mitral regurgitation have lower

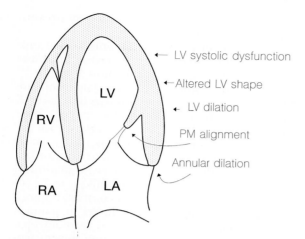

Figure 13·16 Schematic diagram illustrating potential mechanisms of mitral regurgitation in patients with left ventricular dilation and systolic dysfunction. LA, left atrium; LV, left ventricle; PM, papillary muscle; RA, right atrium; RV, right ventricle.

ejection fractions and larger ventricular volumes than those without mitral regurgitation.[128] The prognosis of patients with mitral regurgitation and dilated cardiomyopathy depends on the prognosis of the underlying cardiomyopathy and the severity of ventricular dysfunction.

Mitral regurgitation associated with dilated cardiomyopathy may respond favorably to vasodilator therapy with a decrease in regurgitant volume and improvement in ejection performance.[129, 130] In addition, some investigators suggest that these patients may benefit from surgical placement of an annuloplasty ring to decrease regurgitant severity, despite severe ventricular systolic dysfunction.[126]

MEDICAL THERAPY

Noninvasive Follow-up

In addition to a periodic clinical history and physical examination, noninvasive evaluation is critical for following disease progression in patients with significant mitral regurgitation, specifically for identification of those who may benefit from surgical intervention prior to the onset of overt clinical symptoms. Typically, echocardiography is the preferred method for periodic evaluation as it allows measurement of left ventricular dimensions, volumes, and ejection fraction; measurement of left atrial size; and estimation of pulmonary pressures. Resting and exercise radionuclide ventriculography provide an alternate approach for serial evaluation. Radionuclide studies have the advantage that a quantitative evaluation of right, as well as left, ventricular ejection fractions can be obtained. The disadvantages of the radionuclide approach, compared with echocardiography, are the inability to directly visualize the valve or to evaluate left atrial size, pulmonary pressures, and coexisting valve lesions.

After an initial complete echocardiographic study to define the mechanism and severity of disease, repeat examinations can focus on left ventricular size and function and on secondary changes such as left atrial enlargement and pulmonary pressures. Any significant interim change in clinical status necessitates a more complete examination.

The timing of repeat examinations should be tailored to the specific clinical situation. For the patient with chronic disease, no symptoms, and only mild left ventricular dilation, annual examinations often are appropriate. More frequent examination is warranted for the patient with significant ventricular dilation or evidence of increasing pulmonary pressures. Less frequent evaluation may be adequate for the patient with only mild or moderate regurgitation, depending on the cause of valve dysfunction.

Whenever the optimal timing of sequential studies is unclear, it is helpful to obtain an evaluation at a second time point, for example, in 3 to 6 months, to determine whether the findings are stable or if there is rapid disease progression. This approach is most helpful when a new patient is found to have abnormalities close to the limits that would indicate the need for surgical intervention. If there is no change between the two examinations, subsequent studies can be scheduled at longer intervals, whereas an interval change prompts continued frequent follow-up.

Prevention of Endocarditis and Recurrent Rheumatic Fever

Patients with mitral regurgitation are at high risk for endocarditis and should receive appropriate antibiotic prophylaxis, as discussed in Chapter 6. Patients with rheumatic mitral valve disease also should receive antibiotic treatment to prevent recurrent rheumatic fever.

Vasodilator Therapy

There has been a sustained interest in the concept that afterload (or vasodilator) therapy might favorably impact mitral regurgitant severity, decrease the rate of left ventricular dilation, and improve clinical outcome. There are at least two potential mechanisms of benefit: (1) decreased left ventricular preload might allow more complete mitral valve closure with a reduced regurgitant orifice area, and (2) decreased left ventricular afterload might lead to an increase in antegrade flow across the aortic valve with a corresponding decrease in retrograde flow across the mitral valve. Support for the first of these mechanisms is derived from an animal model of mitral regurgitation, which showed that nitroprusside infusion resulted in a decrease in mitral regurgitant severity in association with a reduction in regurgitant orifice area. Since all pressures decreased to a similar extent, there was no change in the left ventricular to atrial systolic pressure gradient.[22]

The short-term effects of vasodilator administration in patients with chronic mitral regurgitation have been evaluated in a number of studies. Despite heterogeneity and the small numbers of subjects, several conclusions are evident.[29] Treatment with intravenous nitroprusside[131–133] and hydralazine[134, 135] decrease systemic vascular resistance and regurgitant fraction, often with a decrease in ventricular volumes and end-diastolic pressure. Forward cardiac output increases, implying a reduction in the regurgitant fraction.

In general, nitrates reduce end-diastolic volume but do not change regurgitant fraction or forward cardiac output.[136, 137] However, in two studies of patients with severe heart failure due to dilated cardiomyopathy and mitral regurgitation, intravenous nitroglycerin decreased regurgitant volume and increased forward stroke volume in association with a decrease in left ventricular volumes and systemic vascular resistance, but no change in ejection fraction.[25, 138] In addition, a small, randomized trial of oral isosorbide and nifedipine for 14 days in patients with mitral regurgitation showed a reduction in regurgitant fraction, a decrease in ventricular volumes, and an increase in forward cardiac output.[139]

The acute effects of angiotensin-converting enzyme inhibitors are less clear, with discrepant results reported from different studies.[140–143] One clinical study found a decrease in resting left ventricular end-diastolic pressure and an improvement in exercise hemodynamics.[143] In an animal model, enalapril therapy for 3 months led to stabilization of mitral regurgitant severity and left ventricular dimensions compared with controls, suggesting that prevention of ventricular dilation may prevent progressive mitral regurgitation.[144]

One long-term study of patients treated with an angiotensin-converting enzyme inhibitor found a decrease in regurgitant fraction,[144] while another study found no change in ventricular volumes or ejection fraction after 6 months of therapy.[145] To some extent, these apparent differences may be related to the etiology of mitral regurgitation in the study groups. The regurgitant orifice area in patients with rheumatic mitral regurgitation is relatively fixed and, thus, is unlikely to be affected by medical therapy. In contrast, regurgitant orifice area may be reduced in patients with ischemic disease or dilated cardiomyopathy in association with a reduction in ventricular size. This hypothesis is supported by studies showing that, in patients with dilated cardiomyopathy and mitral regurgitation, captopril therapy results in a greater improvement in exercise tolerance, increased forward stroke volume, and decreased ventricular dimensions compared with those without mitral regurgitation.[129] In addition, there was a trend toward a reduction in mitral regurgitant volume at 6 to 12 months of follow-up.[130]

Levine and Gaasch[29] conclude that vasodilators are most effective in patients with mitral regurgitation associated with left ventricular dilation, poor systolic function, and significant symptoms. Less benefit is seen in symptomatic patients with only moderate left ventricular dilation. There is no detectable benefit in asymptomatic patients with only minimal left ventricular enlargement. Currently, while vasodilator therapy is appropriate for patients with significant mitral regurgitation and left ventricular dilation (ie, those with dilated cardiomyopathy or end-stage ischemic disease), the benefits of vasodilator therapy are less clear for patients with moderate regurgitation due to leaflet involvement or regional ventricular dysfunction. Therefore, therapy should be individualized, with objective demonstration of benefit, if possible. Despite the physiologic rationale for afterload reduction to prevent left ventricular dilation in chronic mitral regurgitation, there is no convincing evidence that prophylactic treatment in the asymptomatic patient is beneficial. Medical therapy has not been shown to prevent or delay the time until surgical intervention and is not an alternative to surgical treatment.

Management of Acute Mitral Regurgitation

Acute mitral regurgitation is a medical and surgical emergency. The patient may be stabilized initially by intravenous afterload reduction therapy (eg, nitroprusside) or placement of an intraaortic balloon pump to optimize afterload reduction and maintain coronary blood flow.[22, 131, 133, 146, 147] Surgical intervention is needed to correct both the regurgitant lesion itself and the underlying disease process, when appropriate. Nonsurgical approaches occasionally may be helpful. For example, it has been suggested that ischemic mitral regurgitation might respond to percutaneous revascularization with resolution of regional ischemia.[148] However, when acute mitral regurgitation is caused by papillary muscle rupture, surgical intervention is needed despite the high risk, because outcome with medical therapy alone is dismal.[89, 101, 112, 149]

Surgical risk is related to the clinical status of the patient, overall left ventricular systolic dysfunction, and the etiology of acute regurgitation, with surgical mortality rates as high as 50% for patients with acute mitral regurgitation due to papillary muscle rupture.[89, 101, 112, 149] Surgical risk is lower for patients with acute regurgitation due to myocardial infarction without papillary muscle rupture, mitral valve endocarditis, or chordal rupture with a partial flail leaflet. In addition, the surgical risk is related to the patient's overall clinical status and whether mitral valve repair can be performed.

Timing of Surgical Intervention

For the patient with symptoms from severe mitral regurgitation, surgical intervention improves long-term outcome and relieves symptoms. Surgical treatment of mitral regurgitation due to left ventricular dilation and systolic dysfunction, dilated cardiomyopathy, or end-stage ischemic disease remains more controversial with the major concern being the possibility of worsened left ventricular function postoperatively as a result of increased afterload and loss of normal mitral annular to papillary muscle continuity.[150]

The optimal timing of surgical intervention to prevent left ventricular systolic dysfunction in the *asymptomatic* patient also remains a difficult clinical decision. Predictors of clinical outcome, surgical options, and an approach making decisions about this patient group are presented in Chapter 15.

Other Therapeutic Considerations

Although patients with recent-onset atrial fibrillation are likely to revert to sinus rhythm after surgical intervention for mitral regurgitation, those with atrial fibrillation of longer duration are likely to remain in atrial fibrillation so that the patient remains at increased risk for atrial thrombi and embolic events postoperatively. In one study of more than 300 patients undergoing mitral valve surgery, only 5% of the 216 patients in sinus rhythm were in atrial fibrillation postoperatively. In contrast, of the 97 patients with atrial fibrillation at baseline, 80% were still in atrial fibrillation after mitral valve surgery.[151] Although the 11 patients with recent-onset atrial fibrillation (<3 months) were in sinus rhythm postoperatively in this study, my clinical experience suggests that even with recent-onset atrial fibrillation it may not be possible to restore and maintain sinus rhythm for the long term in all patients.

These data have led to the suggestion that the atrial maze procedure should be considered concurrently with mitral valve surgery to restore sinus rhythm.[151–153] Results with combined mitral valve surgery and the maze procedure have been promising in initial surgical series, with sinus rhythm restored in more than 80% of patients, even when atrial fibrillation had been present for several years before surgical intervention.[154, 155] Sinus rhythm was maintained at follow-up intervals ranging from 1 to 3 years, with evidence of effective atrial contraction.[156, 157] Even among those undergoing repeat mitral valve surgery, sinus rhythm can be restored in 67% of patients using the maze procedure, with Doppler evidence of effective atrial contraction in 75% of those in sinus rhythm.[158] Successful conversion to sinus rhythm is related to age, left atrial size, and cardiothoracic ratio and is most likely in patients with a postoperative atrial dimension of less than 40 mm.[156]

However, despite encouraging results in small series from a few academic medical centers, surgeons continue to be concerned about the combination of mitral valve surgery and the maze procedure. First, the potential benefit is restricted to patients with atrial fibrillation undergoing mitral valve repair, because those undergoing valve replacement need long-term anticoagulation in any case. Few candidates for mitral valve repair are in atrial fibrillation given a trend toward earlier referral for surgical intervention. Second, although reported mortality is no different from that of patients undergoing similar surgery without the maze procedure, cardiopulmonary bypass and cardiac arrest times are almost 50%

greater with the combined procedure.[156] Given these concerns, larger-scale clinical trials of a combined approach to patients with mitral valve disease and atrial fibrillation are needed before this approach is widely utilized.

References

1. Perloff JK, Roberts WC: The mitral apparatus: functional anatomy of mitral regurgitation. Circulation 1972;46:227–239.
2. Roberts WC: Morphologic features of the normal and abnormal mitral valve. Am J Cardiol 1983;51:1005–1028.
3. He S, Fontaine AA, Schwammenthal E, Yoganathan AP, Levine RA: Integrated mechanism for functional mitral regurgitation—leaflet restriction versus coapting force: in vitro studies. Circulation 1997;96:1826–1834.
4. Otsuji Y, Handschumacher MD, Schwammenthal E, et al: Insights from three-dimensional echocardiography into the mechanism of functional mitral regurgitation: direct in vivo demonstration of altered leaflet tethering geometry. Circulation 1997;96:1999–2008.
5. Lee CS, Talbot TL: A fluid-mechanical study of the closure of heart valves. J Fluid Mechanics 1979;91:41–63.
6. Bellhouse BJ, Bellhouse FH: Fluid mechanics of the mitral valve. Nature 1969;224:615.
7. Bellhouse BJ: Fluid mechanics of a model mitral valve and left ventricle. Cardiovasc Res 1972;6:199.
8. Levine RA, Handschumacher MD, Sanfilippo AJ, et al: Three-dimensional echocardiographic reconstruction of the mitral valve, with implications for the diagnosis of mitral valve prolapse. Circulation 1989;80:589–598.
9. Westaby S, Karp RB, Blackstone EH, Bishop SP: Adult human valve dimensions and their surgical significance. Am J Cardiol 1984;53:552–556.
10. Klues HG, Roberts WC, Maron BJ: Morphological determinants of echocardiographic patterns of mitral valve systolic anterior motion in obstructive hypertrophic cardiomyopathy. Circulation 1993;87:1570–1579.
11. Lewis JF, Kuo LC, Nelson JG, Limacher MC, Quinones MA: Pulsed Doppler echocardiographic determination of stroke volume and cardiac output: clinical validation of two methods using the apical window. Circulation 1984;70:425–431.
12. Kunzelman KS, Grande KJ, David TE, Cochran RP, Verrier ED: Aortic root and valve relationships. Impact on surgical repair [published erratum appears in J Thorac Cardiovasc Surg 1994;107:1402]. J Thorac Cardiovasc Surg 1994;107:162–170.
13. Ormiston JA, Shah PM, Tei C, Wong M: Size and motion of the mitral valve annulus in man. I. A two-dimensional echocardiographic method and findings in normal subjects. Circulation 1981;64:113–120.
14. Komoda T, Hetzer R, Uyama C, et al: Mitral annular function assessed by 3D imaging for mitral valve surgery. J Heart Valve Dis 1994;3:483–490.
15. Ormiston JA, Shah PM, Tei C, Wong M: Size and motion of the mitral valve annulus in man. II. Abnormalities in mitral valve prolapse. Circulation 1982;65:713–719.
16. Keren G, Sonnenblick EH, LeJemtel TH: Mitral annulus motion. Relation to pulmonary venous and transmitral flows in normal subjects and in patients with dilated cardiomyopathy. Circulation 1988;78:621–629.
17. Hoglund C, Alam M, Thorstrand C: Atrioventricular valve plane displacement in healthy persons: an echocardiographic study. Acta Med Scand 1988;224:557–562.
18. Simonson JS, Schiller NB: Descent of the base of the left ventricle: an echocardiographic index of left ventricular function. J Am Soc Echocardiogr 1989;2:25–35.
19. Sanfilippo AJ, Abascal VM, Sheehan M, et al: Atrial enlargement as a consequence of atrial fibrillation: a prospective echocardiographic study. Circulation 1990;82:792–797.
20. Tanimoto M, Pai RG: Effect of isolated left atrial enlargement on mitral annular size and valve competence. Am J Cardiol 1996;77:769–774.
21. Mann JM, Davies MJ: The pathology of the mitral valve. *In* Wells FC, Shapiro LM, eds. Mitral Valve Disease. London: Butterworth, 1996:16–27.
22. Yoran C, Yellin EL, Becker RM, Gabbay S, Frater RW, Sonnenblick EH: Mechanism of reduction of mitral regurgitation with vasodilator therapy. Am J Cardiol 1979;43:773–777.
23. Braunwald E: Mitral regurgitation: physiologic, clinical and surgical considerations. N Engl J Med 1969;281:425–433.
24. Eckberg DL, Gault JH, Bouchard RL, Karliner JS, Ross J Jr: Mechanics of left ventricular contraction in chronic severe mitral regurgitation. Circulation 1973;47:1252–1259.
25. Keren G, Bier A, LeJemtel TH: Improvement in forward cardiac output without a change in ejection fraction during nitroglycerin therapy in patients with functional mitral regurgitation. Can J Cardiol 1986;2:206–211.
26. Selzer A, Katayama F: Mitral regurgitation: clinical patterns, pathophysiology and natural history. Medicine (Baltimore) 1972;51:337–366.
27. Pape LA, Price JM, Alpert JS, Ockene IS, Weiner BH: Relation of left atrial size to pulmonary capillary wedge pressure in severe mitral regurgitation. Cardiology 1991;78:297–303.
28. Burwash IG, Blackmore GL, Koilpillai CJ: Usefulness of left atrial and left ventricular chamber sizes as predictors of the severity of mitral regurgitation. Am J Cardiol 1992;70:774–779.
29. Levine HJ, Gaasch WH: Vasoactive drugs in chronic regurgitant lesions of the mitral and aortic valves. J Am Coll Cardiol 1996;28:1083–1091.
30. Urschel CW, Covell JW, Sonnenblick EH, Ross J Jr, Braunwald E: Myocardial mechanics in aortic and mitral valvular regurgitation: the concept of instantaneous impedance as a determinant of the performance of the intact heart. J Clin Invest 1968;47:867–883.
31. Imamura T, McDermott PJ, Kent RL, Nagatsu M, Cooper G, Carabello BA: Acute changes in myosin heavy chain synthesis rate in pressure versus volume overload. Circ Res 1994;75:418–425.
32. Ross J Jr: Applications and limitations of end-systolic measures of ventricular performance. Fed Proc 1984;43:2418–2422.
33. Carabello BA: The changing unnatural history of valvular regurgitation. Ann Thorac Surg 1992;53:191–199.
34. Starling MR, Kirsh MM, Montgomery DG, Gross

MD: Impaired left ventricular contractile function in patients with long-term mitral regurgitation and normal ejection fraction. J Am Coll Cardiol 1993;22:239–250.

35. Starling MR: Effects of valve surgery on left ventricular contractile function in patients with long-term mitral regurgitation. Circulation 1995;92:811–818.

36. Kihara Y, Sasayama S, Miyazaki S, et al: Role of the left atrium in adaptation of the heart to chronic mitral regurgitation in conscious dogs. Circ Res 1988;62:543–553.

37. Roberts WC, Braunwald E, Morrow AG: Acute severe mitral regurgitation secondary to ruptured chordae tendineae: clinical, hemodynamic, and pathologic considerations. Circulation 1966;33:58–70.

38. Braunwald E, Awe WC: The syndrome of severe mitral regurgitation with normal left atrial pressure. Circulation 1963;27:29.

39. Coulshed N, Epstein EJ, McKendrick CS, Galloway RW, Walker E: Systemic embolism in mitral valve disease. Br Heart J 1970;32:26–34.

40. Davison G, Greenland P: Predictors of left atrial thrombus in mitral valve disease. J Gen Intern Med 1991;6:108–112.

41. Blackshear JL, Pearce LA, Asinger RW, et al: Mitral regurgitation associated with reduced thromboembolic events in high-risk patients with nonrheumatic atrial fibrillation. Stroke Prevention in Atrial Fibrillation Investigators. Am J Cardiol 1993;72:840–843.

42. Wanishsawad C, Weathers LB, Puavilai W: Mitral regurgitation and left atrial thrombus in rheumatic mitral valve disease: a clinicopathologic study. Chest 1995;108:677–681.

43. Karatasakis GT, Gotsis AC, Cokkinos DV: Influence of mitral regurgitation on left atrial thrombus and spontaneous echocardiographic contrast in patients with rheumatic mitral valve disease. Am J Cardiol 1995;76:279–281.

44. Movsowitz C, Movsowitz HD, Jacobs LE, Meyerowitz CB, Podolsky LA, Kotler MN: Significant mitral regurgitation is protective against left atrial spontaneous echo contrast and thrombus as assessed by transesophageal echocardiography. J Am Soc Echocardiogr 1993;6:107–114.

45. Shields JP, Watson P, Mielke CH Jr: The right ventricle in mitral regurgitation: evaluation by electron beam tomography. J Heart Valve Dis 1995;4:490–494.

46. Tischler MD, Battle RW, Ashikaga T, Niggel J, Rowen M, LeWinter MM: Effects of exercise on left ventricular performance determined by echocardiography in chronic, severe mitral regurgitation secondary to mitral valve prolapse. Am J Cardiol 1996;77:397–402.

47. Keren G, Katz S, Strom J, Sonnenblick EH, LeJemtel TH: Dynamic mitral regurgitation: an important determinant of the hemodynamic response to load alterations and inotropic therapy in severe heart failure. Circulation 1989;80:306–313.

48. Spain MG, Smith MD, Kwan OL, DeMaria AN: Effect of isometric exercise on mitral and aortic regurgitation as assessed by color Doppler flow imaging. Am J Cardiol 1990;65:78–83.

49. Cohen LS, Mason DT, Braunwald E: Significance of an atrial gallop sound in mitral regurgitation: a clue to the diagnosis of ruptured chordae tendineae. Circulation 1967;35:112–118.

50. Basta LL, Wolfson P, Eckberg DL, Abboud FM: The value of left parasternal impulse recordings in the assessment of mitral regurgitation. Circulation 1973;48:1055–1065.

51. Perloff JK: Physical Examination of the Heart and circulation. Philadelphia: WB Saunders, 1982.

52. Desjardins VA, Enriquez Sarano M, Tajik AJ, Bailey KR, Seward JB: Intensity of murmurs correlates with severity of valvular regurgitation. Am J Med 1996;100:149–156.

53. Sutton GC, Craige E: Clinical signs of severe acute mitral regurgitation. Am J Cardiol 1967;20:141–144.

54. Nellen M, Maurer B, Goodwin JF: Value of physical examination in acute myocardial infarction. Br Heart J 1973;35:777–780.

55. Antman EM, Angoff GH, Sloss LJ: Demonstration of the mechanism by which mitral regurgitation mimics aortic stenosis. Am J Cardiol 1978;42:1044–1048.

56. Merendino KA, Hessel EA: The "murmur on top of the head" in acquired mitral insufficiency: pathological and clinical significance. JAMA 1967;199:892–896.

57. Bentivoglio LG, Urricchio JF, Waldow A, et al: An electrocardiographic analysis of sixty-five cases of mitral regurgitation. Circulation 1958;18:572.

58. Levine RA, Handschumacher MD, Sanfilippo AJ, et al: Three-dimensional echocardiographic reconstruction of the mitral valve, with implications for the diagnosis of mitral valve prolapse. Circulation 1989;80:589–598.

59. Smith MD, Cassidy JM, Gurley JC, Smith AC, Booth DC: Echo Doppler evaluation of patients with acute mitral regurgitation: superiority of transesophageal echocardiography with color flow imaging. Am Heart J 1995;129:967–974.

60. Enriquez Sarano M, Sinak LJ, Tajik AJ, Bailey KR, Seward JB: Changes in effective regurgitant orifice throughout systole in patients with mitral valve prolapse: a clinical study using the proximal isovelocity surface area method. Circulation 1995;92:2951–2958.

61. Stoddard MF, Prince CR, Dillon S, Longaker RA, Morris GT, Liddell NE: Exercise-induced mitral regurgitation is a predictor of morbid events in subjects with mitral valve prolapse. J Am Coll Cardiol 1995;25:693–699.

62. Tischler MD, Battle RW, Saha M, Niggel J, LeWinter MM: Observations suggesting a high incidence of exercise-induced severe mitral regurgitation in patients with mild rheumatic mitral valve disease at rest. J Am Coll Cardiol 1995;25:128–133.

63. Leung DY, Griffin BP, Snader CE, Luthern L, Thomas JD, Marwick TH: Determinants of functional capacity in chronic mitral regurgitation unassociated with coronary artery disease or left ventricular dysfunction. Am J Cardiol 1997;79:914–920.

64. Rosen SE, Borer JS, Hochreiter C, et al: Natural history of the asymptomatic/minimally symptomatic patient with severe mitral regurgitation secondary to mitral valve prolapse and normal right and left ventricular performance. Am J Cardiol 1994;74:374–380.

65. Leung DY, Griffin BP, Stewart WJ, Cosgrove DM, Thomas JD, Marwick TH: Left ventricular function after valve repair for chronic mitral regurgitation: predictive value of preoperative assessment of contractile reserve by exercise echocardiography. J Am Coll Cardiol 1996;28:1198–1205.

66. Kennedy JW, Yarnall SR, Murray JA, Figley MM:

Quantitative angiocardiography. IV. Relationships of left atrial and ventricular pressure and volume in mitral valve disease. Circulation 1970;41:817–824.

67. Fuchs RM, Heuser RR, Yin FC, Brinker JA: Limitations of pulmonary wedge V waves in diagnosing mitral regurgitation. Am J Cardiol 1982;49:849–854.

68. Delahaye JP, Gare JP, Viguier E, Delahaye F, de Gevigney G, Milon H: Natural history of severe mitral regurgitation. Eur Heart J 1991;12(suppl B):5–9.

69. Munoz S, Gallardo J, Diaz Gorrin JR, Medina O: Influence of surgery on the natural history of rheumatic mitral and aortic valve disease. Am J Cardiol 1975;35:234–242.

70. Kennedy JW, Doces JG, Stewart DK: Left ventricular function before and following surgical treatment of mitral valve disease. Am Heart J 1979;97:592–598.

71. Pitarys CJ, Forman MB, Panayiotou H, Hansen DE: Long-term effects of excision of the mitral apparatus on global and regional ventricular function in humans. J Am Coll Cardiol 1990;15:557–563.

72. Crawford MH, Souchek J, Oprian CA, et al: Determinants of survival and left ventricular performance after mitral valve replacement: Department of Veterans Affairs Cooperative Study on Valvular Heart Disease. Circulation 1990;81:1173–1181.

73. David TE, Burns RJ, Bacchus CM, Druck MN: Mitral valve replacement for mitral regurgitation with and without preservation of chordae tendineae. J Thorac Cardiovasc Surg 1984;88:1718–1725.

74. Miki S, Kusuhara K, Ueda Y, Komeda M, Ohkita Y, Tahata T: Mitral valve replacement with preservation of chordae tendineae and papillary muscles. Ann Thorac Surg 1988;45:28–34.

75. Goldman ME, Mora F, Guarino T, Fuster V, Mindich BP: Mitral valvuloplasty is superior to valve replacement for preservation of left ventricular function: an intraoperative two-dimensional echocardiographic study. J Am Coll Cardiol 1987;10:568–575.

76. Rozich JD, Carabello BA, Usher BW, Kratz JM, Bell AE, Zile MR: Mitral valve replacement with and without chordal preservation in patients with chronic mitral regurgitation: mechanisms for differences in postoperative ejection performance. Circulation 1992;86:1718–1726.

77. Corin WJ, Sutsch G, Murakami T, Krogmann ON, Turina M, Hess OM: Left ventricular function in chronic mitral regurgitation: preoperative and postoperative comparison. J Am Coll Cardiol 1995;25:113–121.

78. Enriquez Sarano M, Tajik AJ, Schaff HV, et al: Echocardiographic prediction of left ventricular function after correction of mitral regurgitation: results and clinical implications. J Am Coll Cardiol 1994;24:1536–1543.

79. Ling LH, Enriquez Sarano M, Seward JB, et al: Clinical outcome of mitral regurgitation due to flail leaflet. N Engl J Med 1996;335:1417–1423.

80. Hochreiter C, Niles N, Devereux RB, Kligfield P, Borer JS: Mitral regurgitation: relationship of noninvasive descriptors of right and left ventricular performance to clinical and hemodynamic findings and to prognosis in medically and surgically treated patients. Circulation 1986;73:900–912.

81. Kligfield P, Hochreiter C, Kramer H, et al: Complex arrhythmias in mitral regurgitation with and without mitral valve prolapse: contrast to arrhythmias in mitral valve prolapse without mitral regurgitation. Am J Cardiol 1985;55:1545–1549.

82. Kim S, Kuroda T, Nishinaga M, et al: Relationship between severity of mitral regurgitation and prognosis of mitral valve prolapse: echocardiographic follow-up study. Am Heart J 1996;132:348–355.

83. Zuppiroli A, Rinaldi M, Kramer Fox R, Favilli S, Roman MJ, Devereux RB: Natural history of mitral valve prolapse. Am J Cardiol 1995;75:1028–1032.

84. Hickey AJ, Wilcken DE, Wright JS, Warren BA: Primary (spontaneous) chordal rupture: relation to myxomatous valve disease and mitral valve prolapse. J Am Coll Cardiol 1985;5:1341–1346.

85. Essop MR, Wisenbaugh T, Sareli P: Evidence against a myocardial factor as the cause of left ventricular dilation in active rheumatic carditis. J Am Coll Cardiol 1993;22:826–829.

86. Barlow JB, Marcus RH, Pocock WA, Barlow CW, Essop R, Sareli P: Mechanisms and management of heart failure in active rheumatic carditis. S Afr Med J 1990;78:181–186.

87. Vasan RS, Shrivastava S, Vijayakumar M, Narang R, Lister BC, Narula J: Echocardiographic evaluation of patients with acute rheumatic fever and rheumatic carditis. Circulation 1996;94:73–82.

88. Marcus RH, Sareli P, Pocock WA, Barlow JB: The spectrum of severe rheumatic mitral valve disease in a developing country: correlations among clinical presentation, surgical pathologic findings, and hemodynamic sequelae. Ann Intern Med 1994;120:177–183.

89. Rankin JS, Hickey MS, Smith LR, et al: Ischemic mitral regurgitation. Circulation 1989;79:16–21.

90. Reeder GS: Identification and treatment of complications of myocardial infarction. Mayo Clin Proc 1995;70:880–884.

91. Coma Canella I, Gamallo C, Onsurbe PM, Jadraque LM: Anatomic findings in acute papillary muscle necrosis. Am Heart J 1989;118:1188–1192.

92. Nishimura RA, McGoon MD, Shub C, Miller FA Jr, Ilstrup DM, Tajik AJ: Echocardiographically documented mitral-valve prolapse: long-term follow-up of 237 patients. N Engl J Med 1985;313:1305–1309.

93. Becker AE, Anderson RH: Mitral insufficiency complicating acute myocardial infarction. Eur J Cardiol 1975;2:351–359.

94. Wei JY, Hutchins GM, Bulkley BH: Papillary muscle rupture in fatal acute myocardial infarction: a potentially treatable form of cardiogenic shock. Ann Intern Med 1979;90:149–152.

95. Rankin JS, Feneley MP, Hickey MS, et al: A clinical comparison of mitral valve repair versus valve replacement in ischemic mitral regurgitation. J Thorac Cardiovasc Surg 1988;95:165–177.

96. Killen DA, Reed WA, Wathanacharoen S, Beauchamp G, Rutherford B: Surgical treatment of papillary muscle rupture. Ann Thorac Surg 1983;35:243–248.

97. Clements SD Jr, Story WE, Hurst JW, Craver JM, Jones EL: Ruptured papillary muscle, a complication of myocardial infarction: clinical presentation, diagnosis, and treatment. Clin Cardiol 1985;8:93–103.

98. Nishimura RA, Schaff HV, Shub C, Gersh BJ, Edwards WD, Tajik AJ: Papillary muscle rupture complicating acute myocardial infarction: analysis of 17 patients. Am J Cardiol 1983;51:373–377.

99. Gula G, Yacoub MH: Surgical correction of complete rupture of the anterior papillary muscle. Ann Thorac Surg 1981;32:88–91.

100. Disesa VJ, Cohn LH, Collins JJ Jr, Koster JK Jr, Van-

Devanter S: Determinants of operative survival following combined mitral valve replacement and coronary revascularization. Ann Thorac Surg 1982;34:482–489.

101. Tepe NA, Edmunds LH Jr: Operation for acute post-infarction mitral insufficiency and cardiogenic shock. J Thorac Cardiovasc Surg 1985;89:525–530.

102. Gerbode FL, Hetzer R, Krebber HJ: Surgical management of papillary muscle rupture due to myocardial infarction. World J Surg 1978;2:791–796.

103. Merin G, Giuliani ER, Pluth JR, Wallace RB, Danielson GK: Surgery for mitral valve incompetence after myocardial infarction. Am J Cardiol 1973;32:322–324.

104. Manning WJ, Waksmonski CA, Boyle NG: Papillary muscle rupture complicating inferior myocardial infarction: identification with transesophageal echocardiography. Am Heart J 1995;129:191–193.

105. Buda AJ: The role of echocardiography in the evaluation of mechanical complications of acute myocardial infarction. Circulation 1991;84:109–121.

106. Sharma SK, Seckler J, Israel DH, Borrico S, Ambrose JA: Clinical, angiographic and anatomic findings in acute severe ischemic mitral regurgitation. Am J Cardiol 1992;70:277–280.

107. Tcheng JE, Jackman JD Jr, Nelson CL, et al: Outcome of patients sustaining acute ischemic mitral regurgitation during myocardial infarction. Ann Intern Med 1992;117:18–24.

108. Lehmann KG, Francis CK, Sheehan FH, Dodge HT: Effect of thrombolysis on acute mitral regurgitation during evolving myocardial infarction: experience from the Thrombolysis in Myocardial Infarction (TIMI) trial. J Am Coll Cardiol 1993;22:714–719.

109. Barzilai B, Davis VG, Stone PH, Jaffe AS: Prognostic significance of mitral regurgitation in acute myocardial infarction. The MILIS Study Group. Am J Cardiol 1990;65:1169–1175.

110. Van Dantzig JM, Delemarre BJ, Koster RW, Bot H, Visser CA: Pathogenesis of mitral regurgitation in acute myocardial infarction: importance of changes in left ventricular shape and regional function. Am Heart J 1996;131:865–871.

111. Lehmann KG, Francis CK, Dodge HT: Mitral regurgitation in early myocardial infarction. Incidence, clinical detection, and prognostic implications. TIMI Study Group [published erratum appears in Ann Intern Med 1992;15;117:349]. Ann Intern Med 1992; 117:10–17.

112. Hickey MS, Smith LR, Muhlbaier LH, et al: Current prognosis of ischemic mitral regurgitation. Implications for future management. Circulation 1988;78:51–59.

113. Rankin JS, Hickey MS, Smith LR, et al: Current management of mitral valve incompetence associated with coronary artery disease. J Card Surg 1989;4:25–42.

114. Reinfeld HB, Samet P, Hildner FJ: Resolution of congestive failure, mitral regurgitation, and angina after percutaneous transluminal coronary angioplasty of triple vessel disease. Cathet Cardiovasc Diagn 1985;11:273–277.

115. Heuser RR, Maddoux GL, Goss JE, Ramo BW, Raff GL, Shadoff N: Coronary angioplasty for acute mitral regurgitation due to myocardial infarction: a nonsurgical treatment preserving mitral valve integrity. Ann Intern Med 1987;107:852–855.

116. Leor J, Feinberg MS, Vered Z, et al: Effect of thrombolytic therapy on the evolution of significant mitral regurgitation in patients with a first inferior myocardial infarction. J Am Coll Cardiol 1993;21:1661–1666.

117. Kaul S, Spotnitz WD, Glasheen WP, Touchstone DA: Mechanism of ischemic mitral regurgitation: an experimental evaluation. Circulation 1991;84:2167–2180.

118. Mazeika PK, Nadazdin A, Oakley CM: Influence of haemodynamics and myocardial ischaemia on Doppler transmitral flow in patients undergoing dobutamine echocardiography. Eur Heart J 1994;15:17–25.

119. Heinle SK, Tice FD, Kisslo J: Effect of dobutamine stress echocardiography on mitral regurgitation. J Am Coll Cardiol 1995;25:122–127.

120. Kay GL, Kay JH, Zubiate P, Yokoyama T, Mendez M: Mitral valve repair for mitral regurgitation secondary to coronary artery disease. Circulation 1986;74:88–98.

121. Boltwood CM, Tei C, Wong M, Shah PM: Quantitative echocardiography of the mitral complex in dilated cardiomyopathy: the mechanism of functional mitral regurgitation. Circulation 1983;68:498–508.

122. Izumi S, Miyatake K, Beppu S, et al: Mechanism of mitral regurgitation in patients with myocardial infarction: a study using real-time two-dimensional Doppler flow imaging and echocardiography. Circulation 1987;76:777–785.

123. Waller BF, Howard J, Fess S: Pathology of mitral valve stenosis and pure mitral regurgitation—part I. Clin Cardiol 1994;17:330–336.

124. Waller BF, Howard J, Fess S: Pathology of mitral valve stenosis and pure mitral regurgitation—part II. Clin Cardiol 1994;17:395–402.

125. Kono T, Sabbah HN, Rosman H, et al: Mechanism of functional mitral regurgitation during acute myocardial ischemia. J Am Coll Cardiol 1992;19:1101–1105.

126. Bach DS, Bolling SF: Early improvement in congestive heart failure after correction of secondary mitral regurgitation in end-stage cardiomyopathy. Am Heart J 1995;129:1165–1170.

127. Kono T, Sabbah HN, Rosman H, Alam M, Jafri S, Goldstein S: Left ventricular shape is the primary determinant of functional mitral regurgitation in heart failure. J Am Coll Cardiol 1992;20:1594–1598.

128. Junker A, Thayssen P, Nielsen B, Andersen PE: The hemodynamic and prognostic significance of echo-Doppler-proven mitral regurgitation in patients with dilated cardiomyopathy. Cardiology 1993;83:14–20.

129. Evangelista MA, Bruguera CJ, Serrat SR, et al: Influence of mitral regurgitation on the response to captopril therapy for congestive heart failure caused by idiopathic dilated cardiomyopathy. Am J Cardiol 1992;69:373–376.

130. Keren G, Pardes A, Eschar Y, et al: One-year clinical and echocardiographic follow-up of patients with congestive cardiomyopathy treated with captopril compared with placebo. Isr J Med Sci 1994;30:90–98.

131. Chatterjee K, Parmley WW, Swan HJ, Berman G, Forrester J, Marcus HS: Beneficial effects of vasodilator agents in severe mitral regurgitation due to dysfunction of subvalvar apparatus. Circulation 1973;48:684–690.

132. Goodman DJ, Rossen RM, Holloway EL, Alderman EL, Harrison DC: Effect of nitroprusside on left ventricular dynamics in mitral regurgitation. Circulation 1974;50:1025–1032.

133. Harshaw CW, Grossman W, Munro AB, McLaurin LP: Reduced systemic vascular resistance as therapy for severe mitral regurgitation of valvular origin. Ann Intern Med 1975;83:312–316.

134. Greenberg BH, Massie BM, Brundage BH, Botvinick EH, Parmley WW, Chatterjee K: Beneficial effects of hydralazine in severe mitral regurgitation. Circulation 1978;58:273–279.

135. Greenberg BH, DeMots H, Murphy E, Rahimtoola SH: Arterial dilators in mitral regurgitation: effects on rest and exercise hemodynamics and long-term clinical follow-up. Circulation 1982;65:181–187.

136. Sniderman AD, Marpole DG, Palmer WH, Fallen EL: Response of the left ventricle to nitroglycerin in patients with and without mitral regurgitation. Br Heart J 1974;36:357–361.

137. Elkayam U, Roth A, Kumar A, et al: Hemodynamic and volumetric effects of venodilation with nitroglycerin in chronic mitral regurgitation. Am J Cardiol 1987;60:1106–1111.

138. Hamilton MA, Stevenson LW, Child JS, Moriguchi JD, Walden J, Woo M: Sustained reduction in valvular regurgitation and atrial volumes with tailored vasodilator therapy in advanced congestive heart failure secondary to dilated (ischemic or idiopathic) cardiomyopathy. Am J Cardiol 1991;67:259–263.

139. Kelbaek H, Aldershvile J, Skagen K, Hildebrandt P, Nielsen SL: Pre- and afterload reduction in chronic mitral regurgitation: a double-blind randomized placebo-controlled trial of the acute and 2 weeks' effect of nifedipine or isosorbide dinitrate treatment on left ventricular function and the severity of mitral regurgitation. Br J Clin Pharmacol 1996;41:493–497.

140. Heck I, Schmidt J, Mattern H, Fricke G, Kropp J, Reske S: Reduction of regurgitation in aortic and mitral insufficiency by captopril in acute and long-term trials [in German]. Schweiz Med Wochenschr 1985;115:1615–1618.

141. Wisenbaugh T, Essop R, Sareli P: Short-term vasodilator effect of captopril in patients with severe mitral regurgitation is parasympathetically mediated. Circulation 1991;84: 2049–2053.

142. Rothlisberger C, Sareli P, Wisenbaugh T: Comparison of single dose nifedipine and captopril for chronic severe mitral regurgitation. Am J Cardiol 1994;73:978–981.

143. Schon HR: Hemodynamic and morphologic changes after long-term angiotensin converting enzyme inhibition in patients with chronic valvular regurgitation. J Hypertens Suppl 1994;12:S95–104.

144. Shimoyama H, Sabbah HN, Rosman H, Kono T, Alam M, Goldstein S: Effects of long-term therapy with enalapril on severity of functional mitral regurgitation in dogs with moderate heart failure. J Am Coll Cardiol 1995;25:768–772.

145. Wisenbaugh T, Sinovich V, Dullabh A, Sareli P: Six month pilot study of captopril for mildly symptomatic, severe isolated mitral and isolated aortic regurgitation. J Heart Valve Dis 1994;3:197–204.

146. Sasayama S, Takahashi M, Osakada G, et al: Dynamic geometry of the left atrium and left ventricle in acute mitral regurgitation. Circulation 1979;60:177–186.

147. Horstkotte D, Schulte HD, Niehues R, Klein RM, Piper C, Strauer BE: Diagnostic and therapeutic considerations in acute, severe mitral regurgitation: experience in 42 consecutive patients entering the intensive care unit with pulmonary edema. J Heart Valve Dis 1993;2:512–522.

148. Le Feuvre C, Metzger JP, Lachurie ML, Georges JL, Baubion N, Vacheron A: Treatment of severe mitral regurgitation caused by ischemic papillary muscle dysfunction: indications for coronary angioplasty. Am Heart J 1992;123:860–865.

149. Replogle RL, Campbell CD: Surgery for mitral regurgitation associated with ischemic heart disease: results and strategies. Circulation 1989;79:122–125.

150. Christenson JT, Simonet F, Bloch A, Maurice J, Velebit V, Schmuziger M: Should a mild to moderate ischemic mitral valve regurgitation in patients with poor left ventricular function be repaired or not? J Heart Valve Dis 1995;4:484–488.

151. Chua YL, Schaff HV, Orszulak TA, Morris JJ: Outcome of mitral valve repair in patients with preoperative atrial fibrillation: should the maze procedure be combined with mitral valvuloplasty? J Thorac Cardiovasc Surg 1994;107:408–415.

152. Cox JL: The surgical treatment of atrial fibrillation. IV. Surgical technique. J Thorac Cardiovasc Surg 1991;101:584–592.

153. Cox JL, Schuessler RB, D'Agostino HJ Jr, et al: The surgical treatment of atrial fibrillation. III. Development of a definitive surgical procedure. J Thorac Cardiovasc Surg 1991;101:569–583.

154. Cox JL, Boineau JP, Schuessler RB, Kater KM, Lappas DG: Five-year experience with the maze procedure for atrial fibrillation. Ann Thorac Surg 1993;56:814–823.

155. Sandoval N, Velasco VM, Orjuela H, et al: Concomitant mitral valve or atrial septal defect surgery and the modified Cox-maze procedure. Am J Cardiol 1996;77:591–596.

156. Kawaguchi AT, Kosakai Y, Isobe F, et al: Surgical stratification of patients with atrial fibrillation secondary to organic cardiac lesions. Eur J Cardiothorac Surg 1996;10:983–989.

157. Ueshima K, Hashimoto K, Chiba M, et al: Recovery of atrial function after combined treatment with surgical repair for organic heart disease and maze procedure for atrial fibrillation. J Thorac Cardiovasc Surg 1997;113:214–215.

158. Kobayashi J, Kosakai Y, Isobe F, et al: Rationale of the Cox maze procedure for atrial fibrillation during redo mitral valve operations. J Thorac Cardiovasc Surg 1996;112:1216–1221.

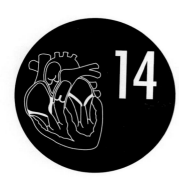

14 Mitral Valve Prolapse

DEFINITION AND DISEASE SPECTRUM

The definition of mitral valve prolapse has evolved as we have learned more about the clinical manifestations of this disease, but interpretation of the literature is confounded by the various definitions and variety of terms used in the past to designate this disease process. The possibility that the same term has been used to refer to different clinical entities or that patients with more than one disease process have been included in the same study group should be considered when comparing clinical studies. Given the overdiagnosis of mitral valve prolapse early in our experience with two-dimensional (2D) echocardiography, it is probable that many early studies included patients who now would be classified as normal. Adding to the confusion are two distinct clinical patterns of disease in patients with mitral valve prolapse.

Most clinical data support the concept that mitral valve prolapse is a genetic connective tissue disorder that primarily affects the mitral leaflets, chordae, and annulus with an autosomal dominant pattern of inheritance and variable penetrance.[1–6] Although the specific gene defect(s) has not been identified, the definition of mitral valve prolapse used throughout this chapter is a primary genetic disorder resulting in anatomic abnormalities of the mitral valve apparatus.

The key features in making a diagnosis of mitral valve prolapse on auscultation are a mid- to late-systolic click and late systolic murmur. Echocardiographic findings include thickened leaflets with marked systolic displacement into the left atrium, often associated with mitral regurgitation.[1, 2] The diagnosis is most secure when both auscultatory and echocardiographic findings are present; however, the diagnosis can be confirmed by echocardiography alone when definitive findings are seen (Figs. 14–1 and 14–2).

There appear to be at least two clinically distinct groups of patients with mitral valve prolapse.[7] The first group consists of younger patients, typically female, with a mid-systolic click and late-systolic murmur on auscultation, in whom the clinical course is benign. This group of patients often is referred to as having mitral valve prolapse "syndrome." The second group consists of older patients, typically male, with marked leaflet thickening and redundancy and chordal rupture, associated with significant mitral regurgitation that often necessitates surgical intervention.[8] The more specific pathologic term, *myxomatous mitral valve disease*, often is used for this group of patients (Table 14–1).

The underlying genetic or environmental reasons for the differences between these two groups of patients remain unclear. One possibility is that closely related, but slightly different genetic defects account for the differences. This situation may be similar to the genetic

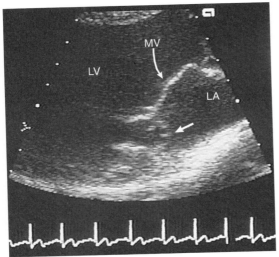

Figure 14·1 Parasternal long-axis echocardiographic view in systole of the mitral valve (MV) shows marked prolapse of the posterior leaflet *(straight arrow)*. LA, left atrium; LV, left ventricle.

TABLE 14·1   CLASSIFICATION OF MITRAL VALVE PROLAPSE

Mitral valve prolapse syndrome
   Younger age (20–50)
   Predominantly female
   Click or click-murmur on examination
   Thin leaflets with systolic displacement on
     echocardiography
   Associated with low blood pressure, orthostatic
     hypotension, palpitations
   Benign long-term outcome
Myxomatous mitral valve disease
   Older age (40–70)
   Predominantly male
   Mitral regurgitation on examination and
     echocardiography
   High likelihood of progressive disease requiring mitral
     valve surgery
Secondary mitral valve prolapse
   Marfan's syndrome
   Hypertrophic cardiomyopathy
   Ehlers-Danlos syndrome

defects in patients with Marfan's syndrome, which all affect the fibrillin gene but which vary between and even within families.[9, 10] Another possibility is that the differences in clinical presentation are gender related. The hypothesis that estrogen or other hormonal effects modulate clinical manifestations is supported by the observation that symptoms in women with mitral valve prolapse typically occur during the reproductive years and that mitral valve prolapse often "resolves" after menopause. A third possibility is related to the difference in ventricular size, geometry, and response to altered hemodynamic states in men and women.[11] Perhaps women gradually "correct" mitral prolapse through a gradual increase in annular size, such that the disproportion between leaflet area and annulus size gradually decreases. In contrast, men may have worsening of prolapse due to a fixed annulus size in conjunction with increased leaflet area. Further clinical and genetic studies are needed to resolve these issues.

Using the definition of mitral valve prolapse as an inherited connective tissue disorder primarily affecting the valve apparatus, it is clear that patients with apparent systolic displacement of normal mitral leaflets do not have mitral valve prolapse. Some investigators have shown that systolic displacement can be induced in individuals with normal mitral valve anatomy when ventricular size is decreased,[12, 13] although another study found no evidence for inducible prolapse with acute volume depletion.[14] In addition, patients with mitral leaflet displacement caused by another disease process (eg, Marfan's syndrome) should not be considered to have mitral valve prolapse syndrome, because the abnormality of the mitral apparatus is a feature of the underlying disease process rather than a primary abnormality of the mitral valve.

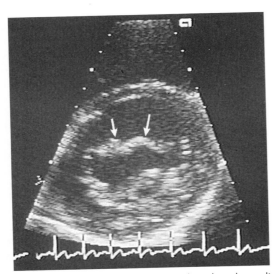

Figure 14·2 Parasternal short-axis diastolic echocardiographic view in the same patient as in Figure 14·1. Thickened mitral leaflets are indicated by an increase in the brightness and thickness of the leaflets on the image. Leaflet redundancy is evidenced by the increased area of the leaflet, resulting in a folded appearance *(arrows)* of the open leaflet in diastole.

In Europe and North America, mitral valve prolapse is probably the most common cause of mitral valve disease, although rheumatic disease accounts for the majority of mitral valve disease worldwide. In surgical series of patients undergoing mitral valve repair or replacement, the prevalence of mitral valve prolapse is 20% to 70%.[15–20] The most reliable clinical estimates suggest that mitral valve prolapse affects about 3% to 6% of adults,[7, 21–23] an estimate confirmed by autopsy series showing a 5% prevalence of mitral valve prolapse.[24, 25] Earlier studies suggesting that mitral valve prolapse affects up to 38% of adults (particularly young women)[26, 27] were based on different definitions of mitral valve prolapse and probably included many normal individuals considering the wide range of normal mitral valve anatomy and the more precise echocardiographic criteria that are now widely accepted.

ANATOMY AND PATHOLOGY

The macroscopic criteria for mitral valve prolapse are an increased leaflet area with opaque and thickened leaflets, chordae elongation and thinning, and dilation of the mitral annulus compared with normal controls.[28, 29] Given the normal variability in mitral valve anatomy and changes with aging, more quantitative criteria often are used; specifically, more than 4 mm of interchordal leaflet hooding into the left atrium involving at least one half of the anterior leaflet or two thirds of the posterior leaflet.[28] The thickness of both leaflets, the length of the posterior leaflet, and annular dimensions increase with age in patients with mitral valve prolapse.[29] In general, severe mitral regurgitation is associated with thicker leaflets, longer posterior leaflet dimensions, and a larger annulus. In patients with mitral valve prolapse, commissural fusion is absent. Calcification is rare, being seen only in elderly patients with superimposed degenerative changes.

In addition to leaflet thickening and redundancy, the mitral chordae are abnormal, with an irregular distribution of chordae,[30] a deficiency of commissural chordae,[30, 31] a relative scarcity of chordae to the middle scallop of the posterior leaflet, an increased frequency of chordal divisions,[28] and a high prevalence of chordal rupture.[8, 32]

On histologic examination, the mitral leaflets show thickening of the spongiosa and disruption of the fibrosa, with fragmentation, splitting, and disarray of collagen fibers and possibly a reduction in the amount of ground substance.[24, 33–36] The distribution of collagen in the chordae also is irregular.[35] Other histologic findings include platelet and fibrin deposits caused by endocardial friction lesions that may involve the chordae as well as the valve leaflets.[37]

The valves from patients with mitral valve prolapse show a higher rate of collagen synthesis than normal valves.[38] A normal valve contains collagen types I, III, and V. Valve tissue from patients with mitral prolapse shows a deficiency of type III collagen[39] and an altered ratio of other collagen types.[40, 41]

Despite the strong evidence that mitral valve prolapse results from a genetic defect,[2–6] the specific abnormal gene has not been identified. Although defects in collagen were thought to be likely factors in the disease process, no abnormalities in the loci encoding the major collagen components have been found.[42, 43] Another possibility is that mitral valve prolapse is caused by a defect in a gene encoding a component of microfibrils, analogous to the defect in Marfan's syndrome.

CLINICAL PRESENTATION

Symptoms

Given the variable definitions of mitral valve prolapse in the literature, the nonspecific symptoms, and the overlap in symptoms between normal subjects, patients with mitral prolapse, and those with other clinical syndromes, it has been somewhat difficult to define which symptoms are truly related to the underlying disease process. Patients with significant mitral regurgitation tend to present with symptoms similar to other patients with mitral regurgitation, particularly exercise limitation and dyspnea, but they may be diagnosed while asymptomatic based on the physical examination finding of a mitral regurgitant murmur (Table 14–2).

Patients with mitral valve prolapse often are asymptomatic. When symptoms do occur, they typically are related to associated arrhythmias or to mitral regurgitation. In natural history studies of mitral valve prolapse, about 65% of patients are asymptomatic at the time of diagnosis. In those with symptoms, the most common symptoms are atypical chest pain, palpitations, dyspnea, fatigue, and dizziness. Due to the nonspecific nature of these symptoms, it remains unclear whether these symptoms are related to mitral valve prolapse or if

TABLE 14·2 CLINICAL MANIFESTATIONS OF MITRAL VALVE PROLAPSE

Primary anatomic abnormality of mitral valve
  Click or click-murmur on auscultation
  Echocardiographic evidence for >2-mm displacement
    of the leaflet into the left atrium in systole in a long-
    axis view
  Pathologic evidence of thickened, redundant leaflets
  Histologic evidence of an increase in the spongiosa
    layer of the leaflet
Hemodynamics
  Mitral regurgitation
  Left atrial and ventricular enlargement
  Eventual left ventricular systolic dysfunction
  Pulmonary hypertension
Clinical complications
  Arrhythmias and sudden death
  Embolic events
  Endocarditis
  Mitral valve surgery

the complaints simply led to a careful cardiac examination that revealed auscultatory evidence of mitral prolapse.

The diagnosis of mitral valve prolapse in asymptomatic individuals often is made because of findings on auscultation, an echocardiogram ordered for unrelated reasons, or findings in family members. Echocardiographic evaluation has a very low yield in adults with nonspecific cardiovascular symptoms and no click detected on physical examination with mitral prolapse found in only 1% to 2% of these patients (less than the estimated prevalence of the disease). In contrast, echocardiographic screening of first-degree family members demonstrates mitral prolapse in about 30% of cases.[23]

Although early studies suggested that mitral valve prolapse is associated with a variety of symptoms, including atypical chest pain, dyspnea, and psychologic symptoms, these associations have not been substantiated by carefully performed, controlled studies.[22, 44–50] In these studies, the prevalence of these symptoms was similar among patients with and without mitral prolapse. As in other patient groups, the possibility of coexisting coronary artery disease should be considered in mitral valve prolapse patients with chest pain, depending on associated risk factors for coronary artery disease.

Physical Examination

The pathognomonic physical examination finding in a patient with mitral valve prolapse is a mid-systolic click and late-systolic murmur on cardiac auscultation (Fig. 14–3). The basis for the mid-systolic click is abrupt tensing of the mitral valve leaflets at their limit of displacement into the left atrium in systole, a motion pattern that is well demonstrated on echocardiography. The murmur is late systolic, rather than holosystolic, because of competency of the valve early in systole, with inadequate leaflet coaptation occurring only after the prolapsed leaflets reach their maximum displacement. As mitral regurgitation becomes more severe, regurgitation becomes holosystolic, and the physical examination findings parallel those in patients with mitral regurgitation due to any cause.

The hallmark of the mid-systolic click in mitral valve prolapse is that its timing varies with changes in left ventricular volume.[51–55] A decrease in left ventricular size leads to earlier prolapse of the leaflets, so that the click is appreciated earlier in systole. With an increase in left ventricular size, prolapse and the click occur later in systole. Auscultation during maneuvers to increase (eg, squatting) and decrease (eg, standing) left ventricular volume enhances recognition of the click, allows demonstration of the dynamic nature of the lesion, and avoids confusion with a normally split S_1 heart sound in association with a benign midsystolic murmur.[23] With mitral valve prolapse, the mitral regurgitant murmur may increase as the patient stands from a squatting position because of the increased regurgitation associated with earlier systolic leaflet prolapse.

In some patients, auscultatory findings may be absent at rest and recognized only with maneuvers to decrease ventricular volume. In addition, the physical examination findings have substantial temporal variation in individual patients, with most patients showing some changes between examinations and up to 10% having diagnostic findings at only one of two examinations.[2] In clinical series of mitral valve prolapse patients, the classic finding of a midsystolic click with a late systolic murmur occurs in 18% to 44% of patients; single or multiple clicks without a murmur are found in 5% to 39%; and a holosystolic murmur with or without a click occurs in 22% to 47%.[2, 56, 57]

Other cardiac physical examination findings depend on the severity of mitral regurgitation. With severe regurgitation, pulmonary congestion and secondary pulmonary hypertension may be evident. The left ventricular apical impulse is hyperdynamic and may be enlarged or displaced if long-standing regurgitation has led to left ventricular dilation. Atrial fibrilla-

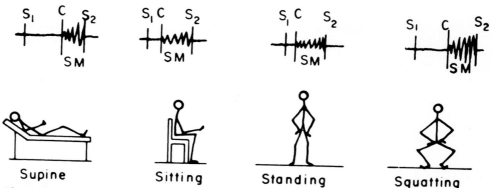

Figure 14·3 Postural changes affect the auscultatory signs of mitral prolapse. On sitting and standing, the systolic click moves closer to S_1, and the murmur is prolonged. On squatting, the click moves toward S_2, and the murmur becomes shorter. These auscultatory variations are related to changes in left ventricular volume and shape. (From Devereux RB, Perloff JK, Reichek N, Josephson ME: Mitral valve prolapse. Circulation 1976;54:3–4; by permission of The American Heart Association.)

tion also may coexist with chronic regurgitation.

Mitral valve prolapse is associated with a relatively low systolic blood pressure and with thoracic bony abnormalities.[44, 50, 58–60] Compared with normal subjects, patients with mitral prolapse have a higher prevalence of pectus excavatum (43%) and straight back (13%).[61] Patients with Marfan's syndrome also have a high prevalence of pectus excavatum, and they also have a very high prevalence of arachnodactyly, scoliosis, and increased arm span to height ratio, none of which is associated with mitral valve prolapse.[61]

Echocardiography

Early 2D echocardiographic criteria for mitral valve prolapse had poor specificity, resulting in overdiagnosis[27, 58] and leading to much of the confusion in the literature about the spectrum of clinical symptoms and outcome with this disease process. More specific echocardiographic criteria[62, 63] have resulted from the recognition of the wide normal range of variability in mitral valve anatomy. For example, isolated systolic chordal motion now is recognized as a normal finding. Demonstration that the three-dimensional shape of the mitral annulus is nonplanar (often described as saddle shaped) led to the realization that the mitral leaflets can appear to be on the left atrial side of the annulus in the apical four-chamber view, even though leaflet closure is normal, and other signs of mitral valve prolapse are absent.[63]

The current echocardiographic criteria for mitral valve prolapse are the presence of at least 2 mm of late-systolic posterior displacement of the leaflets on 2D-guided M-mode echocardiography or at least 2 mm of systolic billowing of one or both leaflets across the annulus plane in a 2D long-axis view.[7, 62, 63] More severe myxomatous disease is associated with leaflet thickening, increased leaflet area that appears as excessive folding or redundancy of the leaflets in diastole, chordal elongation, systolic anterior motion of the chordae, and associated mitral regurgitation (Figs. 14–4 and 14–5). Some investigators have suggested that, in parallel with the clinical distinction between younger patients with benign prolapse and older patients with severe regurgitation, there are two subsets seen on echocardiography: those with dynamic systolic expansion of the annulus causing posterior displacement of the leaflets in systole and those with systolic billowing and leaflet thickening.[11]

Morphologic features of the valve identified on echocardiography are strong predictors of clinical outcome of patients with mitral prolapse. In addition to evaluation of valve anatomy, the echocardiographic examination should include measurements of left ventricular size and systolic function, left atrial size, the degree of pulmonary hypertension, and assessment for myxomatous involvement of the tricuspid or aortic valves. The presence and severity of mitral regurgitation should be evaluated using standard Doppler techniques, as described in Chapter 3.

Prolapse of the tricuspid valve is seen in 9% to 23% of mitral valve prolapse patients.[64] Aortic valve involvement occurs less frequently.

Secondary mitral valve prolapse can be dif-

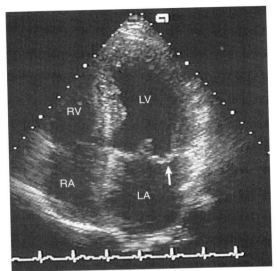

Figure 14·4 Apical four-chamber view in systole shows definite sagging of the enlarged and thickened posterior mitral leaflet *(arrow)* into the left atrium. This appearance can be differentiated from apparent prolapse seen in this view in normal individuals that is related to the saddle shape of the annulus by the definite bowing of the leaflet and the increased leaflet size and thickness. LV, left ventricle; LA, left atrium; RA, right atrium; RV, right ventricle.

ferentiated from primary mitral valve disease by the associated abnormalities, for example, in patients with Marfan's syndrome or hypertrophic cardiomyopathy. Pathologic and echocardiographic studies indicate that the valve anatomy in secondary mitral prolapse often differs strikingly from that in primary mitral valve disease. For example, Marfan's patients have a long, thin anterior leaflet that sags into the left atrium in systole.[65–67] Hypertrophic cardiomyopathy is associated with leaflet elongation and abnormal closure caused by systolic anterior motion, but these anatomic abnormalities are distinct from those seen in mitral valve prolapse.[68, 69]

Other Diagnostic Tests

Patients with mitral valve prolapse have no specific electrocardiographic or chest radiographic findings, other than the associated skeletal abnormalities. Patients with significant mitral regurgitation have electrocardiographic and radiographic changes consistent with mitral regurgitation, rather than mitral valve prolapse per se.

Although mitral valve prolapse can be appreciated on left ventricular angiography, and some cases are dramatic, the interobserver reproducibility of left ventricular angiography for the diagnosis of mitral valve prolapse is low. Thus, this technique is not reliable for confirmation or exclusion of the disease process.[70, 71] Genetic testing is not yet available.

NATURAL HISTORY
Overall Event-Free Survival and Complication Rates

Mitral valve prolapse accounts annually for about 4000 mitral valve operative procedures

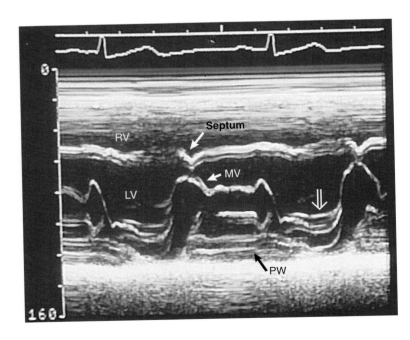

Figure 14·5 M-mode echocardiogram shows increased leaflet thickness *(arrow)* and systolic posterior motion of the leaflets *(open arrow)*. LV, left ventricle; MV, mitral valve; RV, right ventricle; PW, posterior wall.

(25% of all cases), more than 1000 cases of endocarditis (about 10% of all cases), and 4000 cases of sudden death (1% of all cases) in the United States.[23] Despite this significant rate of adverse outcomes, our understanding of the natural history of this disease is confounded by inclusion of patients with mitral valve prolapse syndrome and those with severe mitral regurgitation due to myxomatous mitral valve disease in the same clinical series. Since the clinical course and long-term outcome appear to be quite different for these two groups of patients, it is important to clarify which patient group is described in each study, when possible (Table 14–3).

Overall survival of patients with mitral prolapse is excellent, with survival rates of 97% at 6 years in one study[72] and 88% at 8 years in another series.[57] However, the overall complication rate averages 2% to 4% per year for minimally symptomatic or asymptomatic patients[57, 72, 73] to as high as 88% per year for mitral prolapse patients with severe mitral regurgitation and new symptom onset.[74, 75]

Predictors of Clinical Outcome

Several clinical factors predict the clinical outcome of patients with mitral valve prolapse, including gender, age, and mitral valve morphology. The strongest predictors of outcome are the severity of mitral regurgitation and associated findings of left atrial and left ventricular dilation (Table 14–4).[7, 57, 76]

Gender is an important predictor of clinical outcome for patients with mitral valve prolapse. Men have a cumulative risk for all complications of mitral prolapse of 5% to 10% by age 75, compared with 2% to 5% for women.[7, 21, 76] Women tend to be younger at presentation and have mitral valve prolapse syndrome with a mid-systolic click on auscultation, mild mitral regurgitation, minor skeletal abnormalities, palpitations, and orthostatic hypotension associated with a low body weight and low baseline blood pressure. Men tend to be older at the time of presentation and more often have thickened mitral valve leaflets with significant mitral regurgitation, often prompting surgical intervention.

Age also is predictive of outcome for mitral valve prolapse patients. Older patients have a higher rate of clinical events, even when each gender is evaluated separately.[7, 21, 76] For men with mitral valve prolapse, the cumulative lifetime risk for needing mitral surgery rises from

1 in 220 at age 50, to 1 in 53 at age 60, and to 1 in 28 at age 70 years.[21]

Some investigators suggest that auscultation provides important prognostic data, since patients with single or multiple apical systolic clicks, with or without a systolic murmur, have a low rate of cardiac events compared with those with severe mitral regurgitation.[56]

The morphology of the mitral valve apparatus has been identified as a predictor of outcome in several studies. In general, thicker and more redundant leaflets are associated with a higher likelihood of severe mitral regurgitation and the need for valve surgery.[57, 64, 77] In these studies, the definitions of leaflet thickening and redundancy vary. In the earlier studies, only M-mode echocardiography was available. The M-mode measurement of mitral leaflet "thickness" reflects redundancy as well, since multiple acoustic targets from the same leaflet within the ultrasound beam appear as separate (or thicker) lines on the M-mode tracing. Even with 2D imaging, measurements of leaflet thickness are problematic because of the limitations of ultrasound imaging. A leading edge to leading edge measurement is most accurate but is not feasible with a planar structure, such as a leaflet. Beam width characteristics, transducer frequency, acoustic penetration, and the angle between the ultrasound beam and valve leaflet can affect apparent leaflet thickness. Therefore, the echocardiographer should describe the valve in terms of thickness and redundancy from multiple acoustic windows, and no single numerical value should be used to classify patients as "high risk." It is likely that risk increases gradually as leaflet thickness and redundancy increase, rather than risk suddenly changing from low to high at a specific leaflet thickness.

Mitral Regurgitation

The degree of mitral regurgitation in patients with mitral valve prolapse corresponds roughly to the extent of leaflet thickening and redundancy. The rate of valve replacement for regurgitation in series of patients with mitral valve prolapse varies from 0.4 per 100 patient-years in series of asymptomatic patients to 90% at 10 years in series of patients diagnosed with a flail leaflet segment (Figs. 14–6 and 14–7).[57, 64, 72, 74, 76, 78, 79] Predictors of the need for mitral valve surgery include mitral regurgitant severity, mitral leaflet redundancy and thickening, patient age, male gender, and evidence of left ventricular and left atrial dilation.

TABLE 14-3 NATURAL HISTORY OF MITRAL VALVE PROLAPSE

Study	Definition of MVP	Patients	Percent Female	Mean Age (y)	Symptoms	MR Severity	Mean F/U Duration (y)	Survival	MVR	Endo	Sudden Death	CVA	Predictors of Outcome
Kolibash, 1986[74]	M-mode echo or LV angiography	86	38%	60	85% CHF	All had severe MR	1.0	—	88%	—	—	—	LV-EDD <60 mm Cardiomegaly on CXR Redundant MV-leaflets
Nishimura, 1985[57]	≥3 mm late or holosystolic bowing of mitral leaflets (M-mode)	237	60%	44	None or minimal	Not reported	6.2	88% (8 y)	7.2%	1.3%	2.5%	0.8%	
Duran, 1988[72]	Auscultation plus cine or echo	300	55%	42	Variable	Variable	6.1	97%	9.3%	6%	1%	3.6%	
Marks, 1989[64]	Systolic MV leaflet displacement in PLAX view	456	58%	47	NR	Redundant leaflets: 12% severe MR, 51% none / No leaflet thickening: 0% severe MR, 87% none	Redundant leaflets (n = 319) / No leaflet thickening (n = 137)		6.6%* / 0.7%	3.5%* / 0%		7.5% / 5.8%	Leaflet thickening and redundancy
Tofler, 1990[56]	Mid-systolic click	291	67%		Yes	Murmur on examination: 66%	8	99%	2%	0%	0%		
Zuppiroli, 1995[76]	M-mode echo: ≥2 mm late systolic or ≥3 mm holosystolic posterior leaflet motion	316	70%	42 ± 15	Variable	Variable	8.5		0.4/100 pt-year	0.1/100 pt-year	0.2/100 pt-year	0.3/100 pt-year	Male gender Age >45 years Holosystolic murmur LV-EDD ≥60 mm LA dimension ≥40 mm

*$P < .05$ compared to group with no leaflet thickening.

CHF, congestive heart failure; echo, echocardiography; MR, mitral regurgitation; MVP, mitral valve prolapse; NR, not reported; PLAX, parasternal long-axis; LV, left ventricle; LA, left atrium; EDD, end diastolic dimension; CVA, cerebrovascular accident; MVR, mitral valve replacement; Endo, endocarditis; CXR, chest radiograph; MV, mitral valve.

TABLE 14·4   PREDICTORS OF CLINICAL OUTCOME IN MITRAL VALVE PROLAPSE

Factor	Survival	Valve Surgery	Arrhythmias or Sudden Death	Endocarditis
Age	+ + +*	+ + +	–	–
Gender	+ +	+ +	–	–
Leaflet thickness or redundancy	+ + +	+ + +	+ + + +	+ + + +
Severity of mitral regurgitation	+ + + +	+ + + +	+ + + +	+ + + +
Systolic click	+	–	–	+ + + +
Left ventricular dilation	+	+ + + +	–	–
Left atrial dilation	–	+ +	+ +	–

*The symbols indicate the relative predictive value of each variable for the listed clinical outcomes on a scale of no predictive value (–) to strongly predictive (+ + + +).

The natural history of mitral regurgitation due to mitral prolapse takes two forms. Some patients have a gradual increase in left atrial and left ventricular size associated with progressive annular dilation and increasing mitral regurgitation. The natural history of the disorder in this group of patients is similar to that for chronic mitral regurgitation of any cause.[80–83] The rate of progression of regurgitant severity in patients with mitral prolapse tends to increase with age. In addition, there is marked variability in the rate of progression, with 52% of patients in one series showing an increase in regurgitant severity (as estimated by color flow imaging) over 2 years but the remainder showing no progression.[84] An increase in the severity of mitral regurgitation was more common in those with posterior leaflet prolapse (52% versus 17%, P < .05). Mitral regurgitation, as evidenced by a systolic murmur, is associated with progressive increases in left ventricular and left atrial dimensions in mitral prolapse patients,[85] as expected with chronic mitral regurgitation.

In other mitral valve prolapse patients, disease progression is nonlinear, with an acute increase in mitral regurgitant severity occurring at the time of chordal rupture. These patients may have only mild regurgitation and a stable clinical course for many years, only to present with a rapid deterioration in clinical status or even frank pulmonary edema because of chordal rupture (Fig. 14–8). The prevalence of chordal rupture is 7%[86] to 71%[32] in autopsy series, and the middle scallop of the posterior leaflet is affected most frequently. Not surprisingly, patients with a flail leaflet segment due to chordal rupture have an extremely high rate of symptom onset or left ventricular dilation requiring surgical intervention. By 10 years, 63% ± 8% of these patients have developed heart failure, 30% ± 12% have developed atrial fibrillation, and 90% ± 3% have undergone valve replacement or died (Fig. 14–9). Predictors of death of patients with a flail leaflet segment include older age, more severe symptoms, and a reduced ejection fraction.[79]

Figure 14·6 Relation between development of cardiac events and initial severity of mitral regurgitation in 229 patients with mitral valve prolapse during follow-up study. Mitral regurgitation was found to be nonexistent or trivial in 62 subjects *(dashed line)*, mild in 83 *(thin line)*, moderate in 50 *(medium line)*, and severe in 34 *(thick line)*. *, P < .05 compared with mild regurgitation; **, P < .01 compared with moderate mitral regurgitation. (From Kim S, Kuroda T, Nishinaga M, et al: Relationship between severity of mitral regurgitation and prognosis of mitral valve prolapse: echocardiographic follow-up study. Am Heart J 1996;132:348–355.)

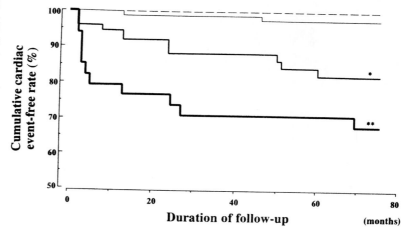

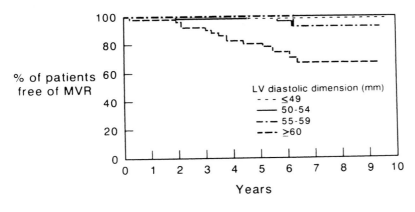

Figure 14·7 Association of initial left ventricular (LV) diastolic dimension with eventual mitral valve replacement (MVR) in 237 initially asymptomatic or minimally symptomatic patients with mitral valve prolapse. (From Nishimura RA, McGoon MD, Shub C, Miller FA Jr, Ilstrup DM, Tajik AJ: Echocardiographically documented mitral-valve prolapse: long-term follow-up of 237 patients. N Engl J Med 1985;313:1305–1309; reprinted by permission from the New England Journal of Medicine.)

Moderate to severe mitral regurgitation occurs in 66% of patients with posterior leaflet prolapse compared with 25% of those with anterior leaflet prolapse.[84] Complications are more common with posterior leaflet involvement. Comparing those with posterior leaflet prolapse and those with anterior leaflet prolapse, atrial fibrillation occurred in 25% and 18%, heart failure in 20% and 10%, and chordal rupture in 15% and 3%, respectively (Table 14–5).[84]

In one study, up to one third of mitral valve prolapse patients with no or minimal regurgitation at rest had significant mitral regurgitation inducible with exercise.[87] Although those with exercise-induced mitral regurgitation had a higher rate of complications, the patients who went on to mitral valve surgery also were older and had evidence of chronic disease (eg, a larger left atrial size)—known risk factors for the need for mitral valve surgery. The change in the right ventricular ejection fraction with exercise also predicts the need for mitral valve surgery in mitral prolapse patients.[78] One explanation may be an excessive rise in pulmonary pressure with exercise. Although these exercise studies suggest that exercise echocardiography in patients with mitral prolapse may have incremental value, the findings require confirmation in other patient groups.

Arrhythmias and Sudden Death

The relationships between mitral valve prolapse and arrhythmias and sudden cardiac death remain debatable.[58, 88–90] However, estimates suggest a 1% to 2.5% risk of sudden death over a 6-year follow-up period.[24, 57, 72] Expressed as a risk ratio, the risk of sudden death is estimated as 10 to 100 times normal,[91, 92] most likely related to frequent and complex ventricular ectopy.[89, 93]

Risk factors for sudden death in mitral prolapse patients are redundant leaflets and moderate to severe mitral regurgitation.[94, 95] It was once postulated that endocardial lesions and thrombus in the angle between the posterior mitral leaflet and left atrial wall might be associated with sudden death,[96] but this relationship has not been confirmed.[97] Complex atrial arrhythmias also occur in mitral prolapse patients, particularly older patients with mitral regurgitation and left atrial and ventricular enlargement.[98]

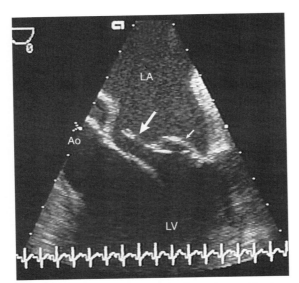

Figure 14·8 Transesophageal echocardiographic view shows severe prolapse of the posterior leaflet with a partial flail segment. The prolapsed segment is curved so that the leaflet tip points toward the left ventricular apex *(small arrow)*. The flail segment is aimed toward the posterior left atrial wall *(large arrow)*. The flail segment showed rapid oscillations in systole on the real-time images. This patient had chronic, mild to moderate mitral regurgitation and a sudden deterioration in clinical status at the time of chordal rupture. Ao, aorta; LA, left atrium; LV, left ventricle.

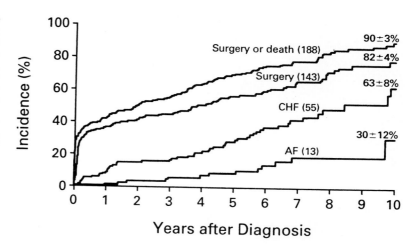

Figure 14·9 Clinical outcome in a series of 229 patients with isolated mitral regurgitation due to a flail leaflet showing the incidence of atrial fibrillation (AF), congestive heart failure (CHF), mitral valve surgery, and surgery or death. A total of 175 patients were initially at risk for atrial fibrillation, and 229 were initially at risk for the other end points. The numbers within parentheses are numbers of events for each end point. The plus-minus values are mean (± SE) event rates at 10 years. (From Ling LH, et al: N Engl J Med 1996; 335:1417–1423; reprinted by permission from the New England Journal of Medicine.)

Embolic Events

Although it has been suggested that mitral valve prolapse is associated with a higher risk of embolic events,[23, 99–103] considerable controversy persists about the risk of embolic events in patients with mitral prolapse. Early studies showed that mitral valve prolapse was found on echocardiography in 2% to 35% of patients with ischemic neurologic events,[100–103] with the apparent variability probably related to specific echocardiographic criteria used in each study. One group of investigators estimate a sixfold increased risk for embolic events in young women with mitral valve prolapse compared with normal controls,[104] whereas other groups suggest that the risk of embolic events due to mitral valve prolapse is very low.[105] The mechanism of embolic events in patients with mitral prolapse but without atrial fibrillation has never been adequately explained. One possible explanation is thrombus formation in the angle between the prolapsed leaflet and the left atrial wall,[96] but this hypothesis has not been fully validated.[97]

Endocarditis

The frequency of endocarditis is 6% to 7% among necropsy cases of mitral valve prolapse[72, 106] and 1% to 6% in clinical series.[57, 72, 76] The risk of endocarditis in mitral valve prolapse patients is estimated to be three to eight times that of the general population[23] and is even higher among those with mitral valve prolapse and a systolic murmur, with an estimated risk of endocarditis of 1 case in 1400 patient-years (Fig. 14–10).[107]

Looking at risk from the point of view of the proportion of all endocarditis cases, the prevalence of mitral valve prolapse as the underlying valve abnormality is 11% to 29% in series of patients with endocarditis.[44, 59, 107–111] As with other lesions predisposing to endocarditis, it is postulated that blood flow turbulence leads to an increased rate of endothelial disruption, and platelet and fibrin deposition on the valve surface with subsequent infection at the time of bacteremia (see Chapter 18).

Other Possible Clinical Associations

Both neuropsychiatric disorders and autonomic dysfunction have been associated with

TABLE 14·5   INCIDENCE OF COMPLICATIONS ASSOCIATED WITH PROLAPSED LEAFLETS IN 229 PATIENTS WITH MITRAL VALVE PROLAPSE

	Leaflet		
Complication	AML (n = 147)	PML (n = 59)	Both (n = 23)
Atrial fibrillation	26 (18%)	15 (25%)	5 (22%)
Congestive heart failure	15 (10%)	12 (20%)	3 (13%)
Chordal rupture	4 (3%)	9 (15%)	1 (4%)
Cerebral embolism	1	1	
Infective endocarditis		1	
Patients with more than one complication	33 (22%)	29* (49%)	7 (30%)

AML, anterior mitral leaflet; PML, posterior mitral leaflet.
    *$P < 0.01$ compared with AML by chi-square analysis.
    From Kim S, Kuroda T, Nishinaga M, et al: Relationship between severity of mitral regurgitation and prognosis of mitral valve prolapse: echocardiographic follow-up study. Am Heart J 1996;132:350.

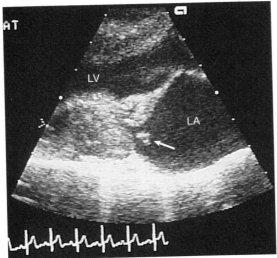

Figure 14·10 This parasternal long-axis echocardiographic image shows mitral valve prolapse with a superimposed valvular vegetation *(arrow)*. In the presence of myxomatous mitral valve disease, it may be difficult to differentiate a vegetation from a partial flail segment solely on the basis of the echocardiographic appearance of the valve. Correlation with clinical features such as fever and with blood culture results is needed for accurate diagnosis. Ao, aorta; LA, left atrium; LV, left ventricle.

mitral valve prolapse in the past.[47] Patients diagnosed as having "panic attacks and mitral valve prolapse" are unlikely to respond to cardiac medications,[49] and many of these patients do not meet strict criteria for a diagnosis of mitral prolapse. More recent, carefully controlled studies suggest that, although there is some overlap in symptoms and while some patients have both disorders, panic disorder is not statistically or biologically related to mitral valve prolapse.[22, 44–50] Indeed, it is difficult to imagine a plausible underlying pathophysiologic mechanism that could incorporate these two entities.

The apparent relationship between autonomic dysfunction and mitral valve prolapse also is unclear.[112–115] The clinical manifestations of autonomic dysfunction—low intravascular volume, orthostatic hypotension, and syncope or presyncope—are similar to mitral valve prolapse symptoms. Moreover, a low intravascular (and intraventricular) volume may lead to systolic displacement of the leaflets into the left atrium, even with a normal valve apparatus. Some investigators think that autonomic dysfunction is a key feature of the mitral valve prolapse syndrome;[116–118] others consider autonomic dysfunction and mitral valve prolapse to be unassociated.[23, 119, 120]

TREATMENT

Management Principles

The most important principle in management of patients with suspected mitral valve prolapse is to avoid overdiagnosis. Strict echocardiographic criteria allow delineation of the extent of leaflet thickening and redundancy, the presence and degree of systolic displacement of the leaflets and coaptation point into the left atrium in the long-axis view, and any associated mitral regurgitation. Transthoracic imaging usually is adequate for diagnosis, and only rarely are high-resolution transesophageal images needed. Diagnosis is based on the combination of clinical and echocardiographic findings.

In my view, mitral valve prolapse can be diagnosed when patients have unequivocal echocardiographic findings, even in the absence of a systolic click on auscultation. In contrast, the diagnosis of mitral valve prolapse cannot be made on the basis of physical examination alone in the absence of confirmatory findings on echocardiography. Since mitral valve prolapse is a primary disease of the valve leaflets, the anatomic abnormalities should be detectable with ultrasound imaging. The apparent finding of a click on examination in the absence of anatomic abnormalities most likely represents a split S_1, and these patients should not be considered to have a disease process. Echocardiographic findings sometimes are borderline or equivocal; normal mitral valve anatomy encompasses a wide range of variability, so that mild anatomic abnormalities may be difficult to differentiate from the extreme of the normal range. When the echocardiographic findings are borderline, clinical follow-up, perhaps with a repeat echocardiographic study in 2 to 3 years, is appropriate.

Estimation of Prognosis

The next step in the management of the patient with mitral valve prolapse is to estimate the risk of complications and the overall prognosis. Key factors in this evaluation include patient age and gender, the extent of leaflet thickening and redundancy, the degree of mitral regurgitation, and left ventricular dimensions and systolic function. Young patients with thin leaflets and little mitral regurgitation are in a low-risk group. Other than endocarditis prophylaxis, therapy consists mainly of reassurance and education about the diagnosis, potential complications, and the low likelihood of an adverse outcome.

Conversely, the older male patient with significant mitral regurgitation is likely to need valve surgery over a relatively short time frame. Management for this group includes frequent periodic clinical and noninvasive evaluation, as well as education about symptoms and complications, and optimal timing of surgical intervention.

Noninvasive Follow-up

Most patients with mitral valve prolapse have a low risk of progressive mitral regurgitation requiring valve surgery. In the absence of a change in clinical symptoms or physical examination findings, only infrequent evaluation is needed. Clinical evaluation with careful auscultation and echocardiography at approximately 5-year intervals is appropriate for this subgroup of mitral prolapse patients.[23] Repeat examination, rather than no follow-up, is recommended, because some of these patients may have progressive leaflet thickening and mitral regurgitation in the interim, switching their status from the low- to intermediate- or high-risk groups.

For the patient with an unclear diagnosis or an intermediate likelihood of complications, evaluation every 2 or 3 years probably is adequate. Again, more frequent evaluation may be warranted if there is a change in clinical status or if new information about the natural history of this disease becomes available.

For the patient with significant mitral regurgitation, the frequency of evaluation parallels that for chronic mitral regurgitation of any cause. Annual echocardiography is appropriate for the stable patient, with more frequent examinations if there is evidence for progressive left ventricular dilation, systolic dysfunction, or a rise in pulmonary pressures. In mitral valve prolapse patients, a sudden deterioration in clinical status due to chordal rupture is relatively common. Repeat echocardiography for suspected chordal rupture is warranted, especially as earlier surgical intervention may be needed.

Medical Therapy

There is no known medical therapy to prevent progression of the underlying disease process in patients with mitral valve prolapse. The basic principles of medical therapy are to prevent complications, identify and treat comorbid diseases, and provide education, reassurance and periodic evaluation.

Patients with mitral valve prolapse and a mitral regurgitant murmur or Doppler echocardiographic evidence of mitral regurgitation should receive endocarditis prophylaxis according to the American Heart Association recommendations (see Chapter 6).[121] Patients with mitral prolapse and no evidence of pathologic mitral regurgitation on echocardiography do not need endocarditis prophylaxis. For the patient with mitral prolapse for whom the status of mitral regurgitation is unknown and evaluation is not possible before a dental or surgical procedure, it is prudent to administer endocarditis prophylaxis and plan on diagnostic evaluation at a later date.

The potential benefits of afterload reduction for decreasing mitral regurgitant severity in patients with mitral prolapse remain unproved. Thus, routine afterload reduction therapy is not indicated for all patients with mitral regurgitation. However, patients with congestive symptoms who are not surgical candidates may benefit from vasodilator therapy. In addition, coexisting systemic hypertension should be treated aggressively to decrease the left ventricular workload and avoid exacerbation of the severity of valvular regurgitation.

Symptomatic arrhythmias may require therapy, but there is no evidence that antiarrhythmic therapy prevents sudden death in mitral prolapse patients. Treatment remains controversial given the proarrhythmic effects of some medications. β-blocking drugs provide relief from symptomatic supraventricular and ventricular arrhythmias in many mitral prolapse patients and should be considered in selected cases.[23] In some cases, the onset of palpitations signals increased mitral regurgitation and the need for surgical intervention.

Chest pain is rarely caused by mitral valve prolapse itself. Anginal symptoms suggest coexisting coronary artery disease, which should be evaluated with appropriate diagnostic tests. If coronary anatomy is normal, a search for treatable noncardiac causes, such as esophageal motility disorder, also is appropriate.

Timing and Choice of Surgical Intervention

The optimal timing of surgical intervention in patients with mitral regurgitation is discussed in Chapter 15. Most patients with mitral valve prolapse have anatomy that is amenable to surgical repair, rather than valve replacement. Because of the lower mortality, improved clinical outcome, absence of a prosthetic valve, and preservation of ventricular function, mitral valve repair is preferred, whenever possible.

References

1. Perloff JK, Child JS, Edwards JE: New guidelines for the clinical diagnosis of mitral valve prolapse. Am J Cardiol 1986;57:1124–1129.
2. Devereux RB, Kramer Fox R, Shear MK, Kligfield P, Pini R, Savage DD: Diagnosis and classification of severity of mitral valve prolapse: methodologic, biologic, and prognostic considerations. Am Heart J 1987;113:1265–1280.
3. Devereux RB, Brown WT, Kramer Fox R, Sachs I: Inheritance of mitral valve prolapse: effect of age and sex on gene expression. Ann Intern Med 1982;97:826–832.
4. Strahan NV, Murphy EA, Fortuin NJ, Come PC, Humphries JO: Inheritance of the mitral valve prolapse syndrome: discussion of a three-dimensional penetrance model. Am J Med 1983;74:967–972.
5. Weiss AN, Mimbs JW, Ludbrook PA, Sobel BE: Echocardiographic detection of mitral valve prolapse: exclusion of false positive diagnosis and determination of inheritance. Circulation 1975;52:1091–1096.
6. Chen WW, Chan FL, Wong PH, Chow JS: Familial occurrence of mitral valve prolapse: is this related to the straight back syndrome? Br Heart J 1983;50:97–100.
7. Devereux RB: Recent developments in the diagnosis and management of mitral valve prolapse. Curr Opin Cardiol 1995;10:107–116.
8. Fukuda N, Oki T, Iuchi A, et al: Predisposing factors for severe mitral regurgitation in idiopathic mitral valve prolapse. Am J Cardiol 1995;76:503–507.
9. Kielty CM, Phillips JE, Child AH, Pope FM, Shuttleworth CA: Fibrillin secretion and microfibril assembly by Marfan dermal fibroblasts. Matrix Biol 1994;14:191–199.
10. Pereira L, Levran O, Ramirez F, et al: A molecular approach to the stratification of cardiovascular risk in families with Marfan's syndrome. N Engl J Med 1994;331:148–153.
11. Pini R, Greppi B, Kramer Fox R, Roman MJ, Devereux RB: Mitral valve dimensions and motion and familial transmission of mitral valve prolapse with and without mitral leaflet billowing. J Am Coll Cardiol 1988;12:1423–1431.
12. Somerville J, Kaku S, Saravalli O: Prolapsed mitral cusps in atrial septal defect: an erroneous radiological interpretation. Br Heart J 1978;40:58–63.
13. Garcia Dorado D, Garcia EJ, Bello L, et al: Mitral valve prolapse secondary to right ventricular enlargement in patients with pulmonary hypertension after toxic rapeseed oil ingestion. Eur Heart J 1985;6:85–90.
14. Konicek S, Guntheroth WG, Sylvester CE, Mack LA, Reichler RJ: Does "physiologic" mitral valve prolapse occur with acute blood loss? Clin Cardiol 1987;10:159–162.
15. Waller BF, McManus BM, Roberts WC: Mitral valve stenosis produced by or worsened by active bacterial endocarditis. Chest 1982;82:498–500.
16. Amlie JP, Langmark F, Storstein O: Pure mitral regurgitation: etiology, pathology and clinical patterns. Acta Med Scand 1976;200:201–208.
17. Falco A, Sante P, Renzulli A, et al: Etiology and incidence of pure mitral insufficiency: a morphological study of 926 native valves. Cardiologia 1990;35:327–330.
18. Hanson TP, Edwards BS, Edwards JE: Pathology of surgically excised mitral valves: one hundred consecutive cases. Arch Pathol Lab Med 1985;109:823–828.
19. Turri M, Thiene G, Bortolotti U, Mazzucco A, Gallucci V: Surgical pathology of disease of the mitral valve, with special reference to lesions promoting valvar incompetence. Int J Cardiol 1989;22:213–219.
20. Olson LJ, Subramanian R, Ackermann DM, Orszulak TA, Edwards WD: Surgical pathology of the mitral valve: a study of 712 cases spanning 21 years. Mayo Clin Proc 1987;62:22–34.
21. Wilcken DE, Hickey AJ: Lifetime risk for patients with mitral valve prolapse of developing severe valve regurgitation requiring surgery. Circulation 1988;78:10–14.
22. Levy D, Savage D: Prevalence and clinical features of mitral valve prolapse. Am Heart J 1987;113:1281–1290.
23. Devereux RB, Kramer Fox R, Kligfield P: Mitral valve prolapse: causes, clinical manifestations, and management. Ann Intern Med 1989;111:305–317.
24. Davies MJ, Moore BP, Braimbridge MV: The floppy mitral valve: study of incidence, pathology, and complications in surgical, necropsy, and forensic material. Br Heart J 1978;40:468–481.
25. Catellier MJ, Waller BF, Clark MA, Pless JE, Hawley DA, Nyhuis AW: Cardiac pathology in 470 consecutive forensic autopsies. J Forensic Sci 1990;35:1042–1054.
26. Savage DD, Levy D, Garrison RJ, et al: Mitral valve prolapse in the general population. 3. Dysrhythmias: the Framingham Study. Am Heart J 1983;106:582–586.
27. Markiewicz W, Stoner J, London E, Hunt SA, Popp RL: Mitral valve prolapse in one hundred presumably healthy young females. Circulation 1976;53:464–473.
28. Virmani R, Atkinson JB, Forman MB: The pathology of mitral valve prolapse. Herz 1988;13:215–226.
29. Weissman NJ, Pini R, Roman MJ, Kramer Fox R, Andersen HS, Devereux RB: In vivo mitral valve morphology and motion in mitral valve prolapse. Am J Cardiol 1994;73:1080–1088.
30. van der Bel Kahn J, Duren DR, Becker AE: Isolated mitral valve prolapse: chordal architecture as an anatomic basis in older patients. J Am Coll Cardiol 1985;5:1335–1340.
31. Becker AE, De Wit AP: Mitral valve apparatus. A spectrum of normality relevant to mitral valve prolapse. Br Heart J 1979;42:680–689.
32. Roberts WC, McIntosh CL, Wallace RB: Mechanisms of severe mitral regurgitation in mitral valve prolapse determined from analysis of operatively excised valves. Am Heart J 1987;113:1316–1323.
33. Renteria VG, Ferrans VJ, Jones M, Roberts WC: Intracellular collagen fibrils in prolapsed ("floppy") human atrioventricular valves. Lab Invest 1976;35:439–443.
34. King BD, Clark MA, Baba N, Kilman JW, Wooley CF: "Myxomatous" mitral valves: collagen dissolution as the primary defect. Circulation 1982;66:288–296.
35. Baker PB, Bansal G, Boudoulas H, Kolibash AJ, Kilman J, Wooley CF: Floppy mitral valve chordae tendineae: histopathologic alterations. Hum Pathol 1988;19:507–512.

36. Whittaker P, Boughner DR, Perkins DG, Canham PB: Quantitative structural analysis of collagen in chordae tendineae and its relation to floppy mitral valves and proteoglycan infiltration. Br Heart J 1987;57:264–269.

37. Edwards WD: Surgical pathology of the aortic valve. *In* Waller BF, ed. Pathology of the Heart and Great Vessels. New York: Churchill Livingstone, 1988:43–100.

38. Henney AM, Parker DJ, Davies MJ: Collagen biosynthesis in normal and abnormal human heart valves. Cardiovasc Res 1982;16:624–630.

39. Hammer D, Leier CV, Baba N, Vasko JS, Wooley CF, Pinnell SR: Altered collagen composition in a prolapsing mitral valve with ruptured chordae tendineae. Am J Med 1979;67:863–866.

40. Lis Y, Burleigh MC, Parker DJ, Child AH, Hogg J, Davies MJ: Biochemical characterization of individual normal, floppy and rheumatic human mitral valves. Biochem J 1987;244:597–603.

41. Cole WG, Chan D, Hickey AJ, Wilcken DE: Collagen composition of normal and myxomatous human mitral heart valves. Biochem J 1984;219:451–460.

42. Wordsworth P, Ogilvie D, Akhras F, Jackson G, Sykes B: Genetic segregation analysis of familial mitral valve prolapse shows no linkage to fibrillar collagen genes. Br Heart J 1989;61:300–306.

43. Henney AM, Tsipouras P, Schwartz RC, Child AH, Devereux RB, Leech GJ: Genetic evidence that mutations in the *COL1A1, COL1A2, COL3A1,* or *COL5A2* collagen genes are not responsible for mitral valve prolapse. Br Heart J 1989;61:292–299.

44. Devereux RB, Kramer Fox R, Brown WT, et al: Relation between clinical features of the mitral prolapse syndrome and echocardiographically documented mitral valve prolapse. J Am Coll Cardiol 1986;8:763–772.

45. Uretsky BF: Does mitral valve prolapse cause nonspecific symptoms? Int J Cardiol 1982;1:435–442.

46. Cowan MD, Fye WB: Prevalence of QTc prolongation in women with mitral valve prolapse. Am J Cardiol 1989;63:133–134.

47. Hartman N, Kramer R, Brown WT, Devereux RB: Panic disorder in patients with mitral valve prolapse. Am J Psychiatry 1982;139:669–670.

48. Hickey AJ, Andrews G, Wilcken DE: Independence of mitral valve prolapse and neurosis. Br Heart J 1983;50:333–336.

49. Margraf J, Ehlers A, Roth WT: Mitral valve prolapse and panic disorder: a review of their relationship. Psychosom Med 1988;50:93–113.

50. Savage DD, Devereux RB, Garrison RJ, et al: Mitral valve prolapse in the general population. 2. Clinical features: the Framingham Study. Am Heart J 1983;106:577–581.

51. Barlow JB, Pocock WA, Marchand P, Denny M: The significance of late systolic murmurs. Am Heart J 1963;66:443–452.

52. Fontana ME, Pence HL, Leighton RF, Wooley CF: The varying clinical spectrum of the systolic click-late systolic murmur syndrome. Circulation 1970;41:807–816.

53. Epstein EJ, Coulshed N: Phonocardiogram and apex cardiogram in systolic click—late systolic murmur syndrome. Br Heart J 1973;35:260–275.

54. Fontana ME, Wooley CF, Leighton RF, Lewis RP: Postural changes in left ventricular and mitral valvular dynamics in the systolic click—late systolic murmur syndrome. Circulation 1975;51:165–113.

55. Devereux RB, Perloff JK, Reichek N, Josephson ME: Mitral valve prolapse. Circulation 1976;54:3–14.

56. Tofler OB, Tofler GH: Use of auscultation to follow patients with mitral systolic clicks and murmurs. Am J Cardiol 1990;66:1355–1358.

57. Nishimura RA, McGoon MD, Shub C, Miller FA Jr, Ilstrup DM, Tajik AJ: Echocardiographically documented mitral-valve prolapse: long-term follow-up of 237 patients. N Engl J Med 1985;313:1305–1309.

58. Savage DD, Garrison RJ, Devereux RB, et al: Mitral valve prolapse in the general population. 1. Epidemiologic features: the Framingham Study. Am Heart J 1983;106:571–576.

59. Hickey AJ, Wilcken DE, Wright JS, Warren BA: Primary (spontaneous) chordal rupture: relation to myxomatous valve disease and mitral valve prolapse. J Am Coll Cardiol 1985;5:1341–1346.

60. Schutte JE, Gaffney FA, Blend L, Blomqvist CG: Distinctive anthropometric characteristics of women with mitral valve prolapse. Am J Med 1981;71:533–538.

61. Roman MJ, Devereux RB, Kramer Fox R, Spitzer MC: Comparison of cardiovascular and skeletal features of primary mitral valve prolapse and Marfan syndrome. Am J Cardiol 1989;63:317–321.

62. Perloff JK, Child JS: Clinical and epidemiologic issues in mitral valve prolapse: overview and perspective. Am Heart J 1987;113:1324–1332.

63. Levine RA, Stathogiannis E, Newell JB, Harrigan P, Weyman AE: Reconsideration of echocardiographic standards for mitral valve prolapse: lack of association between leaflet displacement isolated to the apical four chamber view and independent echocardiographic evidence of abnormality. J Am Coll Cardiol 1988;11:1010–1019.

64. Marks AR, Choong CY, Sanfilippo AJ, Ferre M, Weyman AE: Identification of high-risk and low-risk subgroups of patients with mitral-valve prolapse. N Engl J Med 1989;320:1031–1036.

65. Marsalese DL, Moodie DS, Vacante M, et al: Marfan's syndrome: natural history and long-term follow-up of cardiovascular involvement. J Am Coll Cardiol 1989;14:422–428.

66. Pyeritz RE, McKusick VA: The Marfan syndrome: diagnosis and management. N Engl J Med 1979;300:772–777.

67. Legget ME, Unger TA, O'Sullivan CK, et al: Aortic root complications in Marfan's syndrome: identification of a lower risk group. Heart 1996;75:389–395.

68. Klues HG, Roberts WC, Maron BJ: Morphological determinants of echocardiographic patterns of mitral valve systolic anterior motion in obstructive hypertrophic cardiomyopathy. Circulation 1993;87:1570–1579.

69. Klues HG, Proschan MA, Dollar AL, Spirito P, Roberts WC, Maron BJ: Echocardiographic assessment of mitral valve size in obstructive hypertrophic cardiomyopathy: anatomic validation from mitral valve specimen. Circulation 1993;88:548–555.

70. Kennett JD, Rust PF, Martin RH, Parker BM, Watson LE: Observer variation in the angiocardiographic diagnosis of mitral valve prolapse. Chest 1981;79:146–150.

71. Spindola Franco H, Bjork L, Adams DF, Abrams HL: Classification of the radiological morphology of the mitral valve: differentiation between true and pseudoprolapse. Br Heart J 1980;44:30–36.

72. Duren DR, Becker AE, Dunning AJ: Long-term fol-

low-up of idiopathic mitral valve prolapse in 300 patients: a prospective study. J Am Coll Cardiol 1988;11:42–47.

73. Vered Z, Oren S, Rabinowitz B, Meltzer RS, Neufeld HN: Mitral valve prolapse: quantitative analysis and long-term follow-up. Isr J Med Sci 1985;21:644–648.

74. Kolibash AJ Jr, Kilman JW, Bush CA, Ryan JM, Fontana ME, Wooley CF: Evidence for progression from mild to severe mitral regurgitation in mitral valve prolapse. Am J Cardiol 1986;58:762–767.

75. Kolibash AJ: Progression of mitral regurgitation in patients with mitral valve prolapse. Herz 1988;13:309–317.

76. Zuppiroli A, Rinaldi M, Kramer Fox R, Favilli S, Roman MJ, Devereux RB: Natural history of mitral valve prolapse. Am J Cardiol 1995;75:1028–1032.

77. Grayburn PA, Berk MR, Spain MG, Harrison MR, Smith MD, DeMaria AN: Relation of echocardiographic morphology of the mitral apparatus to mitral regurgitation in mitral valve prolapse: assessment by Doppler color flow imaging. Am Heart J 1990;119:1095–1102.

78. Rosen SE, Borer JS, Hochreiter C, et al: Natural history of the asymptomatic/minimally symptomatic patient with severe mitral regurgitation secondary to mitral valve prolapse and normal right and left ventricular performance. Am J Cardiol 1994;74:374–380.

79. Ling LH, Enriquez Sarano M, Seward JB, et al: Clinical outcome of mitral regurgitation due to flail leaflet. N Engl J Med 1996;335:1417–1423.

80. Hammermeister KE, Fisher L, Kennedy W, Samuels S, Dodge HT: Prediction of late survival in patients with mitral valve disease from clinical, hemodynamic, and quantitative angiographic variables. Circulation 1978;57:341–349.

81. Selzer A, Kelly JJ Jr, Kerth WJ, Gerbode F: Immediate and long-range results of valvuloplasty for mitral regurgitation due to ruptured chordae tendineae. Circulation 1972;45(suppl 1):52–56.

82. Munoz S, Gallardo J, Diaz Gorrin JR, Medina O: Influence of surgery on the natural history of rheumatic mitral and aortic valve disease. Am J Cardiol 1975;35:234–242.

83. Ross J Jr: Left ventricular function and the timing of surgical treatment in valvular heart disease. Ann Intern Med 1981;94:498–504.

84. Kim S, Kuroda T, Nishinaga M, et al: Relationship between severity of mitral regurgitation and prognosis of mitral valve prolapse: echocardiographic follow-up study. Am Heart J 1996;132:348–355.

85. Deng YB, Takenaka K, Sakamoto T, et al: Follow-up in mitral valve prolapse by phonocardiography, M-mode and two-dimensional echocardiography and Doppler echocardiography. Am J Cardiol 1990;65:349–354.

86. Jeresaty RM, Edwards JE, Chawla SK: Mitral valve prolapse and ruptured chordae tendineae. Am J Cardiol 1985;55:138–142.

87. Stoddard MF, Prince CR, Dillon S, Longaker RA, Morris GT, Liddell NE: Exercise-induced mitral regurgitation is a predictor of morbid events in subjects with mitral valve prolapse. J Am Coll Cardiol 1995;25:693–699.

88. Farb A, Tang AL, Atkinson JB, McCarthy WF, Virmani R: Comparison of cardiac findings in patients with mitral valve prolapse who die suddenly to those who have congestive heart failure from mitral regurgitation and to those with fatal noncardiac conditions. Am J Cardiol 1992;70:234–239.

89. Vohra J, Sathe S, Warren R, Tatoulis J, Hunt D: Malignant ventricular arrhythmias in patients with mitral valve prolapse and mild mitral regurgitation. Pacing Clin Electrophysiol 1993;16:1387–1393.

90. Shappell SD, Marshall CE, Brown RE, Bruce TA: Sudden death and the familial occurrence of mid-systolic click, late systolic murmur syndrome. Circulation 1973;48:1128–1134.

91. Kligfield P, Hochreiter C, Niles N, Devereux RB, Borer JS: Relation of sudden death in pure mitral regurgitation, with and without mitral valve prolapse, to repetitive ventricular arrhythmias and right and left ventricular ejection fractions. Am J Cardiol 1987;60:397–399.

92. Kligfield P, Levy D, Devereux RB, Savage DD: Arrhythmias and sudden death in mitral valve prolapse. Am Heart J 1987;113:1298–1307.

93. Kligfield P, Hochreiter C, Kramer H, et al: Complex arrhythmias in mitral regurgitation with and without mitral valve prolapse: contrast to arrhythmias in mitral valve prolapse without mitral regurgitation. Am J Cardiol 1985;55(suppl II):545–549.

94. Winkle RA, Lopes MG, Popp RL, Hancock EW: Life-threatening arrhythmias in the mitral valve prolapse syndrome. Am J Med 1976;60:961–967.

95. DeMaria AN, Amsterdam EA, Vismara LA, Neumann A, Mason DT: Arrhythmias in the mitral valve prolapse syndrome: prevalence, nature, and frequency. Ann Intern Med 1976;84:656–660.

96. Chesler E, King RA, Edwards JE: The myxomatous mitral valve and sudden death. Circulation 1983;67:632–639.

97. Dollar AL, Roberts WC: Morphologic comparison of patients with mitral valve prolapse who died suddenly with patients who died from severe valvular dysfunction or other conditions. J Am Coll Cardiol 1991;17:921–931.

98. Zuppiroli A, Mori F, Favilli S, et al: Arrhythmias in mitral valve prolapse: relation to anterior mitral leaflet thickening, clinical variables, and color Doppler echocardiographic parameters. Am Heart J 1994;128:919–927.

99. Barnett HJ, Jones MW, Broughner D: Cerebral ischemic events associated with prolapsing mitral valve. Trans Am Neurol Assoc 1975;100:84–88.

100. Egeblad H, Soelberg Sorensen P: Prevalence of mitral valve prolapse in younger patients with cerebral ischaemic attacks. A blinded controlled study. Acta Med Scand 1984;216:385–391.

101. Kouvaras G, Bacoulas G: Association of mitral valve leaflet prolapse with cerebral ischaemic events in the young and early middle-aged patient. Q J Med 1985;56:387–392.

102. Adams C, Baubion N, Le Pailleur C, et al: Acute degenerative mitral insufficiency caused by rupture of the chordae in the elderly patient. Ann Med Interne (Paris) 1986;137:391–394.

103. Bogousslavsky J, Regli F: Ischemic stroke in adults younger than 30 years of age: cause and prognosis [published erratum appears in Arch Neurol 1987;44:817]. Arch Neurol 1987;44:479–482.

104. Devereux RB, Kramer Fox R: Gender differences in mitral valve prolapse. Cardiovasc Clin 1989;19:243–258.

105. Kelley RE, Pina I, Lee SC: Cerebral ischemia and mitral valve prolapse: case-control study of associated factors. Stroke 1988;19:443–446.

106. Lucas RV Jr, Edwards JE: The floppy mitral valve. Curr Probl Cardiol 1982;7:1–48.

107. MacMahon SW, Hickey AJ, Wilcken DE, Wittes JT, Feneley MP, Hickie JB: Risk of infective endocarditis in mitral valve prolapse with and without precordial systolic murmurs. Am J Cardiol 1987;59:105–108.

108. Rossi EG, Grinberg M, Mansur AJ, Bellotti G, Pileggi F, Jatene A: Mitral valve prolapse in infective endocarditis. Incidence and characteristics. Arq Bras Cardiol 1990;54:101–104.

109. Clemens JD, Horwitz RI, Jaffe CC, Feinstein AR, Stanton BF: A controlled evaluation of the risk of bacterial endocarditis in persons with mitral-valve prolapse. N Engl J Med 1982;307:776–781.

110. McKinsey DS, Ratts TE, Bisno AL: Underlying cardiac lesions in adults with infective endocarditis: the changing spectrum. Am J Med 1987;82:681–688.

111. Corrigall D, Bolen J, Hancock EW, Popp RL: Mitral valve prolapse and infective endocarditis. Am J Med 1977;63:215–222.

112. Santos AD, Mathew PK, Hilal A, Wallace WA: Orthostatic hypotension: a commonly unrecognized cause of symptoms in mitral valve prolapse. Am J Med 1981;71:746–750.

113. Weissman NJ, Shear MK, Kramer Fox R, Devereux RB: Contrasting patterns of autonomic dysfunction in patients with mitral valve prolapse and panic attacks. Am J Med 1987;82:880–888.

114. Gaffney FA, Karlsson ES, Campbell W, et al: Autonomic dysfunction in women with mitral valve prolapse syndrome. Circulation 1979;59:894–901.

115. Gaffney FA, Bastian BC, Lane LB, et al: Abnormal cardiovascular regulation in the mitral valve prolapse syndrome. Am J Cardiol 1983;52:316–320.

116. Fontana ME, Sparks EA, Boudoulas H, Wooley CF: Mitral valve prolapse and the mitral valve prolapse syndrome. Curr Probl Cardiol 1991;16:309–375.

117. Coghlan HC, Phares P, Cowley M, Copley D, James TN: Dysautonomia in mitral valve prolapse. Am J Med 1979;67:236–244.

118. Boudoulas H, Reynolds JC, Mazzaferri E, Wooley CF: Mitral valve prolapse syndrome: the effect of adrenergic stimulation. J Am Coll Cardiol 1983;2:638–644.

119. Chesler E, Weir EK, Braatz GA, Francis GS: Normal catecholamine and hemodynamic responses to orthostatic tilt in subjects with mitral valve prolapse. Correlation with psychologic testing. Am J Med 1985;78:754–760.

120. Lenders JW, Fast JH, Blankers J, de Boo T, Lemmens WA, Thien T: Normal sympathetic neural activity in patients with mitral valve prolapse. Clin Cardiol 1986;9:177–182.

121. Dajani AS, Taubert KA, Wilson W, et al: Prevention of bacterial endocarditis: recommendations by the American Heart Association. JAMA 1997;277:1794–1801.

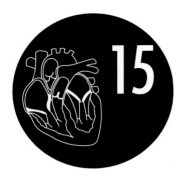

15 Surgical Intervention for Mitral Regurgitation

CLINICAL OUTCOME AFTER SURGERY

Measures of Clinical Outcome

The primary outcome measures for patients undergoing surgical intervention for mitral regurgitation are operative mortality and long-term survival. However, irreversible changes in left ventricular function, the pulmonary vasculature, and cardiac rhythm may occur, particularly with chronic regurgitation, and all of these changes may adversely affect the exercise capacity and quality of life of survivors. In addition, the disease process underlying mitral regurgitation, such as coronary artery disease, may dominate the clinical picture and may be the primary determinant of clinical outcome. Thus, a more complete description of clinical outcome after mitral valve surgery also includes measures of left ventricular function, hemodynamics, and cardiac rhythm. Further,

separate descriptions of outcome for different causes of mitral regurgitation are needed.

Data on functional status and exercise capacity after surgical intervention for mitral regurgitation are limited. Exercise capacity is closely related to left ventricular function, cardiac rhythm, and persistent pulmonary hypertension. However, valvular hemodynamics also affect exercise capacity after valve replacement due to the mild functional stenosis of the prosthetic valve and after valve repair due to residual or recurrent mitral regurgitation.

Overall quality of life after surgery is impacted by other factors that have not been adequately evaluated in clinical studies. These include the risks, cost, and inconvenience of chronic anticoagulation; the need for periodic evaluation of clinical status and valve function; the effects of a surgical scar in terms of body image and increased risk for subsequent cardiac surgery; possible effects of the surgical procedure on cognitive function; valve complications (eg, endocarditis); and the likelihood of future surgical interventions for mitral valve dysfunction. While our knowledge base remains incomplete, a number of studies have provided insight into the complexities of outcome after surgery for mitral regurgitation.

Predictors of Outcome

The five categories of predictors of outcome after surgical intervention for mitral valve regurgitation are clinical factors, comorbid disease, measures of left ventricular systolic function, secondary pathophysiologic abnormalities, and preservation of the chordal apparatus (Table 15–1).

Clinical Factors

As for other cardiac surgical procedures, age and gender are predictors of operative morbidity and mortality[1, 2] with an operative mortality rate of 12.3% for patients older than 75 years of age and 1.1% for younger patients in one series.[3] In addition, preoperative functional status also is a strong predictor of outcome.[1, 3–6]

The etiology of mitral regurgitation predicts operative mortality, with very low operative mortality rates (1% to 3%) reported for series of patients with myxomatous mitral valve dis-

TABLE 15·1 PREDICTORS OF OUTCOME AFTER SURGERY FOR MITRAL REGURGITATION

Demographics
  Age
  Gender
  Functional status
Comorbid disease
  Coronary artery disease
  Other valve involvement
Left ventricular systolic function
  End-systolic volume or dimension
  Ejection fraction
  Wall stress
  Left ventricular sphericity
  Left ventricular maximum change in pressure (dP/dt)
Surgical procedure
  Mitral valve replacement with or without chordal
    preservation
  Mitral valve repair
Other factors
  Left atrial size
  Left ventricular end-diastolic pressure
  Pulmonary artery pressure
  Right ventricular ejection fraction

ease[7–9] compared with those with rheumatic (3% to 7%)[10, 11] or ischemic (9%) mitral regurgitation. Long-term survival also has been better for patients with myxomatous disease than for those with rheumatic or ischemic mitral regurgitation (see Table 15–1).[3, 7–13]

Comorbid Disease

Patients with mitral regurgitation often have other cardiac and noncardiac diseases, and the presence and severity of these comorbid conditions may be the primary determinants of outcome after mitral valve surgery. Many of these patients have coronary artery disease as the primary cause of mitral regurgitation or as a separate disease process. The high rate of coexisting coronary disease even with myxomatous mitral valve disease reflects the high prevalence of coronary disease and the similar age distribution at presentation of these two conditions (Fig. 15–1).[1, 4, 14] Operative mortality for combined mitral valve replacement and coronary artery bypass grafting is much higher than for mitral valve replacement alone (12.1% versus 3.2% for patients <70 years old).[15]

Patients with rheumatic mitral regurgitation may also have rheumatic involvement of the aortic valve, and to a lesser degree, the tricuspid valve. In patients with mitral regurgitation, significant aortic stenosis or regurgitation may necessitate aortic and mitral valve replacement. Concurrent tricuspid annuloplasty may be needed to treat severe tricuspid regurgitation. These more complex surgical procedures bear higher operative mortality rates, ranging from 9% to 18%, and are likely to have worse long-term outcomes because of the risk for dysfunction of more than one valve.[15]

Measures of Left Ventricular Systolic Function

The cumulative clinical experience with mitral valve surgery conclusively demonstrates that patients with excessive left ventricular dilation or contractile dysfunction have worsened left ventricular function and a poor clinical outcome after surgery. The clinical dilemma has been defining the onset of contractile dysfunction in patients with mitral regurgitation, as loading conditions are altered by the regurgitant lesion itself. The ideal measure of left ventricular performance should accurately reflect contractility, regardless of loading conditions, and should be precise, reproducible, and easily measured.

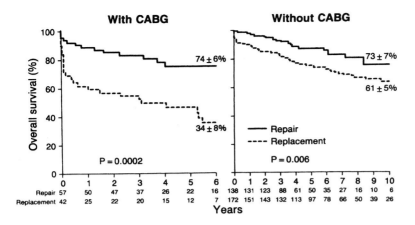

Figure 15·1 Plots of overall survival compared for repair and replacement groups for patients who had *(left)* or did not have *(right)* associated coronary artery bypass graft surgery (CABG). (From Enriquez-Sarano M, Schaff HV, Orszulak TA, Tajik AJ, Bailey KR, Frye RL: Valve repair improves the outcome of surgery for mitral regurgitation: a multivariate analysis. Circulation 1995;91:1022–1028; by permission of The American Heart Association.)

The clinical measures that come closest to meeting these requirements are ejection fraction[2–4, 16] and end-systolic parameters, including end-systolic dimension,[3, 4, 17, 18] volume,[16, 19, 20] and wall stress.[18] The relationship between end-systolic measures and clinical outcome is continuous, and lower ejection fractions or higher end-systolic volumes are associated with a worse prognosis over the entire range of values. However, for clinical decision making, investigators have proposed specific breakpoints that identify groups of patients at risk for poor outcomes to define the optimal timing of surgical intervention. Typical values chosen as breakpoints are an ejection fraction less than 50% or 60%,[2–4] an end-systolic volume index greater than 50 mL/m^2,[19] an echocardiographic end-systolic dimension larger than 45 or 50 mm,[3, 4, 17] and an end-systolic wall stress index greater than 195 mm Hg or an abnormal end-systolic wall stress to volume index.[18, 20] One group of investigators suggested that the ejection fraction and end-systolic volume measured immediately after exercise might be helpful, with a postexercise end-systolic volume index greater than 25 mL/m^2 considered to be more predictive than resting values of postoperative ventricular function (Fig. 15–2).[21]

Other potentially useful measures include an end-diastolic dimension larger than 70 mm or an early systolic ventricular change in pressure (dP/dt) of less than 1343 mm Hg/s, as derived from the Doppler mitral regurgitant jet.[22]

Other Pathophysiologic Indicators

Other pathophysiologic parameters that are predictive of outcome after surgery for mitral regurgitation include increasing left atrial size,[23] an elevated left ventricular end-diastolic pressure,[6, 24] a pulmonary artery mean pressure of more than 20 mm Hg,[16] or a right ventricular ejection fraction less than 30%.[25] The predictive value of right ventricular ejection fraction probably results from the close relationship between pulmonary hypertension and right ventricular function.[26, 27]

Preservation of Chordal Apparatus

The type of mitral valve surgery performed also affects postoperative survival and left ventricular function. Compared with mitral valve

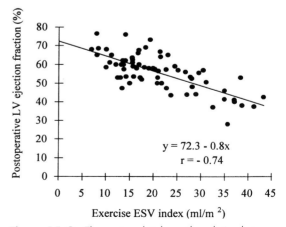

Figure 15·2 The scatter plot shows the relation between the preoperative left ventricular (LV) end-systolic volume (ESV) index at exercise and the postoperative ejection fraction. (From Leung DY, Griffin BP, Stewart WJ, Cosgrove DM III, Thomas JD, Marwick TH: Left ventricular function after valve repair for chronic mitral regurgitation: predictive value of preoperative assessment of contractile reserve by exercise echocardiography. J Am Coll Cardiol 1996;28:1198–1205; reprinted with permission from the American College of Cardiology.)

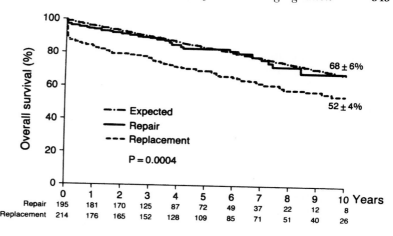

Figure 15·3 Overall survival is compared for valve repair and valve replacement groups (*P* = .0004). The expected survival rate for the total of 409 patients is also represented. The numbers at the bottom indicate the number of patients at risk for each interval. (From Enriquez-Sarano M, Schaff HV, Orszulak TA, Tajik AJ, Bailey KR, Frye RL: Valve repair improves the outcome of surgery for mitral regurgitation: a multivariate analysis. Circulation 1995;91:1022–1028; by permission of The American Heart Association.)

replacement, valve repair has a lower operative mortality rate and better long-term survival.[1, 7–9, 12, 13, 28] In addition, most studies suggest that left ventricular ejection fraction is preserved with chordal preservation either in conjunction with valve replacement or with mitral valve repair (Fig. 15–3).[1, 13, 28–32]

MITRAL VALVE REPLACEMENT
Operative Mortality and Morbidity

Large clinical studies indicate that mitral valve replacement has a higher operative mortality and poorer outcome than surgery for aortic stenosis, aortic regurgitation, or mitral stenosis, particularly when the patient has coexisting coronary artery disease.[15] The overall operative mortality rate for mitral valve replacement is 3% to 29%, with an average rate of 5% to 10% (Table 15–2).[1, 33–44] However, operative mortality depends on the cause of

valvular disease; for example, mortality rates are 27% for ischemic mitral regurgitation and 10% for rheumatic or myxomatous valve disease.[45, 46] Mortality rates for mitral valve repair are considerably lower for these same patient groups.

Long-Term Outcome
Survival

Overall long-term survival after mitral valve replacement has been poor, with reported 5-year survival rates between 50% and 85%.[47–50] To some extent, the poor survival in these studies may be related to patient age, myocardial preservation at surgery, and concealed preoperative left ventricular dysfunction.[51, 52] Survival is better in later series,[3] possibly because of improvements in surgical technique and myocardial preservation. The high prevalence of coexisting coronary artery disease

TABLE 15·2 HOSPITAL MORTALITY AND LONG-TERM OUTCOME AFTER MITRAL VALVE REPAIR

Study	Cause of MR	Patients	Mean Age (y)	Hospital Mortality Rate	Long-Term Survival
Michel, 1991[123]	Myxomatous	156	51	1.3%	84% at 11 y
Jebara, 1992[9]	Myxomatous	79	>70	3.8%	81% at 5 y
David, 1993[7]	Myxomatous	184	57	<1%	94% at 8 y
Fernandez, 1993[10]	Rheumatic	340		6.8%	44 ± 3.7% at 14 y
Bernal, 1993[11]	Rheumatic	327	45 ± 13	3.4%	78% at 16 y
Kay, 1986[107]	Ischemic	101	62 ± 8	~10%	EF > 40%: 58 ± 12% at 10 y EF 21–40%: 33 ± 10% at 10 y EF < 20%: 16 ± 14% at 10 y
Hendren, 1991[12]	Ischemic	65	66 ± 10	9.1%	Restrictive motion: 48% at 3 y Prolapse: 96% at 3 y
Lee, 1996[13]	Mixed	226	63 ± 10	1.8%	71 ± 6% at 7 y

EF, ejection fraction; MR, mitral regurgitation.

also contributes to the poor outcome after mitral valve replacement; an operative mortality rate of 13.4% and a 5-year survival rate of only 76% was reported for a series of patients undergoing combined mitral valve replacement and coronary artery bypass grafting.[53]

Two other key factors affect survival after mitral valve surgery. First, outcome is related to the timing of surgical intervention, with improved survival when surgery is performed before the onset of contractile dysfunction of the left ventricle. Second, ventricular function and survival are improved when at least partial continuity between the mitral annulus and papillary muscles is maintained.

Left Ventricular Function

Left ventricular systolic performance (often expressed as ejection fraction) deteriorates after standard mitral valve replacement. The typical decrease in ejection fraction after surgery is 5 to 10 ejection fraction units (Table 15–3).[4, 16, 21, 28–32, 54, 55] Several mechanisms may contribute to this decline in systolic performance. First, in earlier studies, the adequacy of myocardial preservation during surgery might have been suboptimal. Second, loss of the low impedance pathway for blood flow retrograde across the mitral valve may effectively increase left ventricular afterload, unmasking preexisting contractile dysfunction. While increased afterload may account for deterioration in ventricular function in some patients, recent studies suggest that this factor is of only borderline importance for most patients. Third, disrup-

tion of chordal continuity at the time of mitral valve replacement adversely affects ventricular function, as well as survival, due to abnormal ventricular geometry. The importance of chordal continuity for left ventricular function has led to surgical techniques that allow preservation of some or all of the chordal apparatus when mitral valve replacement is needed and to increased use of mitral valve repair techniques whenever feasible.

Other Outcome Measures

Most mitral prosthetic valves are mechanical given the durability of these valves and because anticoagulation is already needed for atrial fibrillation in most cases. Factors that contribute to postoperative morbidity include the risk of hemorrhage with long-term warfarin therapy and the risk of thromboembolic complications when anticoagulation is inadequate. Even with effective anticoagulation, the rate of thromboembolic complications is 0.6% to 2.3% per patient-year.[56–61] In addition to the presence of a prosthetic valve, atrial fibrillation, left atrial enlargement, and left ventricular systolic dysfunction contribute to the risk of thromboembolism in these patients.

Patients may also have persistent or recurrent heart failure symptoms after surgery. In one study, the incidence of congestive heart failure after valve surgery for mitral regurgitation was 23% ± 2% at 5 years and 33% ± 3% at 10 years.[62] For patients with postoperative heart failure, survival is poor, with an actuarial survival rate of only 44% ± 4% at 5 years. The

TABLE 15·3	LEFT VENTRICULAR FUNCTION AFTER SURGERY FOR MITRAL REGURGITATION				
Study	**Type of Surgery**	**Patients**	**Preop EF (%)**	**Postop EF (%)**	**P Value**
Kennedy, 1979[54]	MVR	7	55 ± 12	43 ± 15	<.05
David, 1984[29]	MVR	15	55 ± 9	48 ± 14	<.01
	MVR + chordal pres	12	53 ± 14	52 ± 16	NS
Goldman, 1987[31]	MVR	8	64 ± 11	40 ± 9	<.0001
	MV repair	10	44 ± 20	49 ± 16	NS
Miki, 1988[30]	MVR	20	54 ± 7	52 ± 8	NS
	MVR + chordal pres	12	54 ± 8	59 ± 8	NS
Crawford, 1990[16]	MVR	48	56 ± 15	45 ± 13	<.001
Rozich, 1992[32]	MVR	7	60 ± 2	36 ± 2	<.05
	MVR + chordal pres	8	63 ± 1	61 ± 2	NS
Enriquez-Sarano, 1995[1]	MVR	214	60 ± 12	49 ± 15	.0001
	MV repair	195	63 ± 9	54 ± 11	.0001
Corin, 1995[28]	MVR	6	60 ± 10	48 ± 10	.01
	MV repair	8	64 ± 5	61 ± 16	NS
Starling, 1995[124]	MV repair	15	58 ± 12	53 ± 16	NS
Leung, 1996[21]	MV repair	74	64 ± 9	55 ± 10	<.001

EF, ejection fraction; MVR, mitral valve replacement; MV, mitral valve; pres, preservation; NS, not significant.

underlying cause of heart failure is impaired ventricular systolic performance in two thirds of patients and heart failure due to valve dysfunction in the remainder. Preoperative predictors of heart failure are ejection fraction, coexisting coronary artery disease, and baseline functional class.

Postoperatively, patients undergoing surgery for mitral regurgitation report a subjective improvement in exercise tolerance, but there have been few objective studies on the degree of improvement in exercise capacity. In one study, postoperative exercise capacity was no different in patients undergoing mitral valve replacement compared with those undergoing repair, with an average exercise duration of 11 minutes on symptom-limited upright bicycle ergometry beginning at a workload of 25 W, with 25-W increases in workload every 3 minutes.[63]

Outcome for Patients With Pulmonary Hypertension

Pulmonary hypertension is a risk factor for a poor outcome after surgery for mitral regurgitation.[6, 16] In the Veterans Affairs Cooperative Study on Valvular Heart Disease, a mean preoperative pulmonary artery pressure of less than 20 mm Hg was a significant predictor of resolution of left ventricular dilation after relief of mitral regurgitation.[16] Overall, mean pulmonary artery pressure declined from 29 $\pm$ 11 to 22 $\pm$ 9 mm Hg ($P <$ .001), and the left ventricular end-diastolic volume index decreased from 117 $\pm$ 51 to 89 $\pm$ 29 mL/m^2 ($P <$ .001).[16]

Studies showing that right ventricular ejection fraction predicts outcome after mitral valve surgery provide further evidence that pulmonary hypertension is associated with a poor prognosis.[25] Since right ventricular ejection fraction tends to be inversely related to pulmonary pressures, it is likely that a reduced right ventricular ejection fraction is a marker of pulmonary hypertension.[26, 27] Taken together, these data suggest that intervention for mitral regurgitation should be considered before significant pulmonary hypertension develops.[16]

In patients with mitral regurgitation operated after the development of pulmonary hypertension, the degree to which pulmonary pressures decline postoperatively affects clinical outcome. If surgery is performed early in the disease course, in addition to relief of the passive elevation in pulmonary pressures due to elevated left atrial pressure, there is a decrease in the reactive component of pulmonary hypertension, which gradually improves during the postoperative period.[64] With more long-standing disease, irreversible changes in the pulmonary vasculature may have occurred, resulting in persistent pulmonary hypertension postoperatively. Some of these patients develop right ventricular dilation and systolic dysfunction, tricuspid regurgitation, and clinical right heart failure.

Homograft Mitral Valve Replacement

Use of a mitral homograft valve has been proposed for selected patients with mitral valve disease. Advantages of a partial or complete homograft mitral valve include preservation of the normal valvular-ventricular interactions, which should preserve ventricular function, and the absence of a need for chronic anticoagulation.[65, 66] Issues that have yet to be addressed include the optimal methods for preparation of the homograft, surgical techniques for implantation, homograft valve hemodynamics, and the long-term durability of this approach. Further studies are needed to define the potential role of homograft mitral valve replacement in patients in whom a mitral valve repair is not technically possible.

MITRAL VALVE REPAIR
Rationale

Mitral valve repair has several potential advantages compared with valve replacement, including avoidance of the suboptimal hemodynamics and potential complications of a prosthetic valve and avoidance of chronic anticoagulation in patients with sinus rhythm or the use of lower intensity anticoagulation in patients with atrial fibrillation. Of even more importance is the role of the mitral valve apparatus in maintaining normal left ventricular geometry and mechanical efficiency.[51, 67] During isovolumic contraction, the ventricle changes shape with a decrease in its long-axis dimension. Long-axis shortening is enhanced by attachments from the papillary muscle tips via the chordae and leaflets to the mitral annulus. The resultant increase in short-axis diameter augments minor-axis shortening during ventricular ejection on the basis of the Frank-Starling mechanism (eg, increased preload).[51] In addition, an intact mitral apparatus helps maintain the normal ellipsoid geometry of the left ventricle, thereby contributing to mechanical efficiency during ventricular ejection. Other effects of an intact mitral apparatus include prevention of ventricular dilation and limitation of increases in end-systolic wall stress by preservation of a normal ratio of wall thickness to ventricular diameter.[68]

A large body of experimental and clinical data support the concept that these potential advantages of mitral valve repair translate into detectable clinical effects. In animal models, chordal interruption leads to a decrease in left ventricular elastance (E_{max}, the end-systolic pressure-volume relationship), an increase in wall stress, and a decrease in the efficiency of ventricular contraction.[69-71] These changes are reversed by reattachment of the chordae.[72, 73] The effect of anterior leaflet chordal severing on left ventricular function is about twice the effect of posterior leaflet chordal disruption.[70] In addition, chordal interruption alters left ventricular geometry with systolic bulging at the site of posteromedial papillary muscle insertion.[70] Fixation of the mitral annulus with a rigid prosthesis leads to further deterioration in ventricular performance, possibly by tethering the posterobasal wall.[71] Overall, the experimental data show that mitral chordal division affects regional wall motion and elastance in association with contraction asynergy and geometric alterations of the left ventricle. In addition, an intact mitral apparatus probably helps support the ventricular free wall in systole, resulting in a low regional afterload and improved contraction synergy.[74]

The findings of clinical series also support the concept that mitral-papillary continuity contributes to left ventricular ejection performance. Even when mitral valve replacement is necessary, preservation of the chordae, so as to not interfere with prosthetic valve function, affects left ventricular systolic performance. In several small, nonrandomized series, left ventricular ejection fraction was preserved in patients undergoing mitral valve replacement with chordal preservation, compared with a decline in ejection fraction in patients undergoing mitral valve replacement with chordal transection (Figs. 15–4 and 15–5).[29, 30, 32] In a small, randomized trial of mitral valve replacement with or without chordal preservation, ventricular function was maintained with chordal preservation based on measurements of radionuclide ejection fraction and preload recruitable stroke work index 3 months and 5 years after surgery.[75] These findings were confirmed in a larger, randomized study of 100 patients undergoing mitral valve replace-

ment with or without chordal preservation with actuarial event-free survival rates at 3 years of 81% versus 68%. Patients with chordal preservation had a higher cardiac output, lower pulmonary pressure, smaller left ventricle, and better exercise capacity compared with those without chordal preservation.[76]

The benefits of chordal preservation for maintenance of left ventricular systolic performance are even more evident in patients undergoing mitral valve repair with preservation of the entire mitral apparatus (Fig. 15–6). Compared with historical controls or concurrent patients at the same institution undergoing mitral valve replacement with chordal disruption, patients undergoing mitral valve repair have higher ejection fractions (Table 15–4).[4, 13, 28, 31] In addition, valve repair for chronic isolated mitral regurgitation results in higher rest and exercise ejection fractions, a lower rest and exercise wall stress, and a more ellipsoid (less spherical) left ventricle compared with matched patients undergoing valve replacement (Figs. 15–7 and 15–8).[63] However, the apparent benefit of valve repair in preserving systolic function may be less apparent as

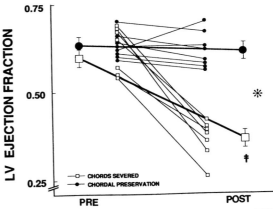

Figure 15·4 The graph shows the preoperative (PRE) and postoperative (POST) left ventricular (LV) ejection fractions for patients undergoing mitral valve replacement (MVR) with chordae tendineae severed *(open squares)* or with chordae tendineae preserved *(closed circles)*. MVR with chords severed resulted in decreased ejection fractions, but MVR with chords preserved did not. Data for individual patients are represented by smaller symbols, and the mean ± SEM is represented by larger symbols. *, $P < .05$ for comparing the two patients groups; ‡, $P < .05$ for comparing PRE and POST status. (From Rozich JD, Carabello BA, Usher BW, Kratz JM, Bell AE, Zile MR: Mitral valve replacement with and without chordal preservation in patients with chronic mitral regurgitation: mechanisms for differences in postoperative ejection performance. Circulation 1992;86:1718–1726; by permission of The American Heart Association.)

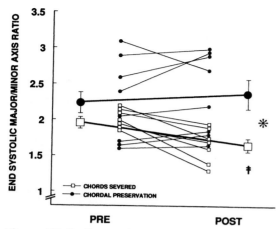

Figure 15·5 The graph shows the preoperative (PRE) and postoperative (POST) ratio of left ventricular end-systolic major (long) axis to minor (short) axis dimensions for patients undergoing mitral valve replacement (MVR) with chordae tendineae severed (open squares) or with chordae tendineae preserved (closed circles). MVR with chords severed resulted in a more spherical geometry. Data for individual patients are represented by smaller symbols, and the mean ± SEM is represented by larger symbols. *, $P < .05$ for comparing the two patient groups; ‡, $P < .05$ for comparing PRE and POST status. (From Rozich JD, Carabello BA, Usher BW, Kratz JM, Bell AE, Zile MR: Mitral valve replacement with and without chordal preservation in patients with chronic mitral regurgitation: mechanisms for differences in postoperative ejection performance. Circulation 1992;86:1718–1726; by permission of The American Heart Association.)

TABLE 15·4	PROPOSED ALGORITHM FOR TIMING OF SURGERY IN PATIENTS WITH ASYMPTOMATIC MITRAL REGURGITATION

Part A

Points	Clinical Variables*	LV Ejection Fraction (%)	LV End-Systolic Dimension (mm)	Feasibility of Valve Repair
0	None	>65	<40	None
1	1	60–65	40–45	Possible
2	≥2	<60	>45	Definite

*Age >60, mean pulmonary artery pressure >20 mm Hg, cardiac index ≤2.0 L/m/m², left ventricular (LV) end-diastolic pressure >12 mm Hg, coronary artery disease, and history of atrial arrhythmias.

Part B

Total Points	Decision Regarding Surgical Intervention
0–1	Delay surgery; recommend clinical and echocardiographic follow-up at 6–12 mo
2	Borderline; recommend clinical and echocardiographic follow-up at 6 mo
≥3	Proceed with surgery

Part C

Additional Predictors of Adverse Outcome in Mitral Regurgitation*

Fractional shortening	<31%
End-systolic volume index	>30 mL/m²
End-systolic stress index	>195 mm Hg
End-diastolic dimension	>70 mm
Doppler dP/dt of MR jet	<1343 mm Hg/s
Right ventricular ejection fraction	<30%

*Add two points for each predictor present.
Algorithm for the timing of surgical intervention in mitral regurgitation (MR):
(A) Assign a point score for each of the four designated categories.
(B) Based on the total score, follow suggested guidelines regarding timing of surgery.
(C) Although not essential for decision analysis, additional predictors of adverse outcome, all of which can be measured by two-dimensional echocardiography, can also be used to support decisions.
From Donovan CL, Starling MR: Role of echocardiography in the timing of surgical intervention for chronic mitral and aortic regurgitation. *In* Otto CM, ed. The Practice of Clinical Echocardiography. Philadelphia: WB Saunders; 1997:327.

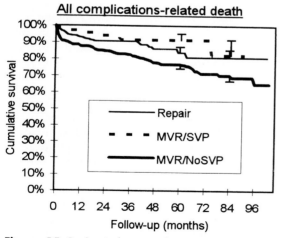

Figure 15·6 Survival curves for complication-related deaths among 612 patients undergoing mitral valve repair (Repair, n = 226), mitral valve replacement with subvalvular preservation (MVR/SVP, n = 68), or mitral valve replacement without subvalvular preservation (MVR/NoSVP, n = 318). (From Lee EM, Shapiro LM, Wells FC: Importance of subvalvular preservation and early operation in mitral valve surgery. Circulation 1996;94:2117–2123; by permission of The American Heart Association.)

more patients undergoing valve replacement have some degree of chordal preservation and as the indications for valve repair are expanded to include a wider range of disease severity. In fact, in two recent large series of patients undergoing mitral valve repair, mean ejection fraction decreased by about 10 ejection fraction units.[1, 21]

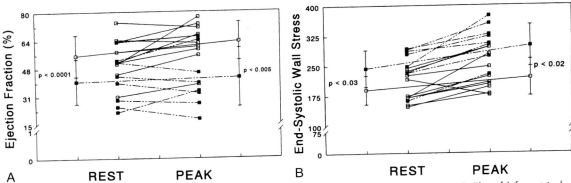

Figure 15·7   *A,* Plot of left ventricular ejection fraction (%) at rest and during peak exercise. *B,* Plot of left ventricular end-systolic circumferential wall stress (kdynes/cm²) at rest and during peak exercise. Both measures are given for patients with mitral valve repair *(open squares)* and for those with mitral valve replacement *(closed squares).* (From Tischler MD, Cooper KA, Rowen M, LeWinter MM: Mitral valve replacement versus mitral valve repair: a Doppler and quantitative stress echocardiographic study. Circulation 1994;89:132–137; by permission of The American Heart Association.)

Even so, on the basis of the experimental and clinical data, a consensus opinion has developed that maintaining chordal continuity is desirable, either as a valve repair procedure or in addition to placement of a prosthetic valve, in order to preserve left ventricular systolic performance.

Technique

Valve Replacement With Chordal Preservation

Chordal preservation in conjunction with placement of a prosthetic valve may include preservation of only the posterior leaflet chordae, the anterior leaflet chordae, or both. The amount of leaflet tissue and number of

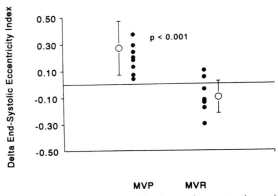

Figure 15·8   The scatter plot shows changes in the end-systolic eccentricity index between rest and peak exercise. (From Tischler MD, Cooper KA, Rowen M, LeWinter MM: Mitral valve replacement versus mitral valve repair: a Doppler and quantitative stress echocardiographic study. Circulation 1994;89:132–137; by permission of The American Heart Association.) MVP, mitral valve repair; MVR, mitral valve replacement.

chordae preserved depends on the underlying disease process and the extent of anatomic valve abnormality. With severe chordal fusion and shortening due to rheumatic disease, excision may be needed to relieve obstruction and allow proper positioning of the prosthesis. Conversely, with severely redundant myxomatous leaflets, leaving excess leaflet tissue may obstruct the outflow tract or impair prosthetic valve function.

Preservation of the posterior leaflet and chordae often is relatively straightforward, since the leaflet tissue sits posterior to the prosthesis and may be left intact without interfering with normal function of the prosthetic valve. The larger anterior leaflet may obstruct inflow across the prosthesis or may show systolic anterior motion into the outflow tract, obstructing left ventricular ejection. These complications may be avoided by resection of the anterior leaflet, however, given the experimental data suggesting that anterior leaflet chordal continuity may be more important than the posterior leaflet, surgical techniques have been developed that allow its preservation. These procedures typically involve division or partial resection of the central portion of the leaflet, with the remaining tissue fixed medially and laterally to prevent valve or outflow obstruction.[30] Another approach includes incising the leaflet parallel to the mitral annulus, removal of excess leaflet tissue, and closure of the remaining leaflet with the annulus using a running suture.[77]

Valve Repair

A wide variety of valve repair techniques have been developed. The most commonly performed repair procedure is quadrilateral resection of the posterior leaflet. A rectangular section of the posterior leaflet containing the excess tissue is resected, the edges are reapproximated, and the annulus is reduced corresponding to the extent of resection, with or without placement of a mitral annuloplasty ring (Fig. 15–9).[33, 78–81] The overall success rate for quadrangular resection in appropriately selected patients is about 90%.[45] While posterior annular calcification makes repair techniques more difficult, one group reports that the success rate for quadrangular resection of the posterior leaflet is high, even in the presence of severe calcification of the annulus or leaflets, although calcium debridement is needed in some cases.[82]

Anterior leaflet repairs tend to be more complicated, involving resection of leaflet tissue, chordal transfers from the posterior leaflet or another section of the anterior leaflet, chordal shortening, papillary muscle shortening, or valve resuspension.[78] Some repair techniques use sutures as "neochordae" to support the valve tissue.[83] Recent data suggest that anterior leaflet repairs can be performed with a high technical success rate and a similar surgical mortality rate and freedom from reoperation at 5 and 10 years compared with results for patients undergoing posterior leaflet repairs.[84–87]

Intraoperative Transesophageal Echocardiographic Monitoring

Most centers performing mitral valve repair procedures use intraoperative transesophageal echocardiography to assess the adequacy of valve repair and detect complications before the surgical procedure is completed. The transesophageal examination typically includes two-dimensional echocardiographic assessment of mitral valve anatomy and motion (Fig. 15–10), color flow imaging of the mitral regurgitant jet in at least two orthogonal views (Fig. 15–11 ; see also color insert), and evaluation of the pattern of pulmonary venous flow (Fig. 15–12). The images and Doppler flows should be recorded at similar loading conditions on the preoperative and postoperative studies to minimize physiologic variability in the assessment of regurgitant severity.

At one large referral center, intraoperative transesophageal echocardiography detected an inadequate repair in 8% of patients with a significant impact on subsequent clinical decisions.[88] Intraoperative monitoring also may provide important prognostic data, as one re-

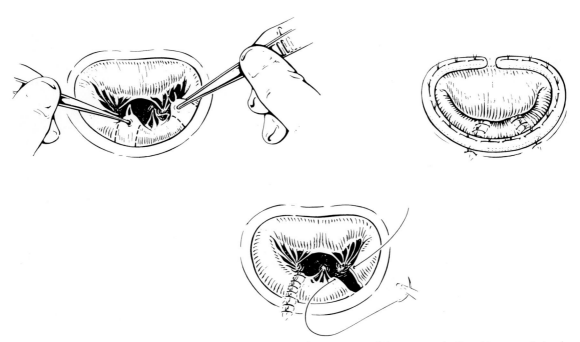

Figure 15·9 Mitral valve repair with quadrilateral resection of two sections of the posterior leaflet with ruptured chordae and placement of an annuloplasty ring. (From Cosgrove DM, Stewart WJ: Mitral valvuloplasty. Curr Probl Cardiol 1989;7:359.)

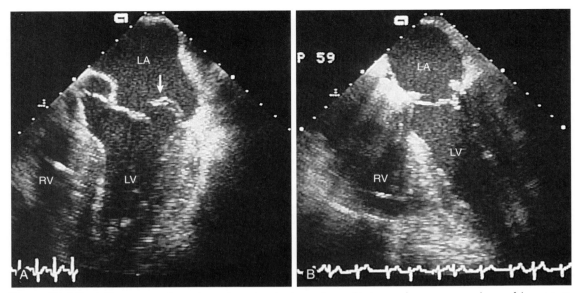

Figure 15·10   *A,* The transesophageal two-dimensional echocardiographic image shows severe prolapse of the posterior mitral valve leaflet *(arrow)* at baseline. *B,* After quadrilateral resection and placement of an annuloplasty ring, leaflet closure is normal. LA, left atrium; LV, left ventricle; RV, right ventricle.

cent study found that, although there was no significant effect on mortality or other morbidity, even mild (1+ or 2+) postoperative mitral regurgitation was associated with a trend toward repeat operation for persistent regurgitation.[89]

Immediate Results

Compared with mitral valve replacement, the operative mortality rate is lower for patients undergoing mitral valve repair. Reported surgical mortality rates for mitral valve

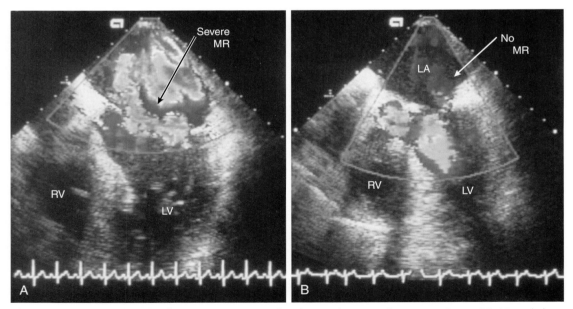

Figure 15·11   Doppler color flow images correspond to the two-dimensional images in Figure 15·10 and show severe mitral regurgitation (MR) with an anteriorly directed jet at baseline *(A)* and no significant regurgitation after mitral valve repair *(B).* The mean arterial pressure was similar during the preoperative and postoperative recordings. LA, left atrium; LV, left ventricle; RV, right ventricle. (These illustrations also occur in the color insert.)

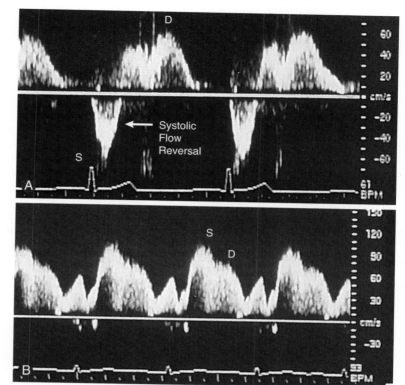

Figure 15·12 Transesophageal Doppler recording of pulmonary venous flow into the left atrium with normal antegrade flow shown above the zero line. *A,* Severe mitral regurgitation is associated with systolic flow reversal in the pulmonary veins *(arrow)* at baseline. *B,* After valve repair, the pattern of systolic flow normalizes, indicating the absence of severe regurgitation. S, systole; D, diastole.

repair average 2% to 4%, ranging from 0% to 7%,[33–44, 90] with higher mortality rates in older patients and those with ischemic mitral regurgitation.[45] These mortality rates are seen despite substantially longer crossclamp and cardiopulmonary bypass times with valve repair compared with valve replacement.[43]

Left ventricular systolic and diastolic function is improved after mitral valve repair compared with valve replacement (Fig. 15–13).[28] Even patients with normal global and regional systolic function have evidence of diastolic dysfunction preoperatively, including an increased peak diastolic filling rate and decreased passive chamber stiffness, which normalize after valve repair.[28]

Complications

An early complication after mitral valve repair is systolic anterior motion of the mitral valve, resulting in dynamic outflow obstruction in 1% to 4% of patients (Fig. 15–14; see also color insert).[88, 91, 92] The incidence of dynamic outflow obstruction has decreased as the surgical technique has been refined, particularly with the use of a flexible or no annuloplasty ring. When dynamic outflow obstruction is de-

tected on the intraoperative echocardiographic study, the obstruction may be relieved by simple alterations in loading conditions, specifically by increasing preload and increasing afterload. If outflow obstruction persists despite these maneuvers, a reduction in the degree of annuloplasty with removal of the ring, or use of the posterior leaflet sliding technique may be needed.[91, 92] Dynamic outflow obstruction after mitral valve repair is most likely to occur in patients with a large redundant posterior leaflet, small left ventricular cavity, and a narrow angle between the closure planes of the mitral and aortic valves, and can be avoided using the sliding leaflet technique.[79, 93, 94]

The other major complication early after mitral valve repair is persistent mitral regurgitation. While a persistent flail segment is seen in only about 1% of patients, about 4% have persistent significant mitral regurgitation detected on the intraoperative transesophageal echocardiogram. Careful evaluation at loading conditions similar to the preoperative baseline, and similar to the expected long-term hemodynamics, is needed to avoid an unnecessary repeat repair procedure or valve replacement. However, given the evidence that even

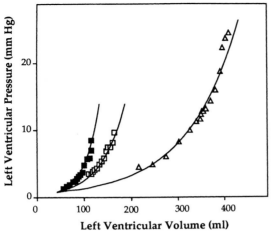

Figure 15·13 Pressure-volume relation for typical control subjects *(closed squares)* and patients before *(open triangles)* and after *(open squares)* mitral valve reconstruction. Compared with control subjects, preoperative patients demonstrated an elevated end-diastolic pressure and decreased diastolic stiffness. After operation, the passive stiffness curves shifted back toward that of the control subjects, with a normalization of end-diastolic pressure. Mathematical analyses demonstrated decreased preoperative and normal postoperative passive chamber stiffness. (From Corin WJ, Sutsch G, Murakami T, Krogmann ON, Turina M, Hess OM: Left ventricular function in chronic mitral regurgitation: preoperative and postoperative comparison. J Am Coll Cardiol 1995;25:113–121; reprinted with permission from the American College of Cardiology.)

mild residual regurgitation is associated with a higher likelihood of reoperation, some groups recommend a second pump run at the initial surgical procedure when more than trivial regurgitation is observed. Using this approach, a second cardiopulmonary bypass procedure is performed in 6% to 8% of their patients.[88, 89] Given the uncertainties involved in clinical decision making in the operating room and the overall low incidence of residual regurgitation long-term,[85] other clinicians prefer to defer a second surgical procedure if the patient is doing well hemodynamically and then reevaluate residual regurgitant severity at a later date.

The operative mortality rate for reoperation after mitral valve repair is 4%, with a 5-year survival rate after repeat surgery of 75%.[95] The indication for reoperation predominantly (in 70%) is severe mitral regurgitation, with hemolytic anemia, mixed mitral stenosis and regurgitation, or mitral stenosis accounting for the remainder. The interval between the initial valve repair and reoperation ranges from 2 months to 25 years. In two thirds of patients, the initial repair is intact, with recurrent mitral regurgitation due to fibrosis and calcification of the annulus, leaflets, or both; recurrent chordal rupture; or valve perforation. In the one third of patients with failure of the initial

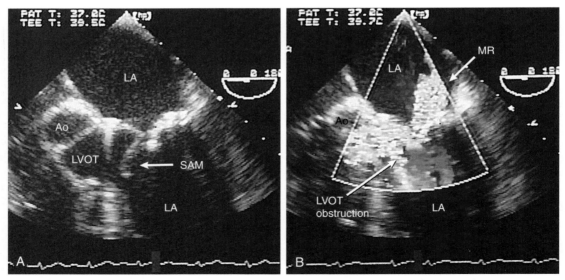

Figure 15·14 *A,* The transesophageal two-dimensional echocardiographic image shows systolic anterior motion (SAM) of the anterior mitral valve leaflet *(arrow)* immediately after mitral valve repair. *B,* The resulting dynamic outflow tract obstruction and mitral regurgitation are seen on color flow imaging. After volume loading, mitral valve motion normalized, and no significant mitral regurgitation or outflow obstruction was evident. At the 6-month follow-up evaluation, the patient had no evidence of outflow obstruction or mitral regurgitation demonstrated by echocardiography. Ao, aorta; LA, left atrium; LVOT, left ventricular outflow tract. (*B* also occurs in the color insert.)

repair, findings included dehiscence of the ring annuloplasty, failure of the commissural repair, and breakdown of the chordal or leaflet repair.[95]

Long-Term Outcome

Mitral valve repair has a long-term survival advantage compared with valve replacement, with reported 5- to 10-year survival rates of 80% to 94% for patients with myxomatous mitral valve disease compared with 40% to 60% survival rates for those with mitral valve replacement.[7, 34, 37, 90] In patients undergoing surgery before development of ventricular dysfunction, predictors of survival include age, functional status, and mitral valve anatomy.[96]

Left ventricular systolic function is maintained at long-term follow-up in those with normal function at baseline.[29, 32, 97, 98] However, for patients with a low postoperative ejection fraction (<50%), the actuarial survival rate is only 38% ± 9% at 8 years.[3]

There is a low incidence of thromboembolic events, with 95% of patients free of cerebrovascular complications 5 to 10 years after mitral valve repair.[7, 99] The risk of endocarditis is low after mitral valve repair, with a rate of 0.4% per year for repair compared with 2.2% per year with a mechanical valve.[33, 99]

Postoperatively, about one third of patients are in atrial fibrillation, so that chronic warfarin anticoagulation is needed, even though valve repair was performed. Atrial fibrillation adversely affects long-term outcome due to the increased risk of embolic events and the lack of atrial contribution to ventricular diastolic filling. As in other patient groups, the duration of atrial fibrillation is the primary determinant of whether sinus rhythm can be achieved and maintained. More than 80% of patients with atrial fibrillation preoperatively remain in atrial fibrillation after surgery.[100] In those with new onset atrial fibrillation within 3 months of surgical intervention, conversion to sinus rhythm is more likely.

Patient Selection

The most important factors affecting whether valve repair is feasible include the cause of valve disease and results of a detailed analysis of mitral valve anatomy and dynamics. In several series, repair has been more successful in patients with myxomatous (also referred to as "degenerative") than in those with rheumatic valve disease.[82] Repair procedures in pa-

tients with ischemic mitral regurgitation or valve incompetence caused by left ventricular dilation and systolic dysfunction must be tailored to the specific clinical setting, coexisting coronary disease, and anatomic features of the mitral leaflets, annulus, and left ventricle. With ischemic mitral regurgitation, evaluation of regurgitant severity by echocardiography is helpful in deciding whether an annuloplasty may be beneficial.[101]

In patients with myxomatous mitral valve disease, echocardiographic evaluation includes assessment of the degree of thickening, redundancy, and prolapse of each leaflet; chordal anatomy and elongation; evidence for ruptured chordae; annular dimensions; and measurements of left atrial and ventricular size and function.[102, 103] The mechanism of mitral regurgitation often can be deduced from analysis of the pattern of leaflet motion (ie, excessive, normal, or restrictive) and the origin and direction of the regurgitant jet.[103] The probability of repair is highest in the case of isolated involvement of the posterior leaflet. Excessive redundancy or elongation of the anterior leaflet may be associated with dynamic outflow obstruction postoperatively, unless a concurrent repair of the anterior leaflet is performed. Anterior leaflet abnormalities are more difficult to repair, although excellent results have been reported by experienced centers.[83–87] Occasionally, prolapse involves one of the mitral valve commissures, which increases the difficulty of repair.

Detailed echocardiographic images of mitral valve anatomy should be carefully reviewed with the surgeon, as the likelihood of valve repair depends not only on valve anatomy, but also on the experience of the surgeon. Both transthoracic and transesophageal echocardiographic images have been shown to be highly predictive of the feasibility of valve repair, with agreement between echocardiography and surgery for 74% to 89% of cases.[102, 104, 105]

As improved techniques for valve repair are developed, more patients will be candidates for this procedure. In the future, it may be possible to customize the approach to valve repair preoperatively using three-dimensional echocardiographic reconstruction of the patient's valve in conjunction with computer modeling of the expected stress-strain relationships after the proposed repair procedure.

Outcome for Specific Patient Groups
Myxomatous Mitral Valve Disease

Mitral valve repair in patients with myxomatous mitral valve disease often produces excellent anatomic and functional results, with little residual mitral regurgitation and no significant inflow obstruction. As seen in Table 15-2, operative mortality is low, and long-term outcome is excellent. Valve repair most often involves quadrilateral resection of a segment of the posterior leaflets, with only a minority of patients requiring more complex repairs or anterior leaflet procedures.

Rheumatic Mitral Valve Disease

In contrast, results of mitral valve repair often are suboptimal in patients with rheumatic mitral regurgitation. Valve repair is technically more difficult and may not be feasible in many cases because of chordal fusion and shortening, in addition to calcification and retraction of leaflet tissue.[17] In clinical series, rheumatic mitral regurgitation is reparable in fewer than 50% of cases.[45, 78]

When mitral valve repair is performed, operative mortality is higher and long-term event-free survival rates are lower compared with those for patients with nonrheumatic mitral regurgitation. Because these patients typically have some component of mitral stenosis in conjunction with regurgitation, the valve repair procedure includes commissurotomy in most cases, annuloplasty in all cases, papillary muscle splitting in about one half of cases, and subvalvular apparatus repair in about one fifth of cases.[11] Concurrent tricuspid valve annuloplasty is needed in one third of patients because of rheumatic involvement of the tricuspid valve.[11]

In one study of patients with rheumatic mitral regurgitation undergoing valve repair or replacement, postoperative death or heart failure was predicted by a preoperative end-systolic dimension larger than 50 mm. Chordal preservation was not a predictor of outcome in this study.[17] Another study found that mortality was higher among those needing tricuspid valve repair, probably because of the higher incidence of pulmonary hypertension and left ventricular systolic dysfunction in this subset.[11]

Ischemic Mitral Regurgitation

Ischemic mitral regurgitation accounts for only about 6% to 10% of patients undergoing mitral valve surgery.[12, 106] Outcome after surgery for ischemic mitral regurgitation is strongly related to baseline ejection fraction, with 10-year survival rates of 58% ± 12% for those with a resting ejection fraction of more than 40%, 33% ± 10% for an ejection fraction between 21% and 40%, and 16% ± 14% for an ejection fraction of less than 20%.[107] In addition, outcome is better with valve repair than with replacement.[106, 107]

Some investigators propose that most patients with moderate to severe regurgitation benefit from mitral valve repair or replacement at the time of coronary bypass surgery[101]; however, the optimal approach to patients with ischemic mitral regurgitation remains controversial. Mitral valve repair is feasible in less than one half of patients with ischemic mitral regurgitation,[106] with the surgical procedure used depending on the exact mechanism of mitral regurgitation.[108] For example, with localized papillary muscle rupture, it may be possible to suture the papillary muscle head in place and use chordal transfer or replacement techniques to provide additional support to the leaflet. However, with extensive necrosis of the papillary muscle and ventricular wall, valve replacement with chordal preservation is preferable. With an old, healed myocardial infarction or with left ventricular dilation and systolic dysfunction, apical displacement of the papillary muscle plus annular dilation leads to incomplete leaflet coaptation, which may be corrected by simple annuloplasty. Annuloplasty alone is sufficient for valve repair in one half to two thirds of patients with ischemic mitral regurgitation. In the remainder, repair techniques include leaflet resection, chordal shortening, and papillary muscle reimplantation or shortening.[12] In some series, the valve repair descriptions suggest that patients with concurrent coronary artery disease and myxomatous mitral valve disease may have been inappropriately diagnosed with ischemic mitral regurgitation.

For intermittent ischemia with episodic mitral regurgitation, several investigations support the concept that revascularization alone may relieve mitral regurgitation in conjunction with a significant improvement in left ventricular ejection fraction.[108–110] Other studies suggest that relief of mitral regurgitation is more complete if an annuloplasty is performed, particularly with moderate to severe regurgitation.[101, 107, 111]

With chronic left ventricular systolic dysfunction leading to mitral regurgitation in patients with coronary artery disease, there is considerable controversy whether mitral regurgitation will resolve with revascularization alone or whether a concurrent annuloplasty is needed. Some investigators have shown an improvement in left ventricular ejection fraction and/or a decrease in mitral regurgitant severity after coronary artery bypass grafting, suggesting that revascularization alone may be effective.[110] Other investigators argue that mitral valve repair at the time of revascularization is needed. In a series of 100 patients older than 65 years, with a baseline ejection fraction of 32% ± 2%, coronary artery bypass grafting plus mitral valve repair (a simple annuloplasty ring in about one half) had an operative mortality rate of 4% and led to a decrease in mitral regurgitant severity from 4+ to 1+ or less in all patients.[112] Further studies addressing the role of surgical intervals for end-stage ischemic mitral regurgitation are needed before this approach is widely disseminated.

Dilated Cardiomyopathy

Although it is evident that moderate to severe mitral regurgitation caused by severe left ventricular dilation and systolic dysfunction exacerbates clinical symptoms and is associated with a worse prognosis than the absence or milder degrees of mitral regurgitation, the potential role of mitral valve repair in these patients is less clear.[113, 114] Traditionally, these patients have been considered poor candidates for surgical intervention due to the presence of severe left ventricular dysfunction and given the concern that systolic function might further deteriorate after relief of mitral regurgitation due to removal of the low-impedance ejection pathway into the left atrium. Recent evidence highlighting the importance of annular-papillary muscle continuity coupled with an increased understanding of the effects of loading conditions on left ventricular performance has led to reconsideration of mitral valve surgery in this patient group.

In preliminary studies of mitral valve repair for severe mitral regurgitation and associated severe left ventricular systolic dysfunction (average baseline ejection fraction of 16% to 18%), operative mortality was low, and the 1-year actuarial survival rate was 70% to 74%.[115–117] These studies showed a decrease in mitral regurgitant severity, an increase in forward cardiac output, and a small decrease in end-diastolic volume after mitral valve repair. In addition, ejection fraction improved by an average of 10 ejection fraction units. The investigators propose that the improvement in ventricular performance can be attributed to changes in the shape of the ventricle and a

lower wall stress, which favorably affects ventricular performance.

Despite these encouraging findings, caution is needed in extrapolating these results to other patients with severe mitral regurgitation and dilated cardiomyopathy. These studies included small numbers of patients, were performed at a single institution, were not randomized, and had no control group to serve as a reference standard. In addition, these patients were high-risk candidates for cardiac surgery, so that more definitive evidence of efficacy in terms of improved clinical outcome is needed before widespread use of mitral valve repair procedures in patients with dilated cardiomyopathy.

OPTIMAL TIMING AND CHOICE OF PROCEDURE

Decisions about the optimal timing of surgical intervention in patients with mitral regurgitation are based on appropriate integration of clinical and physiologic parameters and an understanding of the natural history of the underlying disease process. An estimate of the likelihood that valve repair, rather than replacement, is possible also affects the timing of intervention.

Traditional Indications for Intervention

The clinical decision to refer a patient with mitral regurgitation for mitral valve surgery must consider the relative risks and benefits of continued medical therapy versus surgical intervention. Clearly, surgical intervention was, and continues to be, the treatment of choice for patients with symptoms caused by severe mitral regurgitation.

In asymptomatic patients, however, not only operative mortality and morbidity risks, but also the long-term risks of chronic anticoagulation and the possibility of worsening of left ventricular systolic function postoperatively were important considerations when the primary surgical option was mechanical valve replacement. Thus, traditional indications for mitral valve surgery included significant symptoms due to valvular regurgitation or definite evidence of early contractile dysfunction of the left ventricle. In the asymptomatic patient, valve replacement was deferred until the expected long-term outcome with medical therapy was poor enough to justify a mechanical valve replacement and chronic anticoagulation.

Newer Indications

Recently, our understanding of the pathophysiologic basis for a decline in ventricular function after mitral valve surgery has undergone substantial change. In the past, mitral regurgitation was considered to be a low afterload state, so that valve replacement was thought to simply "unmask" preexisting contractile dysfunction. Now, it is recognized that many patients have a high-normal or high circumferential and meridional wall stress preoperatively (contradicting the traditional idea that mitral regurgitation is a low afterload state), so that the decline in ejection fraction after valve replacement is attributable to other factors.[118] Probably the most important of these factors is the contribution of annular-papillary muscle continuity to ventricular performance.

During the past few years, the balance of risks and benefits for a surgical versus medical approach to chronic mitral regurgitation has shifted. Surgical intervention now is considered earlier in the disease course, even in asymptomatic patients. This change in clinical approach has been based on several considerations. First, the utility of noninvasive end-systolic measures of ventricular size in predicting postoperative contractile dysfunction has been recognized. Second, the option of mitral valve repair or chordal preservation at the time of valve replacement has led to an improvement in postoperative left ventricular function. Third, echocardiographic evaluation of valve anatomy, regurgitant severity, ventricular function, and associated abnormalities allows detailed assessment and follow-up evaluation of individual patients. Fourth, the long-term negative consequences of left atrial enlargement, atrial fibrillation, and pulmonary hypertension suggest that intervention before development of these complications is desirable. Finally, improvements in the surgical approach have resulted in decreased operative mortality and morbidity and improved long-term outcome.

Clinical decision making in the individual patient with mitral regurgitation is complex, requiring the integration of numerous objective and subjective considerations.[52, 119–121] In addition to evaluation of the etiology and severity of valve disease, the left ventricular response to chronic volume overload, and the upstream consequences of an elevated left atrial pressure (eg, pulmonary hypertension, left atrial enlargement, atrial fibrillation), the decision involves consideration of comorbid disease, patient age, functional status, and potential contraindications to long-term anticoagulation. Subjective factors include the patient's preferences regarding surgical intervention, lifestyle considerations relative to chronic anticoagulation, the possibility of a future pregnancy, and the annoyance factor of audible mechanical valve clicks.

Optimally, valve surgery in patients with asymptomatic mitral regurgitation should be performed just before the onset of left ventricular dysfunction or other irreversible complications. Since randomized, prospective studies on the timing of surgical intervention for chronic asymptomatic mitral regurgitation are not available, clinicians instead have extrapolated from surgical series of patients referred for mitral valve surgery with analysis directed toward identification of baseline predictors of postoperative survival and left ventricular function. These preoperative variables are then assumed to be useful indicators for the optimal timing of surgical intervention.

While there is no simple approach that will be applicable to all patients, a framework for decision making in the patient with isolated chronic mitral regurgitation was developed by Donovan and Starling (see Table 15–4). This algorithm incorporates four major factors: clinical variables, left ventricular ejection fraction, left ventricular end-systolic dimension, and the estimated feasibility of valve repair. Using a point scoring system, patients with 3 points or more are predicted to benefit from surgical intervention to prevent left ventricular systolic dysfunction, while those with fewer points can continue to be followed with echocardiography. Other predictors of clinical outcome that may impact this decision are also indicated.

In addition to the predictors in Table 15–4, other factors to consider are the onset of atrial fibrillation, evidence of increasing left atrial size, and increasing pulmonary artery pressures.[120] It is plausible that early intervention may prevent or reverse atrial fibrillation and pulmonary hypertension. While each of these additional factors by itself is only a weak indication for surgery, the combination of several factors makes the case for surgical intervention more compelling.

Although this approach cannot replace clinical judgment in each case and there will be situations in which these guidelines are not helpful, this algorithm provides a useful starting point for clinical decision making for most patients with chronic mitral regurgitation.

Whenever possible, the cardiologist and surgeon should discuss the optimal timing of intervention, review the echocardiographic images together, and present difficult or borderline cases for review at conjoint medical-surgical conferences.

Choice of Procedure

Given the benefits of valve repair compared with valve replacement for mitral regurgitation, every patient should be considered for possible mitral valve repair.[1, 29, 31, 63, 70] If valve anatomy precludes an effective repair or if repair is unsuccessful, valve replacement is appropriate. When valve replacement is necessary, a mechanical valve often is chosen, as many of these patients already require long-term anticoagulation for atrial fibrillation. Mechanical valves have a proven record of long-term durability (see Chapter 17). When possible, most surgeons preserve part or all of the chordal apparatus at the time of mechanical valve replacement. Attempts to use nonstented tissue valves in the mitral position have not been successful, and experience with mitral homografts is limited.[65, 66] If long-term anticoagulation is problematic, a stented porcine valve can be used in the mitral position, although durability is suboptimal compared with a mechanical valve.

When Is Intervention Too Late?

The recent experience with mitral valve repair in patients with dilated cardiomyopathy suggests that surgical risk is acceptable and long-term outcome may be improved even in those with severe left ventricular systolic dysfunction.[115–117] However, if valve repair is not feasible, mitral valve replacement should be approached only with extreme caution if the patient has severe left ventricular dilation or a reduced ejection fraction.[52, 122] These patients have a high operative mortality rate, a very poor long-term outcome, and are likely to have further deterioration in left ventricular function postoperatively.

While a specific point after which it is "too late" for mitral valve replacement is difficult to define, outcome is progressively worse with lower ejection fractions and larger end-systolic volumes.[31, 121] However, given the even poorer prognosis with medical therapy, surgical intervention may still be undertaken after consider-ation of all the clinical parameters, particularly if improved ventricular function is expected with coronary revascularization.[48] For younger patients with severe left ventricular dysfunction and mitral regurgitation, the option of cardiac transplantation also may be considered.

References

1. Enriquez-Sarano M, Schaff HV, Orszulak TA, Tajik AJ, Bailey KR, Frye RL: Valve repair improves the outcome of surgery for mitral regurgitation: a multivariate analysis. Circulation 1995;91:1022–1028.
2. Phillips HR, Levine FH, Carter JE, et al: Mitral valve replacement for isolated mitral regurgitation: analysis of clinical course and late postoperative left ventricular ejection fraction. Am J Cardiol 1981;48:647–654.
3. Enriquez-Sarano M, Tajik AJ, Schaff HV, Orszulak TA, Bailey KR, Frye RL: Echocardiographic prediction of survival after surgical correction of organic mitral regurgitation. Circulation 1994;90:830–837.
4. Enriquez-Sarano M, Tajik AJ. Schaff HV, et al: Echocardiographic prediction of left ventricular function after correction of mitral regurgitation: results and clinical implications. J Am Coll Cardiol 1994;24:1536–1543.
5. Ramanathan KB, Knowles J, Connor MJ, et al: Natural history of chronic mitral insufficiency: relation of peak systolic pressure/end-systolic volume ratio to morbidity and mortality. J Am Coll Cardiol 1984;3:1412–1416.
6. Salomon NW, Stinson EB, Griepp RB, Shumway NE: Mitral valve replacement: long-term evaluation of prosthesis-related mortality and morbidity. Circulation 1977;56:94–101.
7. David TE, Armstrong S, Sun Z, Daniel L: Late results of mitral valve repair for mitral regurgitation due to degenerative disease. Ann Thorac Surg 1993;56:7–12.
8. Acar J, Michel PL, Luxereau P, Vahanian A, Cormier B: Indications for surgery in mitral regurgitation. Eur Heart J 1991;12(suppl B):52–54.
9. Jebara VA, Dervanian P, Acar C, et al: Mitral valve repair using Carpentier techniques in patients more than 70 years old: early and late results. Circulation 1992;86:53–59.
10. Fernandez J, Joyce DH, Hirschfeld KJ, et al: Valve-related events and valve-related mortality in 340 mitral valve repairs: a late phase follow-up study. Eur J Cardiothorac Surg 1993;7:263–270.
11. Bernal JM, Rabasa JM, Vilchez FG, Cagigas JC, Revuelta JM: Mitral valve repair in rheumatic disease: the flexible solution. Circulation 1993;88:746–753.
12. Hendren WG, Nemec JJ, Lytle BW, et al: Mitral valve repair for ischemic mitral insufficiency. Ann Thorac Surg 1991;52:1246–1251.
13. Lee EM, Shapiro LM, Wells FC: Importance of subvalvular preservation and early operation in mitral valve surgery. Circulation 1996;94:2117–2123.
14. Enriquez-Sarano M, Seward JB, Bailey KR, Tajik AJ: Effective regurgitant orifice area: a noninvasive Doppler development of an old hemodynamic concept. J Am Coll Cardiol 1994;23:443–451.
15. Fremes SE, Goldman BS, Ivanov J, Weisel RD, David TE, Salerno T: Valvular surgery in the elderly. Circulation 1989;80(suppl I):77–90.

16. Crawford MH, Souchek J, Oprian CA, et al: Determinants of survival and left ventricular performance after mitral valve replacement: Department of Veterans Affairs Cooperative Study on Valvular Heart Disease. Circulation 1990;81:1173–1181.

17. Wisenbaugh T, Skudicky D, Sareli P: Prediction of outcome after valve replacement for rheumatic mitral regurgitation in the era of chordal preservation. Circulation 1994;89:191–197.

18. Zile MR, Gaasch WH, Carroll JD, Levine HJ: Chronic mitral regurgitation: predictive value of preoperative echocardiographic indexes of left ventricular function and wall stress. J Am Coll Cardiol 1984;3:1235–1242.

19. Borow KM, Green LH, Mann T, et al: End-systolic volume as a predictor of postoperative left ventricular performance in volume overload from valvular regurgitation. Am J Med 1980;68:655–663.

20. Carabello BA, Williams H, Gash AK, et al: Hemodynamic predictors of outcome in patients undergoing valve replacement. Circulation 1986;74:1309–1316.

21. Leung DY, Griffin BP, Stewart WJ, Cosgrove DM III, Thomas JD, Marwick TH: Left ventricular function after valve repair for chronic mitral regurgitation: predictive value of preoperative assessment of contractile reserve by exercise echocardiography. J Am Coll Cardiol 1996;28:1198–1205.

22. Pai RG, Bansal RC, Shah PM: Doppler-derived rate of left ventricular pressure rise: its correlation with the postoperative left ventricular function in mitral regurgitation. Circulation 1990;82:514–520.

23. Reed D, Abbott RD, Smucker ML, Kaul S: Prediction of outcome after mitral valve replacement in patients with symptomatic chronic mitral regurgitation: the importance of left atrial size. Circulation 1991;84:23–34.

24. Pitts WR, Lange RA, Cigarroa JE, Hillis LD: Preoperative left ventricular peak systolic pressure/end-systolic volume ratio and functional status following valve surgery in patients with mitral regurgitation and enlarged end-systolic volumes. Am J Cardiol 1997;79:1493–1497.

25. Hochreiter C, Niles N, Devereux RB, Kligfield P, Borer JS: Mitral regurgitation: relationship of noninvasive descriptors of right and left ventricular performance to clinical and hemodynamic findings and to prognosis in medically and surgically treated patients. Circulation 1986;73:900–912.

26. Grose R, Strain J, Yipintosoi T: Right ventricular function in valvular heart disease: relation to pulmonary artery pressure. J Am Coll Cardiol 1983;2:225–232.

27. Morrison D, Goldman S, Wright AL, et al: The effect of pulmonary hypertension on systolic function of the right ventricle. Chest 1983;84:250–257.

28. Corin WJ, Sutsch G, Murakami T, Krogmann ON, Turina M, Hess OM: Left ventricular function in chronic mitral regurgitation: preoperative and postoperative comparison. J Am Coll Cardiol 1995;25:113–121.

29. David TE, Burns RJ, Bacchus CM, Druck MN: Mitral valve replacement for mitral regurgitation with and without preservation of chordae tendineae. J Thorac Cardiovasc Surg 1984;88:1718–1725.

30. Miki S, Kusuhara K, Ueda Y, Komeda M, Ohkita Y, Tahata T: Mitral valve replacement with preservation of chordae tendineae and papillary muscles. Ann Thorac Surg 1988;45:28–34.

31. Goldman ME, Mora F, Guarino T, Fuster V, Mindich BP: Mitral valvuloplasty is superior to valve replacement for preservation of left ventricular function: an intraoperative two-dimensional echocardiographic study. J Am Coll Cardiol 1987;10:568–575.

32. Rozich JD, Carabello BA, Usher BW, Kratz JM, Bell AE, Zile MR: Mitral valve replacement with and without chordal preservation in patients with chronic mitral regurgitation: mechanisms for differences in postoperative ejection performance. Circulation 1992;86:1718–1726.

33. Duran CG, Pomar JL, Revuelta JM, et al: Conservative operation for mitral insufficiency: critical analysis supported by postoperative hemodynamic studies of 72 patients. J Thorac Cardiovasc Surg 1980;79:326–337.

34. Yacoub M, Halim M, Radley Smith R, McKay R, Nijveld A, Towers M: Surgical treatment of mitral regurgitation caused by floppy valves: repair versus replacement. Circulation 1981;64:210–216.

35. Oliveira DB, Dawkins KD, Kay PH, Paneth M: Chordal rupture. II: Comparison between repair and replacement. Br Heart J 1983;50:318–324.

36. Adebo OA, Ross JK: Surgical treatment of ruptured mitral valve chordae: a comparison between valve replacement and valve repair. Thorac Cardiovasc Surg 1984;32:139–142.

37. Perier P, Deloche A, Chauvaud S, et al: Comparative evaluation of mitral valve repair and replacement with Starr, Bjork, and porcine valve prostheses. Circulation 1984;70:187–192.

38. Orszulak TA, Schaff HV, Danielson GK, et al: Mitral regurgitation due to ruptured chordae tendineae: early and late results of valve repair. J Thorac Cardiovasc Surg 1985;89:491–498.

39. Sand ME, Naftel DC, Blackstone EH, Kirklin JW, Karp RB: A comparison of repair and replacement for mitral valve incompetence. J Thorac Cardiovasc Surg 1987;94:208–219.

40. Angell WW, Oury JH, Shah P: A comparison of replacement and reconstruction in patients with mitral regurgitation. J Thorac Cardiovasc Surg 1987;93:665–674.

41. Cohn LH, Kowalker W, Bhatia S, et al: Comparative morbidity of mitral valve repair versus replacement for mitral regurgitation with and without coronary artery disease. Ann Thorac Surg 1988;45:284–290.

42. Galloway AC, Colvin SB, Baumann FG, et al: A comparison of mitral valve reconstruction with mitral valve replacement: intermediate-term results. Ann Thorac Surg 1989;47:655–662.

43. Craver JM, Cohen C, Weintraub WS: Case-matched comparison of mitral valve replacement and repair. Ann Thorac Surg 1990;49:964–969.

44. Kawachi Y, Oe M, Asou T, Tominaga R, Tokunaga K: Comparative study between valve repair and replacement for mitral pure regurgitation—early and late postoperative results. Jpn Circ J 1991;55:443–452.

45. Cosgrove DM: Mitral valve repair in patients with elongated chordae tendineae. J Card Surg 1989;4:247–252.

46. Tepe NA, Edmunds LH Jr: Operation for acute postinfarction mitral insufficiency and cardiogenic shock. J Thorac Cardiovasc Surg 1985;89:525–530.

47. Rapaport E: Natural history of aortic and mitral valve disease. Am J Cardiol 1975;35:221–227.

48. Hammermeister KE, Fisher L, Kennedy W, Samuels

S, Dodge HT: Prediction of late survival in patients with mitral valve disease from clinical, hemodynamic, and quantitative angiographic variables. Circulation 1978;57:341–349.

49. Munoz S, Gallardo J, Diaz Gorrin JR, Medina O: Influence of surgery on the natural history of rheumatic mitral and aortic valve disease. Am J Cardiol 1975;35:234–242.

50. Delahaye JP, Gare JP, Viguier E, Delahaye F, de Gevigney G, Milon H: Natural history of severe mitral regurgitation. Eur Heart J 1991;12(suppl B):5–9.

51. Carabello BA: The changing unnatural history of valvular regurgitation. Ann Thorac Surg 1992;53:191–199.

52. Carabello BA: The mitral valve apparatus: is there still room to doubt the importance of its preservation [editorial]? J Heart Valve Dis 1993;2:250–252.

53. Ruvolo G, Speziale G, Bianchini R, Greco E, Tonelli E, Marino B: Combined coronary bypass grafting and mitral valve surgery: early and late results. Thorac Cardiovasc Surg 1995;43:90–93.

54. Kennedy JW, Doces JG, Stewart DK: Left ventricular function before and following surgical treatment of mitral valve disease. Am Heart J 1979;97:592–598.

55. Pitarys CJ, Forman MB, Panayiotou H, Hansen DE: Long-term effects of excision of the mitral apparatus on global and regional ventricular function in humans. J Am Coll Cardiol 1990;15:557–563.

56. Thevenet A, Albat B: Long-term follow-up of 292 patients after valve replacement with the Omnicarbon prosthetic valve. J Heart Valve Dis 1995;4:634–639.

57. Nitter-Hauge S, Abdelnoor M, Svennevig JL: Fifteen-year experience with the Medtronic-Hall valve prosthesis: a follow-up study of 1104 consecutive patients. Circulation 1996;94:105–108.

58. Tatoulis J, Chaiyaroj S, Smith JA: Aortic valve replacement in patients 50 years old or younger with the St. Jude medical valve: 14-year experience. J Heart Valve Dis 1996;5:491–497.

59. Godje OL, Fischlein T, Adelhard K, Nollert G, Klinner W, Reichart B: Thirty-year results of Starr-Edwards prostheses in the aortic and mitral position. Ann Thorac Surg 1997;63:613–619.

60. Orszulak TA, Schaff HV, Puga FJ, et al: Event status of the Starr-Edwards aortic valve to 20 years: a benchmark for comparison. Ann Thorac Surg 1997;63:620–626.

61. Hammermeister KE, Henderson WG, Burchfiel CM, et al: Comparison of outcome after valve replacement with a bioprosthesis versus a mechanical prosthesis: initial 5 year results of a randomized trial. J Am Coll Cardiol 1987;10:719–732.

62. Enriquez-Sarano M, Schaff HV, Orszulak TA, Bailey KR, Tajik AJ, Frye RL: Congestive heart failure after surgical correction of mitral regurgitation: a long-term study. Circulation 1995;92:2496–2503.

63. Tischler MD, Cooper KA, Rowen M, LeWinter MM: Mitral valve replacement versus mitral valve repair: a Doppler and quantitative stress echocardiographic study. Circulation 1994;89:132–137.

64. De Gaetano G, Barberis L, Dottori V, et al: Serial Doppler echocardiography follow-up studies in the postoperative evaluation of severe pulmonary hypertension following surgery for mitral and mitral-aortic defects [in Italian]. Minerva Cardioangiol 1993;41:313–317.

65. Acar C, Farge A, Ramsheyi A, et al: Mitral valve replacement using a cryopreserved mitral homograft. Ann Thorac Surg 1994;57:746–748.

66. Acar C, Tolan M, Berrebi A, et al: Homograft replacement of the mitral valve: graft selection, technique of implantation, and results in forty-three patients. J Thorac Cardiovasc Surg 1996;111:367–378.

67. Peterson KL: Timing of cardiac surgery in chronic mitral valve disease: implications of natural history studies and left ventricular mechanics. Semin Thorac Cardiovasc Surg 1989;1:106–117.

68. David TE, Armstrong S, Sun Z: Left ventricular function after mitral valve surgery. J Heart Valve Dis 1995;4(suppl 2):S175–180.

69. Yun KL, Rayhill SC, Niczyporuk MA, et al: Mitral valve replacement in dilated canine hearts with chronic mitral regurgitation: importance of the mitral subvalvular apparatus. Circulation 1991;84:112–124.

70. Hansen DE, Sarris GE, Niczyporuk MA, Derby GC, Cahill PD, Miller DC: Physiologic role of the mitral apparatus in left ventricular regional mechanics, contraction synergy, and global systolic performance. J Thorac Cardiovasc Surg 1989;97:521–533.

71. Spence PA, Peniston CM, David TE, et al: Toward a better understanding of the etiology of left ventricular dysfunction after mitral valve replacement: an experimental study with possible clinical implications. Ann Thorac Surg 1986;41:363–371.

72. Sarris GE, Miller DC: Valvular-ventricular interaction: the importance of the mitral chordae tendineae in terms of global left ventricular systolic function. J Card Surg 1988;3:215–234.

73. Sarris GE, Cahill PD, Hansen DE, Derby GC, Miller DC: Restoration of left ventricular systolic performance after reattachment of the mitral chordae tendineae: the importance of valvular-ventricular interaction. J Thorac Cardiovasc Surg 1988;95:969–979.

74. Sarris GE, Fann JI, Niczyporuk MA, Derby GC, Hansen DE, Miller DC: Global and regional left ventricular systolic performance in the in situ ejecting canine heart: importance of the mitral apparatus. Circulation 1989;80(suppl I):24–42.

75. Komeda M, David TE, Rao V, Sun Z, Weisel RD, Burns RJ: Late hemodynamic effects of the preserved papillary muscles during mitral valve replacement. Circulation 1994;90:190–194.

76. Horstkotte D, Schulte HD, Bircks W, Strauer BE: The effect of chordal preservation on late outcome after mitral valve replacement: a randomized study. J Heart Valve Dis 1993;2:150–158.

77. Rose EA, Oz MC: Preservation of anterior leaflet chordae tendineae during mitral valve replacement. Ann Thorac Surg 1994;57:768–769.

78. Carpentier A: Cardiac valve surgery—the "French correction." J Thorac Cardiovasc Surg 1983;86:323–337.

79. Jebara VA, Mihaileanu S, Acar C, et al: Left ventricular outflow tract obstruction after mitral valve repair: results of the sliding leaflet technique. Circulation 1993;88:30–34.

80. Kay JH, Zubiate P, Mendez MA, Vanstrom N, Yokoyama T: Mitral valve repair for significant mitral insufficiency. Am Heart J 1978;96:253–262.

81. Carpentier A, Deloche A, Dauptain J, et al: A new reconstructive operation for correction of mitral and tricuspid insufficiency. J Thorac Cardiovasc Surg 1971;61:1–13.

82. Grossi EA, Galloway AC, Steinberg BM, et al: Severe calcification does not affect long-term outcome of mitral valve repair. Ann Thorac Surg 1994;58:685–687.

83. David TE, Bos J, Rakowski H: Mitral valve repair by replacement of chordae tendineae with polytetra-fluoroethylene sutures. J Thorac Cardiovasc Surg 1991;101:495–501.

84. Grossi EA, Galloway AC, LeBoutillier M III, et al: Anterior leaflet procedures during mitral valve repair do not adversely influence long-term outcome. J Am Coll Cardiol 1995;25:134–136.

85. Sousa Uva M, Grare P, Jebara V, et al: Transposition of chordae in mitral valve repair: mid-term results. Circulation 1993;88:35–38.

86. Deloche A, Jebara VA, Relland JY, et al: Valve repair with Carpentier techniques: the second decade. J Thorac Cardiovasc Surg 1990;99:990–1001.

87. Smedira NG, Selman R, Cosgrove DM, et al: Repair of anterior leaflet prolapse: chordal transfer is superior to chordal shortening. J Thorac Cardiovasc Surg 1996;112:287–291.

88. Stewart WJ, Currie PJ, Salcedo EE, et al: Intraoperative Doppler color flow mapping for decision-making in valve repair for mitral regurgitation: technique and results in 100 patients. Circulation 1990;81:556–566.

89. Fix J, Isada L, Cosgrove D, et al: Do patients with less than "echo-perfect" results from mitral valve repair by intraoperative echocardiography have a different outcome? Circulation 1993;88:39–48.

90. Akins CW, Hilgenberg AD, Buckley MJ, et al: Mitral valve reconstruction versus replacement for degenerative or ischemic mitral regurgitation. Ann Thorac Surg 1994;58:668–675.

91. Lee KS, Stewart WJ, Lever HM, Underwood PL, Cosgrove DM: Mechanism of outflow tract obstruction causing failed mitral valve repair: anterior displacement of leaflet coaptation. Circulation 1993;88:24–29.

92. Lee KS, Stewart WJ, Savage RM, Loop FD, Cosgrove DM: Systolic anterior motion of mitral valve after the posterior leaflet sliding advancement procedure. Ann Thorac Surg 1994;57:1338–1340.

93. Perier P, Clausnizer B, Mistarz K: Carpentier "sliding leaflet" technique for repair of the mitral valve: early results. Ann Thorac Surg 1994;57:383–386.

94. Mihaileanu S, Marino JP, Chauvaud S, et al: Left ventricular outflow obstruction after mitral valve repair (Carpentier's technique): proposed mechanisms of disease. Circulation 1988;78:78–84.

95. Cerfolio RJ, Orszulak TA, Pluth JR, Harmsen WS, Schaff HV: Reoperation after valve repair for mitral regurgitation: early and intermediate results. J Thorac Cardiovasc Surg 1996;111:1177–1183.

96. Fleischmann KE, Wolff S, Lin CM, Reimold SC, Lee TH, Lee RT: Echocardiographic predictors of survival after surgery for mitral regurgitation in the age of valve repair. Am Heart J 1996;131:281–288.

97. David TE, Uden DE, Strauss HD: The importance of the mitral apparatus in left ventricular function after correction of mitral regurgitation. Circulation 1983;68:76–82.

98. Hennein HA, Swain JA, McIntosh CL, Bonow RO, Stone CD, Clark RE: Comparative assessment of chordal preservation versus chordal resection during mitral valve replacement. J Thorac Cardiovasc Surg 1990;99:828–836.

99. Galloway AC, Colvin SB, Baumann FG, et al: Long-term results of mitral valve reconstruction with Carpentier techniques in 148 patients with mitral insufficiency. Circulation 1988;78:97–105.

100. Chua YL, Schaff HV, Orszulak TA, Morris JJ: Out-come of mitral valve repair in patients with preoperative atrial fibrillation: should the maze procedure be combined with mitral valvuloplasty? J Thorac Cardiovasc Surg 1994;107:408–415.

101. Galloway AC, Grossi EA, Spencer FC, Colvin SB: Operative therapy for mitral insufficiency from coronary artery disease. Semin Thorac Cardiovasc Surg 1995;7:227–232.

102. Hellemans IM, Pieper EG, Ravelli AC, et al: Prediction of surgical strategy in mitral valve regurgitation based on echocardiography. Interuniversity Cardiology Institute of The Netherlands. Am J Cardiol 1997;79:334–338.

103. Griffin BP, Stewart WJ: Echocardiography in patient selection, operative planning, and intraoperative evaluation of mitral valve repair. *In* Otto CM, ed. The Practice of Clinical Echocardiography. Philadelphia: WB Saunders, 1997:355–372.

104. Pieper EP, Hellemans IM, Hamer HP, et al: Additional value of biplane transesophageal echocardiography in assessing the genesis of mitral regurgitation and the feasibility of valve repair. Am J Cardiol 1995;75:489–493.

105. Hellemans IM, Pieper EG, Ravelli AC, et al: Comparison of transthoracic and transesophageal echocardiography with surgical findings in mitral regurgitation. The ESMIR Research Group. Am J Cardiol 1996;77:728–733.

106. Rankin JS, Feneley MP, Hickey MS, et al: A clinical comparison of mitral valve repair versus valve replacement in ischemic mitral regurgitation. J Thorac Cardiovasc Surg 1988;95:165–177.

107. Kay GL, Kay JH, Zubiate P, Yokoyama T, Mendez M: Mitral valve repair for mitral regurgitation secondary to coronary artery disease. Circulation 1986;74:88–98.

108. David TE: Techniques and results of mitral valve repair for ischemic mitral regurgitation. J Card Surg 1994;9:274–277.

109. Christenson JT, Simonet F, Bloch A, Maurice J, Velebit V, Schmuziger M: Should a mild to moderate ischemic mitral valve regurgitation in patients with poor left ventricular function be repaired or not? J Heart Valve Dis 1995;4:484–488.

110. Rankin JS, Hickey MS, Smith LR, et al: Ischemic mitral regurgitation. Circulation 1989;79:116–121.

111. Czer LS, Maurer G, Trento A, et al: Comparative efficacy of ring and suture annuloplasty for ischemic mitral regurgitation. Circulation 1992;86:46–52.

112. Bolling SF, Deeb GM, Bach DS: Mitral valve reconstruction in elderly, ischemic patients. Chest 1996;109:35–40.

113. Kono T, Sabbah HN, Rosman H, Alam M, Jafri S, Goldstein S: Left ventricular shape is the primary determinant of functional mitral regurgitation in heart failure. J Am Coll Cardiol 1992;20:1594–1598.

114. Junker A, Thayssen P, Nielsen B, Andersen PE: The hemodynamic and prognostic significance of echo-Doppler-proven mitral regurgitation in patients with dilated cardiomyopathy. Cardiology 1993;83:14–20.

115. Bolling SF, Deeb GM, Brunsting LA, Bach DS: Early outcome of mitral valve reconstruction in patients with end-stage cardiomyopathy. J Thorac Cardiovasc Surg 1995;109:676–682.

116. Bach DS, Bolling SF: Early improvement in congestive heart failure after correction of secondary mitral regurgitation in end-stage cardiomyopathy. Am Heart J 1995;129:1165–1170.

117. Bach DS, Bolling SF: Improvement following correc-

tion of secondary mitral regurgitation in end-stage cardiomyopathy with mitral annuloplasty. Am J Cardiol 1996;78:966–969.

118. Gaasch WH, Zile MR: Left ventricular function after surgical correction of chronic mitral regurgitation. Eur Heart J 1991;12(suppl B):48–51.

119. Carabello BA: Preservation of left ventricular function in patients with mitral regurgitation: a realistic goal for the nineties [editorial]. J Am Coll Cardiol 1990;15:564–565.

120. Stewart WJ: Choosing the "golden moment" for mitral valve repair [editorial]. J Am Coll Cardiol 1994;24:1544–1546.

121. Donovan CL, Starling MR: Role of echocardiogra-

phy in the timing of surgical intervention for chronic mitral and aortic regurgitation. *In* Otto CM, ed. The Practice of Clinical Echocardiography. Philadelphia: WB Saunders, 1997:327–354.

122. Ross J Jr: Left ventricular function and the timing of surgical treatment in valvular heart disease. Ann Intern Med 1981;94:498–504.

123. Michel PL, Iung B, Blanchard B, Luxereau P, Dorent R, Acar J: Long-term results of mitral valve repair for non-ischaemic mitral regurgitation. Eur Heart J 1991;12(suppl B):39–43.

124. Starling MR: Effects of valve surgery on left ventricular contractile function in patients with long-term mitral regurgitation. Circulation 1995;92:811–818.

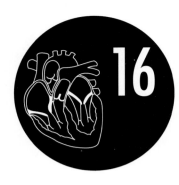

16 Right-Sided Valve Disease

PATHOPHYSIOLOGY OF RIGHT-SIDED VALVE DISEASE

Primary and Secondary Right-Sided Valve Disease

Differentiation of primary valve abnormalities from valve dysfunction caused by pulmonary hypertension is an important first step in the evaluation of patients with tricuspid or pulmonic valve disease. Primary anatomic abnormalities of the tricuspid and pulmonic valves most often are congenital and usually are diagnosed in childhood. In adults, right-sided valve disease more often is the result of pulmonary hypertension, with pulmonary hypertension being due to left-sided heart disease, primary pulmonary disease, or pulmonary vascular disease.

Right Ventricular Response to Pressure or Volume Overload

The right ventricle dilates in the setting of chronic tricuspid or pulmonic regurgitation due to chronic volume overload. Right ventricular dilation caused by volume overload tends to occur predominantly in the short-axis dimension.[1, 2] In addition, right ventricular vol-

ume overload is associated with abnormal motion of the ventricular septum; the septum moves toward the center of the right ventricle in systole and moves rapidly posteriorly in diastole. As this pattern is the opposite of normal, the term *paradoxic septal motion* often is used to refer to this observation.[3–5] In a short-axis image of a patient with volume overload, the reversed curvature of the septum is most apparent at end-diastole (Fig. 16–1). In contrast, the maximal reversed curvature occurs in early diastole and is more evident in patients with pressure overload (Fig. 16–2).[6]

Although right ventricular function initially is normal in patients with chronic right ventricular volume overload, systolic dysfunction occurs at an earlier point in the disease course than is typical for left-sided volume overload conditions.[7, 8] As with left-sided valve disease, right ventricular systolic dysfunction typically improves after intervention for valvular regurgitation unless an irreversible decline in contractility has occurred. Unlike left ventricular volume overload, no specific right ventricular dimensions have been defined as predictors of the onset of contractile dysfunction. The lack of quantitative reference points reflects the difficulties of accurately measuring right ventricular dimensions and volumes given the

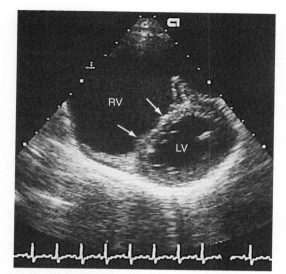

Figure 16·1 Severe right ventricular volume overload due to tricuspid regurgitation resulted in the severe right ventricular dilation seen in this parasternal short-axis echocardiographic view. The septum *(arrows)* is slightly flattened at end-diastole. LV, left ventricle; RV, right ventricle.

complex three-dimensional (3D) anatomy of the right ventricular chamber. In addition, there is no accepted standard of reference for right ventricular systolic dysfunction as it is difficult to accurately measure right ventricular ejection fraction.

The right ventricular response to chronic pressure overload, such as pulmonary hypertension or pulmonic stenosis, also differs somewhat from that of the left ventricle. Although the initial response is an increased wall thickness, ventricular dilation occurs relatively early in the disease course. Further, the response of the right ventricle to pressure overload depends on the acuteness and severity of the pressure overload state. With a gradual onset of increased right ventricular pressure, right ventricular systolic function may remain normal with a compensatory increase in right ventricular wall thickness (Fig. 16–3).[9] With an acute increase in right ventricular pressure, for example with acute pulmonary embolism, decreased right ventricular systolic function and clinical right heart failure may be seen with mean pulmonary pressures of only 20–40 mm Hg.[10] Right ventricular pressure overload often results in right ventricular dilation with secondary annular dilation and tricuspid regurgitation. This engenders a cycle of volume overload leading into more right ventricular dilation and more tricuspid regurgitation.

After interventions to relieve right ventricular pressure overload, an improvement in right ventricular systolic function is expected due to the reduction in right ventricular afterload. Although few studies have analyzed the degree of improvement in right ventricular function

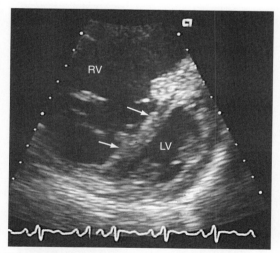

Figure 16·2 Right ventricular pressure overload due to severe pulmonary hypertension results in reversed curvature of the ventricular septum *(arrows)* throughout diastole, which is associated with right ventricular hypertrophy and dilation, seen in this parasternal short-axis echocardiographic view. LV, left ventricle; RV, right ventricle.

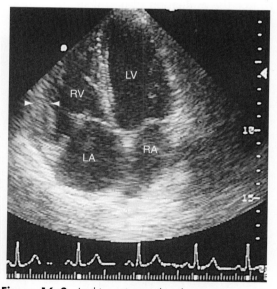

Figure 16·3 In this patient with pulmonic stenosis, the echocardiographic apical four-chamber view shows increased right ventricular wall thickness *(arrowheads)* with preserved systolic function and only mild right ventricular dilation. LA, left atrium; LV, left ventricle; RA, right atrium; RV, right ventricle.

after relief of pulmonic stenosis, the improvement in right ventricular dimensions and systolic function in most patients after lung transplantation supports the concept that systolic function improves with decreased afterload.[11-13]

Principles of Diagnosis

Valve Stenosis and Regurgitation

Echocardiographic evaluation of right-sided valve disease follows the same principles as evaluation of left-sided lesions (see Chapter 3), with two-dimensional (2D) imaging of valve anatomy and dynamics, continuous wave Doppler measurement of the antegrade velocity across the stenotic valve, and color flow imaging of the degree of valvular regurgitation. Transthoracic 2D imaging of the tricuspid valve usually is straightforward with several image planes available, including right ventricular inflow and short-axis views from the parasternal window and four-chamber views from the apical and subcostal windows. On transesophageal imaging, the tricuspid valve is well visualized in the four-chamber view and in a subcostal long-axis view rotated toward the patient's right side.

Evaluation of the degree of tricuspid stenosis includes calculation of the mean pressure gradient and the pressure half-time valve area. Unlike the evaluation of mitral stenosis, short-axis 2D imaging of the valve orifice rarely is feasible. Tricuspid regurgitation is graded by color flow imaging on a 1 to 4+ scale, depending on the extent of the systolic flow disturbance in the right atrium (Fig. 16-4; see also color insert). With severe tricuspid regurgitation, systolic flow reversal also is seen in the hepatic veins. A small degree of tricuspid regurgitation is observed in 65% of normal adults, and some degree of regurgitation is detected in 80% to 90% of those referred for echocardiography.[14]

Clear images of the pulmonic valve are more difficult to obtain in adult patients. Transthoracic views are obtained from the parasternal window in a short-axis view and in a plane parallel to the long axis of the pulmonary outflow tract. In some patients, the pulmonic valve also can be imaged in an anteriorly angulated apical four-chamber view or in a subcostal short-axis view. However, transthoracic views of the pulmonic valve often are limited by poor acoustic access in adults due to adjacent lung tissue.

On transesophageal imaging the pulmonic valve is best visualized in a long-axis plane, typically with the multiplane probe rotated to about 90 degrees, resulting in a long-axis view of the right ventricular outflow tract and pulmonic valve with the aortic valve in an oblique, short-axis orientation. Alternatively, the pulmonic valve can be visualized in a transverse

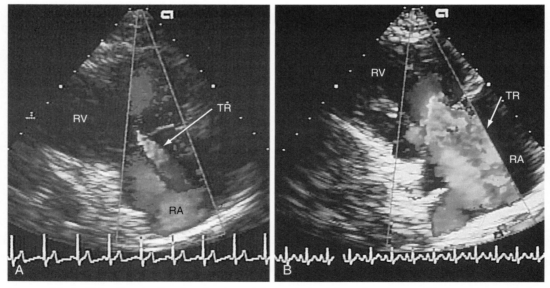

Figure 16·4 Color Doppler flow imaging in a right ventricular inflow view shows mild tricuspid regurgitation (TR) *(A)* and severe tricuspid regurgitation *(B)*. With severe regurgitation, a broad jet of turbulent flow extends to the distal wall of the atrium. RA, right atrium; RV, right ventricle. (This figure also occurs in the color insert.)

plane (0 degrees of rotation) with the probe withdrawn to the level of the pulmonary artery to obtain an image looking straight down the pulmonary artery from the bifurcation to the valve. This view provides a parallel intercept angle for Doppler recordings.

Even from the transesophageal approach, the pulmonic valve may not be well seen due to interposition of the bronchus between the transducer and the pulmonic valve. When pulmonic stenosis is suspected, it is particularly important to evaluate for subvalvular and supravalvular obstruction in addition to valvular stenosis, because right ventricular outflow obstruction may take any one of these forms, which have similar clinical manifestations. Cardiac catheterization may be needed to define the exact level of obstruction when echocardiography is nondiagnostic.

Evaluation of pulmonic stenosis severity relies predominantly on measurement of maximal and mean pressure gradients. In theory, valve area can be calculated using the continuity equation, but this calculation is rarely performed clinically because of the difficulty in measuring the transpulmonic volume flow rate. Pulmonic regurgitation is graded on a 1 to 4+ scale using color Doppler flow imaging. As in evaluation of aortic regurgitation, the most reliable view is a short-axis image of the regurgitant jet as it enters the right ventricular outflow tract. Pulmonic regurgitation is associated with diastolic flow reversal in the pulmonary artery, but this finding has not been used for quantitation of regurgitant severity.

Right Ventricular Size and Function

Right ventricular size and systolic function are evaluated qualitatively in comparison to left ventricular size and function. On transthoracic imaging, the right ventricle is seen well in apical and subcostal four-chamber views. Parasternal right ventricular inflow and short-axis views also are helpful. On transesophageal imaging, right ventricular function is best evaluated using the four-chamber view.

Due to the complex 3D shape of the right ventricle, linear dimensions of right ventricular size are less helpful than linear left ventricular dimensions. For the same reasons, 2D evaluation of right ventricular volumes and ejection fraction has been problematic. However, 3D approaches promise feasible clinical measures of right ventricular size and systolic function in the future. The extent of right ventricular hypertrophy can be assessed qualitatively based on the thickness of the right ventricular free wall. The timing of ventricular septal motion also provides insight into right ventricular function, as previously discussed. While patterns of abnormal septal motion may be appreciated on 2D imaging, the timing and extent of septal motion are best evaluated using M-mode echocardiography.

When right ventricular enlargement and abnormal septal motion are detected, the echocardiographer must ensure that these abnormalities are caused by valvular disease, rather than by congenital intracardiac shunt. In particular, an atrial septal defect results in right-sided chamber enlargement, often with secondary tricuspid regurgitation due to a dilated annulus. Since an atrial septal defect is treatable through surgical closure, special attention to 2D imaging and color flow assessment of the interatrial septum is needed. It is prudent to exclude an intracardiac shunt using echocardiographic contrast (eg, agitated saline) when the patient has right heart enlargement if an atrial septal defect cannot be definitively excluded by 2D and color flow imaging.

Pulmonary Artery Pressures

Estimation of pulmonary pressures is an essential component of the examination in patients with right-sided valve disease. Pulmonary pressures can be estimated noninvasively from the velocity in the tricuspid regurgitant jet and the appearance of the inferior vena cava. Most patients have at least a small amount of tricuspid regurgitation (TR). The velocity (V) of the regurgitant signal is related to the right ventricular to right atrial systolic pressure difference ($\Delta P_{RV\text{-}RA}$) as stated in the Bernoulli equation:

$$\Delta P_{RV\text{-}RA} = 4(V_{TR})^2$$

This pressure gradient then is added to an estimate of right atrial pressure, which is based on the size and respiratory variation in the inferior vena cava (see Chapter 3).

Secondary Echocardiographic Findings

Long-standing pulmonary hypertension results in pulmonary artery dilation, which may be seen on 2D echocardiographic imaging. Although typically of little concern clinically, excessive dilation, often associated with mild to moderate pulmonic stenosis, can lead to pulmonary artery dissection or rupture and may warrant surgical intervention, although the published experience is limited to only a few cases.[15, 16]

With severe right ventricular pressure or volume overload, left ventricular function may be affected in at least two ways. First, left ventricular filling volumes may be reduced because of the low right-sided cardiac output. Second, abnormal diastolic septal motion may further limit left ventricular diastolic filling. Both of these abnormalities may be evident on 2D and Doppler evaluations.

TRICUSPID REGURGITATION

Etiology

Secondary tricuspid regurgitation is much more common than primary valvular disease (Table 16–1). Functional tricuspid regurgitation resulting from pulmonary hypertension is seen in patients with significant left-sided heart disease, those with primary pulmonary hypertension, and those with pulmonary disease leading to cor pulmonale.[17–19] Functional tricuspid regurgitation also occurs in patients with right ventricular dilation, for example, due to right ventricular infarction or an atrial septal defect.[20, 21]

Primary causes of tricuspid regurgitation are less common and include rheumatic valve diseases, trauma, endocarditis, carcinoid, and diet pills.[22–33] Tricuspid involvement occurs in as many as 30% to 50% of patients with rheumatic mitral valve disease.[34] Myxomatous involvement of the tricuspid valve is occasionally seen in patients with mitral valve prolapse.[35, 36] Endocarditis tends to primarily affect the tricuspid valve in intravenous drug users,

leading to significant tricuspid regurgitation despite effective medical therapy in many patients. Endomyocardial fibrosis, which is prevalent in tropical Africa, produces fibrosis of the papillary muscle tip and thickening and shortening of the leaflets and chordae, leading to tricuspid regurgitation. This process may affect both mitral and tricuspid valves.

Although pacer wires traversing the tricuspid valve typically do not interfere with tricuspid valve closure, occasionally a pacer lead in association with thrombus formation produces significant tricuspid regurgitation.[37, 38] Tricuspid regurgitation after cardiac transplantation often results from right ventricular dilation and systolic dysfunction related to rejection, inadequate myocardial preservation at the time of transplantation, or persistent pulmonary hypertension. However, tricuspid valve trauma related to multiple endomyocardial biopsies also has been reported.[39, 40]

Blunt chest injury can cause tricuspid regurgitation through papillary muscle rupture or valve or chordal lacerations. Conduction abnormalities, including right and left bundle branch block and left anterior hemiblock, are common, occurring in more than 90% of patients with traumatic tricuspid regurgitation. In the past, traumatic tricuspid regurgitation often was undetected at the time of the initial injury. Detection has been enhanced with the use of echocardiography to evaluate victims of blunt chest trauma.[28] Most patients are asymptomatic for up to 3 years after trauma. In those with significant symptoms due to acute severe tricuspid regurgitation, valve repair may be attempted,[24, 26] although conservative therapy also is an option.[27–29]

Ebstein's anomaly is a congenital cause of tricuspid regurgitation that often is associated with other congenital defects, particularly ventricular inversion (ie, congenitally corrected transposition of the great vessels). Primary Ebstein's anomaly may occur in isolation or may be associated with a patent foramen ovale, atrial septal defect, pulmonic stenosis, or ventricular septal defect. Ebstein's anomaly is characterized by apical displacement and dysplasia of the septal and posterior leaflets of the tricuspid valve (Fig. 16–5).[41, 42] In one third of cases, the leaflets are adherent to the right ventricular wall, rather than apically displaced, but in all cases, the leaflets are increased in size and dysplastic with abnormal chordal attachments.

A wide range of clinical disease severity is associated with Ebstein's anomaly. Some pa-

TABLE 16·1	CAUSES OF TRICUSPID REGURGITATION

Primary
  Rheumatic
  Mxyomatous
  Ebstein's anomaly
  Endomyocardial fibrosis
  Endocarditis
  Carcinoid
  Traumatic
  Iatrogenic (eg, pacer wire, right ventricular biopsy)
Secondary
  Primary pulmonary hypertension
  Chronic lung disease with pulmonary hypertension
    (eg, cor pulmonale)
  Left heart disease (ventricular or valvular) resulting in
    pulmonary hypertension

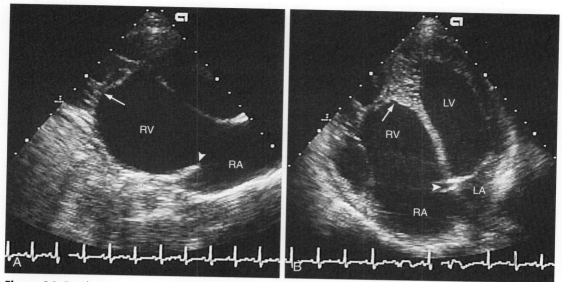

Figure 16·5 Ebstein's anomaly is characterized by apical displacement of the septal leaflet of the tricuspid valve. In the right ventricular inflow view *(A)* and in the apical four-chamber view *(B)*, the insertion of the septal leaflet *(thin arrows)* is markedly apically displaced from the annulus *(arrowheads)*. The segment of right ventricular myocardium between these arrows is "atrialized" in that right atrial pressures are associated with right ventricular electrical activity. Severe tricuspid regurgitation was present as shown in Figure 16·4. LA, left atrium; LV, left ventricle; RA, right atrium; RV, right ventricle.

tients have a poor prognosis due to severe tricuspid regurgitation and a patent foramen ovale with right to left shunting.[43, 44] Others have milder degrees of tricuspid regurgitation. Ebstein's anomaly is associated with ventricular preexcitation in 5% to 10% of cases, and about 33% have a prolonged PR interval. Thus, in adults, the most common (42%) presentation of Ebstein's anomaly is an arrhythmia.[42]

The classic physical examination findings of Ebstein's anomaly are a widely split first heart sound (S_1) because of delayed tricuspid valve closure, a tricuspid regurgitant murmur, and an early systolic click related to the large tricuspid valve leaflet reaching its limit of excursion during systolic closure.[45, 46] At catheterization, the diagnostic finding of Ebstein's anomaly is a right atrial pressure waveform in conjunction with a right ventricular electrocardiographic signal on pull-back into the atrialized segment of the right ventricle.[47]

Carcinoid valve disease is rare, and it is associated only with carcinoid metastatic to the liver. The echocardiographic findings are dramatic, with shortened and thickened tricuspid valve leaflets resulting in a large area of incomplete coaptation (Fig. 16–6).[48, 49] Moderate to severe tricuspid regurgitation occurs in 90% of patients with carcinoid valve disease. In addition, pulmonary valve involvement is seen in

90%, with significant pulmonic regurgitation in 81% and pulmonic stenosis in 53% of patients. Left-sided valve involvement occurs in only 7% of patients with right-sided valve involvement, and nearly all these patients have a patent foramen ovale or lung metastases.

Diagnosis

Tricuspid regurgitation is most often initially diagnosed at the time of echocardiographic evaluation of left-sided heart disease, because symptoms are nonspecific, and physical examination findings are often subtle. Symptoms of severe tricuspid regurgitation may include dyspnea and orthopnea, although it is likely that these symptoms result from left-sided heart disease in many of these patients.[20, 21, 25] With isolated tricuspid regurgitation, patients may complain of fatigue and decreased exercise tolerance due to a low forward cardiac output. Elevated right atrial pressures lead to symptoms of peripheral edema, decreased appetite, and abdominal fullness. However, even moderate to severe tricuspid regurgitation often is well tolerated and produces few overt symptoms.

Physical examination shows jugular venous distention with a visible systolic v wave in 35% to 75% of patients.[20, 21, 25] Hepatomegaly is evi-

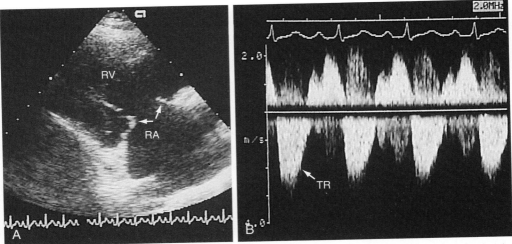

Figure 16·6 *A, Carcinoid heart disease is recognized on two-dimensional echocardiography by the presence of severely shortened and immobile tricuspid valve leaflets (arrows). B, Continuous wave Doppler shows nearly equal intensity of antegrade and retrograde flow across the valve, which is consistent with severe regurgitation. The peak velocity in the tricuspid regurgitant jet is low because pulmonary pressures are not elevated. RA, right atrium; RV, right ventricle.*

dent in 90% of patients, but systolic pulsation of the liver is observed only inconsistently. Classically, the holosystolic murmur of tricuspid regurgitation is heard along the right sternal border with radiation to the hepatic region. Murmur intensity increases with inspiration in association with increased systemic venous return.[25] However, the murmur of tricuspid regurgitation often is inaudible and is heard in fewer than 20% of patients with documented valve dysfunction.[20, 21, 25] Many patients with tricuspid regurgitation are in atrial fibrillation, confounding evaluation of respiratory variation.[18, 20, 21, 25]

The hemodynamic changes in patients with tricuspid regurgitation include an elevated right atrial mean pressure with a systolic v wave, and a decreased cardiac output at rest.[18, 21] These hemodynamic changes depend on the acuteness as well as the severity of the valvular lesion. Right ventriculography rarely is helpful diagnostically, because the catheter across the valve may induce further regurgitation.

Echocardiography now is the reference standard for diagnosis and evaluation of tricuspid regurgitation. The etiology of valve disease is determined from 2D images, with Doppler pulsed, continuous wave, and color flow data used in assessment of regurgitant severity.[50–52]

Natural History

Little information is available on the natural history of tricuspid regurgitation. In adults, this lesion often accompanies other valvular lesions, which may dominate the clinical picture. In patients undergoing tricuspid valve resection for endocarditis, severe regurgitation often is well tolerated initially and for several years.[53, 54] However, in the long term, some of these patients develop symptoms and signs of systemic venous congestion and low cardiac output.[55, 56]

Medical and Surgical Treatment

The medical treatment of tricuspid regurgitation includes efforts to decrease pulmonary pressures (if elevated) and control of systemic congestion using diuretics. Mild or moderate degrees of tricuspid regurgitation usually require no other intervention. However, surgical intervention may be considered for severe regurgitation.

The most common surgical procedure for treatment of tricuspid regurgitation is an annuloplasty, often performed at the time of mitral valve surgery. Annuloplasty can be performed using suture plication of the annulus,[57–60] insertion of a complete ring to distribute tension over the entire annulus,[61–63] or with a semicircular ring.[64] The semicircular ring is reported to maintain annular flexibility and avoid damage to the adjacent conduction system.

When the patient has Ebstein's anomaly, tricuspid valve repair with right ventricular plication, right atrial reduction, and placement of

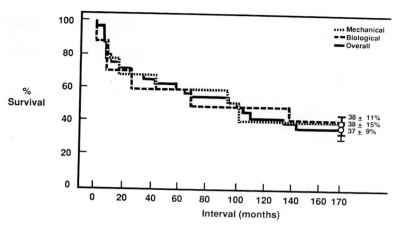

Figure 16·7 Actuarial survival of 60 patients (mean age, 50 ± 15 years) with 28 bioprosthetic and 32 mechanical tricuspid valve replacements performed between January 1978 and June 1993. (From Scully HE, Armstrong CS: Tricuspid valve replacement: fifteen years of experience with mechanical prostheses and bioprostheses. J Thorac Cardiovasc Surg 1995;109:1035–1041.)

an annuloplasty ring often is successful and is preferable to valve replacement.[65] Valves with an elongated, mobile, untethered anterior leaflet are most amenable to repair.[66]

Tricuspid annuloplasty tends to reduce, but not eliminate, tricuspid regurgitation. About 30% to 40% of patients have residual tricuspid regurgitation after a suture annuloplasty. In addition, restriction of the annulus leads to a diastolic pressure gradient in 40% to 50% of patients.[34, 67, 68] Residual tricuspid regurgitation occurs less often with a ring than with semicircular annuloplasty; however, even with a semicircular annuloplasty,[69] only 5% of patients require valve replacement over the next 7 years.[70, 71] Since many of these patients have secondary tricuspid valve dysfunction, improvement in the severity of tricuspid regurgitation is more likely if pulmonary hypertension resolves.[34, 68, 69]

Tricuspid valve replacement is performed only if an annuloplasty is not feasible or fails.[72] The reported operative mortality rate for tricuspid valve replacement is extremely variable, ranging from 7% to 40%, most likely due to differences in patient populations, with impaired myocardial function being a risk factor for undergoing tricuspid valve replacement.[73–85] Postoperative heart block complicates 2% to 45% of reported cases, since the bundle of His is immediately adjacent to the septal cusp of the tricuspid valve. This complication can be avoided by leaving a rim of tricuspid valve tissue at the time of valve replacement. If heart block is a concern, epicardial pacer electrodes are placed at the time of surgery.[73–78]

Five-year survival rates after tricuspid valve replacement range from 55% to 80%, with 10-year actuarial survival rates of 36% to 50%

(Fig. 16–7).[73–84] However, mechanical valves in the tricuspid position have a very high risk of valve thrombosis, ranging from 4% to 30%.[73–78, 86, 87] Of the types of mechanical valves, bileaflet valves have the lowest incidence of clotting but still are prone to thrombosis. With a prosthetic tricuspid valve, the onset of valve thrombosis may be insidious, and a high degree of clinical suspicion is needed to make the diagnosis.[76, 81, 88–90] Despite the risk of rapid calcification, particularly in younger patients,[91–93] bioprosthetic valves have a much lower degree of thrombogenicity in the tricuspid position and therefore may be the valve of choice in some patients (Fig. 16–8).[76–78]

In a series of 146 patients undergoing tricus-

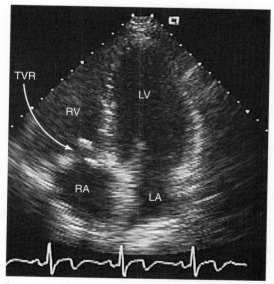

Figure 16·8 This apical four-chamber view shows a calcified porcine tricuspid valve replacement (TVR). LA, left atrium; LV, left ventricle; RA, right atrium; RV, right ventricle.

pid valve replacement, the hospital mortality rate was 16%, and the actuarial survival rate was 74% at 5 years.[94] However, the survival rate was less than 25% at 14 years, largely related to comorbid disease and psychosocial factors in patients needing tricuspid valve replacement. Predictors of long-term outcome were the type of prosthesis, type of surgical myocardial protection, and preoperative functional class. These investigators concluded that, given the poor long-term outcome for this patient group, large bioprosthetic valves are appropriate for most patients with a bileaflet mechanical valve being an alternate choice for patients with longer life expectancies.[94] In contrast, another study found no difference in valve-related complications between those with bioprosthetic or mechanical tricuspid valve replacements. The actuarial survival rate for both groups was 37% ± 9% at 15 years, suggesting a mechanical valve should be considered for younger patients and those needing anticoagulation for other reasons.[82]

TRICUSPID STENOSIS

Etiology

Tricuspid valve stenosis is a rare clinical condition, with rheumatic disease accounting for about 90% of all cases. In patients with rheumatic mitral valve disease, only 3% to 5% have concurrent tricuspid stenosis.[95, 96] Unusual causes of tricuspid stenosis include metastatic carcinoid disease[48] and congenital anomalies of the valve structure. Even more unusual causes include infective endocarditis and Whipple's disease.[97] A right atrial myxoma also can manifest with signs and symptoms mimicking obstruction at the tricuspid valve level.

Diagnosis

Since patients with rheumatic tricuspid stenosis invariably have coexisting mitral valve disease, it is difficult to separate symptoms specific to tricuspid valve obstruction from those of mitral valve stenosis or regurgitation. Reported symptoms include fatigue, dyspnea, and peripheral edema.[95, 98, 99] On physical examination, tricuspid stenosis is characterized by an opening snap, followed by a diastolic rumbling murmur at the right sternal border that varies with respiration.[100] As with tricuspid regurgitation, the physical examination findings may be subtle, and the murmur often is inaudible. Instead, right-

sided involvement may be suspected on the basis of an elevated jugular venous pressure out of proportion to the degree of left-sided failure, or it may be diagnosed initially on echocardiography.

Electrocardiography shows atrial fibrillation in 50% of cases, but right atrial enlargement may be evident in those in sinus rhythm.[95, 98–100] Chest radiography shows an enlarged right atrium but normal pulmonary artery size and clear lung fields. Tricuspid stenosis can be evaluated at catheterization with measurement of the transvalvular pressure gradient and calculation of valve area. Early studies indicated that a tricuspid valve area of less than 1.5 cm^2 is associated with symptoms.[101]

Echocardiography allows definitive diagnosis of the cause and severity of tricuspid stenosis. Rheumatic involvement parallels the changes seen with rheumatic mitral valve disease, including commissural fusion and diastolic doming with thickened and shortened chordae. Even on echocardiography, findings are subtle, and tricuspid valve involvement may be overlooked unless attention is focused on tricuspid valve anatomy and motion in patients with rheumatic mitral valve disease. Doppler evaluation of stenosis severity has largely replaced the need for catheterization in these patients (Fig. 16–9).[50, 102–104]

Natural History

Few data are available on the natural history of tricuspid stenosis, because it typically accompanies rheumatic mitral valve disease. However, like mitral stenosis, tricuspid valve obstruction is the result of a chronic, slowly progressive disease process that correlates with a gradual increase in stenosis severity and gradual symptom onset.

Medical and Surgical Treatment

When tricuspid stenosis is severe, the optimal surgical intervention is direct commissurotomy in conjunction with annuloplasty for any associated tricuspid regurgitation.[57, 105, 106] Most often, tricuspid commissurotomy is performed at the time of mitral valve surgery. Percutaneous balloon valvuloplasty has been described, but experience is limited, and further evaluation of this procedure is needed.[107–109] Medical therapy for tricuspid stenosis usually is ineffective, since diuresis to improve systemic venous congestion further reduces cardiac output. When the patient has

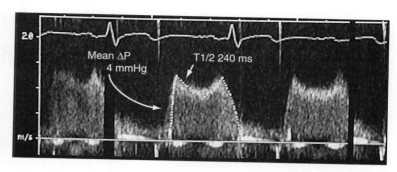

Figure 16·9 Stenosis of a bioprosthetic tricuspid valve replacement with the Doppler velocity curve indicating a mean pressure gradient (mean ΔP) of 4 mm Hg and a pressure half-time (T½) of 240 ms.

significant stenosis, intervention should strongly be considered.

PULMONIC STENOSIS

Etiology

Pulmonary valve stenosis is congenital in 95% of cases; rarer causes include carcinoid syndrome and rheumatic valve disease. Although pulmonic stenosis may be a feature of other types of complex congenital heart disease, such as tetralogy of Fallot, 80% of cases are isolated pulmonary stenosis. The abnormal valve is classified as unicommissural, with prominent systolic doming of the leaflets and an eccentric orifice; bicuspid, with fused commissures; or dysplastic, with severely thickened and deformed valve leaflets. Evaluation of valve morphology is important clinically because dysplastic valves respond poorly to balloon dilation.

Rarely, pulmonic stenosis is associated with an aneurysm of the pulmonary artery. Pulmonary artery aneurysms have been described in patients with only mild pulmonic stenosis and are prone to dissection when excessively large.[15, 16]

Diagnosis

Most patients with mild or moderate pulmonic stenosis are asymptomatic, and even some patients with severe obstruction deny having symptoms. Since typical symptoms include fatigue and dyspnea due to a reduced cardiac output, it is likely that some patients adjust their lifestyle and level of exertion to avoid symptom onset, while not clearly recognizing cardiac limitation.

Physical examination of patients with pulmonic stenosis reveals a crescendo-decrescendo systolic murmur that is loudest at the upper left sternal border and radiates to the suprasternal notch and left neck. A loud and late peaking murmur suggests severe valvular obstruction. As the disease progresses, the second heart sound becomes widely split, with a delayed P_2 resulting from a prolonged right ventricular ejection time. The murmur of pulmonic stenosis is longer in duration than that of aortic stenosis, and the systolic murmur extends beyond A_2. An ejection click with respiratory variation in the loudness of the click may be appreciated at the upper left sternal border. The interval between S_1 and the ejection click increases with greater degrees of valve obstruction, although with severe stenosis, the ejection click may be absent.[110, 111]

On echocardiographic evaluation, the thickened pulmonic leaflets can be visualized with characteristic doming in systole as the leaflets reach their limit of excursion. The severity of pulmonic stenosis is evaluated based on the transpulmonic velocity recorded with continuous wave Doppler ultrasound for calculation of the transvalvular pressure gradient (Fig. 16–10). The elevation in right ventricular systolic pressure also can be confirmed from the tricuspid regurgitant jet velocity, which is elevated as predicted by the Bernoulli equation.

The degree of coexisting pulmonic regurgitation is evaluated using color flow imaging and continuous wave Doppler recordings of signal intensity. The pulmonic regurgitant jet velocity reflects the diastolic pressure difference between the pulmonary artery and right ventricle and thus is expected to be low in the absence of pulmonary hypertension.

Exercise testing is not routinely used for evaluation of pulmonic stenosis. However, while patients maintain a normal oxygen consumption, cardiac output, and right ventricular diastolic pressures when the degree of stenosis is only mild or moderate, a marked increase in right ventricular end-diastolic pressure is seen when pulmonic valve area is less than $0.5 \text{ cm}^2/\text{m}^2$.[112]

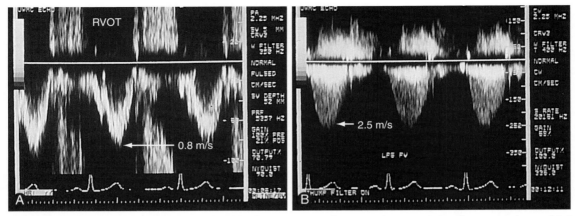

Figure 16·10 Evaluation of a patient with mild pulmonic stenosis shows a right ventricular outflow tract velocity of 0.8 m/s using pulsed Doppler *(A)* and a pulmonary valve velocity of 2.5 m/s using continuous wave Doppler *(B)*, consistent with a peak transpulmonic gradient of only 25 mm Hg.

Typically, cardiac catheterization is not needed in patients with pulmonic stenosis unless the clinical picture and echocardiographic data are discordant. In patients undergoing percutaneous balloon valvuloplasty, pressures on both sides of the pulmonic valve are recorded as the catheter is withdrawn from the pulmonary artery to the right ventricle before and after the procedure.

Natural History

In patients with mild pulmonic stenosis, defined as a gradient less than 50 mm Hg, symptoms are uncommon, and clinical outcome is excellent even without surgical intervention.[113–115] In contrast, patients with severe stenosis (gradient ≥80 mm Hg) are likely to be symptomatic and often have evidence of right heart failure, suggesting that surgical percuta-

neous relief of pulmonic stenosis may be beneficial.[115, 116] Clinical outcome and management of patients with a gradient between 50 and 80 mm Hg has been less clear.

In the second natural history study of congenital heart defects, long-term follow-up was available for 78% of 592 patients enrolled between 1958 and 1969 (Fig. 16–11). Those with a gradient of less than 50 mm Hg were treated medically, those with a gradient of 80 mm Hg or higher underwent surgical intervention, while therapy was individualized for those with intermediate gradients. The overall survival rate at 25 years was 96%. Less than 20% of those initially treated medically required valvotomy at a later date, and reoperation was needed in only 4% of those with initial surgical therapy.[115] The risk of endocarditis appears to be low, and the risk of serious arrhythmias is small. The transpulmonic pressure gradients

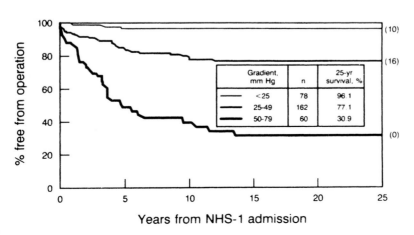

Gradient, mm Hg	n	25-yr survival, %
<25	78	96.1
25-49	162	77.1
50-79	60	30.9

Figure 16·11 Kaplan-Meier curves of the percentage free from surgery for 300 pulmonary stenosis patients managed medically, grouped by gradient at admission to the First Natural History Study (NHS-1). Numbers within parentheses indicate the number of patients remaining under observation 25 years after admission. (From Hayes CJ, Gersony WM, Driscoll DJ, et al: Second natural history study of congenital heart defects: results of treatment of patients with pulmonary valvar stenosis. Circulation 1993;87(suppl I):28–37; by permission of The American Heart Association.)

at follow-up remain low, with a mean gradient of 17.1 ± 11.4 mm Hg for those treated medically and 9.6 ± 6.6 mm Hg for those with prior surgical intervention.[115]

Univariate predictors of a poor clinical outcome include the presence of symptoms (eg, angina, fatigue, dyspnea, syncope), cardiomegaly on chest radiography, an elevated right ventricular end-diastolic pressure, a low cardiac index, electrocardiographic evidence of right ventricular hypertrophy, and a low systolic blood pressure. Multivariate predictors of mortality were age and cardiomegaly. Patients enrolled in the study who were older than 12 years of age and who had evidence of cardiomegaly have a 25-year survival rate of 80%.[115] Event-free survival was closely related to the pressure gradient, with an event-free survival rate of 31% for those with a gradient of 50 to 79 mm Hg, 77% for those with a gradient between 25 and 49 mm Hg, and 96% for those with a gradient of less than 25 mm Hg. These data suggest that relief of pulmonic stenosis should be strongly considered for all patients with a gradient higher than 50 mm Hg.

Medical and Surgical Treatment

Balloon valvuloplasty now is the procedure of choice for children and adults with significant pulmonic stenosis. The procedure is most often performed using a circular balloon, oversized by about 20% to 40% relative to the pulmonic annulus, although double balloon or Inoue balloon approaches also have been described.[16, 117–119] Some investigators suggest that oversizing the balloon diameter is not needed in adults.[16] The mechanism of dilation appears to be separation of congenitally fused commissures. Thus, best results are seen in patients with congenital stenosis with fused but thin leaflets and a normal annulus size. However, the procedure has been performed for acquired pulmonic stenosis due to carcinoid or rheumatic disease.[120, 121] Results are likely to be suboptimal when the valve is dysplastic, the leaflets are excessively thickened, or the annulus is hypoplastic.[121, 122] Of concern, excessive dilation or unfavorable valve morphology may lead to leaflet tearing or avulsion, with consequent severe pulmonic regurgitation.

On average, the transpulmonic gradient decreases by two thirds of its baseline value with little or no increase in pulmonic regurgitant severity (Table 16–2 and Fig. 16–12).[16, 121, 123–128] The morbidity rate is low, with potential complications including perforation with tamponade physiology in 0.1% and worsened tricuspid insufficiency due to right ventricular papillary muscle disruption in 0.2%. Some series report no procedural deaths, while other series report a small risk of death from balloon valvuloplasty of the pulmonic valve in adults.[117, 121, 129]

Pulmonic valve stenosis often is associated with some degree of subvalvular muscular obstruction. In most patients, subvalvular obstruction is due to hypertrophy of the right ventricular myocardium in response to the chronic pressure overload of pulmonic stenosis (Fig. 16–13). After relief of pulmonic stenosis, infundibular hypertrophy tends to regress

TABLE 16·2 PERCUTANEOUS PULMONARY VALVULOPLASTY IN ADULTS

Series	Patients	Mean Age (Range) (y)	Baseline Peak Gradient (mm Hg)	Postprocedure Peak Gradient (mm Hg)	Long-Term Outcome
Sievert, 1989[123]	24	39 (17–72)	92 ± 36	43 ± 19	Subvalvular hypertrophy decreased over 3–12 mo
Fawzy, 1990[124]	22	25 (16–45)	111 ± 33	38 ± 26	Infundibular stenosis decreased from 35 ± 26 to 15 ± 9 mm Hg after 1 y
David, 1993[125]	38	14 (1–63)	97 ± 43	26 ± 17	
Lau, 1993[126]	14	27 (17–47)	102 ± 41	52 ± 19	No restenosis at repeat catheterization in 8 patients (12–30 mo after procedure)
Kaul, 1993[127]	40	28 (18–56)	107 ± 29	37 ± 25	No restenosis at follow-up of 25 ± 12 mo
Chen, 1996[16]	53	26 (13–55)	91 ± 46	38 ± 32	No restenosis at follow-up of 6.9 ± 3.1 y
Teupe, 1997[128]	14	31 (19–65)	82 ± 19	37 ± 14	No restenosis at 5–9 y follow-up with a remaining residual gradient of 25 ± 12 mm Hg

over the next 2 to 12 months, with resolution of subvalvular obstruction.[123, 124, 128] Mid-term follow-up results after pulmonic balloon valvuloplasty have been excellent, with no evidence of restenosis reported in several series with follow-up intervals between 5 and 9 years.[16, 128, 130, 131]

In patients who have poor results with percutaneous valvuloplasty or have unfavorable valve morphology, surgical valvotomy may be considered. In patients with coexisting significant pulmonic regurgitation, valve replacement may be necessary. A homograft valve has the advantages that it is not thrombogenic, and the length of the graft can be used to reconstruct the annulus and outflow tract as needed. Porcine valves generally are avoided due to the risk of valve degeneration, while mechanical valves are thrombogenic, particularly in the low-pressure right side of the heart. Thus, the homograft pulmonic valve often is the best choice when surgical pulmonic valve replacement is needed.

PULMONIC REGURGITATION
Etiology

Pathologic pulmonary regurgitation is rare in adults, although a slight amount of pul-

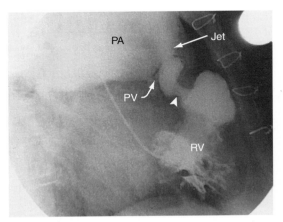

Figure 16·13 This right ventricular angiogram shows doming of a stenotic pulmonic valve and a jet into the markedly dilated pulmonary artery. The dynamic subvalvular obstruction *(arrowhead)* resolved over several months after balloon valvuloplasty. PA, pulmonary artery; PV, pulmonic valve; RV, right ventricle.

monic regurgitation is detectable by Doppler echocardiography in most normal individuals.[14] Pathologic regurgitation is distinguished from this normal regurgitant pattern by a longer duration of flow (typically holodiastolic) and a wider jet as the regurgitant flow crosses the pulmonic valve.

Pulmonic regurgitation in adults most often is caused by pulmonary artery and annular dilation secondary to pulmonary hypertension. Other causes of annular dilation include idiopathic dilation of the pulmonary trunk and, rarely, Marfan's syndrome. Patients with renal failure commonly have a transient pulmonic regurgitant murmur, most likely related to volume overload and pulmonary annular dilation. As the murmur is diminished by extracellular fluid removal, it appears to reflect transient pulmonary hypertension associated with intravascular volume overload.[132]

Pulmonic regurgitation also may be the result of prior surgical interventions for congenital heart disease. For example, although most patients undergoing tetralogy of Fallot repair have excellent long-term outcomes, a potential complication is significant pulmonic regurgitation secondary to the valvotomy used for relief of pulmonic stenosis.[133–135] Other causes of pulmonic regurgitation include rheumatic valve disease, carcinoid, trauma, and endocarditis.[136]

Diagnosis

On physical examination, the murmur of pulmonic regurgitation may be difficult to ap-

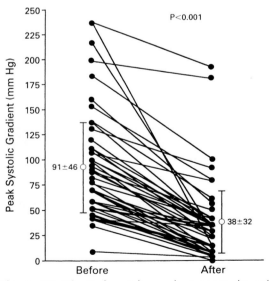

Figure 16·12 Peak systolic gradient across the pulmonic valve before and after balloon valvuloplasty in 53 adolescent or adult patients (age range, 13 to 55; mean age, 26 ± 11 years) with pulmonic valve stenosis. The open circle with bars represents the mean ± SD. (From Chen CR, Cheng TO, Huang T, et al: Percutaneous balloon valvuloplasty for pulmonic stenosis in adolescents and young adults. N Engl J Med 1996;335:21–25; reprinted by permission from the New England Journal of Medicine.)

preciate. Typically, the murmur is a soft, diastolic, decrescendo murmur that is best heard in the left upper parasternal region.

The diagnosis often is initially made by echocardiography (Fig. 16–14; see also color insert). Therefore, echocardiography should be performed periodically for patients at risk for pulmonic regurgitation, including those with a history of repaired tetralogy of Fallot. Color flow imaging shows abnormal diastolic flow in the right ventricular outflow tract. Pulsed Doppler recordings show diastolic flow reversal in the pulmonary artery, which must be differentiated from the more continuous flow of a patent ductus arteriosus. With continuous wave Doppler, the pulmonic regurgitant jet often is best recorded in a parasternal short-axis or right ventricular outflow tract view. The severity of pulmonic regurgitation is graded on a qualitative (0 to 4+) scale based on the extent of the color flow disturbance and the intensity of the continuous wave Doppler signal. More precise direct quantitation of pulmonary regurgitant severity is problematic. Instead, 2D echocardiographic images are used to evaluate right ventricular dilation and systolic dysfunction. Progressive ventricular dilation suggests significant regurgitation in the absence of other causes for this observation.

Cardiac catheterization is only minimally helpful in the diagnosis of pulmonic regurgitation, since angiography must be performed with the catheter across the pulmonic valve. However, catheterization is essential for calculation of pulmonary vascular resistance in patients with pulmonic regurgitation due to pulmonary hypertension.

Natural History

Most patients with mild degrees of pulmonic regurgitation have a benign clinical course and do not develop progressive disease. With moderate to severe regurgitation, chronic volume overload of the right ventricle may lead to right ventricular dilation and systolic dysfunction. Initially, there was concern that transannular patch repair for pulmonic stenosis in patients with tetralogy of Fallot might cause excessive pulmonic regurgitation leading to poor clinical outcomes. However, there was no difference in survival at the 25-year follow-up evaluation of 50 patients with a tetralogy of Fallot repair for those with a transannular patch (89%) or those with a right ventricular outflow patch with intact pulmonary annulus (96%).[137] In addition, there were no group differences in exercise tolerance, quality of life, or functional status.

Medical and Surgical Treatment

No specific therapy is needed for most adults with pulmonic regurgitation as disease severity usually is mild. Surgical intervention should be considered for severe regurgitation and evidence of progressive right ventricular enlargement or the onset of right ventricular systolic dysfunction. A homograft conduit and valve typically are used, although a prosthetic valved conduit may be needed in selected cases. Probably the most common indication for surgical intervention for pulmonic regurgitation in adults is reoperation in tetralogy of Fallot cases.[138]

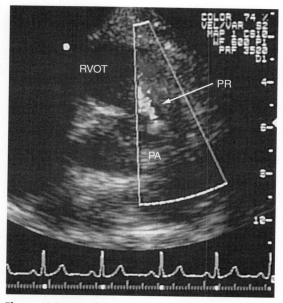

Figure 16·14 This color Doppler image shows mild pulmonic regurgitation in a patient with moderate pulmonic stenosis and mild pulmonic regurgitation (PR). The regurgitant jet is narrow as it crosses the valve plane. Ao, aorta; PA, pulmonary artery; RVOT, right ventricular outflow tract. (This figure also occurs in the color insert.)

References

1. Watanabe T, Katsume H, Matsukubo H, Furukawa K, Ijichi H: Estimation of right ventricular volume with two-dimensional echocardiography. Am J Cardiol 1982;49:1946–1953.
2. Bommer W, Weinert L, Neumann A, et al: Determination of right atrial and right ventricular size by two-dimensional echocardiography. Circulation 1979;60:91–100.
3. Feneley M, Gavaghan T: Paradoxical and pseudopar-

adoxical interventricular septal motion in patients with right ventricular volume overload. Circulation 1986;74:230–238.

4. Pearlman AS, Clark CE, Henry WL, Morganroth J, Itscoitz SB, Epstein SE: Determinants of ventricular septal motion: influence of relative right and left ventricular size. Circulation 1976;54:83–91.

5. Dell'Italia LJ, Walsh RA: Right ventricular diastolic pressure-volume relations and regional dimensions during acute alterations in loading conditions. Circulation 1988;77:1276–1282.

6. Louie EK, Rich S, Levitsky S, Brundage BH: Doppler echocardiographic demonstration of the differential effects of right ventricular pressure and volume overload on left ventricular geometry and filling. J Am Coll Cardiol 1992;19:84–90.

7. Lee FA: Hemodynamics of the right ventricle in normal and disease states. Cardiol Clin 1992;10:59–67.

8. Dell'Italia LJ: The right ventricle: anatomy, physiology, and clinical importance. Curr Probl Cardiol 1991;16:653–720.

9. Spann JFJ, Buccino RA, Sonnenblick EH, Braunwald E: Contractile state of cardiac muscle obtained from cats with experimentally produced ventricular hypertrophy and heart failure. Circ Res 1967;21:341–354.

10. Jardin F, Dubourg O, Gueret P, Delorme G, Bourdarias JP: Quantitative two-dimensional echocardiography in massive pulmonary embolism: emphasis on ventricular interdependence and leftward septal displacement. J Am Coll Cardiol 1987;10:1201–1206.

11. Scuderi LJ, Bailey SR, Calhoon JH, Trinkle JK, Cronin TA, Zabalgoitia M: Echocardiographic assessment of right and left ventricular function after single-lung transplantation. Am Heart J 1994;127:636–642.

12. Kramer MR, Valantine HA, Marshall SE, Starnes VA, Theodore J: Recovery of the right ventricle after single-lung transplantation in pulmonary hypertension. Am J Cardiol 1994;73:494–500.

13. Ritchie M, Waggoner AD, Davila R, Barzilai B, Trulock EP, Eisenberg PR: Echocardiographic characterization of the improvement in right ventricular function in patients with severe pulmonary hypertension after single-lung transplantation. J Am Coll Cardiol 1993;22:1170–1174.

14. Klein AL, Burstow DJ, Tajik AJ, et al: Age-related prevalence of valvular regurgitation in normal subjects: a comprehensive color flow examination of 118 volunteers. J Am Soc Echocardiogr 1990;3:54–63.

15. Lopez Candales A, Kleiger RE, Aleman Gomez J, Kouchoukos NT, Botney MD: Pulmonary artery aneurysm: review and case report. Clin Cardiol 1995;18:738–740.

16. Chen CR, Cheng TO, Huang T, et al: Percutaneous balloon valvuloplasty for pulmonic stenosis in adolescents and young adults. N Engl J Med 1996;335:21–25.

17. Silver MD, Lam JH, Ranganathan N, Wigle ED: Morphology of the human tricuspid valve. Circulation 1971;43:333–348.

18. Hansing CE, Rowe GG: Tricuspid insufficiency: a study of hemodynamics and pathogenesis. Circulation 1972;45:793–799.

19. Cohen SR, Sell JE, McIntosh CL, Clark RE: Tricuspid regurgitation in patients with acquired, chronic, pure mitral regurgitation. I. Prevalence, diagnosis,

and comparison of preoperative clinical and hemodynamic features in patients with and without tricuspid regurgitation. J Thorac Cardiovasc Surg 1987;94:481–487.

20. Muller O, Shillingford J: Tricuspid incompetence. Br Heart J 1954;16:195.

21. Sepulveda G, Lukas DS: The diagnosis of tricuspid insufficiency—clinical features in 60 cases with associated mitral valve disease. Circulation 1955;11:552.

22. Waller BF, Howard J, Fess S: Pathology of tricuspid valve stenosis and pure tricuspid regurgitation—part III. Clin Cardiol 1995;18:225–230.

23. Clawson BJ: Rheumatic heart disease—an analysis of 796 cases. Am Heart J 1940;20:454.

24. Brandenburg RO, McGoon DC, Campeau L, Giuliani ER: Traumatic rupture of the chordae tendineae of the tricuspid valve: successful repair twenty-four years later. Am J Cardiol 1966;18:911–915.

25. Salazar E, Levine HD: Rheumatic tricuspid regurgitation. Am J Med 1962;33:111.

26. Katz NM, Pallas RS: Traumatic rupture of the tricuspid valve: repair by chordal replacements and annuloplasty. J Thorac Cardiovasc Surg 1986;91:310–314.

27. Morgan JR, Forker AD: Isolated tricuspid insufficiency. Circulation 1971;43:559–564.

28. Marvin RF, Schrank JP, Nolan SP: Traumatic tricuspid insufficiency. Am J Cardiol 1973;32:723–726.

29. Cahill NS, Beller BM, Linhart JW, Early RG: Isolated traumatic tricuspid regurgitation: prolonged survival without operative intervention. Chest 1972;61:689–691.

30. Smith WR, Glauser FL, Jemison P: Ruptured chordae of the tricuspid valve: the consequence of flow-directed Swan-Ganz catheterization. Chest 1976;70:790–792.

31. Roberts WC, Sjoerdsma A: The cardiac disease associated with the carcinoid syndrome. Am J Med 1964;36:5.

32. Connolly HM, Crary JL, McGoon MD, et al: Valvular heart disease associated with fenfluramine-phentermine. N Engl J Med 1997;337:581–588.

33. Connolly HM, Nishimura RA, Smith HC, Pellikka PA, Mullany CJ, Kvols LK: Outcome of cardiac surgery for carcinoid heart disease. J Am Coll Cardiol 1995;25:410–416.

34. Duran CM: Tricuspid valve surgery revisited. J Card Surg 1994;9:242–247.

35. Weinreich DJ, Burke JF, Bharati S, Lev M: Isolated prolapse of the tricuspid valve. J Am Coll Cardiol 1985;6:475–481.

36. Chandraratna PN, Lopez JM, Fernandez JJ, Cohen LS: Echocardiographic detection of tricuspid valve prolapse. Circulation 1975;51:823–826.

37. Kendrick MH, Harrington JJ, Sharma GV, Askenazi J, Parisi AF: Ventricular pacemaker wire simulating a right atrial mass. Chest 1977;72:649–650.

38. Zager J, Berberich SN, Eslava R, Klieman C: Dynamic tricuspid valve insufficiency produced by a right ventricular thrombus from a pacemaker. Chest 1978;74:455–456.

39. Votapka TV, Appleton RS, Pennington DG: Tricuspid valve replacement after orthotopic heart transplantation. Ann Thorac Surg 1994;57:752–754.

40. Huddleston CB, Rosenbloom M, Goldstein JA, Pasque MK: Biopsy-induced tricuspid regurgitation after cardiac transplantation. Ann Thorac Surg 1994;57:832–836.

41. Anderson KR, Zuberbuhler JR, Anderson RH, Becker AE, Lie JT: Morphologic spectrum of

Ebstein's anomaly of the heart: a review. Mayo Clin Proc 1979;54:174–180.

42. Celermajer DS, Bull C, Till JA, et al: Ebstein's anomaly: presentation and outcome from fetus to adult. J Am Coll Cardiol 1994;23:170–176.

43. Giuliani ER, Fuster V, Brandenburg RO, Mair DD: Ebstein's anomaly: the clinical features and natural history of Ebstein's anomaly of the tricuspid valve. Mayo Clin Proc 1979;54:163–173.

44. Bialostozky D, Horwitz S, Espino VJ: Ebstein's malformation of the tricuspid valve: a review of 65 cases. Am J Cardiol 1972;29:826–836.

45. Engle MA, Payne TBP, Bruins C, Taussig HB: Ebstein's anomaly of the tricuspid valve: report of 3 cases and analysis of the clinical syndrome. Circulation 1950;1:1246.

46. Fontana ME, Wooley CF: Sail sound in Ebstein's anomaly of the tricuspid valve. Circulation 1972;46:155–164.

47. Hernandez FA, Rochkind R, Cooper HR: The intracavitary electrocardiogram in the diagnosis of Ebstein's anomaly. Am J Cardiol 1958;1:181.

48. Pellikka PA, Tajik AJ, Khandheria BK, et al: Carcinoid heart disease: clinical and echocardiographic spectrum in 74 patients. Circulation 1993;87:1188–1196.

49. Connolly HM, Warnes CA: Ebstein's anomaly: outcome of pregnancy. J Am Coll Cardiol 1994;23:1194–1198.

50. Veyrat C, Kalmanson D, Farjon M, Manin JP, Abitbol G: Non-invasive diagnosis and assessment of tricuspid regurgitation and stenosis using one and two-dimensional echo-pulsed Doppler. Br Heart J 1982;47:596–605.

51. Miyatake K, Okamoto M, Kinoshita N, et al: Evaluation of tricuspid regurgitation by pulsed Doppler and two-dimensional echocardiography. Circulation 1982;66:777–789.

52. DePace NL, Ross J, Iskandrian AS, et al: Tricuspid regurgitation: noninvasive techniques for determining causes and severity. J Am Coll Cardiol 1984;3:1540–1550.

53. Frater RW: Surgical management of endocarditis in drug addicts and long-term results. J Card Surg 1990;5:63–67.

54. Stern HJ, Sisto DA, Strom JA, Soeiro R, Jones SR, Frater RW: Immediate tricuspid valve replacement for endocarditis: indications and results. J Thorac Cardiovasc Surg 1986;91:163–167.

55. Arbulu A, Holmes RJ, Asfaw I: Tricuspid valvulectomy without replacement: twenty years' experience. J Thorac Cardiovasc Surg 1991;102:917–922.

56. Arbulu A, Holmes RJ, Asfaw I: Surgical treatment of intractable right-sided infective endocarditis in drug addicts: 25 years' experience. J Heart Valve Dis 1993;2:129–137.

57. Kay JH, Mendez AM, Zubiate P: A further look at tricuspid annuloplasty. Ann Thorac Surg 1976;22:498–500.

58. Boyd AD, Engelman RM, Isom OW, Reed GE, Spencer FC: Tricuspid annuloplasty: five and one-half years' experience with 78 patients. J Thorac Cardiovasc Surg 1974;68:344–351.

59. Reed GE, Cortes LE: Measured tricuspid annuloplasty: a rapid and reproducible technique. Ann Thorac Surg 1976;21:168–169.

60. Reed GE, Boyd AD, Spencer FC, Engelman RM, Isom OW, Cunningham JNJ: Operative management of tricuspid regurgitation. Circulation 1976;54(suppl III):96–98.

61. Carpentier A, Deloche A, Dauptain J, et al: A new reconstructive operation for correction of mitral and tricuspid insufficiency. J Thorac Cardiovasc Surg 1971;61:1–13.

62. Duran CG, Ubago JL: Clinical and hemodynamic performance of a totally flexible prosthetic ring for atrioventricular valve reconstruction. Ann Thorac Surg 1976;22:458–463.

63. Hecart J, Blaise C, Bex JP, Bajolet A: Technique for tricuspid annuloplasty with a flexible linear reducer: medium-term results. J Thorac Cardiovasc Surg 1980;79:689–692.

64. Meyer J, Bircks W: Predictable correction of tricuspid insufficiency by semicircular annuloplasty. Ann Thorac Surg 1977;23:574–575.

65. Danielson GK, Driscoll DJ, Mair DD, Warnes CA, Oliver WCJ: Operative treatment of Ebstein's anomaly. J Thorac Cardiovasc Surg 1992;104:1195–1202.

66. Seward JB: Ebstein's anomaly: ultrasound imaging and hemodynamic evaluation. Echocardiography 1993;10:641–664.

67. Haerten K, Seipel L, Herzer J, Loogen F, Bircks W: Hemodynamic results after tricuspid valvuloplasty [in German, author's translation]. Z Kardiol 1978;67:661–666.

68. Duran C-MU, Pomar JL, Colman T, Figueroa A, Revuelta JM, Ubago JL: Is tricuspid valve repair necessary? J Thorac Cardiovasc Surg 1980;80:849–860.

69. Rivera R, Duran E, Ajuria M: Carpentier's flexible ring versus De Vega's annuloplasty: a prospective randomized study. J Thorac Cardiovasc Surg 1985;89:196–203.

70. Chidambaram M, Abdulali SA, Baliga BG, Ionescu MI: Long-term results of DeVega tricuspid annuloplasty. Ann Thorac Surg 1987;43:185–188.

71. Mullany CJ, Gersh BJ, Orszulak TA, et al: Repair of tricuspid valve insufficiency in patients undergoing double (aortic and mitral) valve replacement: perioperative mortality and long-term (1 to 20 years) follow-up in 109 patients. J Thorac Cardiovasc Surg 1987;94:740–748.

72. Kaiser GC, Fiore AC: Acquired disease of the tricuspid valve. *In* Baue AE, Geha AS, Hammond GL, Laks H, Naunheim KS, eds. Glenn's Thoracic and Cardiovascular Surgery, ed 6. Stamford, CT: Appleton & Lange; 1996:1931–1942.

73. Kouchoukos NT, Stephenson LW: Indications for and results of tricuspid valve replacement. Adv Cardiol 1976;17:199–206.

74. Stephenson LW, Kouchoukos NT, Kirklin JW: Triple-valve replacement: an analysis of eight years' experience. Ann Thorac Surg 1977;23:327–332.

75. Peterffy A, Henze A, Jonasson R, Bjork VO: Clinical evaluation of the Bjork-Shiley tilting disc valve in the tricuspid position: early and late results in 10 isolated and 51 combined cases. Scand J Thorac Cardiovasc Surg 1978;12:179–187.

76. Thorburn CW, Morgan JJ, Shanahan MX, Chang VP: Long-term results of tricuspid valve replacement and the problem of prosthetic valve thrombosis. Am J Cardiol 1983;51:1128–1132.

77. Gersh BJ, Schaff HV, Vatterott PJ, et al: Results of triple valve replacement in 91 patients: perioperative mortality and long-term follow-up. Circulation 1985;72:130–137.

78. Cohen SR, Sell JE, McIntosh CL, Clark RE: Tricuspid regurgitation in patients with acquired, chronic, pure mitral regurgitation. II. Nonoperative management, tricuspid valve annuloplasty, and tricuspid

valve replacement. J Thorac Cardiovasc Surg 1987;94:488–497.

79. Starr A, Herr R, Wood J: Tricuspid replacement for acquired valve disease. Surg Gynecol Obstet 1966;122:1295–1310.

80. Macmanus Q, Grunkemeier G, Starr A: Late results of triple valve replacement: a 14-year review. Ann Thorac Surg 1978;25:402–406.

81. Singh AK, Feng WC, Sanofsky SJ: Long-term results of St. Jude Medical valve in the tricuspid position. Ann Thorac Surg 1992;54:538–540.

82. Scully HE, Armstrong CS: Tricuspid valve replacement: fifteen years of experience with mechanical prostheses and bioprostheses. J Thorac Cardiovasc Surg 1995;109:1035–1041.

83. Glower DD, White WD, Smith LR, et al: In-hospital and long-term outcome after porcine tricuspid valve replacement. J Thorac Cardiovasc Surg 1995;109:877–883.

84. Singh AK, Christian FD, Williams DO, et al: Follow-up assessment of St. Jude Medical prosthetic valve in the tricuspid position: clinical and hemodynamic results. Ann Thorac Surg 1984;37:324–327.

85. Poveda JJ, Bernal JM, Matorras P, et al: Tricuspid valve replacement in rheumatic disease: preoperative predictors of hospital mortality. J Heart Valve Dis 1996;5:26–30.

86. Sanfelippo PM, Giuliani ER, Danielson GK, Wallace RB, Pluth JR, McGoon DC: Tricuspid valve prosthetic replacement: early and late results with the Starr-Edwards prosthesis. J Thorac Cardiovasc Surg 1976;71:441–445.

87. Jugdutt BI, Fraser RS, Lee SJ, Rossall RE, Callaghan JC: Long-term survival after tricuspid valve replacement: results with seven different prostheses. J Thorac Cardiovasc Surg 1977;74:20–27.

88. Luluaga IT, Carrera D, D'Oliveira J, et al: Successful thrombolytic therapy after acute tricuspid-valve obstruction. Lancet 1971;1:1067–1068.

89. Joyce LD, Boucek M, McGough EC: Urokinase therapy for thrombosis of tricuspid prosthetic valve. J Thorac Cardiovasc Surg 1983;85:935–937.

90. Boskovic D, Elezovic I, Simin N, Rolovic Z, Josipovic V: Late thrombosis of the Bjork-Shiley tilting disc valve in the tricuspid position: thrombolytic treatment with streptokinase. J Thorac Cardiovasc Surg 1986;91:1–8.

91. Geha AS, Laks H, Stansel HCJ, et al: Late failure of porcine valve heterografts in children. J Thorac Cardiovasc Surg 1979;78:351–364.

92. Ishihara T, Ferrans VJ, Boyce SW, Jones M, Roberts WC: Structure and classification of cuspal tears and perforations in porcine bioprosthetic cardiac valves implanted in patients. Am J Cardiol 1981;48:665–678.

93. Cohen SR, Silver MA, McIntosh CL, Roberts WC: Comparison of late (62 to 140 months) degenerative changes in simultaneously implanted and explanted porcine (Hancock) bioprostheses in the tricuspid and mitral valve positions in six patients. Am J Cardiol 1984;53:1599–1602.

94. Van Nooten GJ, Caes FL, Francois KJ, et al: The valve choice in tricuspid valve replacement: 25 years of experience. Eur J Cardiothorac Surg 1995;9:441–446.

95. Kitchin A, Turner R: Diagnosis and treatment of tricuspid stenosis. Br Heart J 1964;16:354.

96. Bousvaros GA, Stubington D: Some auscultatory and phonocardiographic features of tricuspid stenosis. Circulation 1964;29:26.

97. Waller BF, Howard J, Fess S: Pathology of tricuspid valve stenosis and pure tricuspid regurgitation—part III. Clin Cardiol 1995;18:225–230.

98. Gibson R, Wood P: The diagnosis of tricuspid stenosis. Br Heart J 1955;17.

99. Killip TI, Lukas DS: Tricuspid stenosis—clinical features in twelve cases. Am J Med 1958;24:836.

100. El-Sherif N: Rheumatic tricuspid stenosis: a haemodynamic correlation. Br Heart J 1971;33:16–31.

101. Killip TI, Lukas DS: Tricuspid stenosis: physiological criteria for diagnosis and hemodynamic abnormalities. Circulation 1957;16:3.

102. Shimada R, Takeshita A, Nakamura M, Tokunaga K, Hirata T: Diagnosis of tricuspid stenosis by M-mode and two-dimensional echocardiography. Am J Cardiol 1984;53:164–168.

103. Guyer DE, Gillam LD, Foale RA, et al: Comparison of the echocardiographic and hemodynamic diagnosis of rheumatic tricuspid stenosis. J Am Coll Cardiol 1984;3:1135–1144.

104. Perez JE, Ludbrook PA, Ahumada GG: Usefulness of Doppler echocardiography in detecting tricuspid valve stenosis. Am J Cardiol 1985;55:601–603.

105. Carpentier A, Deloche A, Hanania G, et al: Surgical management of acquired tricuspid valve disease. J Thorac Cardiovasc Surg 1974;67:53–65.

106. Grondin P, Lepage G, Castonguay Y, Meere C: The tricuspid valve: a surgical challenge. J Thorac Cardiovasc Surg 1967;53:7–20.

107. Shrivastava S, Goswami KC, Dev V: Concurrent percutaneous balloon valvotomy for combined rheumatic tricuspid and aortic stenosis. Int J Cardiol 1993;38:183–186.

108. Bethencourt A, Medina A, Hernandez E, et al: Combined percutaneous balloon valvuloplasty of mitral and tricuspid valves. Am Heart J 1990;119:1416–1418.

109. Pinto RJ, Loya YS, Desai DM, Sharma S: Concurrent dilation of mitral and tricuspid valve stenosis using a single Inoue balloon: a report of 2 cases. Cathet Cardiovasc Diagn 1993;30:355.

110. Kaplan S, Adolph RJ, Murphy DJ: Pulmonic valve stenosis. *In* Roberts WC, ed. Adult Congenital Heart Disease. Philadelphia: FA Davis, 1987:477–492.

111. Perloff JK: Physical Examination of the Heart and Circulation. Philadelphia: WB Saunders, 1982.

112. Krabill KA, Wang Y, Einzig S, Moller JH: Rest and exercise hemodynamics in pulmonary stenosis: comparison of children and adults. Am J Cardiol 1985;56:360–365.

113. Johnson LW, Grossman W, Dalen JE, Dexter L: Pulmonic stenosis in the adult: long-term follow-up results. N Engl J Med 1972;287:1159–1163.

114. Nugent EW, Freedom RM, Nora JJ, Ellison RC, Rowe RD, Nadas AS: Clinical course in pulmonary stenosis. Circulation 1977;56(suppl I):138–147.

115. Hayes CJ, Gersony WM, Driscoll DJ, et al: Second natural history study of congenital heart defects: results of treatment of patients with pulmonary valvar stenosis. Circulation 1993;87(suppl I):28–37.

116. Nadas AS: Report from the Joint Study on the Natural History of Congenital Heart Defects. IV. Clinical course: introduction. Circulation 1977;56:136–138.

117. Berman AD, McKay RG, Grossman W: Balloon valvuloplasty. *In* Baim DS, Grossman W, eds. Cardiac Catheterization, Angiography, and Intervention, ed 5. Baltimore: Williams & Wilkins, 1996:659–687.

118. Lau K, Hung J, Wu J, Chern M, Yeh K, Fu M: Pul-

monary valvuloplasty in adults using the Inoue balloon catheter. Cathet Cardiovasc Diagn 1994;29:99.

119. Herrmann HC, Hill JA, Krol J, Kleaveland JP, Pepine CJ: Effectiveness of percutaneous balloon valvuloplasty in adults with pulmonic valve stenosis. Am J Cardiol 1991;68:1111–1113.

120. McCrindle BW: Independent predictors of long-term results after balloon pulmonary valvuloplasty. Valvuloplasty and Angioplasty of Congenital Anomalies (VACA) Registry Investigators. Circulation 1994;89:1751–1759.

121. Stanger P, Cassidy SC, Girod DA, Kan JS, Lababidi Z, Shapiro SR: Balloon pulmonary valvuloplasty: results of the Valvuloplasty and Angioplasty of Congenital Anomalies Registry. Am J Cardiol 1990;65:775–783.

122. McCrindle BW: Independent predictors of immediate results of percutaneous balloon aortic valvotomy in children. Valvuloplasty and Angioplasty of Congenital Anomalies (VACA) Registry Investigators. Am J Cardiol 1996;77:286–293.

123. Sievert H, Kober G, Bussman WD, et al: Long-term results of percutaneous pulmonary valvuloplasty in adults. Eur Heart J 1989;10:712–717.

124. Fawzy ME, Galal O, Dunn B, Shaikh A, Sriram R, Duran CM: Regression of infundibular pulmonary stenosis after successful balloon pulmonary valvuloplasty in adults. Cathet Cardiovasc Diagn 1990;21:77–81.

125. David SW, Goussous YM, Harbi N, et al: Management of typical and dysplastic pulmonic stenosis, uncomplicated or associated with complex intracardiac defects, in juveniles and adults: use of percutaneous balloon pulmonary valvuloplasty with eight-month hemodynamic follow-up. Cathet Cardiovasc Diagn 1993;29:105–112.

126. Lau KW, Hung JS: Controversies in percutaneous balloon pulmonary valvuloplasty: timing, patient selection and technique. J Heart Valve Dis 1993;2:321–325.

127. Kaul UA, Singh B, Tyagi S, Bhargava M, Arora R, Khalilullah M: Long-term results after balloon pulmonary valvuloplasty in adults. Am Heart J 1993;126:1152–1155.

128. Teupe CH, Burger W, Schrader R, Zeiher AM: Late (five to nine years) follow-up after balloon dilation of valvular pulmonary stenosis in adults. Am J Cardiol 1997;80:240–242.

129. Pepine CJ, Gessner IH, Feldman RL: Percutaneous balloon valvuloplasty for pulmonic valve stenosis in the adult. Am J Cardiol 1982;50:1442–1445.

130. Masura J, Burch M, Deanfield JE, Sullivan ID: Five-year follow-up after balloon pulmonary valvuloplasty. J Am Coll Cardiol 1993;21:132–136.

131. McCrindle BW, Kan JS: Long-term results after balloon pulmonary valvuloplasty. Circulation 1991;83:1915–1922.

132. Peres JE, Smith CA, Meltzer VN: Pulmonic valve insufficiency: a common cause of transient diastolic murmurs in renal failure. Ann Intern Med 1985;103:497–502.

133. Murphy JG, Gersh BJ, Mair DD, et al: Long-term outcome in patients undergoing surgical repair of tetralogy of Fallot. N Engl J Med 1993;329:593–599.

134. Friedli B, Bolens M, Taktak M: Conduction disturbances after correction of tetralogy of Fallot: are electrophysiologic studies of prognostic value? J Am Coll Cardiol 1988;11:162–165.

135. Rosenthal A, Behrendt D, Sloan H, Ferguson P, Snedecor SM, Schork A: Long-term prognosis (15 to 26 years) after repair of tetralogy of Fallot: I. Survival and symptomatic status. Ann Thorac Surg 1984;38:151–156.

136. Waller BF, Howard J, Fess S: Pathology of pulmonic valve stenosis and pure regurgitation. Clin Cardiol 1995;18:45–50.

137. Miyamura H, Takahashi M, Sugawara M, Eguchi S: The long-term influence of pulmonary valve regurgitation following repair of tetralogy of Fallot: does preservation of the pulmonary valve ring affect quality of life? Surg Today 1996;26:603–606.

138. Waien SA, Liu PP, Ross BL, Williams WG, Webb GD, McLaughlin PR: Serial follow-up of adults with repaired tetralogy of Fallot. J Am Coll Cardiol 1992;20:295–300.

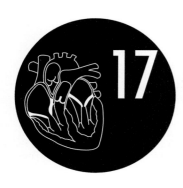

17 Prosthetic Valves

Significant advances in the design and performance of artificial valve substitutes have been made since their introduction in the early 1960s.[1-3] Valve replacement surgery, in conjunction with improvements in surgical technique, optimization of the timing of intervention, and better medical management, has dramatically decreased morbidity and mortality for patients with valvular heart disease. However, implantation of a prosthetic valve still leaves the patient with valvular disease, albeit with a functional prosthetic valve rather than a dysfunctional native valve. Increasingly, surgical approaches that preserve the native valve structure while restoring functional integrity are used whenever possible (see Chapter 8). Implantation of a prosthetic valve is reserved for conditions in which valve-sparing procedures are not feasible or would result in suboptimal hemodynamics compared with a prosthetic valve.

VALVE DESIGN PARAMETERS

Each of the currently available prosthetic valves has certain advantages, but none is ideal for every patient (Table 17–1). The ideal valve substitute should mimic the characteristics of a normal native valve.[4] Hemodynamically, the ideal valve should offer no significant resistance to blood flow, with transvalvular pressure

TABLE 17·1 CHARACTERISTICS OF THE IDEAL VALVE SUBSTITUTE

Permanent
    Durable prosthetic material *or*
    Viable valve with ability to repair and remodel
Hemodynamics equivalent to normal native valve
Nonthrombogenic
Easy to implant, little technical variability
Silent, no patient discomfort

gradients and functional valve areas similar to those of native valves. Depending on valve design, a small degree of backflow may be necessary to prevent valve thrombosis, but the ideal valve should have no significant valvular regurgitation.

The ideal valve should be durable to obviate repeat valve surgery. Implantation should be straightforward to minimize technical variations in valve performance related to surgical experience. The ideal valve should be implantable through a noninvasive or minimally invasive approach.

In addition, the ideal valve should be silent and inapparent to the patient. Many current valve prostheses have audible closing (and sometimes opening) sounds that can be quite loud in some patients, causing considerable patient annoyance and discomfort. Finally, the ideal valve should be nonthrombogenic, so that long-term anticoagulation is not needed, and should be harmless to blood elements.

Currently not any of the available valve prostheses meets all these characteristics, so that selection of a prosthetic valve involves trade-offs between the advantages and disadvantages of each valve type. Ongoing research on possible improvements in valve design includes development of new mechanical valves,[5] heterograft tissue valves with a surface layer of the patient's own endothelial cells,[6–8] and biochemical anticalcification treatments of tissue valves.[9] An intriguing experimental approach is the development of tissue-engineered valves using viable endothelial cells and fibroblasts grown on a biodegradable polymer template.[10]

The two basic types of valve prostheses are mechanical and tissue valves. Tissue valves are described as heterografts if nonhuman valve or pericardial tissue is used to construct a valve prosthesis. The terms homograft and allograft are used interchangeably to describe use of a human valve harvested at the time of death of a different person. Use of the patient's own pulmonic valve to replace a diseased aortic valve is called an autograft valve replacement.

Tissue valves have the advantage of nonthrombogenicity, obviating the need for long-term anticoagulation. The major disadvantage of tissue valves is the limited durability of most available prostheses, although the use of pulmonic autografts and the development of viable heterograft or allograft valve substitutes offer hope that long-term durability will become feasible. The hemodynamics of tissue valves vary considerably with valve type and size; the best hemodynamics are seen with pul-

monic autografts and aortic homografts, and the worst results are seen with small sizes of stented porcine valves.

Mechanical valves are classified as single-disk valves (eg, Bjork-Shiley, Omniscience, Medtronic-Hall), bileaflet valves (eg, St Jude Medical, CarboMedics), and ball-cage valves (eg, Starr-Edwards) (Fig. 17–1). The major advantage of mechanical valves is their durability, and the major disadvantage is the need for long-term anticoagulation. With both tissue and mechanical valves there is an increased risk of endocarditis. Prosthetic valve endocarditis is a devastating complication that often requires surgical intervention and is associated with a very poor clinical outcome (see Chapter 18).

TISSUE VALVES
Stented Heterograft Valves
Hemodynamics

The traditional design of a heterograft valve consists of three valve leaflets that open to

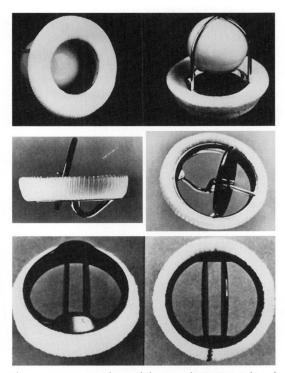

Figure 17·1 Mechanical heart valves: Starr-Edwards *(top)*; Medtronic-Hall *(middle)*; and St. Jude Medical *(bottom)*. (From Nottestad SY, Zabalgoitia M: Echocardiographic recognition and quantitation of prosthetic valve dysfunction. *In* Otto CM, ed. The Practice of Clinical Echocardiography. Philadelphia: WB Saunders, 1997:798.)

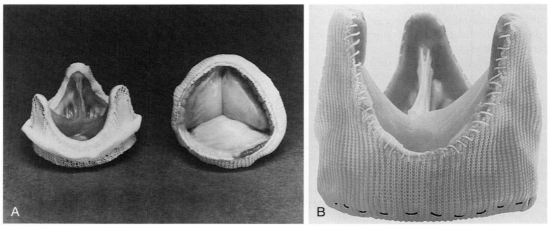

Figure 17·2 Heterograft tissue valves. A, Carpentier-Edwards aortic valve. B, Toronto stentless porcine valve. (Courtesy of St. Jude Medical Heart Valve Division, St. Paul, MN.)

a circular orifice in systole, resembling the anatomy of the native aortic valve (Fig. 17–2). Porcine valves, including Carpentier-Edwards and Hancock valves, use glutaraldehyde-treated porcine aortic leaflets mounted on a semiflexible circular polypropylene stent or on wires shaped to conform to the arch describing the base of each leaflet. Since native porcine valves have two fibrous and one muscular leaflet, care is taken to exclude unsuitable valves, and the muscular leaflet typically is replaced with a fibrous leaflet from a second valve,[11, 12] or the valve is configured to minimize the amount of septal muscle included.[13] Leaflets also have been constructed from bovine pericardial tissue. However, the Ionescu-Shiley bovine pericardial valve was discontinued because of cusp dehiscence.[14]

The rationale for use of a semirigid stent or ring for a tissue valve prosthesis is to maintain the three-dimensional (3D) relationships of the leaflets and to standardize surgical implantation of the valve. However, as experience with these valves has accumulated, it has become evident that the stents produce suboptimal hemodynamics, particularly for small valve sizes, and contribute to high stress-strain relationships that may increase the rate of leaflet deterioration and calcification.

The normal pattern of flow through a stented bioprosthesis is characterized by a circular central flow field with a relatively flat flow velocity profile (Fig. 17–3). For the aortic position, peak velocities of 2 to 3 m/s are typical, and typical antegrade velocities in the mitral position range from 1.5 to 2 m/s. These

Aortic: C–E Porcine (2625)

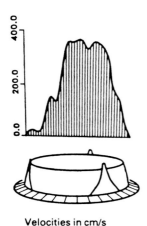

Velocities in cm/s

Aortic: C–E 2625 Porcine

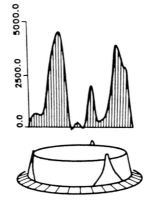

Turbulent shear stresses in dynes/cm²

Figure 17·3 Center line velocity and turbulent shear stress profiles 15 mm downstream of a 27-mm Carpentier-Edwards 2625 porcine valve at peak systole. (From Yoganathan AP, Heinrich RS, Fontaine AA: Fluid dynamics of prosthetic valves. *In* Otto CM, ed. The Practice of Clinical Echocardiography. Philadelphia: WB Saunders, 1997:791.)

correspond to mean antegrade transvalvular pressure gradients of 10 to 15 mm Hg for aortic and 4 to 7 mm Hg for mitral valve implantation (Table 17–2).[15]

A standard approach to describing the hemodynamics of a prosthetic valve is the *performance index*, defined as ratio of the effective orifice area to the area of the sewing ring. Optimal hemodynamics are reflected in a performance index close to 1, with smaller numbers indicating progressively poorer hemodynamics. For stented bioprosthetic valves, the performance index is only 0.3 to 0.4, compared with 0.6 to 0.7 for similarly sized mechanical valves.[16] Possible reasons for these suboptimal hemodynamics include the 3D configuration of the leaflets, the stiffness of the fixed leaflet tissue, impaired opening at the reconstructed commissures, and the presence of semirigid stents.

In vitro fluid dynamic studies show that flow stagnation occurs on the outflow surfaces of the bioprosthetic leaflets during systole. Turbulent and shear stresses are confined to the perimeter of flow stream, but stresses are high enough to potentially cause hemolysis and platelet activation.[16] Although bioprosthetic valves are considered to be relatively nonthrombogenic, turbulence and shear stresses may increase the likelihood of thromboembolic events and tissue overgrowth of the sewing ring.

At valve closure, a small amount of blood, called the *closing volume*, is displaced into the upstream chamber. *Regurgitation* is defined as backflow of blood across the valve in excess of the closing volume. In vitro studies show a closing volume for stented bioprostheses of about 1 mL per beat and almost no valvular regurgitation.[16] A small degree of regurgitation can be detected by color flow imaging in 10% of normally functioning stented bioprostheses.[17]

TABLE 17·2   PROSTHETIC VALVE HEMODYNAMICS

Prosthesis	Peak Velocity (m/s), Mean ± 1 SD	Mean Gradient (mm Hg) Mean ± 1 SD	Valve Area (cm²) Mean (Range)	Performance Index* Mean (Range)	Regurgitant Volume (mL)* Mean (Range)
Aortic Valves					
Mechanical					
Bileaflet					
St. Jude	3.0 ± 0.8	11 ± 6		0.57 (0.43–0.71)	8.5 (6.8–10.8)
CarboMedics				0.54 (0.40–0.65)	7.9 (6.2–9.6)
Tilting disk					
Bjork-Shiley	2.5 ± 0.6	14 ± 5		0.48 (0.38–0.58)	7.0 (5.5–9.2)
Medtronic-Hall	2.6 ± 0.3	12 ± 3		0.58 (0.51–0.64)	5.3 (3.0–7.5)
Ball-Cage					
Starr-Edwards	3.1 ± 0.5	24 ± 4		0.33 (0.30–0.36)	4.1 (2.5–5.5)
Bioprostheses					
Stented					
Hancock	2.4 ± 0.4	11 ± 2	1.8 (1.4–2.3)	0.43 (0.41–0.44)	<2
Carpentier-Edwards	2.4 ± 0.5	14 ± 6	1.8 (1.2–3.1)	0.44 (0.40–0.48)	<2
Nonstented					
SPV-Toronto	2.2 ± 0.4	3 (2–20)	(1.8–2.3)		Trace
Ao-homograft	1.8 ± 0.4	7 ± 3	2.2 (1.7–3.1)		Trace
Mitral Valves					
Mechanical					
Bileaflet					
St. Jude	1.6 ± 0.3	5 ± 2	2.9 (1.8–4.4)	0.49 (0.48–0.51)	11 (9.7–13.1)
Tilting disk					
Bjork-Shiley	1.6 ± 0.3	5 ± 2	2.4 (1.6–3.7)	0.44 (0.42–0.45)	6.7
Medtronic-Hall	1.7 ± 0.3	3 ± 1	2.4 (1.5–3.9)	0.48 (0.45–0.53)	9.0 (7.2–10.0)
Ball-Cage					
Starr-Edwards	1.8 ± 0.4	5 ± 2	2.1 (1.2–2.5)	0.28 (0.27–0.29)	
Bioprostheses					
Hancock	1.5 ± 0.3	4 ± 2	1.7 (1.3–2.7)	0.28 (0.25–0.30)	<2
Carpentier-Edwards	1.8 ± 0.2	7 ± 2	2.5 (1.6–3.5)	0.40 (0.35–0.47)	<2
Homograft	1.8 ± 0.4	7 ± 3	2.2 ± 0.8	—	—

*In vitro data.

Data from references 15, 16, 17, 48, 68, and 277.

Long-Term Outcome

A major advantage of bioprosthetic valves is the low rate of thromboembolism with recent series estimating a rate of thromboembolism of only 1.6% per patient-year in the absence of chronic anticoagulation (Table 17–3).[18]

Traditional stented heterograft valves are subject to progressive calcification, degenerative changes, and tissue failure, with identifiable changes typically beginning 5 to 7 years after valve implantation.[19–23] Excessive calcification leads to increased stiffness of the valve leaflets, resulting in prosthetic valve stenosis. Tissue failure, often rupture in an area of valve thinning adjacent to a calcified area, leads to prosthetic regurgitation.[24] Paraprosthetic regurgitation may occur because of technical difficulties at the time of insertion or because of loss of suture integrity in an area of annular fibrosis, calcification, or infection.

Degeneration of stented bioprosthetic valves is more rapid in children,[25, 26] young adults, and patients with abnormal calcium metabolism (eg, renal failure). It remains controversial whether tissue degeneration is accelerated

TABLE 17·3   LONG-TERM OUTCOME AFTER TISSUE VALVE REPLACEMENT

Valve Type	Years Implanted	Number of Patients	Age (y)	Outcome	
Stented heterograft					
Porcine (Hancock & Carpentier-Edwards)[29]	1971–90	2879	60 ± 15 (AVR)	Actuarial survival	77 ± 1% at 5 y
					54 ± 2% at 10 y
					32 ± 3% at 15 y
				Freedom from thromboembolism	92 ± 1% at 10 y
				Freedom from structural deterioration	78 ± 2% at 10 y
					49 ± 4% at 15 y
			58 ± 13 (MVR)	Actuarial survival	70 ± 1% at 5 y
					50 ± 2% at 10 y
					32 ± 3% at 15 y
				Freedom from thromboembolism	86 ± 1% at 10 y
				Freedom from structural deterioration	69 ± 2% at 10 y
					32 ± 4% at 15 y
Carpentier-Edwards[18]	1975–86	1195	57.3	Actuarial survival	57.4 ± 1.5% at 10 y
				Rate of thromboembolism	1.6%/pt-year
				Rate of structural deterioration	3.3%/pt-year
Stentless heterograft valves					
Toronto SPV valve[48]	1993–94	100	71 ± 7	Survival	96% at 1 y
				No thromboembolism or structural deterioration	
Toronto SPV valve[52]	1987–93	123	61 ± 12	Survival	91 ± 4% at 6 y
				Freedom from thromboembolism	87 ± 7% at 6 y
				Structural deterioration	0%
PRIMA Edwards valve[54]	1991–93	200	68.5 ± 8	Survival	95% at 1 y
				Thromboembolism	3% at 1 y
				AV block requiring pacer	7% at 1 y
				Mild AR	27% at 1 y
Homografts					
Cryopreserved[278]	1973–75	32		Actuarial survival	79% at 10 y
					69% at 13 y
				Thromboembolism	0.4%/pt-year
				Valve failure	3.2%/pt-year
				Endocarditis	0.4%/pt-year
				Reoperation	3.6%/pt-year
Cryopreserved[85]	1981–91	178	46 y (mean)	Survival	85% at 8 y
				Freedom from valve failure	85% at 8 y
Pulmonic autografts[100, 115]	1986–95	195	8 mo–62 y	Freedom from reoperation	95 ± 2% at 2 y
					81 ± 5% at 8 y
	1989–93	33	8–49 y (mean, 31 y)	No deaths at 21 months; no valve failures or endocarditis	

AR, aortic regurgitation; AV, atrioventricular; AVR, aortic valve replacement; MVR, mitral valve replacement; pt-year, patient-year.

during pregnancy or if young pregnant women simply present at a time after surgery when degeneration is likely.[27, 28]

In several large series, the estimated rate of structural deterioration for porcine valve was 3.3% per patient-year, corresponding to a freedom from valve failure at 10 years of 78% ± 2% for aortic valve prostheses and 69 ± 2% for valves in the mitral position (Figs. 17–4 and 17–5).[18, 29, 30] However, the rate of valve deterioration accelerates after 10 years, and only 49% ± 4% of aortic valves and 32% ± 4% of porcine mitral valves remain functional after 15 years.[29]

Stentless Heterograft Valves

Hemodynamics

Although the rigid structures used to support the valve leaflets in traditional bioprosthetic valves may help maintain the 3D relationships of the valve leaflets and provide easier implantation, the rigid sewing ring and stents contribute to suboptimal hemodynamics and increase the mechanical stress on the leaflets, accelerating valve degeneration and calcification. To improve valve hemodynamics and durability while retaining the advantages of a bioprosthetic valve—specifically the ability to reliably provide a wide range of valve sizes and the lack of a need for long-term anticoagulation—several types of stentless bioprosthetic valves have been developed.[31, 32] These valves include the Toronto SPV Stentless valve (St. Jude Medical, St Paul, MN),[33, 34] the Edwards Stentless valve,[35] the Medtronic Freestyle valve,[36–39] and the Cryolife-O'Brien valve (Cryolife International, Atlanta, GA).[40–42] Stentless bioprosthetic valves typically are manufactured from intact porcine aortic valves

processed at low pressures to avoid fixing the collagen fibers in a stretched position. Some stentless valves are impregnated with agents to inhibit calcification, such as α-amino-oleic acid. The addition of a layer of Dacron fabric around the graft adds support and aids implantation.[43, 44] Some of these valves require subcoronary implantation, and others are implanted as an inclusion cylinder, a miniroot, or a total root replacement.[45] Subcoronary implantation has the advantage that coronary reimplantation is not needed but the disadvantages of increased operator variability in surgical technique and a longer aortic crossclamp time.[43] Miniroot or total root replacement requires reimplantation of the coronary arteries, but the normal 3D geometry of the valve apparatus is more easily maintained.

Careful sizing of the patient's outflow tract and root may be more important with stentless bioprosthetic valves than with homografts.[45] Rather than using a valve size equal to the patient's aortic annulus or sinotubular junction diameter, a valve one size larger is used to ensure adequate coaptation of the leaflets in diastole.[43] If the valve is too small, central aortic regurgitation may result from stretching the leaflets. Valve sizing can be performed intraoperatively by the surgeon or can be accurately estimated using transesophageal echocardiography before cardiopulmonary bypass.[46, 47]

Stentless bioprosthetic valves have been used only in the aortic position, and the series have mostly included men with a mean age of 60 to 70 years. After implantation, the echocardiographic appearance mimics a normal aortic valve, other than increased echogenicity in the annulus and aortic root from the surgical procedure and the layer of fabric supporting the

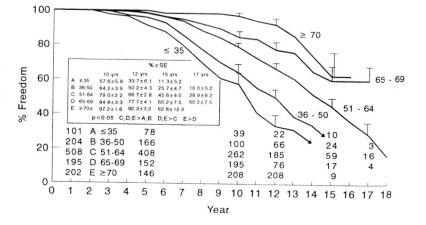

Figure 17·4 Freedom from structural deterioration of Carpentier-Edwards porcine bioprostheses, stratified by age group, for all valve positions. (From Jamieson WR, Munro AI, Miyagishima RT, Allen P, Burr LH, Tyers GF: Carpentier-Edwards standard porcine bioprosthesis: clinical performance to seventeen years. Ann Thorac Surg 1995;60:999–1007; reprinted with permission from the Society of Thoracic Surgeons.)

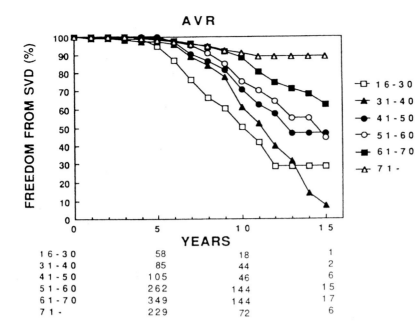

1 6 - 3 0	58	18	1
3 1 - 4 0	85	44	2
4 1 - 5 0	105	46	6
5 1 - 6 0	262	144	1 5
6 1 - 7 0	349	144	1 7
7 1 -	229	72	6

Figure 17·5 Estimates of freedom from structural valve deterioration (SVD) for patients undergoing porcine aortic valve replacement (AVR) are stratified according to age. (From Fann JI, Miller DC, Moore KA, et al: Twenty-year clinical experience with porcine bioprostheses. Ann Thorac Surg 1996;62:1301–1312; reprinted with permission from the Society of Thoracic Surgeons.)

graft.[46] These areas of postoperative thickening and brightness often decrease in prominence over time. In these series, the typical mean transaortic gradient in the early postoperative period is less than 15 mm Hg.[48–51] By the 6-month follow-up, the gradient decreases by about 30%, and the effective orifice area increases by 17% to 35% compared with the immediate postoperative values, probably because of remodeling of the aortic root and regression of left ventricular hypertrophy.[37, 40–43, 52, 53] Despite low transvalvular gradients reported in many series, some studies suggest that hemodynamics are not always optimal. One group reported peak gradients of 11 to 35 mm Hg for 19- to 29-mm valves, and effective orifice areas of only 0.8 to 2.8 over the same size range at the 12-month follow-up evaluation.[54]

More than 95% of patients have no or mild (1+) aortic regurgitation.[55, 56] However, with the Cryolife valve, rare cases of paravalvular regurgitation requiring reoperation have been reported.[42]

Since the experience with the stentless aortic bioprosthetic valve is limited to specialized academic centers, valve performance will need to be further evaluated as more cardiac surgeons use this new approach and as patient selection criteria are expanded. Implantation using the subcoronary technique is of particular concern given the observation with homografts that the technical difficulty of this approach results in considerable variability in postoperative hemodynamics,[57] probably because of distortion of the normal 3D geometry of the valve leaflets relative to the sinuses of Valsalva.

Long-Term Outcome

The operative mortality rate for implantation of stentless bioprosthetic valves in the aortic position is only 3% to 6%.[47, 48, 54, 56] Since most of these patients had aortic stenosis, the surgical mortality appears to be lower than for standard aortic valve replacement. However, the low mortality probably is related to patient selection, as the highest risk patients are excluded from these studies.

The incidence of postoperative complications by 12 months is low but does include endocarditis in 1% to 2%, thromboembolism in 2% to 3%, and hemorrhage in 1.5% of patients.[43, 48, 54] Although several groups have observed a high rate of heart block with stentless compared with stented valves,[51] with up to 7% of patients requiring a permanent pacer by 12 months,[43, 54] other investigators report no episodes of heart block after stentless valve implantation.[58]

There have been no reports of structural valve failure in most of these surgical series, with actuarial survival rates as high as 91% ± 4% at 6 years (see Table 17–3).[43, 52, 54] It is hoped that the lower gradients and larger effective valve areas of stentless, compared with stented, bioprosthetic valves will translate into improved long-term durability. Studies already have shown greater regression of left ventricular hypertrophy and better left ventricular contractile function in patients receiving stentless valves.[59]

Homografts

Hemodynamics of Aortic Homografts

The performance and durability of human heart valves as bioprostheses depend on the specific method of harvesting, preparation, and storage.[60] The early experience in the 1960s with chemically sterilized valves demonstrated a high rate of late cusp rupture.[61–66] Stented homografts were found to have poor hemodynamics.[65, 67] Subsequent results with antibiotic-preserved unstented valves harvested from cadaveric human hearts have been more promising. These valve implants have excellent hemodynamics, are resistant to infection, and do not require long-term anticoagulation.[65, 68] However, concern remains that despite excellent initial results and medium-term durability, the incidence of valve failure increases after 10 years of implantation.[57]

The best results have been obtained with valves harvested within 24 hours of donor death, antibiotic sterilized, and then cryopreserved.[57] Valves harvested and stored in this manner typically contain some viable cells at the time of implantation,[60, 69–71] although the normal endothelium is lost due to the harvesting and preservation process.[72] While the presence of viable cells suggests that the valve may be able to respond normally to ongoing hemodynamic stresses with production of collagen and elastin to maintain the structural integrity of the valve, few studies have examined the long-term cellular activity of implanted homografts.

Histologic examination of explanted homografts tends to show a loss of cellularity over time, although occasional valves show near-normal cellularity.[71, 73, 74] Fibrin deposition is seen on the valve surface and may contribute to decreased elasticity of the leaflets.[75] Calcific fibrosis of the leaflets occasionally is seen, especially in younger patients, possibly related to an immune mechanism.[71, 76] In the long term, the normal layered structure is lost, viable cells are lacking, and progressive calcification occurs.[77, 78]

Typically, donor and recipient matching is not performed, nor is immunosuppression used for aortic homograft valve implantation. Although several lines of evidence suggest there is a host response to the foreign valve,[71, 79–81] there have been no studies to suggest that immunosuppression would improve valve durability. If immunosuppression is considered in the future, the risks of long-term immunosuppression will need to be balanced against the risk (eg, anticoagulation) of a conventional mechanical valve.

Aortic homografts most often are harvested as a block of tissue that includes the ascending aorta, aortic valve, a portion of the ventricular septum, and the anterior mitral leaflet. The tissue block is trimmed as needed at the time of implantation. Several approaches to implantation of homografts have been used, including subcoronary implantation using the valve tissue alone, placing the homograft valve and root as a cylinder within the native aorta (ie, inclusion cylinder), and complete root replacement using the homograft valve and aorta with resection of the corresponding segment of native aorta (Fig. 17–6). Although subcoronary implantation has the advantage that the coronary artery origins are undisturbed, this approach is technically difficult and results in suboptimal hemodynamics if even minor distortion of the 3D anatomy of the valve occurs. Complete root replacement is technically simpler, provides reproducibly excellent hemodynamics, and has become the procedure of choice at most centers, even though reimplantation of the coronaries into the homograft aorta is necessary.[57]

To ensure that an appropriately sized homograft is available, the aortic annulus and sinotubular junction are measured by echocardiography or during angiography preoperatively.[82] The choice of homograft size is based on aortic annulus diameter and the diameter of the aorta at the sinotubular junction.

The antegrade velocities across an aortic homograft are similar to those of a native valve, although slightly increased velocities may occur because of the smaller area of the outflow tract.[68] Hemodynamics and functional valve areas are excellent over the entire range of valve sizes. Typically, little regurgitation is seen.

Long-Term Outcome of Aortic Homografts

Summarizing the data on the long-term outcome with homograft valve replacement is complicated by the differences between centers in harvesting, sterilization, and preserva-

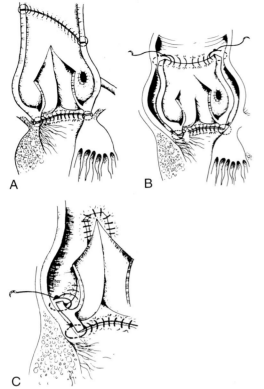

Figure 17·6 The three technical methods for homograft aortic valve insertion. *A,* Root replacement with pedicle coronary artery implantation. *B,* Inclusion cylinder with side-to-side anastomosis. *C,* Subcoronary scalloped implantation. (From O'Brien MF: Homografts and autografts. *In* Baue AE, Geha AS, Hammond GL, Laks H, Naunheim KS, eds. Glenn's Thoracic and Cardiovascular Surgery. Stamford, CT: Appleton & Lange, 1996:2010.)

tion of the homograft and differences in surgical implantation techniques.[60, 71, 83] In early series using antibiotic-stored valves, midterm durability was impressive, with freedom from structural deterioration in 95% of valves at 5 years and 78% of valves at 10 years.[84] However, after 10 years, the rate of deterioration accelerated, with only 42% still functioning normally 15 years after implantation. Similar midterm results, with 85% of valves free from leaflet failure 8 years after implantation, were found using cryopreserved valves at another center.[85]

In another large series of homograft valve replacements, the actuarial survival rate at 12 years was 71% for cryopreserved valves and 62% for valves stored at 4°C.[57, 71, 74] Overall freedom from structural deterioration of the valve at 15 years was 80% ± 5% for cryopreserved and 45% ± 6% for other types of homografts.

The rate of freedom from thromboembolism was 95% at 10 years for isolated aortic homograft valve replacement, with or without concurrent coronary artery bypass grafting, but was only 81% for all homografts, including those with concurrent mitral or other valve surgery.[57, 71, 74] These data emphasize the importance of chronic anticoagulation in patients with bioprosthetic valves if they have other indications for anticoagulation. Endocarditis is rare in patients with homograft valves, with 94% ± 2% of cryopreserved homograft valves free of endocarditis at 15 years.[71, 74, 86]

Mitral Homografts

Recently, the use of mitral homograft valves has been proposed. The mitral homograft consists of the valve leaflets and annulus, chordae, and papillary muscle tips using harvesting and storage techniques similar to those described for aortic homografts. A partial or complete mitral valve replacement can be performed, resulting in excellent hemodynamics in carefully selected cases.[87–90] However, the surgical approach to mitral homograft implantation is complex and requires considerable technical expertise. Issues regarding patient selection and valve sizing have not been fully resolved. Given the known high survival rate and excellent long-term outcome associated with standard mitral valve repair or mechanical valve replacement, the use of mitral homografts will be restricted to a few academic centers until more convincing data regarding the safety and durability of this approach are available.[57]

Autografts
Hemodynamics

The use of the patient's own pulmonic valve to replace an abnormal aortic valve is called a *pulmonic autograft,* or the Ross procedure.[91–100] With this approach, the native pulmonic valve is harvested as a small cylinder consisting of the pulmonic valve, annulus, and proximal main pulmonary artery. The autograft most often is implanted into the aortic position as a complete root replacement with reimplantation of the coronaries, although subcoronary implantation and the inclusion root technique also have been described (Fig. 17–7).[101, 102] Many surgical groups consider that, like homografts, the risk of malinsertion is lowest with the root replacement technique.[40, 103, 104] The

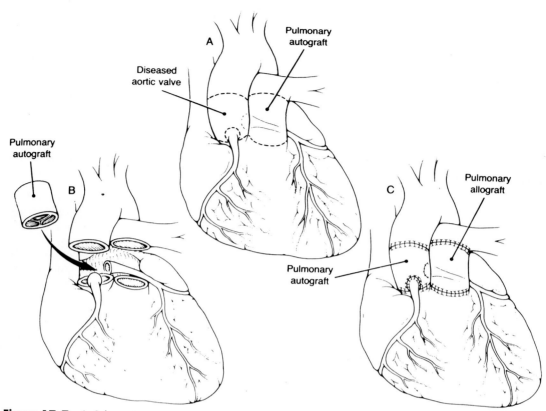

Figure 17·7 *A,* Schematic representation of pulmonic autograft valve replacement. The aortic valve and adjacent aorta are excised, leaving buttons of aortic tissue surrounding the coronary arteries. The pulmonary valve with the small rim of right ventricular muscle and the main pulmonary artery also is excised. *B,* The pulmonary autograft is sutured to the aortic annulus and to the distal aorta, and the coronary arteries are attached to openings in the pulmonary artery. *C,* A pulmonary root autograft is then sutured into the right ventricular outflow tract. (From Kouchoukos NT, D'avila Rom'an VG, Spray TL, Murphy SF, Perrillo JB: Replacement of the aortic root with a pulmonary autograft in children and young adults with aortic-valve disease. N Engl J Med 1994;330:1–6; reprinted by permission from the New England Journal of Medicine.)

pulmonic autograft approach is a double-valve procedure. Since the native pulmonic valve has been removed, this approach necessitates reconstruction of the right ventricular outflow tract using a pulmonary homograft conduit.

Advantages of the pulmonic autograft procedure include excellent hemodynamics, tissue viability, and resistance to infection.[105, 106] The pulmonic autograft is noiseless, nonthrombogenic, and has shown growth potential in children.[98, 107, 108] Even in adults, the size of the pulmonic autograft increased by about 20% after implantation, with most of the increase in size occurring early postoperatively.[109] Histologically, pulmonic autografts show normal valve architecture, with normal cellularity and collagen and elastic fiber orientation.[57]

Disadvantages of the pulmonic autograft procedure include the technical difficulties of harvesting the pulmonic valve. In addition, use of the pulmonic autograft usually is limited to children and young adults (typically <50 years of age, although it has been performed successfully in some older patients) because of changes with age in tissue quality, the relative size of the pulmonic annulus compared to the aortic annulus, and an increasing frequency of comorbid disease. Other concerns about the pulmonic autograft procedure include the need for two valve procedures instead of one, which prolongs the operation and increases the risk of prosthetic valve dysfunction. However, in a randomized trial of pulmonic autograft compared with aortic homograft valve replacement, outcome was similar at 6 months despite longer cardiopulmonary bypass and aortic crossclamp times with the pulmonic autograft procedure.[102]

When considering an individual patient for a pulmonic homograft, there is a relatively wide acceptable range for size matching of the pulmonic valve relative to the aortic annulus. However, the pulmonic autograft should be no smaller than 2 to 3 mm less than the aortic annulus diameter, and insertion is problematic when the aortic annulus is large (>29 mm). Some investigators suggest that when pulmonic to aortic size mismatch is present, surgical reduction of the aortic root may allow use of this procedure.[101]

Long-Term Outcome

In the early experience with pulmonic autografts, the hospital mortality rate was 7.4%, with reoperations occurring for endocarditis and technical reasons at this stage in the learning phase.[91] These explanted valves showed no evidence of leaflet calcification, thinning, or tears.[98] The current operative mortality rate is less than 1% for appropriately selected patients. In addition, the rate of freedom from valve-related death is 82% ± 6% at 14 years after surgery (Fig. 17–8).[110–112]

The major long-term problem with the pulmonic autograft procedure has been degeneration and failure of the right-sided homograft. About 15% to 29% of survivors have required reoperation within 20 years, most often for right-sided valve failure.[95, 110–114] More recent series suggest a lower rate of failure of the autograft or homograft, with a 5-year freedom from reoperation of 89% ± 3%.[115] Failure of the homograft in the pulmonic position

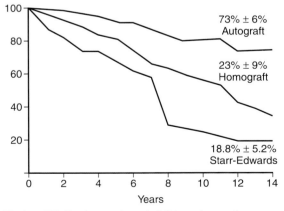

Figure 17·8 Actuarial probabilities of event-free survival after aortic valve replacement with pulmonary autografts in 202 patients compared with outcomes with aortic homografts and Starr-Edwards ball-cage valves. (From Robles A, Vaughan M, Lau JK, Bodnar E, Ross DN: Long-term assessment of aortic valve replacement with autologous pulmonary valve. Ann Thorac Surg 1985;39:238–242; reprinted with permission from the Society of Thoracic Surgeons.)

typically occurs late and is due to obstruction in the distal segment of the homograft conduit.[115] Early autograft failures (within 6 months of implantation) most often are caused by technical errors or persistent endocarditis, with late autograft failures related to aortic annulus dilation, endocarditis, or valve degeneration.

MECHANICAL VALVES

The three basic types of mechanical valve design are bileaflet, single-disk, and ball-cage valves. Each of these designs has specific advantages and disadvantages, and each has unique fluid dynamics and clinical flow characteristics. Most surgical groups use only one type of mechanical valve in all patients, allowing increased surgical expertise and increased awareness of potential complications and long-term outcome for that specific valve type. However, this pattern of clinical use makes direct comparisons between valve types problematic, as it is difficult to separate patient population or institutional differences from differences in valve performance. This problem has been partially alleviated by the development of standards for reporting outcome after valve surgery.[116]

Bileaflet Valves

Available bileaflet valves include the St. Jude Medical and CarboMedics valves. These valves consist of two pyrolytic carbon semicircular disks attached to a rigid valve ring by small hinges. The opening angle of the leaflets relative to the annulus plane is 75 to 90 degrees, with the open valve consisting of three orifices—a small, slitlike central orifice between the two open leaflets and two larger semicircular orifices laterally. Turbulent stresses are most prominent in the leaflet wakes and in the shear layers alongside the three antegrade flow fields (Fig. 17–9).[16]

The hemodynamics of bileaflet valves tend to be better than tilting-disk valves, with a performance index of 0.4 to 0.71, depending on valve size. The average peak velocity is 3.0 ± 0.8 m/s in the aortic position and 1.6 ± 0.3 m/s in the mitral position,[15, 17] although even higher velocities may be recorded in some cases due to the fluid dynamics of the central slitlike orifice.[117] Effective orifice areas, calculated with the continuity equation, range from 0.7 cm^2 for a 19-mm valve to 4.2 cm^2 for a 31-mm valve.[118]

When implanted in the aortic position, there is no clear advantage to a specific orien-

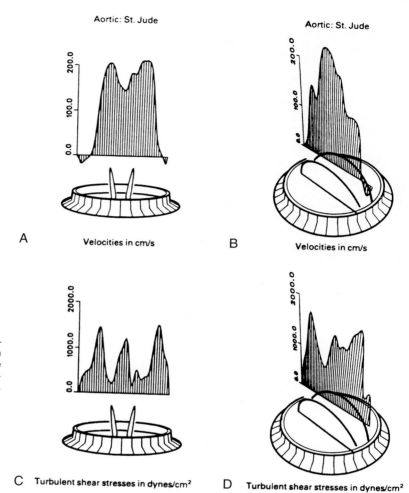

Figure 17·9 Velocity and turbulent shear stress profiles 13 mm downstream of a 27-mm St. Jude Medical bileaflet valve at peak systole. *A and C,* Center line profiles through lateral and central orifices. *B and D,* Profile through the central orifice only. (From Yoganathan AP, Heinrich RS, Fontaine AA: Fluid dynamics of prosthetic valves. *In* Otto CM, ed. The Practice of Clinical Echocardiography. Philadelphia: WB Saunders, 1997:788.)

tation of the leaflet opening plane relative to the aortic root. For the mitral position, some evidence suggests that an orientation perpendicular to the normal plane of mitral valve opening may be optimal, although these findings are not definitive.[16, 119]

Bileaflet valves typically have a small amount (5 to 10 mL/beat) of normal regurgitation. On color flow imaging, two converging jets originating from the pivot points of the valve disks and a smaller central jet often are seen.[120–122] Smaller jets around the closure rim of the leaflets also may be appreciated (Fig. 17–10; see also color insert). This degree of normal regurgitation is designed in part to decrease the risk of valve thrombosis by the increased blood flow motion.

Tilting-Disk Valves

With a tilting-disk valve, a single circular disk rotates within a rigid annulus, with the disk secured by lateral or central metal struts. Available valves include the Medtronic-Hall, Bjork-Shiley, and Omniscience valves, with some older valve designs no longer available because of uneven wear of a nonmetallic disk[123, 124] or strut fracture.[125] The opening angle of the disk relative to the valve annulus ranges from 60 to 80 degrees, resulting in two orifices for antegrade flow. The major orifice is semicircular in cross section, with a typical antegrade velocity of about 2 m/s. Flow though the minor orifice consists of two jets separated by a well-defined wake behind the tilted disk but with a velocity in the minor orifice similar to the major orifice (Fig. 17–11). The wake regions downstream from tilting-disk valves are areas of flow separation and stagnation. In addition, high downstream turbulent stresses reach a magnitude that is associated with platelet activation and red cell hemolysis.[16]

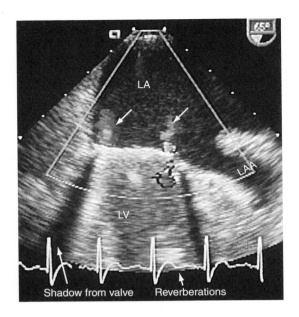

Shadow from valve   Reverberations

Figure 17·10 The transesophageal echocardiographic image of a St. Jude mitral valve shows the normal small regurgitant jets at valve closure. Notice the prominent reverberations *(arrows)* distal to the valve, obscuring evaluation of structures in the far field of the image. LA, left atrium; LAA, left atrial appendage; LV, left ventricle. (This figure also occurs in the color insert.)

Aortic: Medtronic-Hall

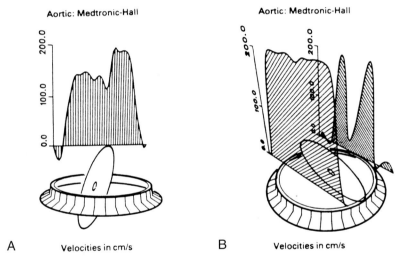

A   Velocities in cm/s

B   Velocities in cm/s

Figure 17·11 Velocity and turbulent shear stress profiles downstream of a 27-mm Medtronic-Hall tilting-disk valve at peak systole. *A and C*, Center line profiles 15 mm downstream across the major and minor orifices. *B and D*, Profile through the major and minor orifices at 13 mm downstream. (From Yoganathan AP, Heinrich RS, Fontaine AA: Fluid dynamics of prosthetic valves. *In* Otto CM, ed. The Practice of Clinical Echocardiography. Philadelphia: WB Saunders, 1997:783.)

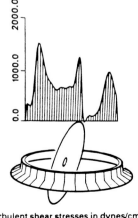

C Turbulent shear stresses in dynes/cm²

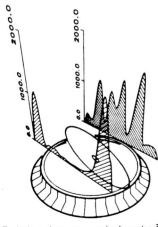

D Turbulent shear stresses in dynes/cm²

The nonperpendicular opening angle of tilting-disk valves is associated with slight resistance to antegrade flow, with typical pressure gradients of 5 to 25 mm Hg in the aortic position and 5 to 10 mm Hg in the mitral position.[15] Effective valve areas range from 1.6 to 3.7 cm^2, with a performance index ranging from 0.40 to 0.65.[16] In the mitral position, the pattern of left ventricular inflow mimics normal physiology most closely if the tilting-disk valve is oriented with the major orifice directed toward the left ventricular free wall.[126]

Tilting-disk valves have a small amount of normal regurgitation (5 to 9 mL/beat), with regurgitation originating from small gaps around the perimeter of the valve.[127, 128] Flow around the central strut also occurs with that specific valve design.[120] Even this normal pattern of regurgitation is associated with high turbulent stresses.

Ball-Cage Valves

The only ball-cage valve in use is the Starr-Edwards 1260, which consists of a Silastic ball with a circular sewing ring and a cage formed by three metal arches located at 120-degree intervals around the sewing ring. Antegrade blood flow occurs around the ball with a typical velocity of 2 m/s.[129] The ball in the center of the flow stream generates a large wake with flow separation and areas of flow reversal (Fig. 17–12).[130] In addition, turbulent and shear stresses reach levels associated with damage to the endothelium and blood cells, factors that contribute to the high thrombogenicity of this valve.[16] The hemodynamic performance of the ball-cage valve is poor, with higher pressure gradients and a lower performance index compared with bileaflet or tilting-disk valves. As the ball seats in the sewing ring during valve closure, a small amount (2 to 5 mL/beat) of low-velocity backflow occurs,[16] which can be visualized on color flow Doppler imaging.

Long-Term Outcome With Mechanical Valves

Currently available mechanical valves are extremely durable (Figs. 17–13 and 17–14). Overall actuarial survival rates range from 94% ± 2% at 10 years for the St. Jude Medical bileaflet valve to 85% ± 3% at 9 years for the Omnicarbon valve and 60% to 70% at 10 years for the Starr-Edwards valve (Table 17–4).[131–135] Of course, survival depends on factors other than valve function, including the underlying disease process, the patient's age, and comorbid conditions. Structural abnormalities of mechanical valves are rare, and when valve dysfunction occurs, it invariably is due to a paravalvular leak, endocarditis, or thrombosis. Since structural failures of mechanical valves have occurred in the past, any new valve design must be rigorously tested before clinical use.[123–125]

Chronic anticoagulation is required with all mechanical valves to prevent valve dysfunction

Aortic: Starr-Edwards

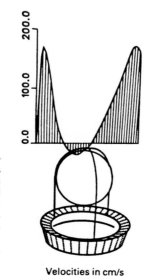

Velocities in cm/s

Figure 17·12 Center line velocity and turbulent shear stress profiles 30 mm downstream of a 27-mm Starr-Edwards ball and cage valve at peak systole. (From Yoganathan AP, Heinrich RS, Fontaine AA: Fluid dynamics of prosthetic valves. *In* Otto CM, ed. The Practice of Clinical Echocardiography. Philadelphia: WB Saunders, 1997:790.)

Aortic: Starr-Edwards

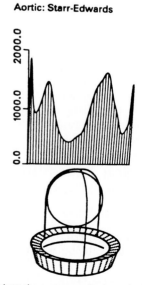

Turbulent shear stresses in dynes/cm^2

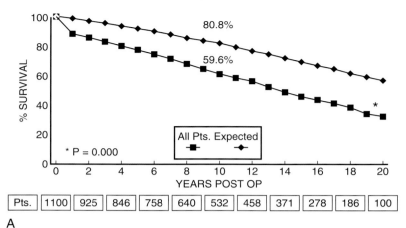

A

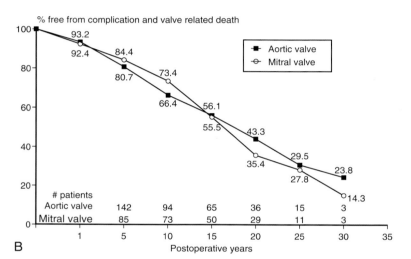

B

Figure 17·13 *A,* Actuarial survival of 1100 patients with Starr-Edwards aortic valve replacements compared with expected survival for an age- and sex-matched population. (From Orszulak TA, Schaff HV, Puga FJ, et al: Event status of the Starr-Edwards aortic valve to 20 years: a benchmark for comparison. Ann Thorac Surg 1997; 63:620–626; reprinted with permission from the Society of Thoracic Surgeons.) *B,* Freedom from all valve-related complications, including valve-related causes of death after aortic and mitral valve replacements in 415 patients with Starr-Edwards prosthetic valves. (From Gödje OL, Fischlein T, Adelhard K, Nollert G, Klinner W, Reichart B: Thirty-year results of Starr-Edwards prostheses in the aortic and mitral position. Ann Thorac Surg 1997;63:613–619; reprinted with permission from the Society of Thoracic Surgeons.)

and thromboembolic events (Table 17–5). Even with appropriate anticoagulation, the rate of thromboembolism is 0.6% to 1.8% per patient-year for bileaflet valves.[131–133] Ball-cage valves have a rate of freedom from thromboembolism of 91% at 5 years.[134, 135] With current dose ranges and monitoring of warfarin therapy, bleeding complications are rare, occurring at a rate of 0.8% to 1.2% per patient-year.[131–133]

MEDICAL MANAGEMENT OF THE PATIENT WITH A PROSTHETIC VALVE

Choice of Valve

In a patient undergoing surgical intervention for valvular heart disease, the type of prosthetic valve chosen for implantation depends on several clinical factors (see Table 17–5). A repair procedure that preserves the patient's native valve while restoring valve function is preferable to implantation of a prosthetic valve. The major considerations in choosing a bioprosthesis or a mechanical valve are the expected durability of the valve and the risks of anticoagulation (Fig. 17–15).

Since there currently are no valve prostheses that have permanent durability without the need for anticoagulation, there often are substantial tradeoffs between these two considerations in each patient. Some decisions are relatively straightforward. For example, in an elderly patient who is a poor candidate for long-term anticoagulation, a bioprosthetic valve may be used if the average durability of the valve exceeds the patient's expected longevity. However, even in the elderly patient, a mechanical valve often is needed given the increased longevity of the U.S. population. Life tables giving the expected additional years of life after a patient has reached her or his

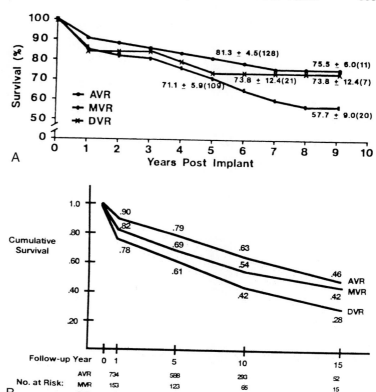

Figure 17·14 *A,* Actuarial survival curves for 1298 patients receiving St. Jude Medical prosthetic valves. (From Arom KV, Nicoloff DM, Kersten TE, Northrup WF III, Lindsay WG, Emergy RW: Ten years' experience with the St. Jude Medical valve prosthesis. Ann Thorac Surg 1989;47:831–837; reprinted with permission from the Society of Thoracic Surgeons.) *B,* Actuarial survival curves for 1104 patients receiving aortic valve replacement (AVR), mitral valve replacement (MVR), or double-valve replacement (DVR) with a Medtronic-Hall valve prosthesis. (From Nitter-Hauge S, Abdelnoor M, Svennevig JL: Fifteen-year experience with the Medtronic-Hall valve prosthesis: a follow-up study of 1104 consecutive patients. Circulation 1996;94(suppl II):105–108; by permission of The American Heart Association.)

current age should be consulted before choosing a specific valve type (Table 17–6). In a younger patient with an expected lifespan longer than the durability of a bioprosthetic valve and no contraindications to chronic anticoagulation, a mechanical valve is most appropriate if a valve-sparing procedure is not possible.

In other cases, the optimal choice of valve is less clear. For example, a young woman desiring a subsequent pregnancy may wish to avoid warfarin anticoagulation, even though the limited durability of a porcine bioprosthetic valve will require reoperation after several years. For these patients, newer approaches such as the pulmonic autograft procedure should be considered. Another difficult decision is the young, physically active adult who wishes to avoid the inconvenience and risk of anticoagulation. For these patients, decision making should include a discussion with the patient of the known durability of a mechanical valve compared with the more limited data on the long-term outcome with the pulmonic autograft procedure. Implantation of a porcine valve should be avoided given the likelihood of poor durability, unless there

are definite contraindications to anticoagulation.

In addition to durability and anticoagulation, other factors that influence the choice of valve type include the expected hemodynamics for a specific valve size, anatomic considerations at the time of surgery, patient preferences and lifestyle, and comorbid diseases that may affect longevity or the risk of anticoagulation.

The specific choice of which porcine valve or which mechanical valve to use depends on an assessment of the hemodynamics and ease of surgical implantation for each valve. Most cardiac surgical centers choose one type of valve in each category (porcine and mechanical), rather than using different valves in each patient. Thus, each cardiac center develops expertise in the implantation and follow-up evaluation of that specific valve type.

Anticoagulation

The basic approach to anticoagulation in patients with prosthetic valves is discussed in Chapter 6. Continuous, effective anticoagulation is essential in patients with mechanical

TABLE 17·4 LONG-TERM OUTCOME AFTER MECHANICAL VALVE REPLACEMENT

Valve Types	Years Implanted	Number of Patients	Mean Age (y)	Outcome	Thromboembolism	Hemorrhage	Endocarditis	Valve Thrombosis	Reference
					Complications (%/Patient-Year)				
Bileaflet				Event-free survival					
St. Jude	1977–87	1298	62 ± 13	67 ± 8% at 9 y	1.5%	0.56%	0.16%	0.09%	279
St. Jude	1978–91	91	39 (range, 15–50)	94 ± 2% at 10 y	0.6%	0.8%	0.4%		133
Omnicarbon	1984–92	292	58	85 ± 3% at 9 y	0.7%	0.8%	0.6%		131
Tilting disk				Actuarial survival					
Medtronic-Hall	1977–87	1104	56	AVR 46 ± 2% at 15 y	1.8%	1.2%		0.05%	132
				MVR 42 ± 4% at 15 y	1.9%			0.19%	
				DVR 28 ± 5% at 15 y	1.9%			0.13%	
Ball-Cage				Event-free survival					
Starr-Edwards	1963–77	362	40 ± 10	AVR 66.4% at 10 y	1.36% (AVR)	1.06%			134
				MVR 73.4%	1.25% (MVR)	0.56%			
Starr-Edwards	1969–91	1100	57	Survival	1.26%	0.18%	0.39%	0.02%	135
				59.6% at 10 y					
				31.2% at 20 y					

AVR, aortic valve replacement; MVR, mitral valve replacement; DVR, double valve replacement.

TABLE 17·5 MEDICAL MANAGEMENT AFTER VALVE SURGERY

Chronic anticoagulation
   Maintain optimal international normalized ratio
   Avoid drug interactions
Prevention of endocarditis
Annual cardiac physical examination
Periodic echocardiographic monitoring

TABLE 17·6 AVERAGE REMAINING LIFETIME AT ANY GIVEN AGE

	Life Expectancy (y)		
Age	*Total Population*	*Men*	*Women*
20–25	56.7	53.5	59.8
25–30	52.0	48.9	55.0
30–35	47.3	44.3	50.1
35–40	42.7	39.8	45.4
40–45	38.1	35.4	40.6
45–50	33.6	31.0	35.9
50–55	29.2	26.7	31.4
55–60	24.9	22.6	27.0
60–65	20.9	18.8	22.8
65–70	17.3	15.3	18.9
70–75	14.0	12.2	15.3
75–80	10.9	9.5	11.9
80–85	8.3	7.1	8.9
≥85	6.0	5.2	6.4

From LEWK93: Abridged Life Tables, United States, 1993. National Center for Health Statistics.

valves. The marked improvements in our ability to closely regulate the therapeutic effect and to avoid complications result from the increased use of the international normalized ratio (INR) and dedicated pharmacist-managed anticoagulation clinics.

Appropriate anticoagulation is particularly important in the perioperative period in patients with mechanical valves undergoing noncardiac surgery. Meticulous management of anticoagulation during pregnancy is necessary to avoid thromboembolic or hemorrhagic complications and to avoid the potential teratogenic effects of warfarin (see Chapter 6).

Prevention of Endocarditis

Appropriate antibiotic prophylaxis for prevention of bacterial endocarditis is essential in patients with prosthetic valves (see Chapter 6). Although the likelihood of endocarditis appears to be lower with homografts and autografts than with other types of prosthetic valves, it still is prudent to recommend endocarditis prophylaxis for these patients, as a

small degree of valvular regurgitation often is present.

Monitoring Valve Function

Periodic evaluation of valve function is recommended in all patients with prosthetic valves to detect early evidence of dysfunction or valve degeneration. The basic modality for periodic follow-up is clinical history and physical examination at no longer than annual intervals.

Most clinicians also perform sequential echocardiography. The appropriate frequency

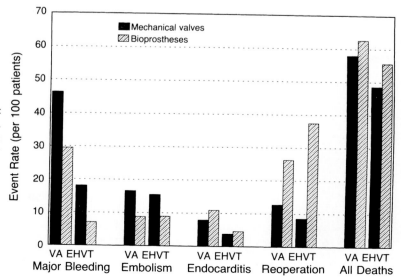

Figure 17·15 A comparison of event rates at 12 years in the Veterans Affairs Cooperative Study on valvular heart disease (VA) and the Edinburgh Heart Valve Trial (EHVT). (From Hammermeister KE, Sethi GK, Henderson WG, Oprian C, Kim T, Rahimtoola S: A comparison of outcomes in men 11 years after heart valve replacement with a mechanical valve or bioprosthesis. N Engl J Med 1993;328:1289–1296; reprinted by permission from the New England Journal of Medicine.)

of echocardiographic examination varies with the type of valve, duration of implantation, and other clinical factors. In general, a baseline echocardiogram is obtained early (within 3 to 4 months) after implantation to serve as the patient's baseline. If there is no clinical or echocardiographic evidence of valve dysfunction, repeat examinations at 2- to 3-year intervals are appropriate, with the frequency of examination increased for older bioprosthetic valves. Because many patients with prosthetic valves have other residual valve lesions, more frequent evaluation may be needed for other indications.

Transesophageal echocardiography has an important role in the evaluation of patients with suspected prosthetic valve dysfunction. Particularly for mechanical valves in the mitral position, transthoracic imaging may be unreliable due to shadowing and reverberations from the valve prosthesis, obscuring the left atrium. However, transesophageal imaging is not a routine procedure and typically is performed only if prosthetic valve dysfunction is suspected based on clinical symptoms, physical examination findings, or abnormalities detected on transthoracic imaging.

Other methods for evaluating prosthetic valve function include fluoroscopic assessment of disk motion, invasive measurement of intracardiac pressures, and left ventricular or aortic root angiography. These approaches are reserved for clinical situations for which noninvasive data are not diagnostic.

Physical Examination

The findings on cardiac auscultation vary with the type of valve prosthesis (Fig. 17–16). Bioprosthetic valves have very soft opening and closing sounds with no distinct valve clicks heard on auscultation, although an ejection type murmur is common with stented porcine valves in the aortic positions.[136]

Bileaflet mechanical valves open silently but have an audible closing click as the disks seat in the valve ring. Tilting-disk valves may have an audible opening, as well as closing sound, due to the disk contacting the restraining strut(s). Ball-cage valves often have multiple sounds during valve opening as the ball moves along the stented cage and also have distinct opening and closing clicks. A systolic ejection murmur is common with all types of mechanical valves in the aortic position. The normal degree of mitral regurgitation seen with mechanical valves rarely is audible on auscultation.

Type of Valve	Aortic Prosthesis		Mitral Prosthesis	
	Normal Findings	Abnormal Findings	Normal Findings	Abnormal Findings
Caged-Ball (Starr–Edwards)	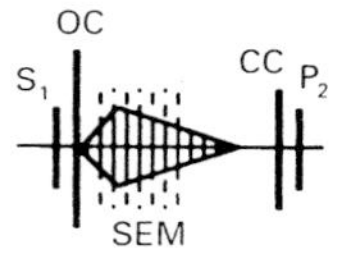 *(schematic)*	Aortic diastolic murmur Decreased intensity of opening or closing click	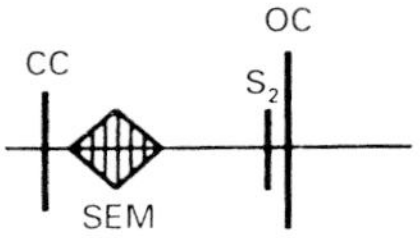 *(schematic)*	Low-frequency apical diastolic murmur High-frequency holosystolic murmur
Single-Tilting-Disk (Bjork–Shiley or Medtronic–Hall)	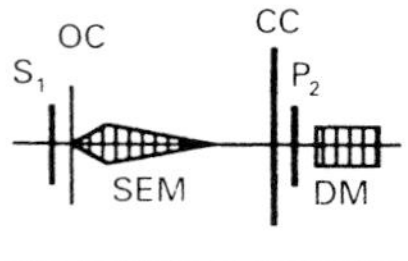 *(schematic)*	Decreased intensity of closing click	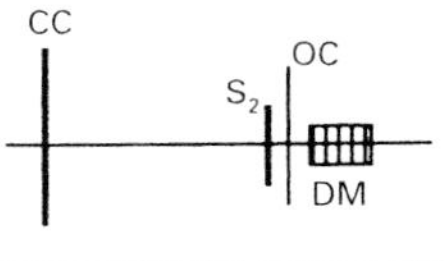 *(schematic)*	High-frequency holosystolic murmur Decreased intensity of closing click
Bileaflet-Tilting-Disk (St. Jude Medical)	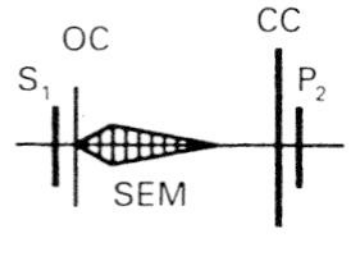 *(schematic)*	Aortic diastolic murmur Decreased intensity of closing click	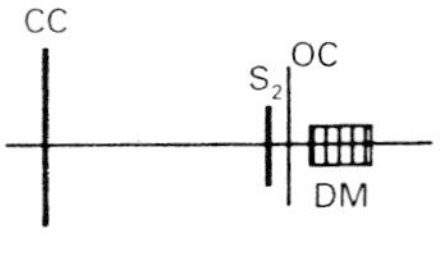 *(schematic)*	High-frequency holosystolic murmur Decreased intensity of closing click
Heterograft Bioprosthesis (Hancock or Carpentier–Edwards)	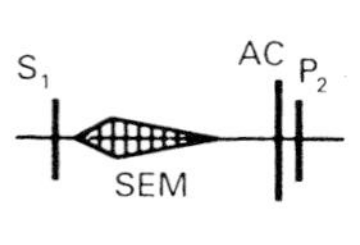 *(schematic)*	Aortic diastolic murmur	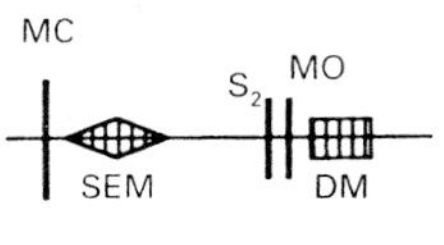 *(schematic)*	High-frequency holosystolic murmur

Figure 17·16 Auscultatory characteristics of various prosthetic valves in the aortic and mitral positions, with schematic diagrams of normal findings and descriptions of abnormal findings. (From Vongpatanasin W, Hillis LD, Lange RA: Prosthetic heart valves. N Engl J Med 1996;335:407; reprinted by permission from the New England Journal of Medicine.)

The presence of an aortic diastolic murmur or a loud systolic murmur is abnormal and suggests prosthetic valve dysfunction with both bioprostheses and mechanical valves. With mechanical valves, muffling of the valve clicks raises the possibility of valve thrombosis or pannus formation. It is important to follow the physical examination sequentially, using each patient's baseline as the reference standard, as a change in physical examination findings raises the possibility of valve dysfunction. A baseline physical examination is particularly important for patients with coexisting valve lesions to distinguish other native valve lesions from prosthetic valve dysfunction.

Echocardiography

Echocardiographic evaluation of prosthetic valves is based on the same principles used for evaluation of native valves, with some important caveats.[15, 137] First, imaging of prosthetic valves is limited by reverberations and shadowing from the metallic components of the valve. Second, the specific fluid dynamics of each type of valve prosthesis are reflected in the Doppler echocardiographic findings. In addition, compared with native valves, the phenomenon of pressure recovery distal to the valve is more prominent with prosthetic valves, particularly with bileaflet mechanical valves.

A complete echocardiographic examination includes two-dimensional (2D) imaging of the prosthetic valve, calculation of the transvalvular pressure gradient and valve area, estimation of the degree of regurgitation, evaluation of left ventricular size and systolic function, and calculation of pulmonary artery systolic pressure. Evaluation of any other coexisting valve disease also is performed during a complete examination. Comparison of the current study with the baseline performed soon after valve implantation is especially helpful.

Echocardiographic imaging of stented bioprosthetic valves is limited by reverberations and shadowing by the rigid stents and sewing ring. However, with good-quality transthoracic images, the valve leaflets can be identified with an appearance similar to the leaflets of the native aortic valve. When transthoracic images are suboptimal, the transesophageal approach can provide improved image quality. When high-quality images are obtained, leaflet thickening and calcification due to valve degeneration and valvular vegetations due to endocarditis can be detected.

Stentless bioprosthetic valves, homografts, and autografts look nearly identical to the native aortic valve on 2D imaging (Fig. 17–17). A slight degree of increased thickness and echogenicity may be seen in the aortic annulus region in the early postoperative period, and

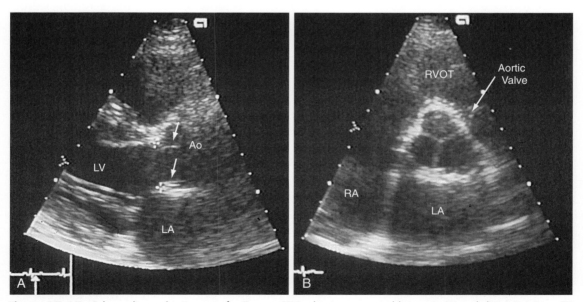

Figure 17·17 Echocardiographic images of a Toronto SPV valve in parasternal long-axis *(A)* and short-axis views *(B)*. Notice the thin leaflets in systole *(arrows)* and the slight increase in echogenicity in the aortic annulus region in the long-axis view and the normal trileaflet appearance of the valve in the short-axis view. Ao, aorta; LA, left atrium; LVOT, left ventricular outflow tract; RA, right atrium; LV, left ventricle.

the increased thickness due to the combined native and prosthetic aorta can be visualized when the intraluminal cylinder approach is used. For aortic root replacement with reimplantation of the coronary arteries, attention should be directed toward imaging the anastomotic sites.

Mechanical valves are difficult to evaluate on 2D transthoracic imaging due to marked reverberations obscuring motion of the disk or ball. However, on multiplane transesophageal imaging, clear views of disk motion can be obtained, allowing recognition of impaired motion caused by pannus or thrombus formation (Fig. 17–18). Transesophageal imaging also is needed if valve thrombosis is suspected as a source of cardiac embolus, since thrombus most often is located on the left atrial side of the mitral sewing ring. Of note, the absence of detectable thrombus by echocardiography does not exclude the valve as a possible embolic source, because the thrombus may be too small for visualization, obscured by technical artifacts, or absent due to recent embolization. In general, given the known risk of systemic embolism with mechanical valves, excluding the valve as a source of embolism is problematic.

Prosthetic valve gradients are calculated based on the antegrade velocity curve using the Bernoulli equation. Numerous studies have shown a close correlation between Doppler and catheterization gradients for most types of valve prostheses.[138–141] Mean gradient calculations are more useful clinically than maximum gradients, as prosthetic valves often have a relatively high maximum instantaneous gradient (and velocity), despite a normal mean gradient, due to a high pressure gradient at the time of valve opening with rapid equilibration of pressures later in the cardiac cycle. For aortic prostheses, this results in an early peaking velocity curve with a more triangular shape than for native aortic stenosis. The proximal velocity should be considered in the evaluation of prosthetic aortic valves to avoid overestimation of the transvalvular pressure gradient.[142] For mitral prostheses, a high opening velocity is followed by rapid deceleration and a short pressure half-time.

Another important factor in Doppler evaluation of prosthetic valve gradients is the phenomenon of pressure recovery. *Pressure recovery* refers to the difference between the pressure immediately distal to a stenotic orifice and the pressure farther downstream. As flow decelerates, pressure gradually rises from its lowest value immediately adjacent to the orifice to a much higher pressure (often close to the prestenotic pressure) at some point downstream. Although this phenomenon is of relatively low magnitude for native valve stenosis, with little impact on the correlation between Doppler and catheter gradients, pressure recovery is more dramatic with prosthetic valves, especially the bileaflet and ball-cage mechanical valves. Thus, the pressure gradient measured across an aortic bileaflet valve is higher if left ventricular pressure is compared with aortic pressure immediately adjacent to the prosthesis compared with more distally in the aorta.[143, 144]

Pressure recovery with bileaflet valves is confounded by the additional effect of local acceleration changes in the slitlike central orifice, resulting in a high localized pressure gradient (and Doppler velocity) compared with the overall pressure gradient across the valve. Therefore, Doppler velocities often appear to overestimate the transvalvular gradient, since the Doppler velocity data reflect the highest pressure drop in the central orifice rather than the overall pressure drop across the valve. In practical terms, overdiagnosis of prosthetic valve stenosis is avoided by using tables of expected velocities for prosthetic valves and obtaining a baseline examination soon after valve replacement to be used as the reference stan-

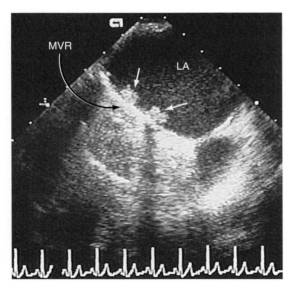

Figure 17·18 This transesophageal echocardiographic image shows pannus or thrombus formation *(arrows)* on the left atrial side of a St. Jude mitral valve replacement (MVR). LA, left atrium.

dard for future Doppler examinations in each patient.

Prosthetic valve areas can be calculated using the continuity equation for aortic and mitral valve prostheses and the pressure half-time method for mitral valve prostheses. Continuity equation valve areas have been compared with invasively obtained data for bioprosthetic[145–147] and mechanical valves.[117, 118] Although it is more accurate to use the measured left ventricular outflow tract diameter in the continuity equation, the known diameter of the sewing ring can be used to obtain an approximation of valve area if image quality is suboptimal. Another method for evaluation of the degree of prosthetic stenosis in the aortic position is the ratio of maximum velocity in the outflow tract to the maximum transvalvular velocity. This ratio eliminates the need for a 2D diameter measurement and, in effect, is already indexed for body size as the normal increase (or "step-up") in velocity across the valve is close to 1, regardless of body size. As the degree of obstruction increases, the velocity ratio decreases, with a ratio of less than 0.25 indicating significant stenosis.[118]

Prosthetic mitral valve areas also can be calculated with the continuity equation using the left ventricular outflow stroke volume and the transmitral flow velocity curve.[146] If the patient has mitral regurgitation, continuity equation valve areas underestimate valve area, as transmitral flow exceeds forward cardiac output. The pressure half-time method also can be used to evaluate prosthetic mitral valve area. For valves with a central flow pattern, such as porcine valves, the constant 220 (used for native valves) can be used to derive functional valve area.[148] For mitral prostheses with more complex fluid dynamics, it remains controversial whether the use of 220 as the constant provides an accurate estimate of valve area. Many clinicians instead report the pressure half-time itself, using evidence of an increased half-time compared with the baseline study as evidence of prosthetic valve stenosis.[138]

The normal degrees and patterns of regurgitation described for each type of prosthetic valve can be detected using color Doppler flow imaging. An awareness of the normal regurgitant flow patterns is needed to avoid misinterpretation of the color flow images.[117, 149] Pathologic valvular regurgitation also can be detected and quantitated using the same approaches as described for native valve regurgitation in Chapter 3 (Fig. 17–19; see also color insert).[150–152] However, because of shadowing of the left atrium by the prosthetic valve from a transthoracic approach, transesophageal imaging is essential when pathologic regurgi-

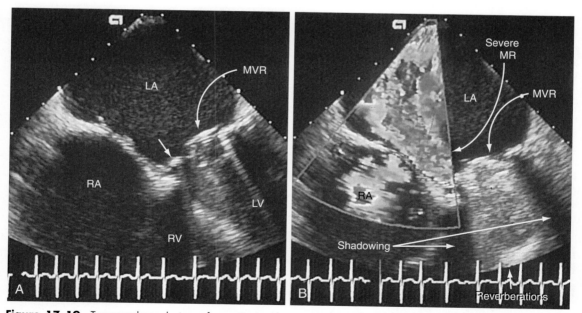

Figure 17·19   Transesophageal view of a patient with suspected prosthetic mitral valve regurgitation. *A,* The two-dimensional image *(A)* showed an area of abnormal motion on real-time imaging at the medial aspect of the sewing ring *(arrow).* *B,* Color flow imaging documented severe paraprosthetic mitral regurgitation (MR) with a large color flow jet filling the entire enlarged left atrium and with systolic flow reversal in the pulmonary veins. LA, left atrium; LV, left ventricle; RA, right atrium; LV, left ventricle; MVR, mitral valve replacement. (Illustration *B* also occurs in the color insert.)

tation of a prosthetic mitral valve is suspected.[153–155] Transesophageal imaging is less valuable for evaluation of prosthetic aortic valve regurgitation.

The cause of prosthetic regurgitation (valvular or paravalvular) often can be deduced from the color flow images. Identification of the location of the proximal flow convergence region is particularly helpful in locating the site of prosthetic regurgitation. The proximal isovelocity approach also may be helpful for quantitation of regurgitant severity.[156]

The examiner must look carefully on the transthoracic echocardiographic study for indirect signs of prosthetic regurgitation, such as persistently elevated pulmonary pressures, a hyperdynamic left ventricle, or an increased antegrade transmitral velocity, reflecting the increased antegrade volume flow rate across the valve. The intensity of the continuous wave Doppler signal compared with antegrade flow also provides a guide to regurgitant severity.[157]

Other Diagnostic Tests

Although the type of prosthetic valve usually is known based on operative records and the patient's valve identification card, the chest radiograph can be used to identify the valve type when an accurate history is unavailable. Fluoroscopy can be used to evaluate the motion of the valve occluder.

Some investigators have suggested that exercise echocardiography may be helpful in evaluating suspected prosthetic valve dysfunction. With the increase in transvalvular flow rate during exercise, corresponding increases in the transvalvular pressure gradient are seen, even with normal valve function. Typically, the aortic gradient increases by 70% (from 15 to 20 or 25 mm Hg), and the mitral gradient increases by over 100% (from 4 to 8 mm Hg).[141, 158–160] Increases in excess of these values or an abnormal increase in pulmonary pressures with exercise raises the possibility of prosthetic valve dysfunction.

EVALUATION AND TREATMENT OF PROSTHETIC VALVE DYSFUNCTION

Primary Structural Failure

Mechanical failure of modern prosthetic valves is rare, although mechanical valve failure has been a limitation of some valve designs in the past, emphasizing the need for rigorous evaluation and testing of all new valve models

(Table 17–7). Examples of mechanical failure in the past that occurred with specific valve models that are no longer used include ball variance in certain models of Starr-Edwards valves, leading to regurgitation or stenosis[161, 162]; uneven wearing of the single disk in the Beall valve, which could lead to regurgitation or disk escape[123, 124, 163]; disk embolization from bileaflet tilting-disk valves; and strut fracture with certain models of single- and double-disk valves.[125, 164]

Structural failure of mechanical valves more often is related to the interface between the valve ring and the native cardiac tissue or to thrombus formation interfering with normal valve motion.[165] Dehiscence of some of the sutures attaching the sewing ring to the annulus probably is the most common cause of mechanical valve dysfunction.[166] Paravalvular regurgitation may occur even with intact sutures soon after implantation due to fibrosis and calcification causing inadequate contact between the sewing ring and annulus. Over time, suture integrity may be disrupted by friction against a calcified annulus or by superimposed infection (see Fig. 17–19). Mechanical valve dysfunction occurs less commonly due to thrombus or tissue overgrowth (eg, pannus) at the annulus that blocks normal opening or

TABLE 17·7   PROSTHETIC VALVE DYSFUNCTION

Primary structural failure
   Mechanical valves
      Paravalvular regurgitation
      Valve dehiscence
      Tissue ingrowth (pannus formation)
      Thrombosis
   Tissue valves
      Tissue degeneration
      Secondary calcification
      Paravalvular regurgitation
Endocarditis
   Vegetations
   Paravalvular abscess
Prosthetic valve stenosis
   Valve thrombosis or pannus (mechanical valves)
   Calcification or pannus (tissue valve)
Prosthetic valve regurgitation
   Paravalvular
   Transvalvular
Thromboembolic complications
   Systemic emboli
   Valve thrombosis
   Spontaneous contrast ("microthrombi")
Hemolytic anemia
Pseudoaneurysm formation
   Aortic root
   Left ventricular
   Mitral-aortic intervalvular fibrosa

closing of the valve disk, resulting either in stenosis or regurgitation. Even small amounts of thrombus formation at the hinges of a tilting-disk valve may impair normal valve function.

Structural failure of tissue valves often is caused by calcification, perforation, or spontaneous tissue degeneration of the valve leaflets, although paravalvular regurgitation also may occur. The overall incidence of bioprosthesis failure is 20% to 30% at 10 years[18, 29, 167] and more than 50% at 15 years. However, the likelihood of primary tissue failure decreases with age, and 90% of elderly patients (>70 years) have not required reoperation 12 to 15 years after valve implantation.[30, 168]

Endocarditis

Implanted prosthetic valves are at higher risk for endocarditis compared with native valves due to the presence of foreign material in combination with abnormal flow patterns. Even with appropriate antibiotic prophylaxis, the estimated risk of prosthetic valve endocarditis is 0.5% per year.[131, 133, 167, 169] Prosthetic valve endocarditis occurring within 2 months of valve implantation is classified as early endocarditis and most often is caused by *Staphylococcus epidermidis*, gram-negative bacteria, or fungi. Endocarditis occurring later after valve implantation has a bacteriologic spectrum similar to that of native valve endocarditis (see Chapter 18).

In patients with endocarditis, the presence of a prosthetic valve is a major risk factor for death.[170] Particularly with mechanical valves, infection typically involves the valve sewing ring and often is associated with conduction abnormalities or paravalvular regurgitation. Development of a paravalvular abscess or fistula formation, resulting from rupture of the abscess into adjacent cardiac chambers, denotes a poor prognosis.[171, 172] Most patients with prosthetic valve endocarditis require surgical intervention for eradication of the infection, with re-replacement of the affected valve.

Accurate diagnosis of prosthetic valve endocarditis depends on transesophageal as well as transthoracic echocardiographic imaging.[173-176] With mechanical valve prostheses, it is rare to visualize vegetations on the disks themselves. A paravalvular abscess is recognized as an echolucent, irregularly shaped area adjacent to the valve sewing ring.[155, 170, 173, 177-180] In some cases, flow into and out of the abscess can be seen on color flow imaging. Rarely, an intracardiac abscess is echo dense, making diagnosis difficult unless the abnormal region of increased thickening adjacent to the valve is recognized. Distinguishing normal postoperative changes and anatomic variants from a pathologic process is facilitated by comparison of the echocardiographic study with a baseline study performed soon after valve implantation.

Prosthetic Valve Stenosis

Prosthetic valve stenosis is most often encountered with bioprosthetic valves that have been implanted for several years. The degree of bioprosthetic valve calcification increases noticeably after 6 years of implantation.[181-185] However, the time interval from valve implantation to significant stenosis is extremely variable. Factors that tend to increase the rate of calcification include younger age, pregnancy, mitral valve position, chronic renal failure, and hypercalcemia.[18, 186-189]

Stenosis of a mechanical prosthesis can occur due to restriction of disk motion by thrombus or pannus formation or due to a restricted annular area with pannus ingrowth. Stenosis due to thrombus formation often is related to inadequate anticoagulation. The likelihood of pannus formation increases with the duration of valve implantation.

Prosthetic valve stenosis may be recognized clinically on the basis of symptoms similar to those characteristic of native valve stenosis. More often, the diagnosis is initially suspected based on physical examination findings or determined during a routine echocardiographic evaluation. On physical examination, the auscultatory findings of prosthetic aortic and mitral stenosis are similar to those of diseased native valves, with the exception of prosthetic valve clicks. The valve clicks typically are crisp, with muffled clicks suggesting valve thrombosis or other interference with the normal opening and closure of the valve. Fluoroscopy may be helpful for defining the extent of normal disk motion. With echocardiography, the diagnosis of prosthetic valve stenosis can be confirmed and the degree of obstruction quantitated, enabling further clinical decisions (Fig. 17–20; see also color insert). The apparent discrepancies between Doppler and catheter data seen with normally functioning bileaflet valves are less evident when prosthetic valve stenosis is present.[143, 144] Indications for reoperation for prosthetic stenosis include symptoms resulting from the prosthetic valve stenosis or incipient valve thrombosis.

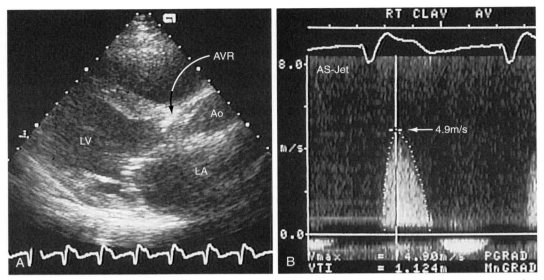

Figure 17·20 *A,* A parasternal long-axis view in a patient with suspected prosthetic porcine aortic valve stenosis shows increased echogenicity in the region of the aortic valve. *B,* The continuous wave Doppler signal shows a velocity of 4.9 m/s, corresponding to a maximum gradient of 96 mm Hg and a mean gradient of 53 mm Hg across the valve. Ao, aorta; AS, aortic stenosis; AVR, aortic valve regurgitation; LA, left atrium; LV, left ventricle. (Illustration *B* also occurs in the color insert.)

Clinically, obstruction at the valvular level may occur with normal prosthetic valve function due to "patient-prosthesis mismatch."[190, 191] As this term implies, functional stenosis may exist, despite normal valve function, due to implantation of a valve that is too small for the patient's body size. Patient-prosthesis mismatch is most likely to occur in elderly women, as the small size of the aortic root allows implantation of only small-sized mechanical or bioprosthetic valves with small functional valve areas. Patient-prosthesis mismatch is recognized by the postoperative persistence of symptoms and secondary hemodynamic changes (eg, left ventricular hypertrophy due to aortic stenosis), with echocardiographic data confirming a relatively high transvalvular gradient and small functional valve area. Patient-prosthesis mismatch may be avoided by use of newer valves with better hemodynamics (when a small valve size is needed). Alternatively, aortic root enlarging techniques to allow implantation of a larger valve may be considered, although the added surgical risk of this approach limits its widespread use.

Prosthetic Valve Regurgitation

With a mechanical valve, pathologic prosthetic regurgitation most often is due to a paravalvular leak. Less commonly, regurgitation is caused by incomplete closure of the valve occluder because of thrombus or pannus formation. With bioprosthetic valves, regurgitation may result from a paravalvular leak or from degeneration and rupture of a valve leaflet. A tear in a bioprosthetic leaflet often occurs adjacent to a region of calcification,[24] although stress-induced structural deterioration of the leaflets also occurs.[186] The prevalence of pathologic regurgitation increases with the duration of valve implantation and is higher for mitral than for aortic bioprostheses.[192]

The clinical presentation of a patient with prosthetic regurgitation ranges from a lack of symptoms despite echocardiographic evidence of pathologic regurgitation to the acute onset of pulmonary edema due to valve cusp rupture. Other patients are diagnosed based on the physical examination finding of a loud mitral regurgitant murmur or an aortic diastolic murmur. The audible characteristic of the murmur may be quite harsh and loud; one of our patients complained about the sudden onset of a "loud honking noise in my chest." Echocardiography showed severe prosthetic regurgitation with cusp rupture adjacent to a region of calcification, and these findings were confirmed at surgery.

Echocardiography allows evaluation of the presence and severity of prosthetic valve regurgitation, with the caveats that care is needed to separate normal from pathologic prosthetic regurgitation and that transesophageal imaging often is needed.[15, 137] Measurements of pressures at cardiac catheterization and aortic or left ventricular angiography are reserved for cases with nondiagnostic echocardiographic data or cases with discrepancies between the clinical and echocardiography findings.

Management of prosthetic regurgitation, in the absence of hemolytic anemia, follows the same principles that guide management of native valve regurgitation. Although reoperation is indicated for severe, symptomatic regurgitation, asymptomatic patients and those with mild or moderate regurgitation often can be managed more conservatively. Medical therapy includes treatment of heart failure symptoms and afterload reduction therapy. Periodic echocardiographic monitoring of valve function and the ventricular response to chronic volume overload is critical, as evidence for progressive ventricular dilation or left ventricular systolic dysfunction suggests that reoperation may be needed to prevent irreversible left ventricular dysfunction. While there are no definitive criteria for the timing of reoperation in patients with prosthetic regurgitation, most clinicians use criteria analogous to those proposed for native aortic and mitral valve regurgitation.

At the time of reoperation, most of these patients require repeat valve replacement. In some cases, a paravalvular leak can be repaired without replacement of the prosthetic valve. Although transcatheter umbrella closure of paravalvular leaks has been described,[193] this procedure has not gained clinical acceptance.

Thromboembolic Complications
Prevalence and Etiology

Thromboembolic complications range from acute valve thrombosis to transient cerebrovascular ischemic events. Thromboemboli are the major cause of morbidity in patients with prosthetic valves with an estimated incidence of clinical events of 0.6% to 2.3% per patient-year.[131–135, 167, 169, 194–196] The incidence of thromboembolism is similar for unanticoagulated patients with bioprosthetic valves and for those with mechanical valves on long-term warfarin therapy.[167, 169] Patients on chronic anticoagulation have an added hemorrhagic risk of about 1% per patient-year.[131–135, 167, 169, 195, 197]

Several pathophysiologic factors contribute to thromboembolic events in patients with prosthetic valves, including the thrombogenicity of the valve materials, flow separation and stagnation, and shear stress damage of blood elements and endothelium with platelet activation and release of thrombogenic factors.[16] Compared to patients with native valve disease, blood elements are damaged at lower shear stress levels in the presence of the foreign surfaces of the valve prosthesis.[198–200] Some investigators have suggested that the finding on transesophageal echocardiography of mobile, linear echoes attached to the valve annulus represents fibrin strands and is associated with a higher risk of embolic events.[201] However, other studies have found no association between the presence of valve strands and the risk of thromboembolic events.[202] Other factors that contribute to a high thromboembolic risk in valve disease patients include concurrent atrial fibrillation, left atrial enlargement, left ventricular dilation, and left ventricular systolic dysfunction. Of course, the risk of thromboembolism is higher when anticoagulation is inadequate.

Valve Thrombosis

Valve thrombosis of a mechanical valve may lead to functional stenosis or regurgitation, and the onset of signs and symptoms may be gradual due to a slowly enlarging thrombus or acute due to abrupt limitation of disk motion by thrombosis of the valve hinges. The risk of valve thrombosis is highest in the tricuspid position, with reported rates as high as 20%,[203] limiting the use of mechanical valves in this position. Valve thrombosis is less likely with left-sided mechanical valves and nearly always occurs in the setting of noncompliance with anticoagulant therapy. If a diagnosis of valve thrombosis is suspected, echocardiographic evaluation can be used to exclude or confirm the diagnosis; transesophageal imaging is needed for valves in the mitral position, as thrombus most often involves the left atrial side of the valve sewing ring.[204–208]

The treatment of valve thrombosis depends on the consequent hemodynamics and overall patient status. If hemodynamics are stable or respond promptly to medical therapy, a conservative approach with reinstitution of appropriate anticoagulation may be tried.[205] With acute hemodynamic compromise, surgical intervention with repeat replacement of the valve is needed even though the risk of surgical intervention is high with an operative mortality of 17% to 40%. Debridement of thrombus, rather than repeat valve replacement, is associated with a high likelihood of repeat thrombosis.[209] Risk factors for operative mortality include coexisting left ventricular systolic dysfunction, coronary artery disease, emergency surgery, and overall functional status.[209, 210]

Thrombolytic therapy has been proposed as an alternate approach, with success rates as high as 70% to 90% in small clinical series. However, in some series the risk of thrombolytic therapy is very high, with death in 20%, systemic emboli in 16%, and the need for urgent surgery in 22% of patients.[207, 211] Given a total complication rate of almost 60%, many clinicians continue to recommend surgical intervention for valve thrombosis with hemodynamic compromise. However, more recent series show better results with thrombolytic therapy, with a low incidence of neurologic complications or death, suggesting that thrombolytic therapy may be appropriate in some cases.[212–214]

Ischemic Neurologic Events

In a patient with a prosthetic valve and an ischemic neurologic event, the valve must be presumed to be the source of embolism unless another definite source is identified. Although echocardiography can be helpful when evidence of valve thrombosis is documented, the absence of echocardiographic evidence for valve thrombosis does not exclude the diagnosis. The accuracy of echocardiography is limited by shadowing and reverberations from the valve prosthesis. Small thrombi may be missed, or the thrombus may no longer be on the valve after the embolic event.

A prudent clinical approach is to assume that the valve is the source of embolism. As a first step, the adequacy of anticoagulation should be carefully reviewed, and the dosage should be adjusted or reinstituted to achieve and maintain a therapeutic effect. Second, if anticoagulation has been adequate, an antiplatelet agent should be added to the regimen (see Chapter 6). Repeat valve replacement for thromboembolic events is problematic because another (usually similar) prosthetic valve needs to be implanted, with a similar thromboembolic risk. Removal of the current valve is likely to be helpful only if definite thrombosis on the valve is documented and if a less thrombogenic valve can be used instead.

Spontaneous Ultrasound Contrast

On echocardiographic evaluation of prosthetic valves, spontaneous contrast often is observed in the left atrium, left ventricle, or both. This contrast effect differs from that seen in low-flow states, such as left atrial blood flow stasis, as there are fewer spontaneous echo targets, and the echos appear larger and brighter, but with a more chaotic motion pattern. Spontaneous contrast is more evident on transesophageal imaging and with the use of a higher-frequency transducer. The spontaneous contrast seen on echocardiographic imaging corresponds to the increased number of "microemboli" observed in these patients on carotid or transcranial Doppler evaluations.[215]

The origin and clinical significance of spontaneous contrast in patients with prosthetic valves remains controversial. Rather than representing aggregates of platelets or red cells, most investigators think this finding represents microcavitation, or small areas of gas formation, related to the forces generated by prosthetic valve closure.[215, 216] One study showed that these signals can be generated in the absence of blood cells.[217] Although some investigators have suggested that there is a higher frequency of "microemboli" on transcranial Doppler among patients with prosthetic valves and ischemic neurologic events,[218] most studies show no significant relationship between Doppler "microemboli" and clinical thromboembolic events.[215, 219–222] These high-intensity echo signals are seen in 50% to 90% of patients with mechanical valves, with some asymptomatic patients showing more than 60 signals per hour on transcranial Doppler studies.[215, 223] The prevalence and frequency of these signals are higher with mechanical compared with bioprosthetic valves, with larger valve sizes, and with a longer duration of implantation.[223–225] Further studies on the significance of "microemboli" in patients with prosthetic valves are needed.

Hemolysis

Although 50% to 95% of patients with mechanical valves have evidence of some intravascular hemolysis, anemia due to hemolysis is rare without prosthetic regurgitation.[191, 226, 227] Clinically evident hemolysis due to mechanical damage of red blood cells occurs more often with valves in the aortic position and noncloth-covered ball-cage valves.[228] Hemolysis may occur with either central or paravalvular regurgitation due to rapid acceleration and deceleration and/or high peak shear rates.[229]

Mild anemia due to prosthetic valve–induced hemolysis often can be treated conservatively with iron and folate replacement therapy. If hemolysis is associated with severe refractory anemia, significant paravalvular regurgitation, or high-output failure, repeat valve replacement or surgical repair of a paraprosthetic leak may be needed.

Other Complications After Prosthetic Valve Surgery

Aortic Root Complications

Aortic valve replacement with a homograft or autograft valve and root occasionally is complicated by stenosis at the distal anastomosis.[103, 230–232] In addition, distortion of the anatomy at the site of coronary reimplantation may lead to myocardial ischemia.

There are several potential complications of aortic root replacement using a composite valve and root with reimplantation of the coronary arteries.[233–238] Modifications of this procedure include the use of a small coronary graft between the coronary artery and aorta, instead of direct reimplantation.[234] The procedure may be performed by excising the native aortic root, using the prosthetic graft as a replacement for that segment of aorta or by retaining the native aorta and wrapping it around the aortic graft.

When the native aorta is retained, dehiscence at a suture line leads to an aortic pseudoaneurysm with passage of blood between the aortic graft and the space between the graft and native aorta. Dehiscence may occur at the proximal or distal suture line or, more often, at the site of coronary reimplantation.[235, 239–242] However, the incidence of coronary dehiscence has been low in recent series.[237, 243, 244] In addition, most cardiac surgeons now resect the native aorta to avoid pseudoaneurysm formation.[236, 237, 242, 245–247]

Patients with aortic pseudoaneurysms have variable symptoms of dyspnea or fatigue or may be asymptomatic. Echocardiography allows detection of the presence, extent, and origin of the pseudoaneurysm (Fig. 17–21; see also color insert).[241, 248–253] Pseudoaneurysms also can be recognized on computed tomography or magnetic resonance imaging, although the lack of dynamic flow information is a disadvantage.[254] In addition, aortic root angiography may be helpful.[255] However, it is important to recognize that blood flow into the pseudoaneurysm with a proximal suture line dehiscence may be only from the left ventricle, thus being missed if only an aortic root injection is performed.[238, 241, 252]

Surgical treatment of a pseudoaneurysm of a composite aortic valve and root is indicated to prevent further dehiscence of the suture line. A pseudoaneurysm that is increasing in size may compress the graft lumen and obstruct blood flow.

Mitral Valve Complications

Left ventricular pseudoaneurysm formation complicates as many as 0.5% to 2.0% of mitral valve replacements.[256–259] The pseudoaneurysm arises at the site of the posterior annular suture line and consists of a disruption in the integrity of the left ventricular wall that allows blood to escape outside the heart. The wall

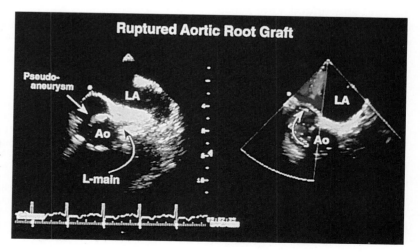

Figure 17·21 Transesophageal echocardiographic imaging in a patient with an ascending aortic graft demonstrates a pseudo-aneurysm around the graft with color flow from the aorta into the pseudo-aneurysm *(arrow).* Ao, aorta; LA, left atrium; L-main, left main coronary artery. (This figure also occurs in the color insert.)

of the pseudoaneurysm consists of pericardial adhesions, resulting in a thin-walled aneurysm at the posterior left ventricular base. In contrast, the wall of a true left ventricular aneurysm consists of thin, scarred myocardium.

A patient with a left ventricular pseudoaneurysm after mitral valve surgery typically presents in the postoperative period with a prolonged recovery and symptoms of chest pain or heart failure. On auscultation, a systolic murmur may be appreciated due to passage of blood into and out of the pseudoaneurysm.[258-260] Some patients are asymptomatic and are diagnosed only by a routine postoperative echocardiographic study. Rarely, a large pseudoaneurysm causes myocardial ischemia by compression of the coronary arteries.[261]

On echocardiography, the definitive features of a pseudoaneurysm are a thin-walled chamber that communicates with the left ventricle through a narrow neck, with a ratio of the diameter of the neck to the maximum aneurysm diameter of less than 0.5, and an abrupt transition from a normal myocardial wall to the opening into the aneurysm.[262-265] This contrasts with a true aneurysm which has a wide neck leading into a bulging area of thinned, dyskinetic myocardium. Doppler flow imaging may show blood flow in and out of the pseudoaneurysm,[261, 266] a feature that is helpful for differentiation from a loculated pericardial effusion or hematoma in the postoperative patient. When transthoracic images are suboptimal, transesophageal echocardiography provides improved image quality.[261, 266, 267] The treatment for a left ventricular pseudoaneurysm is surgical repair, as these structures are prone to further rupture, which often is catastrophic.[268, 269]

Disruptions at other areas around the sewing ring after mitral valve repair can lead to fistula formation between the left ventricle and right atrium or coronary sinus.[270, 271] Another rare complication after mitral valve replacement is a pseudoaneurysm of the mitral aortic intervalvular fibrosa. The small area of normal fibrous tissue between the posterior aortic root and base of the anterior mitral leaflet becomes dilated, creating a blind pouch that lies between the aorta and left atrium that communicates with the left ventricle.[272-275] Most pseudoaneurysms of the mitral-aortic intervalvular fibrosa are caused by infection, and they are most common with prosthetic valves.[276] Rupture of the pseudoaneurysm can lead to aortic or mitral regurgitation or rupture into the pericardial space.[275]

References

1. Harken DE, Soroff MS, Taylor MC: Partial and complete prostheses in aortic insufficiency. J Thorac Cardiovasc Surg 1960;40:744.
2. Starr A, Edwards ML: Mitral replacement: clinical experience with a ball-cage prothesis. Ann Surg 1961;154:726.
3. Braunwald NS, Cooper TS, Morrow AG: Complete replacement of the mitral valve. J Thorac Cardiovasc Surg 1960;40:1.
4. Cohn LH, Lipson W: Selection and complications of cardiac valvular prostheses. *In* Baue AE, Geha AS, Hammond GL, Laks H, Naunheim KS, eds. Glenn's Thoracic and Cardiovascular Surgery. Stamford, CT: Appleton & Lange, 1996:2043–2056.
5. Bhuvaneshwar GS, Muraleedharan CV, Vijayan GA, Kumar RS, Valiathan MS: Development of the Chitra tilting disc heart valve prosthesis. J Heart Valve Dis 1996;5:448–458.
6. Bengtsson L, Ragnarson B, Haegerstrand A: Lining of viable and nonviable allogeneic and xenogeneic cardiovascular tissue with cultured adult human venous endothelium. J Thorac Cardiovasc Surg 1993;106:434–443.
7. Fischlein T, Lehner G, Lante W, et al: Endothelialization of cardiac valve bioprostheses. [published erratum in Int J Artif Organs 1994;17:412]. Int J Artif Organs 1994;17:345–352.
8. Dahm M, Prufer D, Mayer E, Hafner G, Groh E, Oelert H: Effects of surface seeding with vital cells on the calcium uptake of biological materials for heart valve replacement. J Heart Valve Dis 1996;5:148–151.
9. Park KD, Lee WK, Yun JY, et al: Novel anti-calcification treatment of biological tissues by grafting of sulphonated polyethylene oxide. Biomaterials 1997;18:47–51.
10. Shinoka T, Ma PX, Shum Tim D, et al: Tissue-engineered heart valves: autologous valve leaflet replacement study in a lamb model. Circulation 1996;94(suppl II):164–168.
11. Disesa VJ, Allred EN, Kowalker W, Shemin RJ, Collins JJ Jr, Cohn LH: Performance of a fabricated trileaflet porcine bioprosthesis: midterm follow-up of the Hancock modified-orifice valve. J Thorac Cardiovasc Surg 1987;94:220–224.
12. Thomson FJ, Barratt Boyes BG: The glutaraldehyde-treated heterograft valve: some engineering observations. J Thorac Cardiovasc Surg 1977;74:317–321.
13. Silver MD, Wilson GJ: Pathology of mechanical heart valve prostheses and vascular grafts made of artificial materials. *In* Silver MD, ed. Cardiovascular Pathology. New York: Churchill Livingstone, 1991:1487–1546.
14. Gabbay S, Factor SM, Strom J, Becker R, Frater RW: Sudden death due to cuspal dehiscence of the Ionescu-Shiley valve in the mitral position. J Thorac Cardiovasc Surg 1982;84:313–314.
15. Nottestad SY, Zabalgoitia M: Echocardiographic recognition and quantitation of prosthetic valve dysfunction. *In* Otto CM, ed. The Practice of Clinical Echocardiography. Philadelphia: WB Saunders, 1997:797–820.
16. Yoganathan AP, Heinrich RS, Fontaine AA: Fluid dynamics of prosthetic valves. *In* Otto CM, ed. The Practice of Clinical Echocardiography. Philadelphia: WB Saunders, 1997:773–796.
17. Reisner SA, Meltzer RS: Normal values of prosthetic

valve Doppler echocardiographic parameters: a review. J Am Soc Echocardiogr 1988;1:201–210.

18. Jamieson WR, Munro AI, Miyagishima RT, Allen P, Burr LH, Tyers GF: Carpentier-Edwards standard porcine bioprosthesis: clinical performance to seventeen years. Ann Thorac Surg 1995;60:999–1006.

19. Goffin YA, Deuvaert F, Wellens F, Leclerc JL, Kiehm JL, Primo GC: Normally and abnormally functioning left-sided porcine bioprosthetic valves after long-term implantation in patients: distinct spectra of histologic and histochemical changes. J Am Coll Cardiol 1984;4:324–332.

20. Magilligan DJ Jr, Lewis JW Jr, Jara FM, et al: Spontaneous degeneration of bioprosthetic valves. Ann Thorac Surg 1980;30:259–266.

21. Oyer PE, Miller DC, Stinson EB, Reitz BA, Moreno Cabral RJ, Shumway NE: Clinical durability of the Hancock porcine bioprosthetic valve. J Thorac Cardiovasc Surg 1980;80:824–833.

22. Cohn LH, Mudge GH, Pratter F, Collins JJ Jr: Five-to eight-year follow-up of patients undergoing porcine heart-valve replacement. N Engl J Med 1981;304:258–262.

23. Gallo I, Ruiz B, Nistal F, Dur'an CM: Degeneration in porcine bioprosthetic cardiac valves: incidence of primary tissue failures among 938 bioprostheses at risk. Am J Cardiol 1984;53:1061–1065.

24. Schoen FJ: Pathology of bioprostheses and other tissue heart valve replacements. *In* Silver MD, ed. Cardiovascular Pathology. New York: Churchill Livingstone, 1991:1547–1606.

25. Sanders SP, Levy RJ, Freed MD, Norwood WI, Castaneda AR: Use of Hancock porcine xenografts in children and adolescents. Am J Cardiol 1980;46:429–438.

26. Dunn JM: Porcine valve durability in children. Ann Thorac Surg 1981;32:357–368.

27. Sbarouni E, Oakley CM: Outcome of pregnancy in women with valve prostheses. Br Heart J 1994;71:196–201.

28. Lee CN, Wu CC, Lin PY, Hsieh FJ, Chen HY: Pregnancy following cardiac prosthetic valve replacement. Obstet Gynecol 1994;83:353–356.

29. Fann JI, Miller DC, Moore KA, et al: Twenty-year clinical experience with porcine bioprostheses. Ann Thorac Surg 1996;62:1301–1311.

30. Jones EL, Weintraub WS, Craver JM, et al: Ten-year experience with the porcine bioprosthetic valve: interrelationship of valve survival and patient survival in 1,050 valve replacements. Ann Thorac Surg 1990;49:370–383.

31. Sievers HH, Lange PE, Bernhard A: Implantation of a xenogeneic stentless aortic bioprosthesis: first experience. Thorac Cardiovasc Surg 1985;33:225–226.

32. David TE: Heart valve surgery in the '90s: a surgeon's perspective. Can J Cardiol 1990;6:175–179.

33. David TE, Bos J, Rakowski H: Aortic valve replacement with the Toronto SPV bioprosthesis. J Heart Valve Dis 1992;1:244–248.

34. David TE, Ropchan GC, Butany JW: Aortic valve replacement with stentless porcine bioprostheses. J Card Surg 1988;3:501–505.

35. Konertz W, Hamann P, Schwammenthal E, Breithardt G, Scheld HH: Aortic valve replacement with stentless xenografts. J Heart Valve Dis 1992;1:249–252.

36. Kon ND, Westaby S, Amarasena N, Pillai R, Cordell AR: Comparison of implantation techniques using freestyle stentless porcine aortic valve. Ann Thorac Surg 1995;59:857–862.

37. Westaby S, Amarasena N, Long V, et al: Time-related hemodynamic changes after aortic replacement with the freestyle stentless xenograft. Ann Thorac Surg 1995;60:1633–1638.

38. Westaby S, Amarasena N, Ormerod O, Amarasena GA, Pillai R: Aortic valve replacement with the freestyle stentless xenograft. Ann Thorac Surg 1995;60(Suppl 2):S422–427.

39. Yoganathan AP, Eberhardt CE, Walker PG: Hydrodynamic performance of the Medtronic Freestyle Aortic Root Bioprosthesis. J Heart Valve Dis 1994;3:571–580.

40. O'Brien MF: Composite stentless xenograft for aortic valve replacement: clinical evaluation of function. Ann Thorac Surg 1995;60(Suppl 2):S406–409.

41. O'Brien MF: The Cryolife-O'Brien composite aortic stentless xenograft: surgical technique of implantation. Ann Thorac Surg 1995;60(Suppl 2):S410–413.

42. Hvass U, Chatel D, Ouroudji M, et al: The O'Brien-Angell stentless valve: early results of 100 implants. Eur J Cardiothorac Surg 1994;8:384–387.

43. Del Rizzo DF, Goldman BS, David TE: Aortic valve replacement with a stentless porcine bioprosthesis: multicentre trial. Canadian Investigators of the Toronto SPV Valve Trial. Can J Cardiol 1995;11:597–603.

44. Jin XY, Gibson DG, Yacoub MH, Pepper JR: Perioperative assessment of aortic homograft, Toronto stentless valve, and stented valve in the aortic position. Ann Thorac Surg 1995;60(Suppl 2):S395–401.

45. Barratt Boyes BG, Christie GW, Raudkivi PJ: The stentless bioprosthesis: surgical challenges and implications for long-term durability. Eur J Cardiothorac Surg 1992;6(suppl 1):S39–42.

46. Walther T, Falk V, Autschbach R, et al: Hemodynamic assessment of the stentless Toronto SPV bioprosthesis by echocardiography. J Heart Valve Dis 1994;3:657–665.

47. Walther T, Autschbach R, Falk V, et al: The stentless Toronto SPV bioprosthesis for aortic valve replacement. Cardiovasc Surg 1996;4:536–542.

48. Mohr FW, Walther T, Baryalei M, et al: The Toronto SPV bioprosthesis: one-year results in 100 patients. Ann Thorac Surg 1995;60:171–175.

49. Vrandecic MP, Gontijo BF, Fantini FA, et al: The new stentless aortic valve: clinical results of the first 100 patients. Cardiovasc Surg 1994;2:407–414.

50. Hofig M, Nellessen U, Mahmoodi M, et al: Performance of a stentless xenograft aortic bioprosthesis up to four years after implantation. J Thorac Cardiovasc Surg 1992;103:1068–1073.

51. Casabona R, De Paulis R, Zattera GF, et al: Stentless porcine and pericardial valve in aortic position. Ann Thorac Surg 1992;54:681–684.

52. David TE, Feindel CM, Bos J, Sun Z, Scully HE, Rakowski H: Aortic valve replacement with a stentless porcine aortic valve: a six-year experience. J Thorac Cardiovasc Surg 1994;108:1030–1036.

53. Del Rizzo DF, Goldman BS, Christakis GT, David TE: Hemodynamic benefits of the Toronto Stentless Valve. J Thorac Cardiovasc Surg 1996;112:1431–1445.

54. Dossche K, Vanermen H, Daenen W, Pillai R, Konertz W: Hemodynamic performance of the PRIMA Edwards stentless aortic xenograft: early results of a multicenter clinical trial. Thorac Cardiovasc Surg 1996;44:11–14.

55. Goldman BS, David TE, Del Rizzo DF, Sever J, Bos J: Stentless porcine bioprosthesis for aortic valve replacement. J Cardiovasc Surg 1994;35(Suppl 1):105–110.

56. Wong K, Shad S, Waterworth PD, Khaghani A, Pepper JR, Yacoub MH: Early experience with the Toronto stentless porcine valve. Ann Thorac Surg 1995;60(Suppl 2):S402–405.

57. O'Brien MF: Homografts and autografts. *In* Baue AE, Geha AS, Hammond GL, Laks H, Naunheim KS, eds. Glenn's Thoracic and Cardiovascular Surgery. Stamford, CT: Appleton & Lange, 1996:1981–2004.

58. Goldman BS, del Rizzo D, Christakis GT, Sever J, Fremes SE: Aortic valve replacement with a stentless porcine bioprosthesis (TSPV). Isr J Med Sci 1996;32:846–848.

59. Jin XY, Pepper JR, Gibson DG: Effects of incoordination on left ventricular force-velocity relation in aortic stenosis. Heart 1996;76:495–501.

60. Grunkemeier GL, Bodnar E: Comparison of structural valve failure among different "models" of homograft valves. J Heart Valve Dis 1994;3:556–560.

61. Beall AC, Morris GC, Cooley DA, et al: Homotransplantation of the aortic valve. J Thorac Cardiovasc Surg 1961;42:497.

62. Duran CG, Gunning AJ: A method for placing a total homologous aortic valve in the subcoronary position. Lancet 1962;2:488.

63. Ross DW: Homograft replacement of the aortic valve. Lancet 1962;2:487.

64. Barratt Boyes BG: Homograft aortic valve replacement in aortic incompetence and stenosis. Thorax 1964;19:131.

65. Barratt Boyes BG, Roche AHG, Whitlock RML: Six year review of the results of freehand aortic valve replacement using an antibiotic sterilized homograft valve. Circulation 1977;55:353–361.

66. Paneth M, O'Brien MF: Transplantation of human homograft aortic valve. Thorax 1966;21:115–117.

67. Angell WW, Shumway NE, Kosek JC: A five-year study of viable aortic valve homografts. J Thorac Cardiovasc Surg 1972;64:329–339.

68. Jaffe WM, Coverdale HA, Roche AH, Brandt PW, Ormiston JA, Barratt Boyes BG: Doppler echocardiography in the assessment of the homograft aortic valve. Am J Cardiol 1989;63:1466–1470.

69. Watts LK, Duffy P, Field RB, Stafford EG, O'Brien MF: Establishment of a viable homograft cardiac valve bank: a rapid method of determining homograft viability. Ann Thorac Surg 1976;21:230–236.

70. McGiffin DC, O'Brien MF, Stafford EG, Gardner MA, Pohlner PG: Long-term results of the viable cryopreserved allograft aortic valve: continuing evidence for superior valve durability. J Card Surg 1988;3:289–296.

71. O'Brien MF, Stafford G, Gardner M, et al: The viable cryopreserved allograft aortic valve. J Card Surg 1987;2:153–167.

72. Lupinetti FM, Lemmer JH Jr: Comparison of allografts and prosthetic valves when used for emergency aortic valve replacement for active infective endocarditis. Am J Cardiol 1991;68:637–641.

73. Kosek JC, Iben AB, Shumway NE, Angell WW: Morphology of fresh heart valve homografts. Surgery 1969;66:269–274.

74. O'Brien MF, McGiffin DC, Stafford EG, et al: Allograft aortic valve replacement: long-term comparative clinical analysis of the viable cryopreserved and

antibiotic 4 degrees C stored valves. J Card Surg 1991;6:534–543.

75. Christie GW, Barratt Boyes BG: On stress reduction in bioprosthetic heart valve leaflets by the use of a flexible stent. J Card Surg 1991;6:476–481.

76. Clarke DR, Campbell DN, Hayward AR, Bishop DA: Degeneration of aortic valve allografts in young recipients. J Thorac Cardiovasc Surg 1993;105:934–941.

77. Mitchell RN, Jonas RA, Schoen FJ: Structure-function correlations in cryopreserved allograft cardiac valves. Ann Thorac Surg 1995;60(Suppl 2):S108–112.

78. Schoen FJ, Levy RJ: Pathology of substitute heart valves: new concepts and developments. J Card Surg 1994;9:222–227.

79. Zhao XM, Green M, Frazer IH, Hogan P, O'Brien MF: Donor-specific immune response after aortic valve allografting in the rat. Ann Thorac Surg 1994;57:1158–1163.

80. Lang SJ, Giordano MS, Cardon Cardo C, Summers BD, Staiano Coico L, Hajjar DP: Biochemical and cellular characterization of cardiac valve tissue after cryopreservation or antibiotic preservation. J Thorac Cardiovasc Surg 1994;108:63–67.

81. Yankah AC, Wottge HU, Muller Ruchholtz W: Prognostic importance of viability and a study of a second set allograft valve: an experimental study. J Card Surg 1988;3:263–270.

82. Bartzokis T, St Goar F, DiBiase A, Miller DC, Bolger AF: Freehand allograft aortic valve replacement and aortic root replacement: utility of intraoperative echocardiography and Doppler color flow mapping. J Thorac Cardiovasc Surg 1991;101:545–553.

83. Crescenzo DG, Hilbert SL, Messier RH Jr, et al: Human cryopreserved homografts: electron microscopic analysis of cellular injury. Ann Thorac Surg 1993;55:25–30.

84. Barratt Boyes BG, Roche AH, Subramanyan R, Pemberton JR, Whitlock RM: Long-term follow-up of patients with the antibiotic-sterilized aortic homograft valve inserted freehand in the aortic position. Circulation 1987;75:768–777.

85. Kirklin JK, Smith D, Novick W, et al: Long-term function of cryopreserved aortic homografts: a ten-year study. J Thorac Cardiovasc Surg 1993;106:154–165.

86. Haydock D, Barratt Boyes B, Macedo T, Kirklin JW, Blackstone E: Aortic valve replacement for active infectious endocarditis in 108 patients: a comparison of freehand allograft valves with mechanical prostheses and bioprostheses. J Thorac Cardiovasc Surg 1992;103:130–139.

87. Pomar JL, Mestres CA, Pare JC, Miro JM: Management of persistent tricuspid endocarditis with transplantation of cryopreserved mitral homografts. J Thorac Cardiovasc Surg 1994;107:1460–1463.

88. Acar C, Farge A, Ramsheyi A, et al: Mitral valve replacement using a cryopreserved mitral homograft. Ann Thorac Surg 1994;57:746–748.

89. Kumar AS, Trehan H: Homograft mitral valve replacement—a case report. J Heart Valve Dis 1994;3:473–475.

90. Vetter HO, Dagge A, Liao K, et al: Mitral allograft with chordal support: echocardiographic evaluation in sheep. J Heart Valve Dis 1995;4:35–39.

91. Ross DN: Replacement of aortic and mitral valves with a pulmonary autograft. Lancet 1967;2:956–958.

92. Somerville J, Saravalli O, Ross D, Stone S: Long-

term results of pulmonary autograft for aortic valve replacement. Br Heart J 1979;42:533–540.

93. Ross D: The versatile homograft and autograft valve. Ann Thorac Surg 1989;48(Suppl 3):S69–70.

94. Ross D, Jackson M, Davies J: The pulmonary autograft—a permanent aortic valve. Eur J Cardiothorac Surg 1992;6:113–116.

95. Ross DN: Aortic root replacement with a pulmonary autograft—current trends. J Heart Valve Dis 1994;3:358–360.

96. Stelzer P, Jones DJ, Elkins RC: Aortic root replacement with pulmonary autograft. Circulation 1989;80(suppl II):209–213.

97. Oury JH, Angell WW, Eddy AC, Cleveland JC: Pulmonary autograft—past, present, and future. J Heart Valve Dis 1993;2:365–375.

98. Gerosa G, McKay R, Davies J, Ross DN: Comparison of the aortic homograft and the pulmonary autograft for aortic valve or root replacement in children. J Thorac Cardiovasc Surg 1991;102:51–60.

99. Sievers HH, Leyh R, Loose R, Guha M, Petry A, Bernhard A: Time course of dimension and function of the autologous pulmonary root in the aortic position. J Thorac Cardiovasc Surg 1993;105:775–780.

100. Kouchoukos NT, D'avila Rom'an VG, Spray TL, Murphy SF, Perrillo JB: Replacement of the aortic root with a pulmonary autograft in children and young adults with aortic-valve disease. N Engl J Med 1994;330:1–6.

101. David TE, Omran A, Webb G, Rakowski H, Armstrong S, Sun Z: Geometric mismatch of the aortic and pulmonary roots causes aortic insufficiency after the Ross procedure. J Thorac Cardiovasc Surg 1996;112:1231–1237.

102. Santini F, Dyke C, Edwards S, et al: Pulmonary autograft versus homograft replacement of the aortic valve: a prospective randomized trial. J Thorac Cardiovasc Surg 1997;113:894–899.

103. Pacifico AD, Kirklin JK, McGiffin DC, Matter GJ, Nanda NC, Diethelm AG: The Ross operation—early echocardiographic comparison of different operative techniques. J Heart Valve Dis 1994;3:365–370.

104. Hurvitz RJ: The Ross procedure: to do or not to do [letter]. Ann Thorac Surg 1994;58:1565–1566.

105. McKay R, Ross DN: Primary repair and autotransplantation of cardiac valves. Annu Rev Med 1993;44(suppl P):181–188.

106. Oury JH: Clinical aspects of the Ross procedure: indications and contraindications. Semin Thorac Cardiovasc Surg 1996;8:328–335.

107. Walls JT, McDaniel WC, Pope ER, et al: Documented growth of autogenous pulmonary valve translocated to the aortic valve position [letter]. J Thorac Cardiovasc Surg 1994;107:1530–1531.

108. Elkins RC, Knott Craig CJ, Razook JD, Ward KE, Overholt ED, Lane MM: Pulmonary autograft replacement of the aortic valve in the potential parent. J Card Surg 1994;9:198–203.

109. Hokken RB, Bogers AJ, Taams MA, et al: Does the pulmonary autograft in the aortic position in adults increase in diameter? An echocardiographic study. J Thorac Cardiovasc Surg 1997;113:667–674.

110. Robles A, Vaughan M, Lau JK, Bodnar E, Ross DN: Long-term assessment of aortic valve replacement with autologous pulmonary valve. Ann Thorac Surg 1985;39:238–242.

111. Wain WH, Greco R, Ignegeri A, Bodnar E, Ross DN: Fifteen years' experience with 615 homograft and autograft aortic valve replacements. Int J Artif Organs 1980;3:169–172.

112. Oury JH, Eddy AC, Cleveland JC: The Ross procedure: a progress report. J Heart Valve Dis 1994;3:361–364.

113. O'Brien MF: Aortic valve implantation techniques—should they be any different for the pulmonary autograft and the aortic homograft? J Heart Valve Dis 1993;2:385–387.

114. Bodnar E, Wain WH, Martelli V, Ross DN: Long-term performance of homograft and autograft valves. Artif Organs 1980;4:20–23.

115. Elkins RC, Lane MM, McCue C: Pulmonary autograft reoperation: incidence and management. Ann Thorac Surg 1996;62:450–455.

116. Edmunds LH Jr, Clark RE, Cohn LH, Grunkemeier GL, Miller DC, Weisel RD: Guidelines for reporting morbidity and mortality after cardiac valvular operations. The American Association for Thoracic Surgery, Ad Hoc Liaison Committee for Standardizing Definitions of Prosthetic Heart Valve Morbidity. Ann Thorac Surg 1996;62:932–935.

117. Baumgartner H, Khan S, DeRobertis M, Czer L, Maurer G: Effect of prosthetic aortic valve design on the Doppler-catheter gradient correlation: an in vitro study of normal St. Jude, Medtronic-Hall, Starr-Edwards and Hancock valves. J Am Coll Cardiol 1992;19:324–332.

118. Chafizadeh ER, Zoghbi WA: Doppler echocardiographic assessment of the St. Jude Medical prosthetic valve in the aortic position using the continuity equation. Circulation 1991;83:213–223.

119. Van Rijk Zwikker GL, Delemarre BJ, Huysmans HA: The orientation of the bi-leaflet CarboMedics valve in the mitral position determines left ventricular spatial flow patterns. Eur J Cardiothorac Surg 1996;10:513–520.

120. Hixson CS, Smith MD, Mattson MD, Morris EJ, Lenhoff SJ, Salley RK: Comparison of transesophageal color flow Doppler imaging of normal mitral regurgitant jets in St. Jude Medical and Medtronic Hall cardiac prostheses. J Am Soc Echocardiogr 1992;5:57–62.

121. Lange HW, Olson JD, Pedersen WR, et al: Transesophageal color Doppler echocardiography of the normal St. Jude Medical mitral valve prosthesis. Am Heart J 1991;122:489–494.

122. Chambers J, Cross J, Deverall P, Sowton E: Echocardiographic description of the CarboMedics bileaflet prosthetic heart valve. J Am Coll Cardiol 1993;21:398–405.

123. Joob AW, Kron IL, Craddock GB, Mentzer RL Jr, Nolan SP, Crosby IK: A decade of experience with the Model 103 and 104 Beall valve prostheses. J Thorac Cardiovasc Surg 1985;89:444–447.

124. Conti VR, Nishimura A, Coughlin TR, Farrell RW: Indications for replacement of the Beall 103 and 104 disc valves. Ann Thorac Surg 1986;42:315–320.

125. Grunkemeier GL, Starr A, Rahimtoola SH: Prosthetic heart valve performance: long-term follow-up. Curr Probl Cardiol 1992;17:329–406.

126. Jones M, McMillan ST, Eidbo EE, Woo YR, Yoganathan AP: Evaluation of prosthetic heart valves by Doppler flow imaging. Echocardiography 1986;3:513–525.

127. Baldwin JT, Deutsch S, Geselowitz DB, Tarbell JM: LDA measurements of mean velocity and Reynolds stress fields within an artificial heart ventricle. J Biomech Eng 1994;116:190–200.

128. Kohler J, Wirtz R, Fehske W: In vitro steady leakage jet formation of technical heart valve prostheses: a photo video optical and color Doppler study. *In* Liepschs D, ed. Third International Symposium on Biofluid Mechanics. Munich, Germany: VDI-Verlag GmbH Publishers, 1994:315–323.

129. Alton ME, Pasierski TJ, Orsinelli DA, Eaton GM, Pearson AC: Comparison of transthoracic and transesophageal echocardiography in evaluation of 47 Starr-Edwards prosthetic valves. J Am Coll Cardiol 1992;20:1503–1511.

130. Yoganathan AP, Reamer HH, Corcoran WH, Harrison EC, Shulman IA, Parnassus W: The Starr-Edwards aortic ball valve: flow characteristics, thrombus formation, and tissue overgrowth. Artif Organs 1981;5:6–17.

131. Thevenet A, Albat B: Long-term follow up of 292 patients after valve replacement with the Omnicarbon prosthetic valve. J Heart Valve Dis 1995;4:634–639.

132. Nitter-Hauge S, Abdelnoor M, Svennevig JL: Fifteen-year experience with the Medtronic-Hall valve prosthesis: a follow-up study of 1104 consecutive patients. Circulation 1996;94(suppl II):105–108.

133. Tatoulis J, Chaiyaroj S, Smith JA: Aortic valve replacement in patients 50 years old or younger with the St. Jude Medical valve: 14-year experience. J Heart Valve Dis 1996;5:491–497.

134. Gödje OL, Fischlein T, Adelhard K, Nollert G, Klinner W, Reichart B: Thirty-year results of Starr-Edwards prostheses in the aortic and mitral position. Ann Thorac Surg 1997;63:613–619.

135. Orszulak TA, Schaff HV, Puga FJ, et al: Event status of the Starr-Edwards aortic valve to 20 years: a benchmark for comparison. Ann Thorac Surg 1997;63:620–626.

136. Vongpatanasin W, Hillis LD, Lange RA: Prosthetic heart valves. N Engl J Med 1996;335:407–416.

137. Otto CM, Pearlman AS: Echocardiographic evaluation of prosthetic valve dysfunction. *In* Otto CM, Pearlman AS, eds. Textbook of Clinical Echocardiography. Philadelphia: WB Saunders, 1995:279–304.

138. Wilkins GT, Gillam LD, Kritzer GL, Levine RA, Palacios IF, Weyman AE: Validation of continuous-wave echocardiographic measurements of mitral and tricuspid prosthetic valve gradients: a simultaneous Doppler-catheter study. Circulation 1986;74:786–795.

139. Burstow DJ, Nishimura RA, Bailey KR, et al: Continuous wave Doppler echocardiographic measurement of prosthetic valve gradients: a simultaneous Doppler-catheter correlative study. Circulation 1989;80:504–514.

140. Leavitt JI, Coats MH, Falk RH: Effects of exercise on transmitral gradient and pulmonary artery pressure in patients with mitral stenosis or a prosthetic mitral valve: a Doppler echocardiographic study. J Am Coll Cardiol 1991;17:1520–1526.

141. van den Brink RB, Verheul HA, Visser CA, Koelemay MJ, Dunning AJ: Value of exercise Doppler echocardiography in patients with prosthetic or bioprosthetic cardiac valves. Am J Cardiol 1992;69:367–372.

142. Stewart SF, Nast EP, Arabia FA, Talbot TL, Proschan M, Clark RE: Errors in pressure gradient measurement by continuous wave Doppler ultrasound: type, size and age effects in bioprosthetic aortic valves. J Am Coll Cardiol 1991;18:769–779.

143. Baumgartner H, Khan S, DeRobertis M, Czer L, Maurer G: Discrepancies between Doppler and catheter gradients in aortic prosthetic valves in vitro: a manifestation of localized gradients and pressure recovery. Circulation 1990;82:1467–1475.

144. Baumgartner H, Schima H, Tulzer G, Kuhn P: Effect of stenosis geometry on the Doppler-catheter gradient relation in vitro: a manifestation of pressure recovery. J Am Coll Cardiol 1993;21:1018–1025.

145. Rothbart RM, Castriz JL, Harding LV, Russo CD, Teague SM: Determination of aortic valve area by two-dimensional and Doppler echocardiography in patients with normal and stenotic bioprosthetic valves. J Am Coll Cardiol 1990;15:817–824.

146. Dumesnil JG, Honos GN, Lemieux M, Beauchemin J: Validation and applications of indexed aortic prosthetic valve areas calculated by Doppler echocardiography. J Am Coll Cardiol 1990;16:637–643.

147. Chambers JB, Cochrane T, Black MM, Jackson G: The Gorlin formula validated against directly observed orifice area in porcine mitral bioprostheses. J Am Coll Cardiol 1989;13:348–353.

148. Kapur KK, Fan P, Nanda NC, Yoganathan AP, Goyal RG: Doppler color flow mapping in the evaluation of prosthetic mitral and aortic valve function. J Am Coll Cardiol 1989;13:1561–1571.

149. Flachskampf FA, O'Shea JP, Griffin BP, Guerrero L, Weyman AE, Thomas JD: Patterns of normal transvalvular regurgitation in mechanical valve prostheses. J Am Coll Cardiol 1991;18:1493–1498.

150. Come PC: Pitfalls in the diagnosis of periprosthetic valvular regurgitation by pulsed Doppler echocardiography. J Am Coll Cardiol 1987;9:1176–1179.

151. Nellessen U, Masuyama T, Appleton CP, Tye T, Popp RL: Mitral prosthesis malfunction: comparative Doppler echocardiographic studies of mitral prostheses before and after replacement. Circulation 1989;79:330–336.

152. Nellessen U, Schnittger I, Appleton CP, et al: Transesophageal two-dimensional echocardiography and color Doppler flow velocity mapping in the evaluation of cardiac valve prostheses. Circulation 1988;78:848–855.

153. Khandheria BK, Seward JB, Oh JK, et al: Value and limitations of transesophageal echocardiography in assessment of mitral valve prostheses. Circulation 1991;83:1956–1968.

154. Karalis DG, Chandrasekaran K, Ross JJ Jr, et al: Single-plane transesophageal echocardiography for assessing function of mechanical or bioprosthetic valves in the aortic valve position. Am J Cardiol 1992;69:1310–1315.

155. Daniel WG, Mugge A, Grote J, et al: Comparison of transthoracic and transesophageal echocardiography for detection of abnormalities of prosthetic and bioprosthetic valves in the mitral and aortic positions. Am J Cardiol 1993;71:210–215.

156. Yoshida K, Yoshikawa J, Akasaka T, Nishigami K, Minagoe S: Value of acceleration flow signals proximal to the leaking orifice in assessing the severity of prosthetic mitral valve regurgitation. J Am Coll Cardiol 1992;19:333–338.

157. Cohen GI, Davison MB, Klein AL, Salcedo EE, Stewart WJ: A comparison of flow convergence with other transthoracic echocardiographic indexes of prosthetic mitral regurgitation. J Am Soc Echocardiogr 1992;5:620–627.

158. Wiseth R, Skjaerpe T, Hatle L: Rapid systolic intraventricular velocities after valve replacement for aortic stenosis. Am J Cardiol 1993;71:944–948.

159. Reisner SA, Lichtenberg GS, Shapiro JR, Schwarz KQ, Meltzer RS: Exercise Doppler echocardiography in patients with mitral prosthetic valves. Am Heart J 1989;118:755–759.

160. Tatineni S, Barner HB, Pearson AC, Halbe D, Woodruff R, Labovitz AJ: Rest and exercise evaluation of St. Jude Medical and Medtronic Hall prostheses: influence of primary lesion, valvular type, valvular size, and left ventricular function. Circulation 1989;80(suppl II):16–23.

161. Grunkemeier GL, Starr A: Late ball variance with the Model 1000 Starr-Edwards aortic valve prosthesis: risk analysis and strategy of operative management. J Thorac Cardiovasc Surg 1986;91:918–923.

162. McHenry MM, Smeloff EA, Fong WY, Miller GE Jr, Ryan PM: Critical obstruction of prosthetic heart valves due to lipid absorption by Silastic. J Thorac Cardiovasc Surg 1970;59:413–425.

163. Silver MD, Wilson GJ: The pathology of wear in the Beall model 104 heart valve prosthesis. Circulation 1977;56(suppl II):1617–1622.

164. Lindblom D, Rodriguez L, Bjork VO: Mechanical failure of the Bjork-Shiley valve: updated follow-up and considerations on prophylactic rereplacement. J Thorac Cardiovasc Surg 1989;97:95–97.

165. Silver MD: Infective endocarditis. *In* Silver MD, ed. Cardiovascular Pathology. New York: Churchill Livingstone, 1991:895–932.

166. Joassin A, Edwards JE: Causes of death within 30 days of mitral valvular replacement: analysis of 93 cases. Cardiovasc Clin 1973;5:169–184.

167. Bloomfield P, Wheatley DJ, Prescott RJ, Miller HC: Twelve-year comparison of a Bjork-Shiley mechanical heart valve with porcine bioprostheses. N Engl J Med 1991;324:573–579.

168. Cohn LH, Collins JJ Jr, Disesa VJ, et al: Fifteen-year experience with 1678 Hancock porcine bioprosthetic heart valve replacements. Ann Surg 1989;210:435–442.

169. Hammermeister KE, Henderson WG, Burchfiel CM, et al: Comparison of outcome after valve replacement with a bioprosthesis versus a mechanical prosthesis: initial 5-year results of a randomized trial. J Am Coll Cardiol 1987;10:719–732.

170. Jaffe WM, Morgan DE, Pearlman AS, Otto CM: Infective endocarditis, 1983–1988: echocardiographic findings and factors influencing morbidity and mortality. J Am Coll Cardiol 1990;15:1227–1233.

171. Arnett EN, Roberts WC: Prosthetic valve endocarditis: clinicopathologic analysis of 22 necropsy patients with comparison observations in 74 necropsy patients with active infective endocarditis involving natural left-sided cardiac valves. Am J Cardiol 1976;38:281–292.

172. Buchbinder NA, Roberts WC: Left-sided valvular active infective endocarditis: a study of forty-five necropsy patients. Am J Med 1972;53:20–35.

173. Mugge A, Daniel WG, Frank G, Lichtlen PR: Echocardiography in infective endocarditis: reassessment of prognostic implications of vegetation size determined by the transthoracic and the transesophageal approach. J Am Coll Cardiol 1989;14:631–638.

174. Taams MA, Gussenhoven EJ, Bos E, et al: Enhanced morphological diagnosis in infective endocarditis by transoesophageal echocardiography. Br Heart J 1990;63:109–113.

175. Daniel WG, Mugge A, Martin RP, et al: Improvement in the diagnosis of abscesses associated with endocarditis by transesophageal echocardiography. N Engl J Med 1991;324:795–800.

176. Yvorchuk KJ, Chan KL: Application of transthoracic and transesophageal echocardiography in the diagnosis and management of infective endocarditis. J Am Soc Echocardiogr 1994;7:1294–1308.

177. Shively BK, Gurule FT, Roldan CA, Leggett JH, Schiller NB: Diagnostic value of transesophageal compared with transthoracic echocardiography in infective endocarditis. J Am Coll Cardiol 1991;18:391–397.

178. Pedersen WR, Walker M, Olson JD, et al: Value of transesophageal echocardiography as an adjunct to transthoracic echocardiography in evaluation of native and prosthetic valve endocarditis. Chest 1991;100:351–356.

179. Shapiro SM, Young E, De Guzman S, et al: Transesophageal echocardiography in diagnosis of infective endocarditis. Chest 1994;105:377–382.

180. Schiller NB: Clinical decision making in patients with endocarditis: the role of echocardiography. *In* Otto CM, ed. The Practice of Clinical Echocardiography. Philadelphia: WB Saunders, 1997.

181. Cipriano PR, Billingham ME, Oyer PE, Kutsche LM, Stinson EB: Calcification of porcine prosthetic heart valves: a radiographic and light microscopy study. Circulation 1982;66:1100–1104.

182. Gallucci V, Bortolotti U, Milano A, Valfre C, Mazzucco A, Thiene G: Isolated mitral valve replacement with the Hancock bioprosthesis: a 13-year appraisal. Ann Thorac Surg 1984;38:571–578.

183. Gallo I, Nistal F, Cay'on R, Arbe E, Blasquez R, Artinano E: Long-term performance of porcine heart valve bioprostheses. Eur J Cardiothorac Surg 1988;2:273–281.

184. Gallo I, Nistal F, Arbe E, Artinano E: Comparative study of primary tissue failure between porcine (Hancock and Carpentier-Edwards) and bovine pericardial (Ionescu-Shiley) bioprostheses in the aortic position at five- to nine-year follow-up. Am J Cardiol 1988;61:812–816.

185. Gallo I, Nistal F, Blasquez R, Arbe E, Artinano E: Incidence of primary tissue valve failure in porcine bioprosthetic heart valves. Ann Thorac Surg 1988;45:66–70.

186. Ishihara T, Ferrans VJ, Boyce SW, Jones M, Roberts WC: Structure and classification of cuspal tears and perforations in porcine bioprosthetic cardiac valves implanted in patients. Am J Cardiol 1981;48:665–678.

187. Silver MM, Pollock J, Silver MD, Williams WG, Trusler GA: Calcification in porcine xenograft valves in children. Am J Cardiol 1980;45:685–689.

188. Ayhan A, Yapar EG, Yuce K, Kisnisci HA, Nazli N, Ozmen F: Pregnancy and its complications after cardiac valve replacement. Int J Gynaecol Obstet 1991;35:117–122.

189. Badduke BR, Jamieson WR, Miyagishima RT, et al: Pregnancy and childbearing in a population with biologic valvular prostheses. J Thorac Cardiovasc Surg 1991;102:179–186.

190. Rahimtoola SH: The problem of valve prosthesis-patient mismatch. Circulation 1978;58:20–24.

191. Lund O, Emmertsen K, Nielsen TT, et al: Impact of size mismatch and left ventricular function on performance of the St. Jude disc valve after aortic valve replacement. Ann Thorac Surg 1997;63:1227–1234.

192. Jamieson WR, Tyers GF, Janusz MT, et al: Age as a determinant for selection of porcine bioprostheses for cardiac valve replacement: experience with Carpentier-Edwards standard bioprosthesis. Can J Cardiol 1991;7:181–188.

193. Hourihan M, Perry SB, Mandell VS, et al: Transcatheter umbrella closure of valvular and paravalvular leaks. J Am Coll Cardiol 1992;20:1371–1377.

194. Edmunds LH Jr: Thromboembolic complications of current cardiac valvular prostheses. Ann Thorac Surg 1982;34:96–106.

195. Cannegieter SC, van der Meer FJ, Briet E, Rosendaal FR: Warfarin and aspirin after heart-valve replacement. N Engl J Med 1994;330:507–508.

196. Deb'etaz LF, Ruchat P, Hurni M, et al: St. Jude Medical valve prosthesis: an analysis of long-term outcome and prognostic factors. J Thorac Cardiovasc Surg 1997;113:134–148.

197. Lieberman A, Hass WK, Pinto R, et al: Intracranial hemorrhage and infarction in anticoagulated patients with prosthetic heart valves. Stroke 1978;9:18–24.

198. Mohandas N, Hochmuth RM, Spaeth EE: Adhesion of red cells to foreign surfaces in the presence of flow. J Biomed Mater Res 1974;8:119–136.

199. Blackshear PL Jr, Forstrom RJ, Dorman FD, Voss GO: Effect of flow on cells near walls. Fed Proc 1971;30:1600–1611.

200. Sutera SP, Mehrjardi MH: Deformation and fragmentation of human red blood cells in turbulent shear flow. Biophys J 1975;15:1–10.

201. Isada LR, Torelli JN, Stewart WJ, Klein AL: Detection of fibrous strands on prosthetic mitral valves with transesophageal echocardiography: another potential embolic source. J Am Soc Echocardiogr 1994;7:641–645.

202. Stoddard MF, Dawkins PR, Longaker RA: Mobile strands are frequently attached to the St. Jude Medical mitral valve prosthesis as assessed by two-dimensional transesophageal echocardiography. Am Heart J 1992;124:671–674.

203. Thorburn CW, Morgan JJ, Shanahan MX, Chang VP: Long-term results of tricuspid valve replacement and the problem of prosthetic valve thrombosis. Am J Cardiol 1983;51:1128–1132.

204. Habib G, Cornen A, Mesana T, Monties JR, Djiane P, Luccioni R: Diagnosis of prosthetic heart valve thrombosis: the respective values of transthoracic and transoesophageal Doppler echocardiography. Eur Heart J 1993;14:447–455.

205. Gueret P, Vignon P, Fournier P, et al: Transesophageal echocardiography for the diagnosis and management of nonobstructive thrombosis of mechanical mitral valve prosthesis. Circulation 1995;91:103–110.

206. Lanzieri M, Michaelson S, Cohen IS: Transesophageal echocardiography in the diagnosis of mitral bioprosthetic obstruction. Crit Care Med 1991;19:979–981.

207. Dzavik V, Cohen G, Chan KL: Role of transesophageal echocardiography in the diagnosis and management of prosthetic valve thrombosis. J Am Coll Cardiol 1991;18:1829–1833.

208. Young E, Shapiro SM, French WJ, Ginzton LE: Use of transesophageal echocardiography during thrombolysis with tissue plasminogen activator of a thrombosed prosthetic mitral valve. J Am Soc Echocardiogr 1992;5:153–158.

209. Martinell J, Jimenez A, Rabago G, Artiz V, Fraile J, Farre J: Mechanical cardiac valve thrombosis: is thrombectomy justified? Circulation 1991;84(suppl III):70–75.

210. Christakis GT, Weisel RD, David TE, Salerno TA, Ivanov J: Predictors of operative survival after valve replacement. Circulation 1988;78:2125–2134.

211. Ledain LD, Ohayon JP, Colle JP, Lorient Roudaut FM, Roudaut RP, Besse PM: Acute thrombotic obstruction with disc valve prostheses: diagnostic considerations and fibrinolytic treatment. J Am Coll Cardiol 1986;7:743–751.

212. Reddy NK, Padmanabhan TN, Singh S, et al: Thrombolysis in left-sided prosthetic valve occlusion: immediate and follow-up results. Ann Thorac Surg 1994;58:462–470.

213. Silber H, Khan SS, Matloff JM, Chaux A, DeRobertis M, Gray R: The St. Jude valve: thrombolysis as the first line of therapy for cardiac valve thrombosis. Circulation 1993;87:30–37.

214. Vitale N, Renzulli A, Cerasuolo F, et al: Prosthetic valve obstruction: thrombolysis versus operation. Ann Thorac Surg 1994;57:365–370.

215. Deklunder G, Lecroart JL, Savoye C, Coquet B, Houdas Y: Transcranial high-intensity Doppler signals in patients with mechanical heart valve prostheses: their relationship with abnormal intracavitary echoes. J Heart Valve Dis 1996;5:662–667.

216. Georgiadis D, Mackay TG, Kelman AW, Grosset DG, Wheatley DJ, Lees KR: Differentiation between gaseous and formed embolic materials in vivo: application in prosthetic heart valve patients. Stroke 1994;25:1559–1563.

217. Mackay TG, Georgiadis D, Grosset DG, Lees KR, Wheatley DJ: On the origin of cerebrovascular microemboli associated with prosthetic heart valves. Neurol Res 1995;17:349–352.

218. Tong DC, Albers GW: Transcranial Doppler-detected microemboli in patients with acute stroke. Stroke 1995;26:1588–1592.

219. Reisner SA, Rinkevich D, Markiewicz W, Adler Z, Milo S: Spontaneous echocardiographic contrast with the CarboMedics mitral valve prosthesis. Am J Cardiol 1992;70:1497–1500.

220. Kort A, Kronzon I: Microbubble formation: in vitro and in vivo observation. J Clin Ultrasound 1982;10:117–120.

221. Sherrington C, Bamford J: Diagnostic pitfall and the reporting of cerebrovascular events in patients with prosthetic heart valves. J Heart Valve Dis 1994;3:607–610.

222. Eicke BM, Barth V, Kukowski B, Werner G, Paulus W: Cardiac microembolism: prevalence and clinical outcome. J Neurol Sci 1996;136:143–147.

223. Braekken SK, Russell D, Brucher R, Svennevig J: Incidence and frequency of cerebral embolic signals in patients with a similar bileaflet mechanical heart valve. Stroke 1995;26:1225–1230.

224. Grosset DG, Cowburn P, Georgiadis D, Dargie HJ, Faichney A, Lees KR: Ultrasound detection of cerebral emboli in patients with prosthetic heart valves. J Heart Valve Dis 1994;3:128–132.

225. Grosset DG, Georgiadis D, Kelman AW, et al: Detection of microemboli by transcranial Doppler ultrasound. Tex Heart Inst J 1996;23:289–292.

226. Skoularigis J, Essop MR, Skudicky D, Middlemost SJ, Sareli P: Frequency and severity of intravascular hemolysis after left-sided cardiac valve replacement with Medtronic-Hall and St. Jude Medical prostheses and influence of prosthetic type, position, size and number. Am J Cardiol 1993;71:587–591.

227. Barmada H, Starr A: Clinical hemolysis with the St. Jude heart valve without paravalvular leak. Med Prog Technol 1994;20:191–194.

228. Santinga JT, Kirsh MM: Hemolytic anemia in series 2300 and 2310 Starr-Edwards prosthetic valves. Ann Thorac Surg 1972;14:539–544.

229. Garcia MJ, Vandervoort P, Stewart WJ, et al: Mechanisms of hemolysis with mitral prosthetic regurgitation: study using transesophageal echocardiography and fluid dynamic simulation. J Am Coll Cardiol 1996;27:399–406.

230. Joyce F, Tingleff J, Aagaard J, Pettersson G: The Ross operation in the treatment of native and prosthetic aortic valve endocarditis. J Heart Valve Dis 1994;3:371–376.

231. Joyce F, Tingleff J, Pettersson G: Expanding indications for the Ross operation. J Heart Valve Dis 1995;4:352–363.

232. Joyce F, Tingleff J, Pettersson G: The Ross operation: results of early experience including treatment for endocarditis. Eur J Cardiothorac Surg 1995;9:384–391.

233. Bentall H, De Bono A: A technique for complete replacement of the ascending aorta. Thorax 1968;23:338–339.

234. Cabrol C, Pavie A, Gandjbakhch I, et al: Complete replacement of the ascending aorta with reimplantation of the coronary arteries: new surgical approach. J Thorac Cardiovasc Surg 1981;81:309–315.

235. Kouchoukos NT, Marshall WG Jr, Wedige Stecher TA: Eleven-year experience with composite graft replacement of the ascending aorta and aortic valve. J Thorac Cardiovasc Surg 1986;92:691–705.

236. Kouchoukos NT: Composite graft replacement of the ascending aorta and aortic valve with the inclusion-wrap and open techniques. Semin Thorac Cardiovasc Surg 1991;3:171–176.

237. Gott VL, Cameron DE, Pyeritz RE, et al: Composite graft repair of Marfan aneurysm of the ascending aorta: results in 150 patients. J Card Surg 1994;9:482–489.

238. Zoghbi WA: Echocardiographic recognition of unusual complications after surgery on the great vessels and cardiac valves. *In* Otto CM, ed. The Practice of Clinical Echocardiography. Philadelphia: WB Saunders, 1997:821–836.

239. Donaldson RM, Ross DN: Composite graft replacement for the treatment of aneurysms of the ascending aorta associated with aortic valvular disease. Circulation 1982;66(suppl II):16–21.

240. Marvasti MA, Parker FB Jr, Randall PA, Witwer GA: Composite graft replacement of the ascending aorta and aortic valve: late follow-up with intra-arterial digital subtraction angiography. J Thorac Cardiovasc Surg 1988;95:924–928.

241. Barbetseas J, Crawford ES, Safi HJ, Coselli JS, Quinones MA, Zoghbi WA: Doppler echocardiographic evaluation of pseudoaneurysms complicating composite grafts of the ascending aorta. Circulation 1992;85:212–222.

242. Carrel T, Pasic M, Jenni R, Tkebuchava T, Turina MI: Reoperations after operation on the thoracic aorta: etiology, surgical techniques, and prevention. Ann Thorac Surg 1993;56:259–268.

243. Westaby S, Parry A, Pillai R: Aortic root replacement: modifications of technique with improvements in technology. Eur J Cardiothorac Surg 1992;6(suppl 1):S44–48.

244. Gott VL, Gillinov AM, Pyeritz RE, et al: Aortic root replacement: risk factor analysis of a seventeen-year experience with 270 patients. J Thorac Cardiovasc Surg 1995;109:536–544.

245. Coselli JS, Crawford ES: Composite valve-graft replacement of aortic root using separate Dacron tube for coronary artery reattachment. Ann Thorac Surg 1989;47:558–565.

246. Lewis CT, Cooley DA, Murphy MC, Talledo O, Vega D: Surgical repair of aortic root aneurysms in 280 patients. Ann Thorac Surg 1992;53:38–45.

247. Finkbohner R, Johnston D, Crawford ES, Coselli J, Milewicz DM: Marfan syndrome: long-term survival and complications after aortic aneurysm repair. Circulation 1995;91:728–733.

248. Wendel CH, Cornman CR, Dianzumba SB: Diagnosis of pseudoaneurysm of the ascending aorta by pulsed Doppler cross sectional echocardiography. Br Heart J 1985;53:567–570.

249. Rice MJ, McDonald RW, Reller MD: Diagnosis of coronary artery dehiscence and pseudoaneurysm formation in postoperative Marfan patient by color flow Doppler echocardiography. J Clin Ultrasound 1989;17:359–365.

250. Hoadley SD, Hartshorne MF: Noninvasive diagnosis of pseudoaneurysm of the ascending aorta. J Clin Ultrasound 1987;15:325–332.

251. Shioi K, Nagata Y, Tsuchioka H: Usefulness of echocardiography in the long-term follow-up study after surgical treatment of annuloaortic ectasia. Jpn J Surg 1988;18:636–640.

252. Rosenzweig BP, Donahue T, Attubato M, Feit F, Kronzon I: Left ventricle-to-ascending aorta communication complicating composite graft repair undetected by aortography: diagnosis by transesophageal echocardiography. J Am Soc Echocardiogr 1991;4:639–644.

253. Lasorda DM, Power TP, Dianzumba SB, Incorvati RL: Diagnosis of aortic pseudoaneurysm by echocardiography. Clin Cardiol 1992;15:773–776.

254. Pucillo AL, Schechter AG, Kay RH, Moggio R, Herman MV: Identification of calcified intracardiac lesions using gradient echo MR imaging. J Comput Assist Tomogr 1990;14:743–747.

255. Nath PH, Zollikofer C, Castaneda Zuniga WR, et al: Radiological evaluation of composite aortic grafts. Ann Thorac Surg 1979;131:43–51.

256. Roberts WC, Morrow AG: Causes of early postoperative death following cardiac valve replacement. Clinico-pathologic correlations in 64 patients studied at necropsy. J Thorac Cardiovasc Surg 1967;54:422–437.

257. Roberts WC, Morrow AG: Late postoperative pathological findings after cardiac valve replacement. Circulation 1967;35(suppl I):48–62.

258. Bjork VO, Henze A, Rodriguez L: Left ventricular rupture as a complication of mitral valve replacement. J Thorac Cardiovasc Surg 1977;73:14–22.

259. Karlson KJ, Ashraf MM, Berger RL: Rupture of left ventricle following mitral valve replacement. Ann Thorac Surg 1988;46:590–597.

260. Azariades M, Lennox SC: Rupture of the posterior wall of the left ventricle after mitral valve replacement: etiological and technical considerations. Ann Thorac Surg 1988;46:491–494.

261. Baker WB, Klein MS, Reardon MJ, Zoghbi WA: Left ventricular pseudoaneurysm complicating mitral valve replacement: transesophageal echocardiographic diagnosis and impact on management. J Am Soc Echocardiogr 1993;6:548–552.

262. Catherwood E, Mintz GS, Kotler MN, Parry WR, Segal BL: Two-dimensional echocardiographic recognition of left ventricular pseudoaneurysm. Circulation 1980;62:294–303.

263. Roelandt JR, Sutherland GR, Yoshida K, Yoshikawa J: Improved diagnosis and characterization of left ventricular pseudoaneurysm by Doppler color flow imaging. J Am Coll Cardiol 1988;12:807–811.

264. Kupari M, Verkkala K, Maamies T, Hartel G: Value of combined cross sectional and Doppler echocardiography in the detection of left ventricular pseudoaneurysm after mitral valve replacement. Br Heart J 1987;58:52–56.

265. Olalla JJ, Vazquez de Prada JA, Duran RM, Villarroel MT, Otero Fernandez M: Color Doppler diagnosis of left ventricular pseudoaneurysm. Chest 1988;94:443–444.

266. Alam M, Glick C, Garcia R, Lewis JW Jr: Transesophageal echocardiographic features of left ventricular pseudoaneurysm resulting after mitral valve replacement surgery. Am Heart J 1992;123:226–228.

267. Esakof DD, Vannan MA, Pandian NG, Cao QL, Schwartz SL, Bojar RM: Visualization of left ventricular pseudoaneurysm with panoramic transesophageal echocardiography. J Am Soc Echocardiogr 1994;7:174–178.

268. Vlodaver Z, Coe JI, Edwards JE: True and false left ventricular aneurysms: propensity for the latter to rupture. Circulation 1975;51:567–572.

269. Stewart S, Huddle R, Stuard I, Schreiner BF, DeWeese JA: False aneurysm and pseudo-false aneurysm of the left ventricle: etiology, pathology, diagnosis, and operative management. Ann Thorac Surg 1981;31:259–265.

270. Yee GW, Naasz C, Hatle L, Pipkin R, Schnittger I: Doppler diagnosis of left ventricle to coronary sinus fistula: an unusual complication of mitral valve replacement. J Am Soc Echocardiogr 1988;1:458–462.

271. Watanabe A, Kazui T, Tsukamoto M, Komatsu S: Left ventricular pseudoaneurysm and intracardiac fistulas after replacement of mitral valve prosthesis. Ann Thorac Surg 1993;55:1236–1239.

272. Chesler E, Korns ME, Porter GE, Reyes CN, Edwards JE: False aneurysm of the left ventricle secondary to bacterial endocarditis with perforation of the mitral-aortic intervalvular fibrosa. Circulation 1968;37:518–523.

273. Edward JE, Burchell HB: The pathological anatomy of deficiencies between the ring and the heart including aortic sinus aneurysms. Thorax 1957;12:125–139.

274. Layman TE, January LE: Mycotic left ventricular aneurysm involving the fibrous atrioventricular body. Am J Cardiol 1967;20:423–427.

275. Qizilbash AH, Schwartz CJ: False aneurysm of left ventricle due to perforation of mitral-aortic intervalvular fibrosa with rupture and cardiac tamponade: rare complication of infective endocarditis. Am J Cardiol 1973;32:110–113.

276. Afridi I, Apostolidou MA, Saad RM, Zoghbi WA: Pseudoaneurysms of the mitral-aortic intervalvular fibrosa: dynamic characterization using transesophageal echocardiographic and Doppler techniques. J Am Coll Cardiol 1995;25:137–145.

277. Alam M, Rosman HS, Lakier JB, et al: Doppler and echocardiographic features of normal and dysfunctioning bioprosthetic valves. J Am Coll Cardiol 1987;10:851–858.

278. Angell WW, Angell JD, Oury JH, Lamberti JJ, Grehl TM: Long-term follow-up of viable frozen aortic homografts: a viable homograft valve bank. J Thorac Cardiovasc Surg 1987;93:815–822.

279. Arom KV, Nicoloff DM, Kersten TE, Northrup WF III, Lindsay WG, Emergy RW: Ten years' experience with the St. Jude Medical valve prosthesis. Ann Thorac Surg 1989;47:831–837.

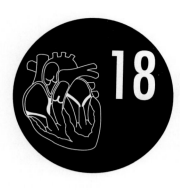

18 Infective Endocarditis

Infective endocarditis is defined as an inflammation of the endocardium caused by microorganisms.[1] The infection usually involves a valve, but other native and prosthetic intracardiac surfaces also can be affected. The diagnosis of infective endocarditis is most firmly established by pathologic criteria, specifically by histologic examination of an intracardiac or embolized vegetation or demonstration of an intracardiac abscess at surgery or autopsy. Clinical series based on a strict pathologic definition of endocarditis have provided essential data on the clinical features, diagnostic criteria, natural history, and prognosis of this disease. However, a pathologic definition is less useful for making decisions about individual patients, because the diagnosis is made too late in the clinical course (ie, at surgery or autopsy) to affect patient management.

During the past two decades, various clinical criteria have been proposed and subsequently modified for the diagnosis of infective endocarditis. The current clinical criteria are based predominantly on evidence of typical infective organisms and echocardiographic demonstration of a valvular vegetation or intracardiac abscess. Secondary clinical criteria include the systemic, vascular, and immunologic consequences of the disease process.

The most useful classifications of infective endocarditis are those based on the etiology of disease and the anatomy of the affected cardiac structures. Even though the large number of specific organisms that can cause endocarditis results in a large number of etiologic subgroups, the disease course and expected complications do differ substantially based on the organism involved. For example, the clinical course and optimal treatment for *Streptococcus viridans* endocarditis differ dramatically from those for fungal endocarditis.

Alternatively, an anatomic classification

scheme distinguishes between prosthetic valve and native valve endocarditis and between right- and left-sided heart involvement. These groupings are helpful given the different causes and outcomes for these patient groups. Classification of endocarditis as acute or subacute has largely been superseded by these etiologic and anatomic classifications, as the rapidity of the disease course basically is a function of the virulence of the causative organism and the specific cardiac structures affected. This chapter uses primarily an anatomic classification of infective endocarditis, but differences based on etiologic agents also are described.

PATHOPHYSIOLOGY AND DISEASE COURSE

The hallmark of infective endocarditis is development of a vegetation (an infected fibrin-platelet mass) at the infected site, typically on a valve, with continuous release of organisms into the blood (Fig. 18–1). Local tissue destruction by the infective process leads to valvular dysfunction, heart failure, and abscess formation. Persistent bacteremia is associated with systemic symptoms, vascular phenomena, and immune complex disease. Macroscopic embolization of all or part of the infected vegetation results in metastatic infection and ischemic events.

Valvular Vegetations

The initial step in the pathogenesis of endocarditis is thought to be formation of a sterile fibrin-platelet thrombus at a site of endothelial disruption. This process typically occurs on the upstream side of the valve (ie, atrial side of mitral valve or ventricular side of aortic valve), probably related to the effects of shear stress on endothelial integrity. Endothelial disruption is most likely when underlying structural heart disease is present, particularly lesions resulting in high-velocity, turbulent blood flow patterns, such as valvular regurgitation or stenosis. Prosthetic material also provides a site for initiation of this cycle due to microthrombi formation on the valve sewing ring at the junction between the prosthetic material and the endocardium. However, even in the absence of structural heart disease, small, noninfected thrombi are seen along the valve closure line in 1% to 2% of all autopsies.[1] These small, sterile vegetations are seen most often on the ventricular side of the aortic valve, followed in frequency by the atrial surfaces of the mitral and tricuspid valves. It is plausible that small thrombi form frequently on valve surfaces but only become infected if there is superimposed bacteremia with or without impaired immune mechanisms.

Substantial experimental and clinical data support the concept that transient bacteremia is an essential step in the pathogenesis of endocarditis. Specifically, both animal models of the disease process and the association of organisms known to cause transient bacteremia with endocarditis support this theory of the disease process.[2–5] After seeding of the thrombus occurs, subsequent cycles of bacterial proliferation and repetitive thrombus formation lead to formation of the vegetation. Microscopically, vegetations are masses of platelets, fibrin, and other matrix proteins with a high concentration of infective organisms. The mi-

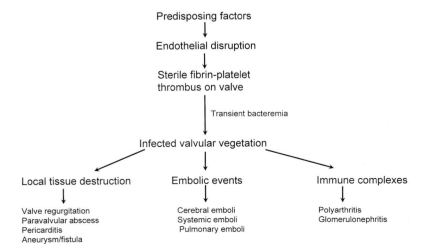

Figure 18·1 Flow chart of the pathophysiology of infective endocarditis.

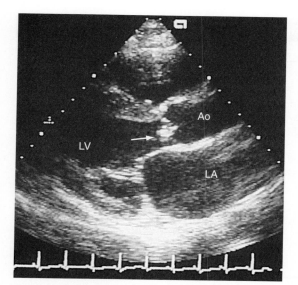

Figure 18·2 This parasternal long-axis echocardiographic image shows a typical aortic valve vegetation. An echodense mass is attached to the ventricular side of the aortic valve *(arrow)*, prolapses into the outflow tract in diastole, and shows rapid oscillations independent of valve motion. Ao, aorta; LA, left atrium; LV, left ventricle.

croorganisms may be relatively quiescent, limiting the action of some antibiotics. In addition, the platelet-fibrin layers impair antibiotic penetration into the vegetation.

Grossly, vegetations typically are attached to a valve but also may be seen on other endothelial surfaces, particularly in the path of a high-velocity jet or turbulent flow stream (Figs. 18–2 and 18–3). Valvular vegetations often have a small attachment point relative to the size of the mass, resulting in oscillating motion of the vegetation separate from the normal pattern of valve motion. However, there is considerable variation in the size and shape of vegetations, and some have a broad base with only limited mobility. While the vegetation itself contains variable numbers of leukocytes, the adjacent valve tissue shows an accumulation of large numbers of leukocytes and associated tissue destruction. Infection can spread to structures continuous with the valve leaflets, including the valve annulus, the adjacent myocardium, and the pericardium.

In untreated or inadequately treated cases of endocarditis, vegetations may increase in size. The fragile vegetation may fragment or separate from the valve tissue, resulting in embolization of the infected mass. With effective treatment, valvular vegetations tend to decrease in size as the mass organizes, although persistent "healed" vegetations may still be detectable on echocardiography, at surgery, or at autopsy months to years after the acute episode.[6]

Microbiology

Although any microorganism potentially can cause endocarditis, infection is most common with specific organisms, depending on the type of endocarditis (Table 18–1). These

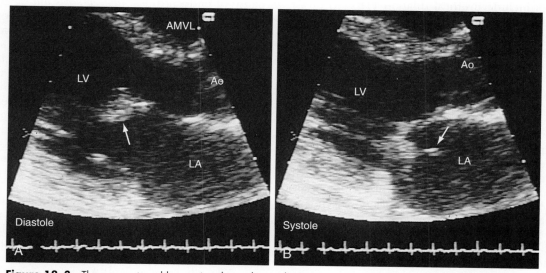

Figure 18·3 These parasternal long-axis echocardiographic images at end-diastole *(A)* and end-systole *(B)* show a typical mitral valve vegetation. An echogenic mass *(arrow)* is attached to the left atrial side of the anterior mitral valve leaflet (AMVL) and prolapses into the left atrium in systole. Ao, aorta; LA, left atrium; LV, left ventricle.

TABLE 18·1 MICROORGANISMS CAUSING INFECTIVE ENDOCARDITIS

	Approximate Prevalence			
			Prosthetic Valves (%)	
Organism	Native Valve Endocarditis (%)	IVDUs (%)	EARLY	LATE
Streptococci				
Viridans	25–40	<5	5–10	15–60
Enterococcus	10–20	8	5–15	10–15
S. bovis	10			
β-hemolytic	4–5	10–25 (group A)		
Pneumococcus	1–3			
Staphylococci				
S. aureus	15–35	>50	10–44	10–25
S. epidermidis	3–5		15–57	3–33
HACEK organisms	3–5		18	7
Gram-negative bacilli	5–10	10	8–37	5–25
Polymicrobial	2	5	6–22	2–4
Fungi	1–5		9–13	4–6
Culture negative	5–15	5	3	4

IVDUs, intravenous drug users.

causative organisms share at least two properties: an association with frequent bacteremia and an ability to adhere to the valve or thrombus surface. Transient bacteremia, which is a necessary step in the development of infective endocarditis, occurs frequently, even in normal individuals. Minor gum bleeding, such as that associated with teeth brushing or dental procedures, results in transient bacteremia in 18% to 85% of cases; even chewing candy leads to bacteremia in 17% to 51% of cases. Medical procedures that invade nonsterile areas also result in transient bacteremia. Examples include urethral dilation (18% to 33%), transurethral prostatic resection (12% to 46%), normal vaginal delivery (0% to 11%), and barium enema (11%).[7]

In some cases, adhesion to the valve appears to be mediated by specific extracellular polysaccharides produced by the microorganism, for example, dextran formation by oral streptococci. In other cases, tissue factors released by damaged endothelium or the nonbacterial thrombotic lesion may be important. Potential mediators of adherence of microorganisms include fibronectin, fibrinogen, laminin, and type IV collagen.[8] However, the role of these factors in the pathogenesis of endocarditis remains controversial.[9]

Streptococci are the most common group of organisms causing endocarditis, particularly the viridans group of streptococci, including *Streptococcus sanguis*, *Streptococcus oralis*, *Streptococcus salivarius*, and *Streptococcus mutans*. Infection with *Streptococcus bovis*, a nonenterococcal

group D streptococcus, has been associated with colon carcinoma. Enterococci, gram-positive gastrointestinal tract flora, tend to cause subacute infection in older men after gastrointestinal procedures or in younger women after obstetric procedures. Other streptococci that cause endocarditis include nutritionally variant strains that require special media for growth and are seen most often in patients with impaired immune function from diabetes, cancer, alcohol use, or hepatic failure.[8]

Coagulase-positive and coagulase-negative staphylococci are an increasingly frequent cause of endocarditis. *Staphylococcus aureus* endocarditis leads to extensive tissue destruction and a high prevalence of local and distal complications when the left heart is involved, so that mortality rates are high (25% to 40%). In contrast, right-sided *S. aureus* endocarditis in intravenous drug users has a more benign clinical course and often responds to a relatively short course of antibiotic therapy. Although *Staphylococcus epidermidis* can be a contaminant organism identified in blood cultures, it also can cause endocarditis. Prosthetic valves are particularly prone to methicillin-resistant *S. epidermidis* infection.

A group of slow-growing, fastidious, gram-negative bacilli is increasingly recognized as causing endocarditis. It is designated the HACEK group: *Haemophilus* species, *Actinobacillus actinomycetemcomitans*, *Cardiobacterium hominis*, *Eikenella corrodens*, and *Kingella* species.

Other microorganisms that can cause endocarditis include fungi (*Candida, Aspergillus,* and

Torulopsis species), which are most common in patients with indwelling lines, in those with prosthetic valves, or in immunosuppressed patients. Fungal infections are characterized by large vegetations and associated with a high rate of embolic complications. Blood cultures may be negative, and the diagnosis may depend on isolation of the organism from removed emboli or at the time of cardiac surgery. Outcome is poor, with a mortality rate approaching 50%.[10]

Predisposing Conditions

While 20% to 30% of patients in clinical series of infective endocarditis have no identifiable predisposing risk factor, most patients have known underlying valvular disease (about 50%), congenital heart disease (4% to 18%), a prosthetic valve (12% to 17%), or a history of intravenous drug use (about 30%) (Table 18–2). Structural heart disease that results in abnormal intracardiac flow patterns, particularly those characterized by high-velocity and turbulent flow streams, is associated with a high risk for endocarditis development. In contrast, structural heart disease associated with relatively laminar, low-velocity flow patterns is not associated with an increased risk. Similarly, intravascular prosthetic material is a risk factor only if associated with abnormal adjacent flow patterns.

Valvular and Congenital Heart Disease

Patients with any type of valvular stenosis or regurgitation are at increased risk for endocarditis (see Table 18–2). A bicuspid aortic valve is a particularly high-risk lesion; about one third of all cases of aortic valve endocarditis occur on bicuspid valves. Degenerative aortic valve disease accounts for an additional 15% of aortic valve endocarditis cases.[11] Mitral valve endocarditis often (in ⅔ of cases) involves a previously normal valve, although patients with myxomatous mitral valve disease, rheumatic disease, or congenital abnormalities of the valve leaflets are at higher risk.

The site of infection tends to be the upstream side of the valve in patients with no evidence for underlying heart disease and in those with valvular regurgitation. However, calcific aortic stenosis is associated with development of vegetations on the aortic side of the leaflets, little aortic regurgitation, and a high prevalence of paravalvular abscess formation. One autopsy series demonstrated ring abscesses in 21 (84%) of 25 cases of aortic valve endocarditis superimposed on a previously stenotic valve, compared with 37 (52%) of 71 cases with a nonstenotic valve.[11] The prevalence of multivalve involvement by endocarditis is estimated to be as high as 24%.

Congenital heart disease characterized by high-velocity or turbulent flow patterns is a risk factor for infective endocarditis. Both patent ductus arteriosus and ventricular septal defects are associated with a high risk of endocarditis, while atrial septal defects are not a risk factor. Vegetations typically are seen in the path of the jet stream—the right ventricular side of a ventricular septal defect (often affecting the tricuspid valve) and the pulmonary artery side of a patent ductus arteriosus. Given the high risk of endocarditis and the low morbidity and mortality rates for surgical or percutaneous closure of a patent ductus arteriosus, most clinicians recommend prophylactic closure of this defect. Although a ventricular septal defect is associated with a risk of infective endocarditis of 1.45 cases per 1000 patient-years,[12] closure of the defect solely to decrease the risk of endocarditis is controversial and is not recommended by most clinicians due to

TABLE 18·2 CONDITIONS PREDISPOSING TO INFECTIVE ENDOCARDITIS		
Condition	**Estimated Risk (per 1000 pt-yrs)**	**Percent of Endocarditis Cases**
Native valve disease		
Aortic stenosis	0.73	10–18%
Aortic regurgitation (often bicuspid valve)	0.4	17–30%
Mitral stenosis	0.17	<1%
Mitral regurgitation (includes mitral valve prolapse)	1.3	21–33%
Pulmonic stenosis	0.09	
Congenital heart disease		4–18%
Ventricular septal defect	1.5	
Patent ductus arteriosus	1.4	
Aortic coarctation	0.7	
Cyanotic congenital disease	8.2	
Tetralogy of Fallot	2.3	
Eisenmenger's syndrome	1.2	
Atrial septal defect	~0	
Hypertrophic cardiomyopathy	Low	
Prosthetic valve		12–17%
IVDU		30–50%

IVDU, intravenous drug use.
Data from references 6, 12, 68, 119, 146, 147, and 148.

the higher surgical mortality and morbidity for this intracardiac repair compared with the less risky extracardiac closure of a patent ductus arteriosus. Some clinicians do recommend closure of a small ventricular septal defect after an episode of endocarditis to decrease the risk of recurrent infection,[13] but this approach is not uniformly accepted.

Patients with surgically repaired valvular or congenital heart disease remain at risk for endocarditis if residual high-velocity or turbulent flow patterns are present, for example, persistent valvular regurgitation. Surgical systemic to pulmonary shunts are prone to infection, and implantation of a prosthetic valve or other prosthetic material substantially increases the risk of endocarditis of this patient group.

Prosthetic Valves and Other Prosthetic Material

Infections of mechanical prosthetic valves typically affect the sewing ring and paravalvular region. Adherence of organisms or thrombus to the metal leaflets or struts is unusual. In contrast, tissue prosthetic valves may show typical valvular vegetations with associated leaflet destruction, often on the downstream side of the valve, although the infection also may affect the sewing ring and paravalvular region. Valved conduits may become infected at the proximal or distal anastomosis and at the valvular level. Homograft valve replacements appear to be relatively resistant to infection, a feature that makes them particularly valuable in the surgical management of endocarditis.

Other types of prosthetic intravascular tissue, such as ascending aortic grafts, mitral annuloplasty rings, permanent pacer leads, and septal defect patches, may become infected, but the risk is quite low. Endocarditis prophylaxis is not generally recommended for these types of prosthetic materials.

Infection of temporary percutaneously inserted intravascular devices, such as central venous lines, temporary pacers, and Swan-Ganz catheters, may result in superimposed endocarditis. Differentiation of transient bacteremia that responds promptly to removal of the device and antibiotics versus endocarditis that requires prolonged antibiotic therapy remains a difficult clinical problem.

Intravenous Drug Use

The use of unprescribed intravenous drugs is associated with a high risk of endocarditis.

Although about one fourth of affected individuals have underlying valve disease, most have no evidence of preexisting structural heart disease. The presumed mechanism of risk in this patient group is numerous episodes of bacteremia, related to poor sterile technique, combined with microvalvular damage from particulates in the injected substances. Infection most often is caused by *S. aureus* and predominantly affects the tricuspid valve.

Systemic Diseases With Impaired Immunologic Function

Immunocompromised patients do not appear to have an increased risk of endocarditis, although when endocarditis does occur, the etiologic agent is more likely to be atypical.[8] Endocarditis is rare in neutropenic, febrile patients, and other explanations for fever often are readily apparent in this group. Endocarditis in patients with acquired immunodeficiency syndrome (AIDS) most often is related to concurrent intravenous drug use.[14] The disease course is different from that of other patients with right-sided endocarditis in that pneumonia and hemodynamic compromise due to sepsis are more common.[15] Patients with diabetes may be at increased risk for endocarditis, possibly related to the increased incidence of bacteremia due to skin, soft tissue, and urinary tract infections.[16]

Valve Destruction and Local Complications

The clinical outcome of patients with infective endocarditis is directly related to the extent of valve destruction and extension of the infective process into adjacent tissues.

Valve Dysfunction

Destruction of valve tissue may lead to regurgitation because of perforation of a valve leaflet, deformity of the coaptation zone, rupture of chordae, or loss of the normal annular and commissural support structures (Fig. 18–4; see also color insert). Even with only minimal tissue destruction, presence of the vegetation may impede normal valve closure and lead to valvular regurgitation. The relatively acute onset of significant valvular regurgitation in patients with endocarditis is poorly tolerated, as the time course of disease precludes the normal adaptive responses of the ventricle and vasculature to volume overload. Clinical evidence of heart failure is common, especially with aortic valve involvement. Al-

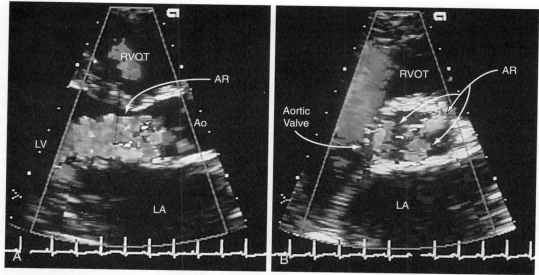

Figure 18·4   Color flow Doppler images in the same patient as in Figure 18·2 show severe aortic regurgitation (AR) due to valve destruction by infective endocarditis in long-axis *(A)* and short-axis *(B)* views. Ao, aorta; LA, left atrium; LV, left ventricle; RVOT, right ventricular outflow tract. (This figure also occurs in the color insert.)

though valvular regurgitation is the norm, rarely, a large vegetation partially occludes the valve orifice and results in functional valvular stenosis,[17] particularly in cases of fungal infection and other organisms associated with extremely large vegetations.

Paravalvular Abscess

Extension of the infectious process into the adjacent valve annulus leads to abscess formation. Paravalvular abscesses are seen most commonly in patients with aortic valve endocarditis and may involve the base of the ventricular septum, including the conduction system (Fig. 18–5). Thus, heart block in a patient with aortic valve endocarditis suggests the possibility of a paravalvular abscess. Extension of aortic annular infection into the contiguous base of the anterior mitral valve leaflet may result in a pseudoaneurysm of the mitral leaflet or an abscess in the mitral-aortic fibrosa.[18–21]

Pericarditis

Paravalvular infection involving the mitral or tricuspid annulus may extend into the adjacent pericardium. Purulent pericarditis also may be caused by a mycotic aneurysm of the proximal aorta, a septic coronary embolus, or a myocardial abscess. Although a rare complication of bacterial endocarditis, pericarditis is associated with an extremely high mortality

rate.[22, 23] A sterile pericardial effusion may result from pericardial inflammation due to an adjacent annular abscess, myocardial abscess, or aortic root abscess.

Aneurysm and Fistula Formation

Rather than forming an abscess, some patients with aortic valve endocarditis develop a

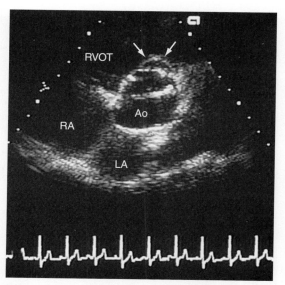

Figure 18·5   This transthoracic short-axis echocardiographic image shows a small, crescentic, echolucent area *(arrows)* adjacent to the aortic valve consistent with a paravalvular abscess. Ao, aorta; LA, left atrium; RA, right atrium; RVOT, right ventricular outflow tract.

sinus of Valsalva aneurysm because of loss of structural integrity in the aortic wall. With continued tissue destruction, aneurysm or abscess formation may culminate in rupture with development of an intracardiac fistula (Fig. 18–6; see also color insert). Aortic annular abscesses may rupture into the right ventricular outflow tract from the right coronary sinus of Valsalva, into the left atrium from the left coronary cusp region, or into the right atrium from the noncoronary cusp region. Acute development of a fistula from the high-pressure aorta into a low-pressure atrium or right ventricle is poorly tolerated hemodynamically.

Embolic Events

In addition to local tissue destruction and direct extension of the infectious process, endocarditis is characterized by systemic manifestations that fall into three broad categories: vascular events, immunologic phenomena, and nonspecific signs of systemic infection.

Valvular vegetations are fragile, mobile masses, often with only a small area of attachment to the valve leaflet, so it is not surprising that fragments or entire vegetations can embolize to the systemic vascular bed in cases of left-sided endocarditis or the pulmonary vascular bed in cases of right-sided endocarditis. Detectable embolization to the cerebral circulation, resulting in transient ischemic attacks

or cerebrovascular accidents, occurs in 10% to 30% of patients with endocarditis. Embolization to the coronary circulation resulting in myocardial ischemia or infarction, particularly to the left coronary artery from an aortic valve vegetation, occurs in 10% of patients.[11] Coronary embolization may be recognized initially by the finding of a regional wall motion abnormality on echocardiography. Embolization to other organs (eg, spleen) may be clinically silent or may result in significant symptoms, sometimes requiring emergent surgical intervention, as in cases of ischemic bowel syndrome or a peripheral arterial occlusion.

There has been substantial interest in defining which patients are at highest risk for embolic events in the hope that embolic events could be prevented in high-risk patents. Although data combined from multiple studies suggest that large, mobile vegetations on the mitral valve are at most risk for embolization, surgical intervention based on vegetation size and appearance alone remains controversial. The risk of embolization with fungal endocarditis is very high, and most clinicians recommend early surgical intervention in this situation to avoid systemic embolic events.[10]

Embolization also may spread the infection and produce a cerebral or peripheral mycotic aneurysm, which can rupture unexpectedly later in the disease course. Renal infarction due to embolism may lead to renal insuffi-

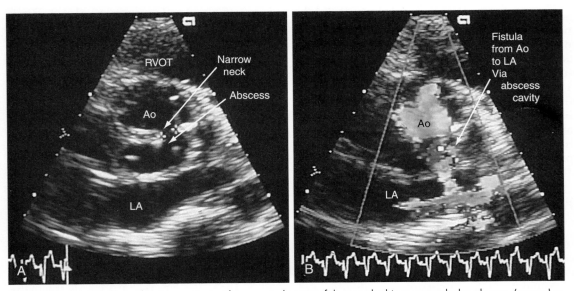

Figure 18·6   *A,* Endocarditis in a patient with an aortic homograft has resulted in a paravalvular abscess *(arrows)* as seen in a parasternal short-axis transthoracic echocardiographic image. *B,* In the same image plane, color flow imaging shows a fistula from the aortic root into the left atrium via the abscess cavity *(arrow).* Ao, aorta; LA, left atrium; RVOT, right ventricular outflow tract. (Illustration *B* also occurs in the color insert.)

ciency. Other causes of renal dysfunction in patients with endocarditis include antibiotic toxicity, focal or diffuse glomerulonephritis related to immune complex deposition, and low renal blood flow due to heart failure. Right-sided embolic events result in localized areas of pulmonary infarction with associated lung abscess formation. In some cases, the course is complicated by development of an empyema.

Immunologic Phenomena

In addition to direct tissue destruction at the site of intracardiac infection and embolization of the valvular vegetations, immune complex–mediated tissue injury is a key component of infective endocarditis. Circulating immune complexes are found in 84% to 100% of patients with infective endocarditis, with levels of circulating immune complexes correlating with disease duration and hypocomplementemia.[24–27] The available evidence suggests that circulating immune complexes are formed during episodes of antibody excess and are then deposited in skin, synovium, and the glomerular basement membrane,[28, 29] rather than being the consequence of antigen-antibody complexing within the tissue.[30] The circulating immune complexes most likely originate in the valvular vegetations and may contribute to local destruction of the valve.[31] The presence of IgM and polymeric IgA rheumatoid factors in patients with infective endocarditis may contribute to persistent bacteremia by exerting an antiphagocytic effect by blocking the IgG Fc terminus or by impairing complement fixation to the complexed IgG molecule.[32]

The predominant clinical manifestations of immune-mediated injury include polyarthritis and glomerulonephritis. Typically, IgG and early complement components (C1q, C4, C3) are deposited in the glomerular basement membrane in an irregular pattern typical of immune complex injury,[33] with the IgG antibody being specific for the infecting bacterial organism.[34] An early autopsy study indicated that 33% of untreated patients had diffuse glomerulonephritis, and 48% had focal glomerulonephritis.[35] In a later series of patients dying despite antibiotic therapy, focal glomerulonephritis was seen in 8%, and diffuse glomerulonephritis was seen in 14% of cases.[36] Both forms of renal involvement are immune mediated, and the presence and pattern of glomerulonephritis are related to the specific organism (eg, higher prevalence among patients infected with *S. aureus*) and duration of disease.[32]

The levels of circulating immune complexes fall with effective therapy, whereas persistent or recurrent elevations in circulating immune complexes suggest the failure of medical therapy.[32] Although plasmapheresis can decrease circulating immune complex levels and ameliorate systemic immune-mediated injury, the primary treatment for the extracardiac manifestations of infective endocarditis is effective medical and surgical therapy of the primary intracardiac infection. With effective therapy, immune complexes decrease, and the systemic signs of immune-mediated injury resolve.[32]

DIAGNOSIS

History

Fever, the most common presenting symptom of patients with endocarditis, occurs in 90% to 100% of all cases. The prevalence of other nonspecific symptoms varies widely in different series, with malaise in 12% to 94% of patients, anorexia in about 75%, weight loss in 50%, and back pain in about 40%.[37–40] A neurologic event or mental status change is the presenting symptom of 15% of subjects.[41]

Physical Examination

Nonspecific signs are common on physical examination of patients with endocarditis. Findings at presentation include splinter hemorrhages in 15%, splenomegaly in 20% to 30%, and petechiae in 15% to 50%.[8] The classic finding of a change in murmur or new murmur is found in only 10% to 25% of patients. However, a preexisting, unchanged murmur is found in 85% to 95% of subjects, emphasizing the potential for endocarditis in patients with preexisting valvular disease.[42, 43] The absence of a murmur does not exclude the diagnosis of endocarditis; 5% to 15% of patients have no murmur detected on auscultation despite later confirmation of a diagnosis of endocarditis.[42, 43]

Systemic Signs and Laboratory Data

In addition to fever, evidence of embolic events or of immunologic phenomena supports a diagnosis of endocarditis. Historically, peripheral findings were helpful in establishing the diagnosis of endocarditis. However, these findings tend to occur late in the disease course, and with earlier diagnosis and more effective treatment, the classic peripheral manifestations of endocarditis are seen infrequently. Osler's nodes are seen in only 10% to 15%, Janeway lesions in 3% to 5%, and Roth spots in 2% to 10% of patients.[44–46] Even so, these findings appear to be specific, if not sensitive, for the diagnosis of endocarditis. Osler's nodes can be recognized on the fingertips as a painful, pea-size, bluish nodule with an erythematous base. Janeway lesions are painless, small, pink macules on the fingertips. Roth spots are small areas of retinal bleeding with a central pale area seen on funduscopic examination. It remains controversial whether these classic manifestations of endocarditis represent embolic events or immunologic phenomena.[32]

Laboratory examination of patients with infective endocarditis frequently reveals nonspecific signs of a systemic disease, including an elevated erythrocyte sedimentation rate in 90%, hematuria in 25%, a positive rheumatoid factor in 25% to 50%, anemia in 50% to 80%, and circulating immune complexes in more than 95% of patients.[26]

Blood Cultures

One of the major criteria for the diagnosis of endocarditis is blood cultures persistently positive for organisms typical for endocarditis. To document bacteremia, identify the causative agent, and determine antibiotic sensitivities, a minimum of three sets of blood cultures are drawn from different sites over a 24-hour period prior to antibiotic therapy.[8] Although the causative organism is isolated from the first two sets in 98% of cases,[47] additional samples may be needed if the patient has received prior antibiotic therapy. Arterial blood samples have no advantage over venous blood cultures.

In addition to standard blood culture techniques (ie, trypticase soy and thioglycollate broth bottles), routine subcultures should be performed. Special media may be needed for growth of nutritionally variant streptococci. A prolonged incubation period (at least 3 weeks) should be allowed for apparently negative cultures.[8]

About 10% to 20% of cases that are later proved to be endocarditis at surgery or autopsy have negative blood cultures. Culture-negative endocarditis is more likely if the patient receives any antibiotic therapy (even oral) before cultures are obtained,[48] underlining the importance of drawing blood cultures

in febrile patients with risk factors for endocarditis. Other factors associated with negative blood cultures are fungal infection, uremia, infection with nutritionally deficit organisms, and advanced disease. Some rare forms of endocarditis, such as Q fever, can only be diagnosed by serology.

Echocardiography

Echocardiography is central to the evaluation of the patient with suspected or known endocarditis. In the patient with suspected endocarditis, echocardiography, particularly the transesophageal approach, has a high sensitivity and specificity for detection of valvular vegetations. In addition, differentiation of infective endocarditis from other cardiac structural abnormalities is possible.

Detection of Valvular Vegetations

The reported sensitivity of transthoracic echocardiography for detection of valvular vegetations varies from 36% to 90% in series of patients with suspected endocarditis using surgical or autopsy findings as the standard of reference.[49–55] This degree of variability reflects the fact that detection of vegetations depends on a meticulous examination with the use of nonstandard echocardiographic image planes, optimal instrument settings, adequate examination time, and an experienced operator. Image quality is limited in some individuals due to poor ultrasound tissue penetration related to body habitus, interposed lung tissue, or shadowing by prosthetic valves and conduits. The transesophageal approach offers superior image quality, particularly for posterior cardiac structures such as the mitral valve, and has a much higher sensitivity for detection of valvular vegetations, ranging from 82% to 100% in different series (Fig. 18–7).[49, 52–56]

The specificity of echocardiography for detection of valvular vegetations is more difficult to ascertain since most series include only subjects with documented endocarditis. In addition, the presence or absence of a vegetation can only be confirmed in subjects who die or undergo valvular surgery. To avoid this selection and ascertainment bias, other studies have included all patients with suspected endocarditis, using subsequent clinical outcome over a defined follow-up period as the reference standard for the absence of endocarditis. Using this approach, the specificity of echocardiography is estimated to be 91% to 98% for trans-

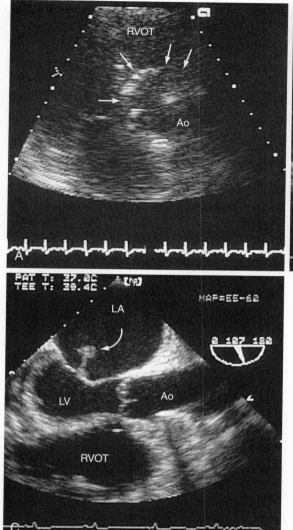

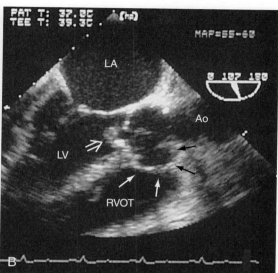

Figure 18·7 The improved image quality of transesophageal compared with transthoracic echocardiography is illustrated by this examination. *A,* Transthoracic images were of limited quality, although distortion and irregularity of the right coronary sinus of Valsalva was observed *(arrows). B,* Transesophageal images clearly show an abscess cavity in the region of the right coronary sinus of Valsalva *(arrows)* and an aortic valve vegetation with prolapse of the leaflet because of valve destruction *(open arrow). C,* With slight angulation of the transesophageal probe, a small, mobile mitral valve vegetation *(curved arrow)* is seen. Ao, aorta; LA, left atrium; LV, left ventricle; RVOT, right ventricular outflow tract.

thoracic and 91% to 100% for transesophageal imaging.[51–53, 55, 57]

By echocardiography, an intracardiac mass is diagnosed as a vegetation based on its shape, location, echogenicity, and motion. Typically, a vegetation is an irregularly shaped mass, with an ultrasound signal intensity less than that of myocardium, attached to the upstream side of a valve. This mass shows rapid oscillating motion that is independent of the motion of the valve itself. Vegetations vary in length and width from a few millimeters to several centimeters. Most vegetations have a narrow attachment point and are longer than wide, but there is wide variation in the size and shape of vegetations. Occasional vegetations have a broad base and are relatively immobile.[58]

Other echocardiographic findings that may be mistaken for an infected valvular vegetation include ultrasound imaging artifacts, variations of normal anatomy, other intracardiac masses (eg, tumor, thrombus), nonbacterial thrombotic endocarditis, and old, healed valvular vegetations (Fig. 18–8). Careful imaging technique and interpretation by an experienced observer limit the misidentification of beam width artifacts, reverberations, and multipath artifacts. Imaging the suspected structure in at least two imaging planes, preferably from different acoustic windows, minimizes the likelihood of imaging artifacts.

Numerous variations of normal intracardiac anatomy are increasingly recognized as the resolution of our imaging techniques improves.

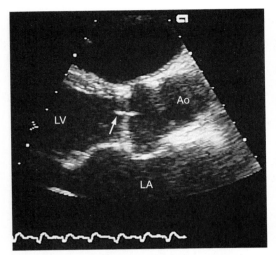

Figure 18·8 This parasternal long-axis view shows a Lambl's excrescence *(arrow)* at the aortic valve closure line during diastole. This normal structure may be mistaken for a valvular vegetation. Ao, aorta; LA, left atrium; LV, left ventricle.

Normal anatomic variants that move chaotically, including a right atrial Eustachian valve or Chiari network, or a Lambl's excrescence on the aortic or mitral valve, are especially likely to be mistaken for vegetations.[59]

Since endocarditis occurs most often in patients with preexisting valvular disease, the underlying structural abnormalities of the valve may mask the presence of valvular vegetations (eg, shadowing by calcification in degenerative valve disease) or may simulate a vegetation (eg, partial flail leaflet in myxomatous mitral valve disease). Comparing the current echocardiographic examination with previous studies may help resolve these issues. Alternatively, the superior image quality of transesophageal imaging may provide definitive differentiation of underlying valve disease from superimposed infection. In some cases, even with all these approaches, a clear distinction cannot be made, and clinical decision making must rely on other diagnostic criteria.

Intracardiac thrombi and tumors may have shapes and echogenicity patterns similar to those of valvular vegetations. However, intracardiac thrombus formation occurs most often in the ventricular apex or in the left atrium and rarely exhibits the chaotic motion characteristic of a valvular vegetation. While most cardiac tumors are readily differentiated from valvular vegetations by their location and appearance, a papillary fibroelastoma may be indistinguishable from a valvular vegetation. In

this situation, bacteriologic results and other clinical findings are key to the correct diagnosis.

The valvular lesions of nonbacterial thrombotic endocarditis (ie, Libman-Sacks vegetations) differ from infected vegetations in size, shape, and location; they are small (3–4 mm), verrucose, sessile masses typically located at the valve closure line (Fig. 18–9).[60, 61] A definitive diagnosis for an individual patient depends on correlation with other clinical findings and the results of blood cultures.

Echocardiographic evaluation of prosthetic valves for endocarditis is particularly difficult due to shadowing and reverberations from the valve prosthesis. Transesophageal imaging is especially helpful for evaluation of prosthetic mitral valves, offering posterior views of the valve apparatus that allow detection of paravalvular infection. Aortic valve prostheses are best evaluated using a combination of transthoracic and transesophageal views, since the posterior sewing ring is obscured on the transthoracic views while the anterior sewing ring is obscured on the transesophageal views. Normal postoperative changes with prosthetic valves, including prominent pledgets and mobile suture material, may make interpretation problematic. With a prosthetic conduit, images may be suboptimal from all approaches because of masking of the conduit lumen. Even so, transesophageal echocardiography should be

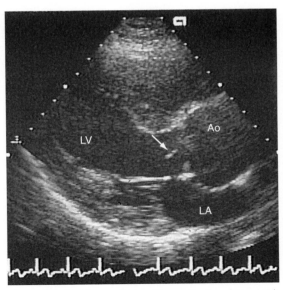

Figure 18·9 This parasternal long-axis view during mid-diastole shows the typical appearance of nonbacterial thrombotic endocarditis *(arrow)*. Ao, aorta; LA, left atrium; LV, left ventricle.

considered in these cases, as improved image quality and a different acoustic window may allow acquisition of diagnostic images.

Serial echocardiographic studies in patients being treated for endocarditis have shown that vegetations tend to decrease in size and increase in echogenicity during the healing process.[58, 62] However, residual vegetations still may be seen months to years after the active infection. Although the relative immobility and increased echogenicity of these healed vegetations helps differentiate them from active disease, exclusion of the possibility of active infection depends on blood cultures and clinical criteria.

Evaluation of Valvular and Ventricular Dysfunction

Besides identification of valvular vegetations, echocardiography is essential for evaluating the degree of valve destruction and consequent valve regurgitation in patients with infective endocarditis. The combined use of two-dimensional echocardiography and pulsed, continuous wave, and color flow Doppler enables reliable evaluation of hemodynamic severity (see Chapter 3), and this information can be used for making decisions regarding the need for and timing of cardiac surgery. Cardiac catheterization rarely is performed in patents with active endocarditis, as adequate data can be obtained noninvasively

and given the potential risk of dislodging a valvular vegetation. Echocardiography also allows evaluation of global and regional left and right ventricular systolic function, and estimation of pulmonary pressures and other intracardiac hemodynamics.

Role in Clinical Decision Making

Given the high sensitivity and specificity of echocardiography for detection of valvular vegetations, it has become an essential component of the diagnostic evaluation of patients with suspected endocarditis. Transthoracic echocardiography and blood cultures should be performed whenever the diagnosis of endocarditis is suspected on clinical grounds (Fig. 18–10). Results from one series suggest that a definite diagnosis of infective endocarditis is confirmed in only about 25% of patients with suspected endocarditis,[52] and prompt exclusion of the diagnosis may reduce costs and direct attention toward alternate diagnoses.

Transesophageal imaging should be performed promptly in patients with suspected prosthetic valve endocarditis, given the low accuracy of transthoracic imaging in this situation.[58] However, the role of transesophageal echocardiography in diagnosing patients with suspected native valve endocarditis is more controversial. Some investigators insist that transesophageal imaging is needed in all suspected cases.[63] At the other extreme, some

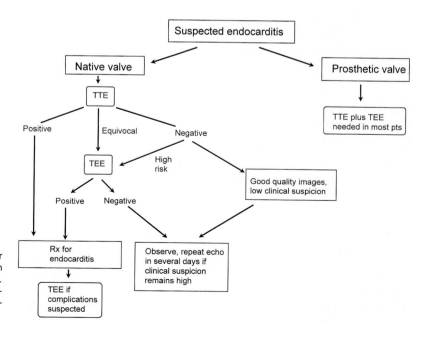

Figure 18·10 Flow chart for the role of echocardiography in the diagnosis (Rx) of endocarditis. TEE, transesophageal echocardiography; TTE, transthoracic echocardiography.

investigators suggest transesophageal echocardiography is needed only if the transthoracic study is technically inadequate or indicates an intermediate probability of disease.[64] In my view, the decision to perform transesophageal imaging in patients with suspected native valve endocarditis should be based on the results of the transthoracic study and the pretest likelihood of disease. An estimate of the probability that the echocardiographic findings represent a vegetation (ie, low probability, possible, probable, or almost certain) is more useful than a bivariate (ie, yes or no) description.[52]

A high-quality transthoracic study with definite evidence of valvular vegetations confirms the diagnosis of endocarditis. Transesophageal imaging can be reserved for evaluation of high-risk patients or those with suspected paravalvular abscess. If a meticulously performed transthoracic study with good to excellent image quality shows no evidence of valvular vegetations or valve dysfunction and the clinical likelihood of disease is low (eg, negative blood cultures, no embolic events), clinical observation is warranted. If the clinical features continue to support the possibility of endocarditis, transesophageal imaging is appropriate. Alternatively, a repeat transthoracic study may be performed to reevaluate the possibility of valvular vegetations or valve destruction.

If the pretest likelihood of endocarditis is high (eg, positive blood cultures, embolic events), and the transthoracic study is negative, transesophageal imaging is indicated because of its higher sensitivity for detecting valvular vegetations. Exclusion of the possibility of endocarditis in these patients avoids unnecessary delays in evaluating other diagnostic possibilities and avoids unnecessary treatment. In one study, the negative predictive value of transesophageal echocardiography for native valve endocarditis was 100% (40 patients), and the results led to a 60% reduction in total antibiotic therapy.[65] Another prospective study of 105 patients with suspected endocarditis[57] also demonstrated the high negative predictive value of transesophageal echocardiography (92%). Three of the five missed cases did have evidence of endocarditis found on a subsequent study, suggesting that repeat evaluation after several days is appropriate if the pretest likelihood of disease remains high.

When the transthoracic study is poor quality, equivocal, or nondiagnostic, transesophageal imaging should be strongly considered. While research studies define an echocardiographic study as positive or negative, the study result often is not so definitive when evaluating individual patients. Sometimes, the echocardiographic appearance suggests a vegetation but is somewhat atypical. In other cases, it is unclear whether a valvular vegetation is superimposed on underlying valvular disease or the primary valve disease has progressed without infection. More importantly, the quality of the transthoracic images must be taken into account. Excellent images allow high diagnostic certainty, and inadequate images produce a nondiagnostic study. In between, the level of diagnostic certainty depends on the clarity with which each valve is seen. In all these situations, transesophageal imaging provides high-quality images that provide more definitive clinical data, allowing efficient and accurate patient management decisions.

Clinical Diagnostic Criteria

The clinical diagnosis of infective endocarditis can be difficult because of the protean but often nonspecific manifestations of disease and the wide variability in the clinical presentation. In the early 1980s, strict clinical criteria for the diagnosis of endocarditis were proposed by Pelletier and Petersdorf,[39] with later modification by von Reyn and associates.[66] These criteria (or minor variations) are the basis for inclusion of subjects in nearly all published clinical and surgical series of infective endocarditis.

In brief, these clinical criteria diagnosed endocarditis as *definite* if histologic evidence of intracardiac endothelial infection was found at cardiac surgery, by embolectomy, or at autopsy. Endocarditis was *probable* if uniformly positive blood cultures were documented for a patient with a new regurgitant murmur or for a patient with underlying heart disease and evidence of embolic events. If blood cultures were negative or intermittently positive, the combination of fever, a new regurgitant murmur, and embolic events was required for a diagnosis of probable endocarditis. Endocarditis was considered to be *possible* if only some of these criteria were met.

One of the limitations of these clinical criteria for the diagnosis of endocarditis was the difficulty in demonstrating endocardial infection directly in a living patient other than at the time of surgery. This limitation now can be remedied by the high accuracy of noninvasive echocardiographic techniques for demonstration of valvular vegetations and the secondary consequences of infection. New criteria for the clinical diagnosis of endocarditis that incorporate echocardiographic findings have been developed by the Duke Endocarditis Service (Table 18–3).[67] These criteria still include pathologic demonstration of typical infected lesions as being diagnostic for infective endocarditis. In the absence of pathologic material, the clinical diagnosis is based on a combination of major and minor criteria.

Major criteria for the diagnosis of infective endocarditis are (1) persistently positive blood cultures with typical microorganisms and (2) echocardiographic evidence of endocarditis, defined as an oscillating valvular vegetation, intracardiac abscess, prosthetic valve de-

hiscence, or new valvular regurgitation. The presence of both major criteria excludes patients with other explanations for an abnormal echocardiographic examination and patients with bacteremia but without echocardiographic evidence for endocarditis.

Minor criteria for the diagnosis of infective endocarditis include a predisposing cardiac condition or intravenous drug use, fever, vascular events, immunologic phenomena, other microbiologic evidence, and echocardiographic findings that are consistent with (but not definitive for) a diagnosis of endocarditis. Meeting both major criteria, one major and three minor, or five minor criteria supports the diagnosis of definite infective endocarditis.

TABLE 18·3 DUKE CRITERIA FOR DEFINITE INFECTIVE ENDOCARDITIS

Pathologic Criteria

Microorganisms: demonstrated by culture or histology in a vegetation, *or* in a vegetation that has embolized, *or* in an intracardiac abscess, *or*

Pathologic lesions: vegetation or intracardiac abscess present, confirmed by histology showing active endocarditis

Clinical Criteria

Major criteria

Positive blood culture for infective endocarditis

Typical microorganism for infective endocarditis from two separate blood cultures

Viridans streptococci,* *Streptococcus bovis*, HACEK group, *or*

Community-acquired *Staphylococcus aureus* or enterococci in the absence of a primary focus, *or*

Persistently positive blood culture, defined as recovery of a microorganism consistent with infective endocarditis from

(i) Blood cultures drawn more than 12 hours apart, *or*

(ii) All of three or a majority of four or more separate blood cultures, with first and last drawn at least 1 hour apart

Evidence of endocardial involvement

Positive echocardiogram for infective endocarditis

(i) Oscillating intracardiac mass, on valve or supporting structures, *or* in the path of regurgitant jets, *or* on implanted material, in the absence of an alternative anatomic explanation, *or*

(ii) Abscess, *or*

(iii) New partial dehiscence of prosthetic valve, *or*

New valvular regurgitation (increase or change in preexisting murmur not sufficient)

Minor criteria

Predisposition: predisposing heart condition *or* intravenous drug use

Fever: ≥38.0°C (100.4°F)

Vascular phenomena: major arterial emboli, septic pulmonary infarcts, mycotic aneurysm, intracranial hemorrhage, conjunctival hemorrhages, Janeway lesions

Immunologic phenomena: glomerulonephritis, Osler's nodes, Roth spots, rheumatoid factor

Microbiologic evidence: positive blood culture but not meeting major criterion as noted previously† *or* serologic evidence of active infection with organism consistent with infective endocarditis

Echocardiogram: consistent with infective endocarditis but not meeting major criterion as noted previously

Diagnosis

2 major criteria *or*

1 major and 3 minor criteria *or*

5 minor criteria

HACEK, *Haemophilus* spp., *Actinobacillus actinomycetemcomitans, Cardiobacterium hominis, Eikenella* spp., and *Kingella kingae.*

*Including nutritional variant strains.

†Excluding single positive cultures for coagulase-negative staphylococci and organisms that do not cause endocarditis.

Reprinted by permission of the publisher from Durack DT, Lukes AS, Bright DK: New criteria for diagnosis of infective endocarditis: utilization of specific echocardiographic findings. Duke Endocarditis Service. Am J Med 1994;96:200–209. Copyright 1994 by Excerpta Medica Inc.

Patients with lesser numbers of criteria still may have endocarditis (ie, possible cases), but the diagnosis is less certain. The diagnosis of endocarditis can be rejected if there is a clear alternate cause for the clinical symptoms and signs, the clinical abnormalities resolve after 4 days or fewer of antibiotic therapy, or if surgery or pathologic examination fails to reveal evidence of endocarditis after up to 4 days of antibiotic therapy.

The clinical validity of the Duke criteria in a series of 405 consecutive cases of suspected endocarditis was high, with 80% (55/69) of cases confirmed by pathology classified as definite endocarditis, compared with only 51% (35/69) of confirmed cases using the older clinical criteria.[67] In a separate clinical series of patients who did not have pathologic confirmation, the Duke criteria classified significantly more suspected cases as definite endocarditis than the older von Reyn criteria (30 of 51 versus 10 of 51).[68] Of the 10 patients with pathologic demonstration of vegetations at surgery, all 10 (100%) were correctly diagnosed by the Duke criteria, but only 5 (50%) of 10 were correctly diagnosed by the von Reyn criteria. In addition, the negative predictive value of the Duke criteria has been estimated as 92% or higher based on subsequent clinical outcomes of 48 patients for whom the diagnosis was rejected.[69]

Differential Diagnosis

Adherence to the Duke criteria eliminates most other clinical presentations that may initially suggest endocarditis. Although the possibility of endocarditis always must be considered, most febrile episodes in patients with underlying heart disease result from other discernible causes. Nonbacterial thrombotic endocarditis is differentiated from infective endocarditis by the clinical setting (ie, patients with immune-mediated or malignant disease) and by no evidence of infection. In patients with embolic or cerebrovascular events, other causes should be sought when blood cultures and echocardiography demonstrate no evidence of endocarditis. Although endocarditis remains in the differential diagnosis of patients with fever of unknown origin, the use of transthoracic and transesophageal echocardiography nearly always identifies cases of fever due to infective endocarditis.

A common clinical dilemma is the patient with positive blood cultures and a transcutaneously inserted indwelling catheter. If bacteremia resolves with removal of the device and brief antibiotic therapy, endocarditis is unlikely. If the clinical situation requires treatment without removal of the intravascular device, diagnosis may be more difficult, but echocardiographic imaging in conjunction with the Duke criteria usually permits a reliable diagnosis.[67, 69]

LEFT-SIDED NATIVE VALVE DISEASE

Disease Course and Prognosis

The disease course in patients with left-sided native valve endocarditis is directly related to the specific etiologic agent and the degree of valve destruction (Fig. 18–11). A poor outcome usually is caused by heart failure, renal failure, embolic events, or rupture of a mycotic aneurysm. With prompt initiation of appropriate antibiotic therapy, defervescence occurs in 3 to 7 days, although blood cultures may remain positive for 1 or 2 weeks even with effective therapy.[70]

Elderly subjects often have an atypical presentation of endocarditis, with a lower incidence of fever and leukocytosis than younger patients,[71] which may lead to delay in making the correct diagnosis and instituting treatment.[72] Although the infecting organisms and echocardiographic findings are similar in elderly and younger patients, several studies have shown that the higher prevalence of prosthetic valves and comorbid disease, in conjunction with the delay in diagnosis, lead to a worse outcome for elderly patients.[73, 74]

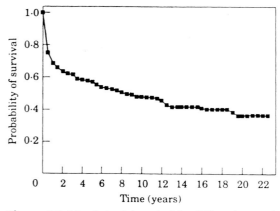

Figure 18·11 Actuarial survival for 330 patients with infective endocarditis hospitalized between 1970 and 1982 in Hôpital Cardiologique, Lyon, France. (From Delahaye F, Ecochard R, deGevigney G, et al: The long-term prognosis of infective endocarditis. Eur Heart J 1995;161:48.)

With current combined medical and surgical therapy for endocarditis, traditional clinical predictors of outcome, such as severe regurgitation and heart failure, have become indications for surgical intervention and are less useful for predicting death. Several studies have reexamined clinical and echocardiographic predictors of outcome of patients with infective endocarditis in the surgical era. Risk factors for in-hospital death include age, aortic valve involvement, abscess formation, systemic embolism, mycotic aneurysm formation, and infection with *S. aureus*.[50, 75–77]

Valve Dysfunction and Heart Failure

Valvular vegetations typically lead to valvular regurgitation through destruction of the valve apparatus or impairment of valve closure. However, the degree of regurgitation varies, and just as not all patients with endocarditis have a detectable murmur, about 1% to 5% of patients with definite endocarditis have no echocardiographic evidence of valvular regurgitation. The absence of regurgitation despite valve infection most often results from a vegetation at the base of the leaflet without associated leaflet perforation. When present, regurgitation of the affected valve is mild (in about 10% to 25%) or moderate (in about 25% of patients) initially, with severe regurgitation in only about one third of patients at presentation.[50, 52, 62]

No data have been published on the use of afterload reduction therapy to decrease the degree of valvular regurgitation in patients with infective endocarditis. While these agents may be helpful for immediate hemodynamic stabilization, a significant effect on outcome is unlikely since the underlying problem is progressive valve destruction. In addition, the short time frame of an endocarditis episode makes demonstration of a substantial effect on left ventricular size and systolic function or clinical outcome unlikely.

The primary causes of death of patients with infective endocarditis include heart failure secondary to valvular regurgitation, consequences of embolic events, rupture of a mycotic aneurysm, and renal failure.[16] The reported incidence of heart failure varies from 20% to 80% in different clinical series.[39, 50, 78, 79] Some of the reported variability in the diagnosis of heart failure may reflect the different clinical definitions or patient populations in the studies.

The diagnosis of heart failure is straightforward, relying on typical symptoms, physical examination, and chest radiographic findings. The diagnosis is confirmed by an echocardiographic examination demonstrating severe valvular regurgitation. Associated left ventricular systolic dysfunction is uncommon and may be related to the acute volume overload state, although myocarditis rarely complicates infective endocarditis.

The onset of heart failure, even mild in severity, mandates careful consideration of surgical intervention, given the poor prognosis with medical therapy alone once there is significant valvular regurgitation (the predominant cause of heart failure).[50, 77, 80] Acute, severe heart failure prompts consideration of acute structural failure, such as rupture of a paravalvular abscess, which also can be diagnosed by echocardiography. While decisions regarding surgical management are in progress, heart failure can be managed with standard medical therapy, including diuretics and afterload reduction, although severe cases may require invasive hemodynamic monitoring. In patients with acute mitral regurgitation, placement of an intraaortic balloon counterpulsation device may allow stabilization before surgery. With aortic regurgitation, the focus is on intravenous pharmacologic therapy, as counterpulsation may worsen the backflow across the aortic valve. In either case, valve surgery should be performed promptly, regardless of the response to medical therapy, as the onset of heart failure indicates extensive valve destruction and predicts a poor outcome without surgical therapy.[80, 81]

Embolic Events

The disease course of native left-sided endocarditis is complicated by systemic embolization in about 30% of cases.[49, 50, 82–84] The risk of embolization decreases over time during antimicrobial therapy from 13 cases per 1000 patient-days in the first week of therapy to less than 1.2 cases per 1000 patient-days after the second week (Fig. 18–12).[85]

Potential predictors of systemic embolization include the etiologic agent, the valve affected, and the size, shape, and mobility of the vegetation on echocardiography. Even when there is good agreement between observers about the characteristics of the vegetation,[86] it has been difficult to assess the importance of these potential predictors because of the small sample sizes in most series. In addition, there may be a bias against demonstrating a relationship between echocardiographic findings and

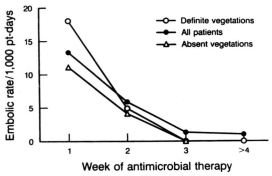

Figure 18·12 Incidence of embolic events among patients with infective endocarditis. (From Steckelberg JM, Murphy JG, Ballard D, et al: Emboli in infective endocarditis: the prognostic value of echocardiography. Ann Intern Med 1991;114:637.)

embolic events when the echocardiogram is performed after the event, since the vegetation is no longer on the affected valve but instead is at the site of embolization. While some studies suggest that vegetation size is not a risk factor for embolization,[85] the overall published data comparing vegetation size on echocardiography with subsequent embolic events do appear to support a relationship between vegetation size and embolic events, with emboli occurring in 19% of those with a vegetation 10 mm or smaller in size and in 33% of those with larger vegetations (Table 18–4).[49, 50] Embolism also appears to be associated with mitral (versus aortic) valve vegetations.[49, 50] The risk of embolization with a specific microorganism is less clear, as different organisms appear to be risk factors in different series.[50, 85]

In an echocardiographic study of 204 patients with endocarditis (148 with native valve infection), echocardiographic predictors of complications (ie, persistent infection, embolism, heart failure, surgery, and death) on multivariate analysis were vegetation size, extent, and mobility and not patient age, gender, vegetation site, or the infecting microorganism (Fig. 18–13).[82]

Persistent Infection and Paravalvular Abscess

Persistent clinical evidence of infection indicates inadequate medical therapy, with possible development of a paravalvular abscess. In autopsy series, paravalvular abscess complicates up to 60% of cases of aortic valve endocarditis,[11] and mitral annular abscess occurs in about 16% of mitral endocarditis cases (Fig. 18–14).[87] Although the incidence of paravalvular abscess may be overestimated in autopsy series, clinical series also suggest a high incidence of paravalvular aortic abscess formation (23% in one prospective series) and a lower rate of mitral annular abscess formation (15%).[88] Again, these estimates may be high since only patients with surgical or autopsy confirmation of the diagnosis were included. The outcome of patients with endocarditis and paravalvular abscess is poor with a hospital mortality rate of 23%, compared with 14% for those without an abscess.[88]

Abscess formation is suspected clinically

TABLE 18·4   SIZE OF VEGETATION BY TWO-DIMENSIONAL ECHOCARDIOGRAPHY AND RISK OF EMBOLISM

| Study | Patients | Number of Emboli | Patients With Embolism | | P Value |
			No Veg or ≤10 mm	Veg >10 mm	
Lutas et al.	76	17	16% (8/50)	45% (9/26)	0.06‡
Buda et al.*	42	14	26% (8/31)	55% (6/11)	0.08‡
Wann et al.†	21	7	21% (3/14)	57% (4/7)	0.16§
Wong et al.	31	6	20% (3/15)	19% (3/16)	0.64§
Jaffe et al.	50	10	11% (2/18)	26% (8/32)	0.19§
Total	251	56	19% (24/128)	33% (30/92)	0.018‡

*Excludes patients with right-sided endocarditis.
†Vegetation size graded qualitatively on 1+ to 3+ scale; 3+ was considered >10 mm.
‡Chi square analysis.
§Fisher's exact test.
Data from Lutas et al: Am Heart J 1986;112:107; Buda et al: Am Heart J 1986;112:1291; Wann et al: Circulation 1979;60:728; Wong et al: Arch Intern Med 1983;143:1874.
From Jaffe WM, Morgan DE, Pearlman AS, Otto CM: Infective endocarditis, 1983–1988: echocardiographic findings and factors influencing morbidity and mortality. J Am Coll Cardiol 1990;15:1227–1233; reprinted with permission from the American College of Cardiology.

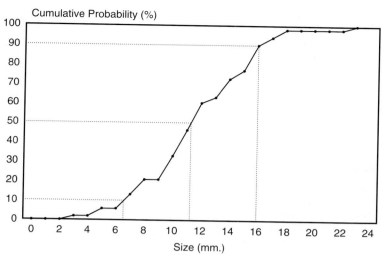

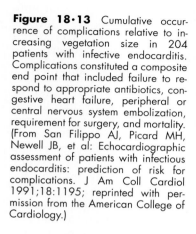

Figure 18·13 Cumulative occurrence of complications relative to increasing vegetation size in 204 patients with infective endocarditis. Complications constituted a composite end point that included failure to respond to appropriate antibiotics, congestive heart failure, peripheral or central nervous system embolization, requirement for surgery, and mortality. (From San Filippo AJ, Picard MH, Newell JB, et al: Echocardiographic assessment of patients with infectious endocarditis: prediction of risk for complications. J Am Coll Cardiol 1991;18:1195; reprinted with permission from the American College of Cardiology.)

when there is evidence of persistent infection despite adequate antibiotic therapy (eg, fever, persistent positive blood cultures). With aortic valve endocarditis, involvement of the base of the septum by the abscess may lead to first-degree or higher grades of atrioventricular block. With mitral valve endocarditis, a pericardial effusion suggests involvement of the adjacent mitral annulus. In many cases, the diagnosis of paravalvular abscess is made at the time of echocardiographic evaluation, often before the onset of obvious clinical signs.

Paravalvular abscess may be recognized on transthoracic echocardiography in some cases (sensitivity of 28% to 43%, specificity of 99%), but is best evaluated by transesophageal imaging (sensitivity of 87% to 90%, specificity of 95%).[20, 88] An abscess is recognized echocardio-

graphically as an abnormal echo-lucent deformity of the paravalvular region or sometimes as a relatively echo-dense paravalvular mass. (See Figs. 18–5, 18–6, and 18–7.) There may or may not be evidence of blood flow in the abscess cavity. When blood flow is observed, the abscess cavity may appear pulsatile, particularly if located in the intervalvular fibrosa.[20] Although it sometimes is difficult to distinguish between paravalvular deformities due to an abscess and normal anatomic structures seen in oblique image planes, interobserver variability for detection of abscess by echocardiography is only 3% to 4%.[21, 58, 88, 89] The accuracy of echocardiographic evaluation is likely to improve as three-dimensional imaging and reconstruction techniques become more widely available.

An aortic root abscess may lead to formation of a sinus of Valsalva aneurysm due to weakening of the structural integrity of the aortic wall. These aneurysms may rupture into adjacent cardiac chambers, particularly the right ventricular outflow tract, the right atrium, or the left atrium. Sinus of Valsalva aneurysms and the presence of a fistula can easily be demonstrated by echocardiography. An aortic annular abscess also may extend into the base of the contiguous anterior mitral leaflet, leading to pseudoaneurysm formation, which appears as a deformity of the anterior leaflet protruding into the left atrium. This deformity may be associated with mitral leaflet perforation, mitral valve vegetations, and mitral regurgitation.[20, 21] Rupture of the aortic-mitral intervalvular fibrosa with a fistula formed from the aortic root to left atrium also has been described.

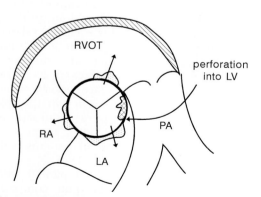

Figure 18·14 This schematic diagram shows the close relationship between the aortic valve and adjacent structures. An aortic annular abscess can rupture into the left ventricle (LV), left atrium (LA), right atrium (RA), or right ventricular outflow tract (RVOT).

A mitral annular abscess is much less likely to rupture because of its anatomic location. Mitral annular involvement can result in purulent pericarditis, a largely fatal complication, by direct extension of infection into the pericardial space or by rupture of the abscess into the pericardium. Aortic and mitral annular abscesses are best treated surgically, unless the extent of tissue destruction is so wide as to preclude surgical debridement.

Medical Therapy

The basic principles for medical therapy of infective endocarditis include the use of high doses of parenteral antibiotics effective against the specific microorganism. After isolation of the etiologic agent, the minimal inhibiting concentration (MIC) and minimal bactericidal concentration (MBC) are determined for the standard antibiotics used.[8] Guidelines for antibiotic treatment of the most common agents causing infective endocarditis in adults have been developed by the American Heart Association and are summarized in Table 18–5.[75]

Antibiotic therapy is monitored based on the clinical response to treatment. Measurement of the serum bacterial titer (ie, the highest dilution of the patient's serum that kills a standard inoculum of the organism in vitro) is not well standardized and is not recommended for routine use.[75] Repeat blood cultures during and following the course of therapy, particularly with *S. aureus* endocarditis, are needed to ensure eradication of the infection. Persistently positive blood cultures indicate paravalvular abscess or metastatic infection and require appropriate evaluation and possible surgical intervention.

The time course for resolution of fever with effective therapy varies, but most patients defervesce with 3 to 7 days of effective medical therapy.[70] Recurrent fever suggests paravalvular abscess formation.[90] Serial transesophageal echocardiographic studies during medical therapy for endocarditis show that, compared with patients with decreasing vegetation size, a stable or increasing vegetation size is associated with a higher risk of valve replacement, embolic events, paravalvular abscess formation, and mortality (10% versus 0%),[62] suggesting that echocardiography may be helpful in monitoring the effectiveness of antibiotic therapy.

Surgical Therapy

The decision to perform cardiac surgery in a patient with infective endocarditis is never trivial and must be based on the specific disease course, degree of tissue destruction, hemodynamics, and complications in each individual (Table 18–6). In addition, other factors, such as comorbid disease, must be considered in this difficult clinical decision. However, the advantages of surgical intervention are generally accepted in three clinical situations. First, persistent infection (most often caused by paravalvular abscess) that is unresponsive to appropriate antibiotic therapy requires surgical debridement of the abscess and adjacent infected tissue. Second, surgical intervention also is needed when heart failure supervenes, because these clinical symptoms indicate hemodynamic compromise due to severe valvular regurgitation. Third, patients with recurrent embolic events may benefit from valvular surgery to prevent further embolic episodes. Recently, earlier and more aggressive surgical intervention has been recommended by some groups given that these standard criteria lead to intervention only after irreversible consequences of the disease process have occurred (Fig. 18–15).[80, 81, 91] It is hoped that clinical or echocardiographic identification of patients at high risk will allow intervention before irreversible complications have occurred and result in better long-term clinical outcomes.

The surgical mortality rate for patients undergoing intervention for native valve infective endocarditis is as low as 5% for clinically stable patients to as high as 30% for patients with complex pathology.[80, 91–96] Surgical mortality does not appear to be related to the timing of surgery; surgery during active infection has the same risk as surgery performed late after the acute episode, although there may be a higher risk of recurrent endocarditis with active aortic valve disease.[94, 95] An important observation, emphasized in several surgical series, is that surgical mortality is closely related to the clinical status of the patient at the time of surgery.[95] Patients with hemodynamic compromise, multiorgan failure, or extensive intracardiac tissue destruction fare poorly, while those undergoing surgery earlier in the disease course have lower operative mortality rates and better clinical outcomes, supporting earlier surgical intervention in patients with appropriate indications (Table 18–7).[93]

The surgical procedure in a patient with infective endocarditis may be quite complex, depending on the extent of destruction of the valve apparatus and surrounding tissue. Often, reconstruction of the aortic or mitral annulus is necessary in addition to valve replacement

TABLE 18·5 AMERICAN HEART ASSOCIATION RECOMMENDATIONS FOR ANTIBIOTIC TREATMENT OF INFECTIVE ENDOCARDITIS IN ADULTS

Cause of Endocarditis	Antibiotic	Dosage and Route	Duration (wk)	Comments
Native valve endocarditis due to penicillin-susceptible viridans streptococci and *Streptococcus bovis* (MIC ≤0.1 µg/mL)[1]	Aqueous crystalline penicillin G sodium or	12–18 million U/24 h IV, either continuously or in six equally divided doses	4	Preferred in most patients older than 65 y and in those with impairment of the eighth nerve or renal function
	Ceftriaxone sodium	2 g once daily IV or IM[2]	4	
	Aqueous crystalline penicillin G sodium	12–18 million U/24 h IV; either continuously or in six equally divided doses	2	When obtained 1 h after a 20–30 min IV infusion or IM injection, serum concentration of gentamicin of approximately 3 µg/mL is desirable; trough concentration should be <1 µg/mL
	With gentamicin sulfate[3]	1 mg/kg IM or IV every 8 h	2	
	Vancomycin hydrochloride[4]	30 mg/kg per 24 h IV in two equally divided doses, not to exceed 2 g/24 h unless serum levels are monitored	4	Vancomycin therapy is recommended for patients allergic to β-lactams; peak serum concentrations of vancomycin should be obtained 1 h after completion of the infusion and should be in the range of 30–45 µg/mL for twice-daily dosing
Native valve endocarditis due to strains of viridans streptococci and *Streptococcus bovis* relatively resistant to penicillin G (MIC >0.1 µg/mL and <0.5 µg/mL)[1]	Aqueous crystalline penicillin G sodium	18 million U/24 h IV, either continuously or in six equally divided doses	4	Cefazolin or other first-generation cephalosporins may be substituted for penicillin in patients whose penicillin hypersensitivity is not of the immediate type
	With gentamicin sulfate[3]	1 mg/kg IM or IV every 8 h	2	
	Vancomycin hydrochloride[4]	30 mg/kg per 24 h IV in two equally divided doses, not to exceed 2 g/24 h unless serum levels are monitored	4	Vancomycin therapy is recommended for patients allergic to β-lactams
Endocarditis due to enterococci[5]	Aqueous crystalline penicillin G sodium	18–30 million U/24 h IV, either continuously or in six equally divided doses	4–6	4-wk therapy recommended for patients with symptoms <3 mo in duration; 6-wk therapy recommended for patients with symptoms >3 mo in duration
	With gentamicin sulfate[3]	1 mg/kg IM or IV every 8 h	4–6	
	Ampicillin sodium	12 g/24 h IV either continuously or in six equally divided doses	4–6	4-wk therapy recommended for patients with symptoms <3 mo in duration; 6-wk therapy recommended for patients with symptoms >3 mo in duration
	With gentamicin sulfate[3]	1 mg/kg IM or IV every 8 h	4–6	

Table continued on next page

TABLE 18·5   AMERICAN HEART ASSOCIATION RECOMMENDATIONS FOR ANTIBIOTIC TREATMENT OF INFECTIVE ENDOCARDITIS IN ADULTS *Continued*

Cause of Endocarditis	Antibiotic	Dosage and Route	Duration (wk)	Comments
Endocarditis due to enterococci[5]	Vancomycin hydrochloride[4]	30 mg/kg per 24 h IV in two equally divided doses, not to exceed 2 g/24 h unless serum levels are monitored	4–6	Vancomycin therapy is recommended for patients allergic to β-lactams; cephalosporins are not acceptable alternatives for patients allergic to penicillin
	With gentamicin sulfate[3]	1 mg/kg IM or IV every 8 h	4–6	
Methicillin-susceptible staphylococci				
Endocarditis due to staphylococcus in the absence of prosthetic material[6]	Regimens for non-β-lactam–allergic patients Nafcillin sodium or oxacillin sodium	2 g IV every 4 h	4–6 wk	Benefit of additional aminoglycosides has not been established
	With optional addition of gentamicin sulfate[3]	1 mg/kg IM or IV every 8 h	3–5 d	
	Regimens for β-lactam–allergic patients Cefazolin (or other first-generation cephalosporins in equivalent dosages)	2 g IV every 8 h	4–6 wk	Cephalosporins should be avoided in patients with immediate-type hypersensitivity to penicillin
	With optional addition of gentamicin[3]	1 mg/kg IM or IV every 8 h	3–5 d	
	Vancomycin hydrochloride[4]	30 mg/kg per 24 h IV in two equally divided doses, not to exceed 2 g/24 h unless serum levels are monitored	4–6 wk	Recommended for patients allergic to penicillin
Methicillin-resistant staphylococci				
	Vancomycin hydrochloride[4]	30 mg/kg per 24 h IV in two equally divided doses, not to exceed 2 g/24 h unless serum levels are monitored	4–6 wk	
Endocarditis due to HACEK microorganisms (*Haemophilus parainfluenzae, Haemophilus aphrophilus, Actinobacillus actinomycetemcomitans, Cardiobacterium hominis, Eikenella corrodens,* and *Kingella kingae*)[6]	Ceftriaxone sodium[2]	2 g once daily IV or IM[2]	4	Cefotaxime sodium or other third-generation cephalosporins may be substituted
	Ampicillin sodium[7]	12 g/24 h IV, either continuously or in 6 equally divided doses	4	
	With gentamicin sulfate[3]	1 mg/kg IM or IV every 8 h	4	

TABLE 18·5   AMERICAN HEART ASSOCIATION RECOMMENDATIONS FOR ANTIBIOTIC TREATMENT OF INFECTIVE ENDOCARDITIS IN ADULTS *Continued*

Cause of Endocarditis	Antibiotic	Dosage and Route	Duration (wk)	Comments
Staphylococcal endocarditis in the presence of a prosthetic valve or other prosthetic material[6]	**Regimen for methicillin-resistant staphylococci**			
	Vancomycin hydrochloride[4]	30 mg/kg per 24 h IV in 2 or 4 equally divided doses, not to exceed 2 g/24 h unless serum levels are monitored	≥6	
	With rifampin[8] And with gentamicin sulfate[3, 9]	300 mg orally every 8 h 1.0 mg/kg IM or IV every 8 h	≥6 2	Rifampin increases the amount of warfarin sodium required for antithrombotic therapy
	Regimen for methicillin-susceptible staphylococci			
	Nafcillin sodium or oxacillin sodium With rifampin[8] And with gentamicin sulfate[3, 9]	2 g IV every 4 h 300 mg orally every 8 h 1.0 mg/kg IM or IV every 8 h	≥6 ≥6 2	First-generation cephalosporins or vancomycin should be used in patients allergic to β-lactams Cephalosporins should be avoided in patients with immediate-type hypersensitivity to penicillin or with methicillin-resistant staphylococci

IM, intramuscular; IV, intravenous; MIC, minimum inhibitory concentration.

[1]Dosages recommended are for patients with normal renal function.

[2]Patients should be informed that IM injection of ceftriaxone is painful.

[3]Dosing of gentamicin on a mg/kg basis produces higher serum concentrations in obese patients than in lean patients. In obese patients, dosing should be based on ideal body weight. (Ideal body weight for men is 50 kg + 2.3 kg per 1 inch over 5 feet, and ideal body weight for women is 45.5 kg + 2.3 kg per 1 inch over 5 feet.) Relative contraindications to the use of gentamicin are age >65 y, renal impairment, or impairment of the eighth nerve. Other potentially nephrotoxic agents (eg, nonsteroidal antiinflammatory drugs) should be used cautiously in patients receiving gentamicin.

[4]Vancomycin dosage should be reduced in patients with impaired renal function. Vancomycin given on a mg/kg basis produces higher serum concentrations in obese patients than in lean patients. In obese patients, dosing should be based on ideal body weight. Each dose of vancomycin should be infused over at least 1 h to reduce the risk of the histamine-release "red man" syndrome.

[5]All enterococci causing endocarditis must be tested for antimicrobial susceptibility to select optimal therapy. This table is for endocarditis due to gentamicin- or vancomycin-susceptible enterococci, viridans streptococci with a minimum inhibitory concentration of >0.5 μg/mL, nutritionally variant viridans streptococci, or prosthetic valve endocarditis caused by viridans streptococci or *Streptococcus bovis*.

[6]For treatment of endocarditis due to penicillin-susceptible staphylococci (minimum inhibitory concentration ≤0.1 μg/mL), aqueous crystalline penicillin G sodium can be used for 4 to 6 wk instead of nafcillin or oxacillin. Shorter antibiotic courses have been effective in some drug addicts with right-sided endocarditis due to *Staphylococcus aureus*.

[7]Ampicillin should not be used if laboratory tests show β-lactamase production.

[8]Rifampin plays a unique role in the eradication of staphylococcal infection involving prosthetic material; combination therapy is essential to prevent emergence of rifampin resistance.

[9]Use during initial 2 wk.

Adapted from Wilson WR, Karchmer AW, Dajani AS, et al: Antibiotic treatment of adults with infective endocarditis due to streptococci, enterococci, staphylococci, and HACEK microorganisms. JAMA 1995;274:1706–1713; Copyright 1995, American Medical Association.

(Fig. 18–16).[97] The choice of prosthetic valve is based on the same criteria used for other patients undergoing valve surgery: durability, hemodynamics, and anticoagulation issues. Careful debridement of all infected tissue and obliteration of abscess cavities is important to avoid the low (12%) but definite risk of recurrent endocarditis on the newly implanted prosthesis.[93] This risk is similar for mechanical and heterograft tissue valves, but it may be less for homograft valve replacements.[98] Although surgery should not be unnecessarily delayed for extracardiac sites of infection, preoperative evaluation should include evaluation and treatment of dental sites of active infection when possible.

TABLE 18·6   INDICATIONS FOR SURGICAL INTERVENTION IN INFECTIVE ENDOCARDITIS

Pathologic Process	Clinical Criteria	Echocardiographic Criteria
Persistent infection	Positive blood cultures, fever, atrioventricular block	Paravalvular abscess
Tissue destruction	Heart failure	Severe valvular regurgitation
Emboli	Recurrent embolic events	Large, mobile vegetations

Among patients undergoing surgery for infective endocarditis, 14% have preoperative acute neurologic deficits, including embolic cerebrovascular accidents (80%), ruptured mycotic aneurysms (9%), transient ischemic attacks (6%), and meningitis (6%).[99] Evaluation with computed tomography often provides useful information. These patients may do well after cardiac surgery (operative mortality rate of 6%), but the procedure preferably should be delayed for 2 to 3 weeks after an embolic cerebrovascular accident or mycotic aneurysm rupture to avoid worsening of the neurologic status. Even with delayed surgery, worsening neurologic status has been reported in up to 19% of patients.[100]

Increasingly, surgical options other than standard valve replacement are employed in patients with infective endocarditis. Homo-graft aortic valves offer several advantages, including resistance to infection, no anticoagulation, and hemodynamics similar to a native valve.[98] In addition to the valve itself, the graft typically includes the aortic root and anterior mitral leaflet, allowing repair of associated lesions such as a septal abscess, a fistula, or involvement of the anterior mitral leaflet.[96, 98]

The long-term outcome of patients after surgical intervention for endocarditis depends on the adequacy of the debridement and the degree of residual cardiac damage. Antibiotics are continued until the planned duration of medical therapy (4 to 6 weeks) is completed. Long-term survival after surgery for infective endocarditis at 10 years was 66%, with 85% of the survivors free of recurrent episodes in one series.[91] For patients treated with combined medical and surgical compared with those treated with medical therapy alone (not randomized), the survival rate at 5 years was 75% for the combined treatment group (n = 57) and only 54% for the medical group (n = 83).[80] Another group reported a 5-year survival rate after surgery of 81% ± 3% for aortic valve endocarditis and 83% ± 4% for mitral valve endocarditis.[94]

Given recent improvements in surgical technique and outcome, the persistently poor outcome with medical therapy alone, and the improved diagnostic data available with echocardiography, some groups of investigators advocate earlier surgical intervention in selected patients with infective endocarditis who do not meet traditional surgical criteria.[101] In one se-

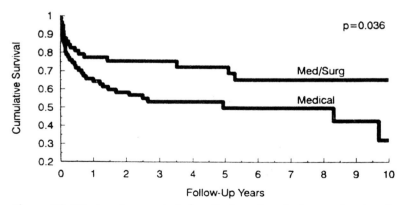

Figure 18·15 Long-term survival of medically and surgically treated patients in 140 consecutive patients with infective endocarditis, based on the von Reyn criteria, was significantly better than that of medically treated patients by Kaplan-Meier log rank method (P = .036). The 5-year survival rate was 75% for the medical plus surgical group and 53% for the medical treatment group. (From Vlessis AA, Hovaguimian H, Jaggers J, Ahmad A, Starr A: Infective endocarditis: ten-year review of medical and surgical therapy. Ann Thorac Surg 1996;61:1219; reprinted with permission from the Society of Thoracic Surgeons.)

TABLE 18·7	INFECTIVE ENDOCARDITIS: THE UNIVERSITY OF WASHINGTON MEDICAL CENTER EXPERIENCE	

Factor	Pre-Echo, 1963–72[39]	2D Echo, 1983–88[50]
Number of patients	125	70
Mean age (y)	43 (73% male)	47 (57% male)
Predisposing conditions		
Valve disease	27%	24%
Prosthetic valve	12%	16%
Congenital	26%	6%
IVDU	15%	29%
Causative organism		
Staphylococcus aureus	30%	34%
Streptococcus viridans	28%	26%
Mortality	38%	10%
Embolic events	50%	43%
Cardiac surgery	22%	51%
Operative mortality	52%	6%
Risk factors for early mortality	CHF Embolism Mycotic aneurysm Prosthetic valve	Embolism *S. aureus* Prosthetic valve

CHF, congestive heart failure; Echo, echocardiography; IVDU, intravenous drug use; 2D, two dimensional.

ries of 203 patients selected for early surgical intervention (average of 10 days from admission), the hospital mortality rate was only 4%, with an additional 6% incidence of late death within 2 years.[81]

Using an early surgical approach, intervention is indicated at the onset of heart failure symptoms, providing echocardiography confirms severe valve regurgitation, rather than waiting until the patient develops refractory heart failure. Echocardiographic demonstration of an abscess is convincing evidence for persistent infection requiring surgical intervention, avoiding the delay associated with demonstration of persistently positive blood cultures and thus preventing more widespread tissue destruction. Some clinicians advocate surgical intervention if vegetation size on transesophageal echocardiography fails to decrease after 1 week of therapy, as this finding suggests failure to control the infectious process.[58]

An early surgical approach to prevent systemic emboli is more problematic. Although some investigators are convinced that larger vegetations (>1 cm in diameter) are associated with a higher risk of embolism, others remain unconvinced. Even if vegetation size is a risk factor, two thirds of patients with large vegetations do not suffer embolic events, making it difficult to advocate surgery in all these cases. Conversely, about 20% of patients with smaller vegetations also have embolic complications. A pragmatic approach is to consider vegetation size, mobility, and location along with other echocardiographic and clinical factors in the decision-making process. For example, a large vegetation in a patient with significant valve regurgitation may prompt earlier surgical intervention, because valve surgery for the regurgitant lesion will be needed at some point and early surgery may prevent embolic events. Few clinicians advocate surgical intervention based on vegetation size alone.

RIGHT-SIDED ENDOCARDITIS IN INTRAVENOUS DRUG USERS

Disease Course

Endocarditis in intravenous drug users affects the right heart in about 75% of patients.[102–104] In the 25% to 33% with left heart

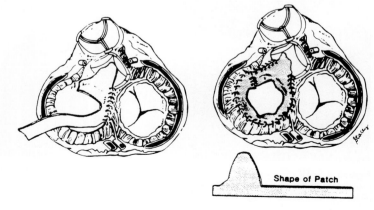

Figure 18·16 Example of the complex reconstructive surgery often needed in patients with extensive destruction due to endocarditis. A pericardial patch is used to reconstruct the mitral annulus and the intervalvular trigone, allowing insertion of mitral and aortic replacement valves. From Davia TE, Feindel CM: Reconstruction of the mitral annulus. Circulation 76(Suppl III):III102–107, 1987, with permission.

Shape of Patch

involvement, the disease course, prognosis, and treatment are similar to that for other types of left-sided endocarditis.[105] More than 50% of cases of right-sided endocarditis in intravenous drug users are caused by *S. aureus;* other common etiologic agents include group A streptococci, *S. viridans,* and enterococcus.[106, 107]

Clinical recognition of endocarditis in intravenous drug users is problematic. Only 6% to 13% of febrile drug users have endocarditis. Because the classic signs and symptoms often are absent in those with endocarditis,[108] blood cultures and echocardiography are central for diagnosis.

The mean age of patients with right-sided endocarditis is about 30 to 35 years, and about one third have a previous history of endocarditis or underlying heart disease.[103, 105] The tricuspid valve is infected in nearly all cases of right-sided endocarditis, although recognition of pulmonary valve involvement has increased based on the high-quality images obtained with transesophageal echocardiography.

Typical presenting symptoms are fever (>90% of patients), nonspecific complaints, and pulmonary or pleural symptoms. The initial differential diagnosis typically includes pneumonia or other pulmonary infections. Even when tricuspid regurgitation is present, a murmur often is difficult to appreciate by auscultation.[109] Chest radiography is abnormal at presentation in 75% of patients. Findings include nodular densities consistent with septic pulmonary emboli in 45%, infiltrates in 70%, and pleural effusions in 33% of patients. About 20% of intravenous drug users have extracardiac-associated infections, including osteomyelitis, empyema, septic arthritis, meningitis, and epidural abscess. Renal insufficiency is seen is 3% to 4% of cases.[103, 105]

Transthoracic echocardiography provides useful diagnostic and prognostic data in intravenous drug users with endocarditis.[109, 110] One of the primary goals of echocardiographic imaging in this situation is exclusion of left-sided valve involvement. If transthoracic images are nondiagnostic or left-sided valve involvement is strongly suspected, transesophageal imaging is needed (Fig. 18–17).

Prognosis

The prognosis for right-sided endocarditis due to *S. aureus* is relatively benign, with an in-hospital mortality rate of only 3% to 9%.[105, 109, 111] Tricuspid regurgitation tends to be well tolerated clinically, at least in the short term. Although 30-day mortality for endocarditis in drug users is low, long-term outcome remains poor, with a 5- to 10-year survival rate of only 10% due to recurrent drug use, other chronic

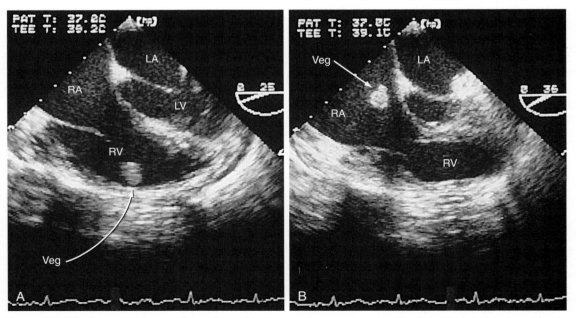

Figure 18·17 Transesophageal echocardiographic images show a vegetation (Veg) attached to the tricuspid valve prolapsing in the right ventricle (RV) during diastole *(A)* and into the right atrium (RA) during systole *(B)* in a patient with a history of intravenous drug use. LA, left atrium; LV, left ventricle.

medical problems, and the social problems prevalent among these patients.[102, 111]

Medical Therapy

In a series of 50 cases selected to include only patients with isolated right heart *S. aureus* infection and no evidence of extracardiac infectious complications, treatment with a 2-week course of combined medical therapy with an antistaphylococcal penicillin plus an aminoglycoside was effective in 94% of episodes.[103, 112] However, other studies suggest that prolonged fever and complications lead to a longer duration of therapy for a substantial number of cases.[105] When extracardiac sites of infection are present, treatment duration is based on the need for appropriate eradication of infection at the extracardiac, as well as cardiac, sites of involvement. Since a substantial number of patients with presumed right-sided endocarditis have left-sided heart involvement, echocardiography is mandatory for determining the appropriate duration of medical therapy (Fig. 18–18).

Evidence of persistent infection (eg, persistent fever) in drug users with endocarditis may indicate refractory endocardial infection. However, a careful search for extracardiac sites of infection also is needed.

Surgical Therapy

Surgical intervention is needed less frequently for right-sided than left-sided endocarditis. Even large vegetations respond well to medical therapy, often without further complications,[73, 111, 113] and tricuspid annular abscess formation is rare. Tricuspid regurgitation may result in peripheral edema and other signs of right heart failure but generally is better tolerated than left-sided acute valvular regurgitation. Embolization to the lungs results in less severe clinical consequences than systemic emboli from left-sided endocarditis.

Surgical intervention is needed in right-sided endocarditis for persistent infection or abscess formation in 6% to 25% of cases,[73, 105, 111] with a reported operative mortality rate of 12%.[91] It has been suggested that a vegetation larger than 1 cm in diameter is predictive of a poor response to medical therapy.[109, 114]

If feasible, valve debridement or repair is preferable when surgical intervention is needed. If repair is not possible, most surgical groups recommend removal of the tricuspid valve for control of infections refractory to medical therapy, as the consequent severe tricuspid regurgitation is well tolerated initially if pulmonary pressures are low.[115, 116] Although removal of the tricuspid valve eventually may lead to symptoms of peripheral edema and a low output syndrome, only about one third of patients subsequently require valve replacement for these symptoms.[113, 115] Early tricuspid valve replacement is undesirable because of the likelihood of reinfection in this patient group and the high 30-day mortality with early valve replacement.[115]

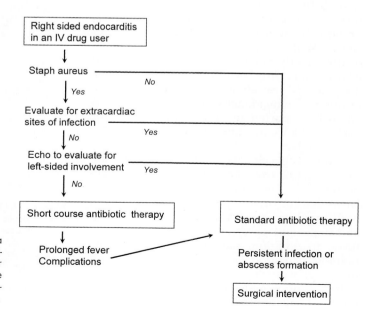

Figure 18·18 The flow chart illustrates a treatment approach to right-sided endocarditis. This approach provides a guideline for patient management, but treatment must be individualized according to other clinical factors and the disease course for each patient.

PROSTHETIC VALVE ENDOCARDITIS
Disease Course

Prosthetic valve endocarditis is classified as early (within 60 days of surgical implantation) or late (more than 60 days after surgery), given the different mechanisms of infection and types of etiologic agents in these two situations. Early prosthetic valve endocarditis, which accounts for about one third of cases, probably is related to infection at the time of surgery and typically is caused by staphylococci, fungi, or gram-negative bacilli. Late prosthetic valve endocarditis is a consequence of transient bacteremia and has a prevalence of etiologic agents similar to that for native valve endocarditis.[92, 117, 118] The source of infection in late prosthetic valve endocarditis most often is a dental procedure (20%), followed in frequency by urosepsis and urologic procedures (14%) and indwelling central lines for venous access or hemodynamic monitoring in the intensive care unit setting (7%).[119, 120]

The clinical presentation and diagnostic criteria for prosthetic valve endocarditis are no different than for native valve endocarditis, as previously described. However, transthoracic echocardiography has a much lower sensitivity for detection of prosthetic valve endocarditis due to reverberations and shadowing from the prosthesis or sewing ring. Transesophageal echocardiography has a far greater diagnostic accuracy in this setting and should be considered whenever prosthetic valve endocarditis is suspected.[53, 72, 121, 122]

With bioprosthetic valves, the infectious process affects the valve leaflets, the annulus, or both in approximately equal numbers of cases.[87] With mechanical valves, the site of infection nearly always is the sewing ring and adjacent annulus, because metal and Pyrolyte materials do not allow adherence of bacteria or fungi. The incidence of paravalvular abscess has been reported to be as high as 63% for aortic and 25% for mitral valve prostheses.[88]

Although endocarditis related to permanent intravenous pacemakers is rare, early and late infections of the pacer wire have been reported.[123–126] The clinical presentation is similar to that for other types of prosthesis-related endocarditis, with fever, systemic symptoms and signs, and persistently positive blood cultures. In addition, patients may have septic pulmonary emboli. Vegetations associated with the pacer wire or tricuspid valve are seen in only 23% of patients on transthoracic imaging but can be demonstrated with transesophageal imaging in 94% of patients.[127] Recognition of involvement of the pacer wire by endocarditis is crucial, because complete removal of the system and prolonged antibiotic therapy are needed to eradicate the infection.[127, 128]

Prognosis

The long-term outcome for patients with prosthetic valve endocarditis is worse than for those with native valve endocarditis because of the difficulty in eradicating infection in the implanted foreign body and because of the high prevalence of complications (Fig. 18–19). Mortality rates for early prosthetic valve endocarditis are as high as 80%,[129] and the mortality rate for late prosthetic valve endocarditis is 30% to 50%.[119, 129] Important prognostic factors include the infectious agent, heart failure symptoms, systemic embolic events, and persistent sepsis.[119, 129, 130] Outcome is poor when infection is caused by staphylococci, HACEK group organisms, and with culture-negative endocarditis.[131]

Medical Therapy

The basic principles of medical therapy for prosthetic valve endocarditis are identical to those for native valve endocarditis: bactericidal antibiotics at high doses for a prolonged period with the goal of eradicating the intracar-

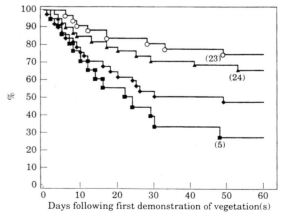

Figure 18·19 Cumulative freedom from thromboembolic complications *(solid diamonds)* of prosthetic mitral valve endocarditis. The influence of vegetation size is demonstrated by transesophageal echocardiography: vegetations of 1 to 4 mm *(open circles)*, 5 to 9 mm *(solid triangles)*, larger than 10 mm *(solid squares)*. (From Horstkotte D, Piper C, Niehues R, Wiemer M, Schultheiss HP: Late prosthetic valve endocarditis. Eur Heart J 1995;16(suppl B):44.)

diac site of infection. However, despite optimal medical therapy, eradication of infection is difficult with an implanted foreign device, and complications requiring surgical intervention occur frequently, including a high incidence of paravalvular abscess formation. Only 40% to 50% of prosthetic valve endocarditis cases are cured with medical therapy alone. Even when surgical intervention is deferred in the acute phase of the infection, late surgery often is needed for paravalvular regurgitation.

Surgical Therapy

In earlier series, surgical mortality rates for prosthetic valve endocarditis were high, possibly related to surgical technique. In addition, delay in referral for surgery leads to excessive tissue destruction, making repair difficult or impossible.[93] Recent series report lower operative mortality rates of 10% to 13% (Fig. 18–20).[92, 118]

Long-term survival has been reported to be as high as 82% at 5 years and 60% at 10 years after surgery for prosthetic valve endocarditis.[118] In a smaller series comparing medical and surgical therapy, the survival rate at 6 months was 77% for the group treated with medical and surgical therapy and 44% for those treated with medical therapy alone.[92] Although no randomized trials have compared medical with surgical therapy for prosthetic valve endocarditis, the known dismal progno-

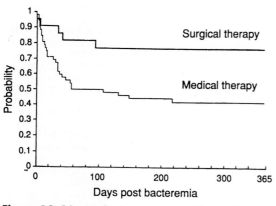

Figure 18·20 Medical versus surgical therapy for prosthetic valve endocarditis. Comparison of Kaplan-Meier curves shows that the survival of patients treated with surgical valve replacement was significantly better than that of patients treated with medical therapy only ($P = .01$ by Mantel-Cox test). (From Yu VL, Fang FD, Keys TF, et al: Prosthetic valve endocarditis: superiority of surgical valve replacement versus medical therapy only. Ann Thorac Surg 1994;58:1076; reprinted with permission from the Society of Thoracic Surgeons.)

sis with medical therapy alone, the presence of an implanted foreign body, and our increased understanding of the impact of intracardiac tissue destruction on short- and long-term outcome support early surgical intervention in many patients with prosthetic valve endocarditis.

However, there is one subset of patients that does well with medical therapy alone. This low-risk group can be identified by a rapid response to antibiotic therapy; no evidence of large vegetations, significant valvular dysfunction, or annular abscess on transesophageal echocardiography; and no clinical signs of heart failure or systemic embolization.

NONBACTERIAL THROMBOTIC ENDOCARDITIS

The differential diagnosis of infective endocarditis includes nonbacterial thrombotic endocarditis.[132–134] This disease process is characterized by sterile valvular vegetations and a high risk of embolic events. It occurs predominantly in patients with an underlying malignancy or with systemic lupus erythematosus. Vegetations due to nonbacterial thrombotic endocarditis typically are small (<1 cm in diameter), broad based, and irregularly shaped, and they occur most often on the aortic and mitral valves.[135] Although the appearance of the vegetations differs somewhat from the vegetations seen in infective endocarditis, these two conditions cannot be reliably differentiated on imaging studies, so that careful bacteriologic and clinical evaluation is needed (see Fig. 18–9).[136, 137] As with infective endocarditis, vegetations are diagnosed more accurately using transesophageal than transthoracic echocardiographic imaging.

In a series of 200 patients with underlying malignancies, nonbacterial thrombotic endocarditis was detected by echocardiography in 19% of patients and in only 2% of control subjects.[138] Vegetations were most common in patients with a lymphoma or with carcinoma of the pancreas or lung. The disease course was complicated by thromboembolism in 11% of all patients, including 24% of those with valvular vegetations and 8% of those without valvular vegetations.

In patients with systemic lupus erythematosus, valve disease may be due either to nonspecific fibrotic changes of the leaflets or to nonbacterial thrombotic endocarditis and is seen in the majority (about ¾) of patients.[139] While earlier studies suggested that the presence of valvular vegetations correlated with antiphospholipid levels,[140] this observation has not been confirmed in subsequent studies.[139] Valvular involvement in patients with systemic lupus erythematosus is not benign. Complications include significant valvular regurgitation in about one fourth of patients. Over a 5-year follow-up period, the combined incidence of thromboembolic events, heart failure, and valve replacement was 22% in one series.[141]

The treatment of nonbacterial thrombotic endocarditis remains controversial. While therapy should be directed at the underlying disease process, the role of anticoagulation in preventing neurologic events is less clear.[142-145] Some investigators recommend anticoagulation with heparin to prevent embolic events when vegetations are detected, but no controlled studies have examined this therapeutic approach.[144] The role of long-term warfarin anticoagulation also is unclear. Given the lack of randomized trials, most clinicians individualize therapy based on the overall clinical situation, the occurrence of embolic events, the risk of anticoagulation, and the echocardiographic findings.

References

1. Silver MD: Infective endocarditis. *In* Silver MD, ed. Cardiovascular Pathology. New York: Churchill Livingstone, 1991:895–932.
2. Ferguson DJ, McColm AA, Ryan DM, Acred P: A morphological study of experimental staphylococcal endocarditis and aortitis. II. Inter-relationship of bacteria, vegetation and cardiovasculature in established infections. Br J Exp Pathol 1986;67:679–686.
3. Durack DT, Beeson PB: Experimental bacterial endocarditis. I. Colonization of a sterile vegetation. Br J Exp Pathol 1972;53:44–49.
4. Baddour LM, Christensen GD, Lowrance JH, Simpson WA: Pathogenesis of experimental endocarditis. Rev Infect Dis 1989;11:452–463.
5. Durack DT: Experimental bacterial endocarditis. IV. Structure and evolution of very early lesions. J Pathol 1975;115:81–89.
6. Roberts WC, Buchbinder NA: Healed left-sided infective endocarditis: a clinicopathologic study of 59 patients. Am J Cardiol 1977;40:876–888.
7. Everett ED, Hirschmann JV: Transient bacteremia and endocarditis prophylaxis: a review. Medicine (Baltimore) 1977;56:61–77.
8. Scheld WM, Sande MA: Endocarditis and intravascular infections. *In* Mandell GL, Bennet JE, Dolin R, eds. Prinicples and Practice of Infectious Disease. New York: Churchill-Livingstone, 1994:740–783.
9. Flock JI, Hienz SA, Heimdahl A, Schennings T: Reconsideration of the role of fibronectin binding in endocarditis caused by *Staphylococcus aureus*. Infect Immun 1996;64:1876–1878.
10. Rubinstein E, Lang R: Fungal endocarditis. Eur Heart J 1995;16(suppl B):84–89.
11. Roberts WC, Oluwole BO, Fernicola DJ: Compari-
son of active infective endocarditis involving a previously stenotic versus a previously nonstenotic aortic valve. Am J Cardiol 1993;71:1082–1088.
12. Gersony WM, Hayes CJ, Driscoll DJ, et al: Bacterial endocarditis in patients with aortic stenosis, pulmonary stenosis, or ventricular septal defect. Circulation 1993;87:121–126.
13. L'Ecuyer TJ, Embrey RP: Closure of hemodynamically insignificant ventricular septal defect after infective endocarditis. Am J Cardiol 1993;72:1093–1094.
14. Currie PF, Sutherland GR, Jacob AJ, Bell JE, Brettle RP, Boon NA: A review of endocarditis in acquired immunodeficiency syndrome and human immunodeficiency virus infection. Eur Heart J 1995;16(suppl B):15–18.
15. Acierno LJ: Cardiac complications in acquired immunodeficiency syndrome (AIDS): a review. J Am Coll Cardiol 1989;13:1144–1154.
16. Karchmer AW: Infective endocarditis. *In* Braunwald E, ed. Heart Disease: a Textbook of Cardiovascular Medicine. Philadelphia: WB Saunders, 1997:1077–1104.
17. Roberts WC, Ewy GA, Glancy DL, Marcus FI: Valvular stenosis produced by active infective endocarditis. Circulation 1967;36:449–451.
18. Layman TE, January LE: Mycotic left ventricular aneurysm involving the fibrous atrioventricular body. Am J Cardiol 1967;20:423–427.
19. Qizilbash AH, Schwartz CJ: False aneurysm of left ventricle due to perforation of mitral-aortic intervalvular fibrosa with rupture and cardiac tamponade: rare complication of infective endocarditis. Am J Cardiol 1973;32:110–113.
20. Afridi I, Apostolidou MA, Saad RM, Zoghbi WA: Pseudoaneurysms of the mitral-aortic intervalvular fibrosa: dynamic characterization using transesophageal echocardiographic and Doppler techniques. J Am Coll Cardiol 1995;25:137–145.
21. Karalis DG, Bansal RC, Hauck AJ, et al: Transesophageal echocardiographic recognition of subaortic complications in aortic valve endocarditis: clinical and surgical implications. Circulation 1992;86:353–362.
22. Petitalot JP, Allal J, Thomas P, et al: Cardiac complications of infectious endocarditis [in French]. Ann Med Interne (Paris) 1985;136:539–546.
23. Klacsmann PG, Bulkley BH, Hutchins GM: The changed spectrum of purulent pericarditis: an 86 year autopsy experience in 200 patients. Am J Med 1977;63:666–673.
24. Bayer AS, Theofilopoulos AN, Eisenberg R, Friedman SG, Guze LB: Thrombotic thrombocytopenic purpura-like syndrome associated with infective endocarditis: a possible immune complex disorder. JAMA 1977;238:408–410.
25. Hooper DC, Bayer AS, Karchmer AW, Theofilopoulos AN, Swartz MN: Circulating immune complexes in prosthetic valve endocarditis. Arch Intern Med 1983;143:2081–2084.
26. Bayer AS, Theofilopoulos AN, Tillman DB, Dixon FJ, Guze LB: Use of circulating immune complex levels in the serodifferentiation of endocarditic and nonendocarditic septicemias. Am J Med 1979;66:58–62.
27. Cabane J, Godeau P, Herreman G, Acar J, Digeon M, Bach JF: Fate of circulating immune complexes in infective endocarditis. Am J Med 1979;66:277–282.

28. Davis JA, Weisman MH, Dail DH: Vascular disease in infective endocarditis: report of immune-mediated events in skin and brain. Arch Intern Med 1978;138:480–483.

29. Nast CC, Colodro IH, Cohen AH: Splenic immune deposits in bacterial endocarditis. Clin Immunol Immunopathol 1986;40:209–213.

30. Sindrey M, Barratt J, Hewitt J, Naish P: Infective endocarditis-associated glomerulonephritis in rabbits: evidence of a pathogenetic role for antiglobulins. Clin Exp Immunol 1981;45:253–260.

31. Williams RC Jr, Kilpatrick K: Immunofluorescence studies of cardiac valves in infective endocarditis. Arch Intern Med 1985;145:297–300.

32. Bayer AS, Theofilopoulos AN: Immune complexes in infective endocarditis. Semin Immunopathol 1989;11:457–469.

33. Gutman RA, Striker GE, Gilliland BC, Cutler RE: The immune complex glomerulonephritis of bacterial endocarditis. Medicine (Baltimore) 1972;51:1–25.

34. Levy RL, Hong R: The immune nature of subacute bacterial endocarditis (SBE) nephritis. Am J Med 1973;54:645–652.

35. Spain DM, King DW: The effect of penicillin on the renal lesions of subacute bacterial endocarditis. Ann Intern Med 1952;36:1086.

36. Neugarten J, Gallo GR, Baldwin DS: Glomerulonephritis in bacterial endocarditis. Am J Kidney Dis 1984;3:371–379.

37. Lerner PI, Weinstein L: Infective endocarditis in the antibiotic era. N Engl J Med 1966;274:259–266.

38. Venezio FR, Westenfelder GO, Cook FV, Emmerman J, Phair JP: Infective endocarditis in a community hospital. Arch Intern Med 1982;142:789–792.

39. Pelletier LL, Petersdorf RG: Infective endocarditis: a review of 125 cases from the University of Washington hospitals. Medicine (Baltimore) 1977;56:287–313.

40. Weinstein L, Rubin RH: Infective endocarditis—1973. Prog Cardiovasc Dis 1973;16:239–274.

41. Tunkel AR, Kaye D: Neurologic complications of infective endocarditis. Neurol Clin 1993;11:419–440.

42. Terpenning MS, Buggy BP, Kauffman CA: Infective endocarditis: clinical features in young and elderly patients. Am J Med 1987;83:626–634.

43. Weinstein L, Schlesinger JJ: Pathoanatomic, pathophysiologic and clinical correlations in endocarditis [second of two parts]. N Engl J Med 1974;291:1122–1126.

44. Yee J, McAllister CK: The utility of Osler's nodes in the diagnosis of infective endocarditis. Chest 1987;92:751–752.

45. Kerr A Jr, Tan JS: Biopsies of the Janeway lesion of infective endocarditis. J Cutan Pathol 1979;6:124–129.

46. Silverberg HH: Roth's spots. Mt Sinai J Med 1970;37:77–79.

47. Werner AS, Cobbs CG, Kaye D, Hook EW: Studies on the bacteremia of bacterial endocarditis. JAMA 1967;202:199–203.

48. Pesanti EL, Smith IM: Infective endocarditis with negative blood cultures: an analysis of 52 cases. Am J Med 1979;66:43–50.

49. Mugge A, Daniel WG, Frank G, Lichtlen PR: Echocardiography in infective endocarditis: reassessment of prognostic implications of vegetation size determined by the transthoracic and the transesophageal approach. J Am Coll Cardiol 1989;14:631–638.

50. Jaffe WM, Morgan DE, Pearlman AS, Otto CM: Infective endocarditis, 1983–1988: echocardiographic findings and factors influencing morbidity and mortality. J Am Coll Cardiol 1990;15:1227–1233.

51. Burger AJ, Peart B, Jabi H, Touchon RC: The role of two-dimensional echocardiography in the diagnosis of infective endocarditis [published erratum appears in Angiology 1991;42:765]. Angiology 1991;42:552–560.

52. Shively BK, Gurule FT, Roldan CA, Leggett JH, Schiller NB: Diagnostic value of transesophageal compared with transthoracic echocardiography in infective endocarditis. J Am Coll Cardiol 1991;18:391–397.

53. Pedersen WR, Walker M, Olson JD, et al: Value of transesophageal echocardiography as an adjunct to transthoracic echocardiography in evaluation of native and prosthetic valve endocarditis. Chest 1991;100:351–356.

54. Daniel WG, Mugge A, Grote J, et al: Comparison of transthoracic and transesophageal echocardiography for detection of abnormalities of prosthetic and bioprosthetic valves in the mitral and aortic positions. Am J Cardiol 1993;71:210–215.

55. Shapiro SM, Young E, De Guzman S, et al: Transesophageal echocardiography in diagnosis of infective endocarditis. Chest 1994;105:377–382.

56. Yvorchuk KJ, Chan KL: Application of transthoracic and transesophageal echocardiography in the diagnosis and management of infective endocarditis. J Am Soc Echocardiogr 1994;7:1294–1308.

57. Sochowski RA, Chan KL: Implication of negative results on a monoplane transesophageal echocardiographic study in patients with suspected infective endocarditis. J Am Coll Cardiol 1993;21:216–221.

58. Schiller NB: Clinical decision making in patients with endocarditis: the role of echocardiography. *In* Otto CM, ed. The Practice of Clinical Echocardiography. Philadelphia: WB Saunders, 1997.

59. Otto CM, Pearlman AS: The role of echocardiography in suspected or definite endocarditis. *In* Otto CM, Pearlman AS, eds. Textbook of Clinical Echocardiography. Philadelphia: WB Saunders, 1995:305–321.

60. Hogevik H, Olaison L, Andersson R, Lindberg J, Alestig K: Epidemiologic aspects of infective endocarditis in an urban population: a 5-year prospective study. Medicine (Baltimore) 1995;74:324–339.

61. Nihoyannopoulos P, Gomez PM, Joshi J, Loizou S, Walport MJ, Oakley CM: Cardiac abnormalities in systemic lupus erythematosus: association with raised anticardiolipin antibodies. Circulation 1990;82:369–375.

62. Rohmann S, Erbel R, Darius H, et al: Prediction of rapid versus prolonged healing of infective endocarditis by monitoring vegetation size. J Am Soc Echocardiogr 1991;4:465–474.

63. Khandheria BK: Suspected bacterial endocarditis: to TEE or not to TEE [editorial; comment]. J Am Coll Cardiol 1993;21:222–224.

64. Lindner JR, Case RA, Dent JM, Abbott RD, Scheld WM, Kaul S: Diagnostic value of echocardiography in suspected endocarditis: an evaluation based on the pretest probability of disease. Circulation 1996;93:730–736.

65. Lowry RW, Zoghbi WA, Baker WB, Wray RA, Quinones MA: Clinical impact of transesophageal echocardiography in the diagnosis and management of infective endocarditis. Am J Cardiol 1994;73:1089–1091.

66. von Reyn CF, Levy BS, Arbeit RD, Friedland G, Crumpacker CS: Infective endocarditis: an analysis based on strict case definitions. Ann Intern Med 1981;94:505–517.

67. Durack DT, Lukes AS, Bright DK: New criteria for diagnosis of infective endocarditis: utilization of specific echocardiographic findings. Duke Endocarditis Service. Am J Med 1994;96:200–209.

68. Bayer AS, Ward JI, Ginzton LE, Shapiro SM: Evaluation of new clinical criteria for the diagnosis of infective endocarditis. Am J Med 1994;96:211–219.

69. Dodds GA, Sexton DJ, Durack DT, Bashore TM, Corey GR, Kisslo J: Negative predictive value of the Duke criteria for infective endocarditis. Am J Cardiol 1996;77:403–407.

70. Lederman MM, Sprague L, Wallis RS, Ellner JJ: Duration of fever during treatment of infective endocarditis. Medicine (Baltimore) 1992;71:52–57.

71. Werner GS, Schulz R, Fuchs JB, et al: Infective endocarditis in the elderly in the era of transesophageal echocardiography: clinical features and prognosis compared with younger patients. Am J Med 1996;100:90–97.

72. Erbel R, Liu F, Ge J, Rohmann S, Kupferwasser I: Identification of high-risk subgroups in infective endocarditis and the role of echocardiography. Eur Heart J 1995;16:588–602.

73. Robbins MJ, Frater RW, Soeiro R, Frishman WH, Strom JA: Influence of vegetation size on clinical outcome of right-sided infective endocarditis. Am J Med 1986;80:165–171.

74. Watanakunakorn C, Burkert T: Infective endocarditis at a large community teaching hospital, 1980–1990: a review of 210 episodes. Medicine (Baltimore) 1993;72:90–102.

75. Wilson WR, Karchmer AW, Dajani AS, et al: Antibiotic treatment of adults with infective endocarditis due to streptococci, enterococci, staphylococci, and HACEK microorganisms. JAMA 1995;274:1706–1713.

76. Malquarti V, Saradarian W, Etienne J, Milon H, Delahaye JP: Prognosis of native valve infective endocarditis: a review of 253 cases. Eur Heart J 1984;5(suppl C):11–20.

77. Mansur AJ, Grinberg M, Cardoso RH, da Luz PL, Bellotti G, Pileggi F: Determinants of prognosis in 300 episodes of infective endocarditis. Thorac Cardiovasc Surg 1996;44:2–10.

78. Woo KS, Lam YM, Kwok HT, Tse LK, Vallance Owen J: Prognostic index in prediction of mortality from infective endocarditis. Int J Cardiol 1989;24:47–54.

79. Varma MP, McCluskey DR, Khan MM, Cleland J, O'Kane HO, Adgey AA: Heart failure associated with infective endocarditis: a review of 40 cases. Br Heart J 1986;55:191–197.

80. Vlessis AA, Hovaguimian H, Jaggers J, Ahmad A, Starr A: Infective endocarditis: ten-year review of medical and surgical therapy. Ann Thorac Surg 1996;61:1217–1222.

81. Middlemost S, Wisenbaugh T, Meyerowitz C, et al: A case for early surgery in native left-sided endocarditis complicated by heart failure: results in 203 patients. J Am Coll Cardiol 1991;18:663–667.

82. Sanfilippo AJ, Picard MH, Newell JB, et al: Echocardiographic assessment of patients with infectious endocarditis: prediction of risk for complications. J Am Coll Cardiol 1991;18:1191–1199.

83. Erbel R, Rohmann S, Drexler M, et al: Improved diagnostic value of echocardiography in patients with infective endocarditis by transoesophageal approach. A prospective study. Eur Heart J 1988;9:43–53.

84. Lutas EM, Roberts RB, Devereux RB, Prieto LM: Relation between the presence of echocardiographic vegetations and the complication rate in infective endocarditis. Am Heart J 1986;112:107–113.

85. Steckelberg JM, Murphy JG, Ballard D, et al: Emboli in infective endocarditis: the prognostic value of echocardiography. Ann Intern Med 1991;114:635–640.

86. Heinle S, Wilderman N, Harrison JK, et al: Value of transthoracic echocardiography in predicting embolic events in active infective endocarditis. Duke Endocarditis Service. Am J Cardiol 1994;74:799–801.

87. Fernicola DJ, Roberts WC: Frequency of ring abscess and cuspal infection in active infective endocarditis involving bioprosthetic valves. Am J Cardiol 1993;72:314–323.

88. Daniel WG, Mugge A, Martin RP, et al: Improvement in the diagnosis of abscesses associated with endocarditis by transesophageal echocardiography. N Engl J Med 1991;324:795–800.

89. Leung DY, Cranney GB, Hopkins AP, Walsh WF: Role of transoesophageal echocardiography in the diagnosis and management of aortic root abscess. Br Heart J 1994;72:175–181.

90. Douglas A, Moore Gillon J, Eykyn S: Fever during treatment of infective endocarditis. Lancet 1986;1:1341–1343.

91. Larbalestier RI, Kinchla NM, Aranki SF, Couper GS, Collins JJ Jr, Cohn LH: Acute bacterial endocarditis: Optimizing surgical results. Circulation 1992;86:68–74.

92. Yu VL, Fang GD, Keys TF, et al: Prosthetic valve endocarditis: superiority of surgical valve replacement versus medical therapy only. Ann Thorac Surg 1994;58:1073–1077.

93. Colombo T, Lanfranchi M, Passini L, et al: Active infective endocarditis: surgical approach. Eur J Cardiothorac Surg 1994;8:15–24.

94. Aranki SF, Adams DH, Rizzo RJ, et al: Determinants of early mortality and late survival in mitral valve endocarditis. Circulation 1995;92:143–149.

95. Aranki SF, Santini F, Adams DH, et al: Aortic valve endocarditis. Determinants of early survival and late morbidity. Circulation 1994;90:175–182.

96. Glazier JJ, Verwilghen J, Donaldson RM, Ross DN: Treatment of complicated prosthetic aortic valve endocarditis with annular abscess formation by homograft aortic root replacement. J Am Coll Cardiol 1991;17:1177–1182.

97. Frater RWM: Surgery for bacterial endocarditis. *In* Baue AE, Geha AS, Laks H, Hammond GL, Naunheim KS, eds. Glenn's Thoracic and Cardiovascular Surgery. Stamford, CT: Appleton & Lange, 1996:1915–1930.

98. Lupinetti FM, Lemmer JH Jr: Comparison of allografts and prosthetic valves when used for emergency aortic valve replacement for active infective endocarditis. Am J Cardiol 1991;68:637–641.

99. Gillinov AM, Shah RV, Curtis WE, et al: Valve replacement in patients with endocarditis and acute neurologic deficit. Ann Thorac Surg 1996;61:1125–1129.

100. Eishi K, Kawazoe K, Kuriyama Y, Kitoh Y, Kawashima Y, Omae T: Surgical management of infective

endocarditis associated with cerebral complications: multi-center retrospective study in Japan. J Thorac Cardiovasc Surg 1995;110:1745–1755.

101. Cormier B, Vahanian A: Echocardiography and indications for surgery. Eur Heart J 1995;19:68–71.

102. Cherubin CE, Sapira JD: The medical complications of drug addiction and the medical assessment of the intravenous drug user: 25 years later. Ann Intern Med 1993;119:1017–1028.

103. Chambers HF, Miller RT, Newman MD: Right-sided *Staphylococcus aureus* endocarditis in intravenous drug abusers: two-week combination therapy. Ann Intern Med 1988;109:619–624.

104. Reisberg BE: Infective endocarditis in the narcotic addict. Prog Cardiovasc Dis 1979;22:193–204.

105. Faber M, Frimodt Moller N, Espersen F, Skinhoj P, Rosdahl V: *Staphylococcus aureus* endocarditis in Danish intravenous drug users: high proportion of left-sided endocarditis. Scand J Infect Dis 1995;27:483–487.

106. Levine DP, Crane LR, Zervos MJ: Bacteremia in narcotic addicts at the Detroit Medical Center. II. Infectious endocarditis: a prospective comparative study. Rev Infect Dis 1986;8:374–396.

107. Barg NL, Kish MA, Kauffman CA, Supena RB: Group A streptococcal bacteremia in intravenous drug abusers. Am J Med 1985;78:569–574.

108. Weisse AB, Heller DR, Schimenti RJ, Montgomery RL, Kapila R: The febrile parenteral drug user: a prospective study in 121 patients. Am J Med 1993;94:274–280.

109. Hecht SR, Berger M: Right-sided endocarditis in intravenous drug users. Prognostic features in 102 episodes. Ann Intern Med 1992;117:560–566.

110. San Roman JA, Vilacosta I, Zamorano JL, Almeria C, Sanchez Harguindey L: Transesophageal echocardiography in right-sided endocarditis. J Am Coll Cardiol 1993;21:1226–1230.

111. Frater RW: Surgical management of endocarditis in drug addicts and long-term results. J Card Surg 1990;5:63–67.

112. DiNubile MJ: Short-course antibiotic therapy for right-sided endocarditis caused by *Staphylococcus aureus* in injection drug users. Ann Intern Med 1994;121:873–876.

113. Stern HJ, Sisto DA, Strom JA, Soeiro R, Jones SR, Frater RW: Immediate tricuspid valve replacement for endocarditis: indications and results. J Thorac Cardiovasc Surg 1986;91:163–167.

114. Robbins MJ, Soeiro R, Frishman WH, Strom JA: Right-sided valvular endocarditis: etiology, diagnosis, and an approach to therapy. Am Heart J 1986;111:128–135.

115. Arbulu A, Holmes RJ, Asfaw I: Surgical treatment of intractable right-sided infective endocarditis in drug addicts: 25 years' experience. J Heart Valve Dis 1993;2:129–137.

116. Arbulu A, Holmes RJ, Asfaw I: Tricuspid valvulectomy without replacement. Twenty years' experience. J Thorac Cardiovasc Surg 1991;102:917–922.

117. Sett SS, Hudon MP, Jamieson WR, Chow AW: Prosthetic valve endocarditis: experience with porcine bioprostheses. J Thorac Cardiovasc Surg 1993;105:428–434.

118. Lytle BW, Priest BP, Taylor PC, et al: Surgical treatment of prosthetic valve endocarditis. J Thorac Cardiovasc Surg 1996;111:198–207.

119. Horstkotte D, Piper C, Niehues R, Wiemer M, Schultheiss HP: Late prosthetic valve endocarditis. Eur Heart J 1995;16(suppl B):39–47.

120. Fang G, Keys TF, Gentry LO, et al: Prosthetic valve endocarditis resulting from nosocomial bacteremia: a prospective, multicenter study. Ann Intern Med 1993;119:1560–1567.

121. Morguet AJ, Werner GS, Andreas S, Kreuzer H: Diagnostic value of transesophageal compared with transthoracic echocardiography in suspected prosthetic valve endocarditis. Herz 1995;20:390–398.

122. Vered Z, Mossinson D, Peleg E, Kaplinsky E, Motro M, Beker B: Echocardiographic assessment of prosthetic valve endocarditis. Eur Heart J 1995;16(suppl B):63–67.

123. Conklin EF, Gianelli S, Nealon T: Four hundred consecutive patients with permanent transvenous pacemaker. J Thorac Cardiovasc Surg 1975;69:1–7.

124. Loffler S, Kasper J, Postulka J, et al: Septic complications in patients with permanent pacemakers. Cor Vasa 1988;30:400–404.

125. Choo MH, Holmes DRJ, Gersh BJ, et al: Permanent pacemaker infections: characterization and management. Am J Cardiol 1981;48:559–564.

126. Lewis AB, Hayes DL, Holmes DRJ, Vlietstra RE, Pluth JR, Osborn MJ: Update on infections involving permanent pacemakers: characterization and management. J Thorac Cardiovasc Surg 1985;89:758–763.

127. Klug D, Lacroix D, Savoye C, et al: Systemic infection related to endocarditis on pacemaker leads. Circulation 1997;95:2098–2107.

128. Harjula A, Jarvinen A, Virtanen KS, Mattila S: Pacemaker infections—treatment with total or partial pacemaker system removal. Thorac Cardiovasc Surg 1985;33:218–220.

129. Gagliardi C, Di Tommaso L, Mastroroberto P, Stassano P, Spampinato N: Bioprosthetic valve endocarditis: factors affecting bad outcome. J Cardiovasc Surg Torino 1991;32:800–806.

130. Wolff M, Witchitz S, Chastang C, Regnier B, Vachon F: Prosthetic valve endocarditis in the ICU: prognostic factors of overall survival in a series of 122 cases and consequences for treatment decision. Chest 1995;108:688–694.

131. Soma Y, Handa S, Iwanaga S: Medical treatment or surgical intervention? A cooperative retrospective study on infective endocarditis—timing of operation. Jpn Circ J 1991;55:799–803.

132. Libman E: Characterization of various forms of endocarditis. JAMA 1923;80:813–818.

133. MacDonald RA, Robbins SL: The significance of non-bacterial thrombotic endocarditis: an autopsy and clinical study of 78 cases. Ann Intern Med 1957;46:255.

134. Chino F, Kodama A, Otake M: Non-bacterial thrombotic endocarditis in a Japanese autopsy sample. Am Heart J 1975;90:190.

135. Roldan CA, Shively BK: Echocardiographic findings in systemic diseases characterized by immune-mediated injury. *In* Otto CM, ed. The Practice of Clinical Echocardiography. Philadelphia: WB Saunders, 1997;585–601.

136. Lopez JA, Fishbein MC, Siegel RJ: Echocardiographic features of nonbacterial thrombotic endocarditis. Am J Cardiol 1987;59:478–480.

137. Blanchard DG, Ross RS, Dittrich HC: Nonbacterial thrombotic endocarditis: assessment by transesophageal echocardiography. Chest 1992;102:954–956.

138. Edoute Y, Haim N, Rinkevich D, Brenner B, Reisner SA: Cardiac valvular vegetations in cancer patients: a prospective echocardiographic study of 200 patients. Am J Med 1997;102:252–258.

139. Roldan CA, Shively BK, Lau CC, Gurule FT, Smith EA, Crawford MH: Systemic lupus erythematosus valve disease by transesophageal echocardiography and the role of antiphospholipid antibodies. J Am Coll Cardiol 1992;20:1127–1134.

140. Hojnik M, George J, Ziporen L, Shoenfeld Y: Heart valve involvement (Libman-Sacks endocarditis) in the antiphospholipid syndrome. Circulation 1996;93:1579–1587.

141. Roldan CA, Shively BK, Crawford MH: An echocardiographic study of valvular heart disease associated with systemic lupus erythematosus. N Engl J Med 1996;335:1424–1430.

142. Bessis D, Sotto A, Viard JP, et al: Trousseau's syndrome with nonbacterial thrombotic endocarditis: pathogenic role of antiphospholipid syndrome. Am J Med 1995;98:511–513.

143. Rogers LR, Cho ES, Kempin S, Posner JB: Cerebral infarction from non-bacterial thrombotic endocarditis: clinical and pathological study including the effects of anticoagulation. Am J Med 1987;83:746–756.

144. Lopez JA, Ross RS, Fishbein MC, Siegel RJ: Nonbacterial thrombotic endocarditis: a review. Am Heart J 1987;113:773–784.

145. Biller J, Challa VR, Toole JF, Howard VJ: Nonbacterial thrombotic endocarditis. A neurologic perspective of clinicopathologic correlations of 99 patients. Arch Neurol 1982;39:95–98.

146. Delahaye JP, Leport C: Consensus development conference: apropos of prophylaxis of bacterial endocarditis [in French]. Arch Mal Coeur Vaiss 1992;85:257–258.

147. Corone P, Levy A, Hallali P, Davido A, Wyler Y, Corone A: Fifty-four cases of infectious endocarditis seen in 32 years in a population of 2038 congenital heart diseases [in French]. Arch Mal Coeur Vaiss 1989;82:779–784.

148. Loire R, Madonna O, Tabib A: Cardiac abscess in infectious endocarditis: apropos of 25 anatomo-clinical cases [in French]. Arch Mal Coeur Vaiss 1985;78:1216–1222.

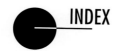

INDEX

Note: Page numbers in *italics* refer to illustrations; page numbers followed by t refer to tables.

ISBN 0-7216-7139-X

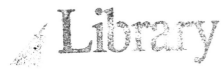